Immunodiffusion

Second Edition

Immunodiffusion

SECOND EDITION

ALFRED J. CROWLE

Webb-Waring Lung Institute, and Department of Microbiology
University of Colorado School of Medicine
Denver, Colorado

ACADEMIC PRESS New York and London   1973

A Subsidiary of Harcourt Brace Jovanovich, Publishers

To My Parents

Contents

Preface to the First Edition

In the past decade immunology has enjoyed an obvious rise in popular medical and biochemical thinking, growing from a subject regarded with only moderate interest by the average physician and biochemist of a few years ago to one now often occupying their foremost thoughts. In the author's opinion, there are two reasons for this rise. The first is that allergy is being implicated as a complicating or causative factor in increasing numbers of human diseases, most interestingly those of auto- or isohypersensitization. The second, and that directly relating to the subject of this book, is that by the recent prodigious developments of immunodiffusion serologic techniques, biological research has been provided with a type of analytic tool the like of which in specificity, resolution, and simplicity has never before been known; with it researchers are performing serologic analyses which would have astounded the immunologist of a decade ago. Immunodiffusion as an analytic method has developed from something of a laboratory curiosity, misunderstood and mistrusted, into a well-accepted technique now often employed by non-serologists than by those who rightly can think of it as a proud development of their own field. Believing that its infancy is passing away and its maturation is beginning, the author thinks that the time has arrived to document basic knowledge of immunodiffusion, formally record the history of its development, demonstrate how usefully it has been employed, introduce its techniques to potential new users, and gather into one reference work various sorts of knowledge on these techniques, often obscure and overlooked, which will aid those who already utilize immunodiffusion.

The theory of antigen–antibody reactions in semisolid media still is rather poorly developed, and its mathematical details will not interest most users of immunodiffusion. Moreover, a discussion of the mathematics of this theory would be excessively lengthy for a book of this size. Hence, theory is approached in Chapters II and III in a general, nonmathematical manner. In Chapter IV, the writer has striven to prepare a compendium of uses to which immunodiffusion has been put, but this summary must be acknowledged incomplete: immunodiffusion now is being applied in so many different fields, often being mentioned only obscurely, that completeness in any such survey is impossible. Chapter V describes in detail principal and accessory immunodiffusion techniques which in the author's opinion will best serve the reader. For those who are already users of immunodiffusion, this chapter includes descriptions of the latest improvements on established techniques. For the novice, it presents not only general methods but also details on subjects related to immunodiffusion techniques so often hard to find, such as how to photograph or stain antigen–antibody precipitin bands. Appendixes have been composed to supplement this chapter as a handy formulary, and a glossary is appended of terms commonly used in connection with immunodiffusion which might confuse the uninitiated.

The author wishes to thank several of his associates who have contributed to him their most valued assistance in preparing this book: Mrs. Lyle B. McMurry and Mrs. Peggy Braun for their secretarial work; Mr. David C. Lueker who with patience and enthusiasm has set up numerous experiments used to prepare photographic illustrations and to help answer a multitude of technical and theoretical questions which have arisen during preparation of this manuscript; the author's wife Clarice M. Crowle for her encouragement and her faithful help in many particulars, large and small; Dr. James J. Waring for his helpful suggestions on composition. To several others who have participated in lesser extent also goes the author's sincere thanks.

Preparation of this handbook has been greatly facilitated by financial assistance given to the author by the United States Department of Health, Education, and Welfare (Grants E-2283 and E-3697), the National Science Foundation (Grant G-4025), and the New York Tuberculosis and Health Association (James Alexander Miller Fellowship awarded the author, 1959–1960).

ALFRED J. CROWLE

Introduction

In the decade since the first edition of this book was published, immunodiffusion has become accepted as a primary bioanalytic technique. More publications mentioning its application now appear in one year than appeared in the decade 1950–1960. Well-standardized and widely employed immunodiffusion diagnostic tests exist.

Perhaps one of the surest signs of its acceptance as a routine tool is its commercialization as evidenced by the concerns developed to market the instruments, materials, and antisera that it employs. Explanatory comments no longer must preface presentation of an immunodiffusion pattern as evidence for the purity or nature of complex macromolecules for the general scientific public now understands and accepts such data. The technique has been essential in following step by step degradation of macromolecules in analyses of their ultrastructure, and then the opposite in their resynthesis. Immunodiffusion is used to monitor manufacturing processes, detect fraudulent products, standardize biologicals, prepare reagents for use with it and with other immunological techniques, classify plants and animals, study the epidemiology of disease, monitor human physiology and pathology, and indicate genetically determined disease risks before the disease develops. It can be used whenever antigens or antibodies need to be quantitated or characterized and, indirectly, to study simpler substances which are neither antigen nor antibody. In its more exotic forms (e.g., two-dimensional single electroimmunodiffusion) it has even become a form of art: students have been known to hang "portraits" of their own serum patterns on walls, and there has been at least one report of discard stained electroimmunodiffusograms disappearing from the laboratory and reappearing elsewhere in the city for sale as a novel form of artistic expression.

The tremendous growth and popular acceptance of immunodiffusion technology during the past ten years has necessitated considerable enlargement and change of this book. It has been written to answer the average user's most common questions: "Can my problem be elucidated by utilizing this technique? Is the substance I am studying an antigen and, if so, what is an antigen? How can I prepare proper antibodies to it? What kind of immunodiffusion test will be the best for me?" Consequently, much more space is used for practical than for theoretical discussion. Whenever possible, the first question is answered by example, and unusual examples have been chosen whenever they have been available because including a chapter solely on applications of immunodiffusion techniques, as was done in the first edition, has not been practical. Hence, the examples have been selected to serve a dual purpose: to be illustrative and a general guide to the literature.

The second and third questions concern a large body of information which though essential to is not directly part of immunodiffusion, namely, the nature of antigens and antibodies and characteristics of their interaction in semisolid media. Because this information is not readily found in immunology textbooks or in manuals on general immunologic techniques because of their much broader orientation, an attempt has been made to provide it in Chapters 1 and 2. Especially important, and inadequately discussed in other sources of information, is the question of how to make antibodies for use in immunodiffusion tests. The question is much more complex than it might appear to be on the surface. Different animals make antibodies of differing characteristics; different antigens elicit different kinds of antibody response in a given animal; the nature of antibodies obtained depends upon the time at which they are taken, even within one animal given just one exposure to antigen; the nature of antibodies also depends vitally on how and how much of the antigen is given. Precipitins usually are used for immunodiffusion tests, but if precipitins cannot be raised other kinds of antibodies can be substituted. Antibodies from one species of animal may be better than those from another because, for example, they can be used at high salt concentration for an antigen which is insoluble at low salt concentration. Some species of animal will readily make antibodies to some antigen or antigenic determinant which other species treat as nonantigenic. The precipitins from a horse may be better for qualitative analyses than those from a rabbit and *vice versa*. Whole antiserum may be superior to purified, concentrated precipitins. Points such as these are discussed extensively, because using immunodiffusion to its fullest potential depends on preparing and selecting the best possible antiserum (i.e., analytic reagent) for a given task.

Although antiserum is centrally important in immunodiffusion techniques, other seemingly minor factors may be equally important in determining the outcome of a test. For instance, a reaction can be overlooked for lack of adequate lighting; it may be difficult to photograph; a permanent record of it may be lost because of inappropriate staining and preserving methods. In addition to its extensive discussion of antigens and antibodies, Chapter 2 therefore includes ancillary information necessary to avoid or solve problems such as these. An unusually large number of footnotes appear in this chapter to provide, unobtrusively, valuable explanatory and technical information directly connected with subjects discussed in the text.

In the early days of immunodiffusion, test nomenclature was simply and logically established by the mode in which antigen and antiserum were mixed. Thus, if only one reactant diffused significantly, the technique was called "single diffusion"; both diffused in the "double diffusion" test; and if antigen first was electrophoresed and later analyzed immunologically, "immunoelectrophoresis" was being employed. In the last ten years new ways for intermingling antigen and antiserum have been discovered and exploited. Sometimes their naming has been haphazard; sometimes it has conformed to the descriptive logic of precedent. Chapters 3 through 7 attempt to answer the last question of our average immunodiffusion user ("What kind of immunodiffusion test will be the best for me?") and to explain immunodiffusion techniques in a sequence based on differences in antigen–antiserum mixing techniques. Thus, Chapters 3, 4, and 5 discuss single diffusion, double diffusion, and immunoelectrophoresis, respectively; Chapter 6 discusses the exciting but still relatively little used technique of electroimmunodiffusion; and Chapter 7 describes several even less used techniques in analogous sequence (e.g., two-dimensional single and double immunoelectrophoresis, immunochromatography, immunosedimentation, immunorheophoresis).

The chapter on the history of immunodiffusion is presented last in this edition rather than first as it was in the last edition because today it probably will be of more incidental than essential interest to the average reader and because historical developments in this subject during the past decade are more appropriately described in other chapters to indicate how a technique was conceived of and developed.

The Glossary explains itself. The Appendixes include only technical information deemed essential for general use in immunodiffusion techniques. For example, only the best all-purpose stains for immunodiffusion patterns are included; and only those buffer and electrolyte formulas which are the most efficient, have special utility, or by tacit acceptance have become standards are recorded. This selectiveness does not mean that formulas for stains, buffers, electrolyte solutions, or vehicles of immunization which are not included have all been tested in our laboratory and found inferior or that alternate formulas and techniques are not likely to be useful. Its purpose, as was stated above, is simply to provide the average user of immunodiffusion with the least ambiguous and most useful answers to his problems. One very conspicuous lack in the Appendix is a formulary and list of procedures for special stains and indicators. But this lack is intended because such a formulary could not be prepared adequately without undue use of space and because for these specialized procedures the reader usually will want to refer to an original description (appropriate references are given in Chapter 2) to understand the rationale as well as technical details of application.

For what interest it may be to the reader, composing the second edition of this book required approximately fivefold more time and energy than writing the first edition. The literature analyzed was larger by equal proportion. Nevertheless, the task has been satisfying and, in the end, inspiring. Surprising as it may seem, my impression is that the most exciting and rewarding immunodiffusion experiments are yet to come; I refer particularly to the tremendous opportunities for new research provided by recent developments in electroimmunodiffusion. My work in composing this second edition has been greatly eased by several individuals to whom I offer my most sincere gratitude, notably my secretary Ada M. Harrison, my wife and literary critic Clarice M. Crowle, and my technical associate Karen S. Jarrett.

ALFRED J. CROWLE

Chapter 1

Basic Information

The purposes of this chapter are to introduce the reader to the two principal reagents of immunodiffusion tests, antiserum and antigen, and to explain the basic physical events and processes of these tests so as to prepare him for using and understanding immunodiffusion techniques.

Antiserum

Antiserum is the fundamental reagent of immunodiffusion and provides its great versatility and high specificity. It is used to detect, characterize, and quantitate antigens. Antiserum is produced by animals exposed appropriately to antigen (Weiser *et al.*, 1969). An animal's lymphoid system, recognizing antigen as a foreign substance and an implied biological threat (e.g., infection, tumor), manufactures proteins that react selectively with this foreign "body" and therefore are known as "antibodies." The antibodies used in immunodiffusion tests are most commonly obtained by drawing blood from the antigen-immunized animal, allowing the blood to clot, centrifuging out the clot and accompanying blood cells, and drawing off the clear, amber-colored supernatant antiserum.

Antibodies

Serum contains many kinds of dissolved macromolecules, most of them proteins. These are classified electrophoretically into major groups by increasing isoelectric point (i.e., decreasing electrophoretic mobility) as prealbumins, albumin, α-globulins, β-globulins, γ-globulins, and basic proteins. In turn, these are subclassified by function, molecular size,

1

solubility, and antigenic composition (Weiser *et al.*, 1969). Most antiserum antibodies are γ-globulins termed, collectively, "immunoglobulins" because of their functions, and referred to by formula as "Ig" with a following letter to indicate class (e.g., IgA: Weiser *et al.*, 1969; Smith, 1966). Antiserum contains several different classes of immunoglobulin which may or may not be antibodies against the immunizing antigen. Those that are antibodies usually are heterogeneous, differing in how they react with the same antigen and in what effect they consequently produce.

Solubility in distilled water distinguishes between two major varieties of immunoglobulin. Those precipitating when dialyzed against distilled water are euglobulins; those remaining in solution are pseudoglobulins (Boyd, 1966). Against protein antigens, rabbits produce primarily euglobulins, whereas horses form principally pseudoglobulins. But each species of animal also can, and usually does, produce small amounts of the other type of antibody (Siskind, 1966; Johnston and Allen, 1968). The principal euglobulin antibodies are electrophoretically classed as γ_2- or Ig_2-globulins because they are more cathodic than the pseudoglobulins, which, correspondingly, are γ_1-globulins. Though obsolescent, the terms euglobulin and pseudoglobulin remain useful for indicating whether or not antibodies can be used in distilled water, which may be important in some immunodiffusion tests.

Different classes of antibody molecules share many chemical, physical, and biological characteristics. But because of differences in amino acid constitution they can be distinguished from each other immunologically (Abramoff and La Via, 1970). For instance, rabbit antiserum specific for one class of human immunoglobulin will not cross-react with another class of human immunoglobulin. By this and associated criteria, characterized human immunoglobulins have been classified as IgG, IgM, IgA, IgD, and IgE (Abramoff and La Via, 1970). Such nomenclatural systematization for immunoglobulins is relatively recent. Although it is being applied to antisera of lower animals as quickly as data accumulate and are interpreted, most classes of lower animal immunoglobulins have not yet been identified with their human serum counterparts. Consequently, other interim designations for antibody classes which only suggest similarities to human serum immunoglobulins are frequently used. For example, a 19 S animal immunoglobulin may be called γ_{1M} because it is a macromolecular γ-globulin with a γ_1 mobility in the immunoelectrophoretic pattern for that animal's serum. But it should not be called IgM without considerable proof of its homology with human serum IgM.

The term "19 S" above refers to the physical characteristic of molecular size as estimated by ultracentrifugal sedimentation, in which "S" signifies "Svedberg" (Boyd, 1966). The class of antibody most frequently used in immunodiffusion tests is an antigen-precipitating 7 S immunoglobulin (precipitin) of molecular weight approximately 175,000 (Tran Van Ky *et al.*, 1966a; Remington *et al.*, 1962). Other classes of antibody may be larger because of attached accessory structures (e.g., 11 S secretory IgA in man, of molecular weight 400,000; Dayton *et al.*, 1971), because they polymerize (e.g., 11 S and 14 S chicken precipitins: Kubo and Benedict, 1969; Van Orden and Treffers, 1968a; Hersh and Benedict, 1966), or because they are manufactured by the body in pentamers (e.g., 19 S IgM antibodies of molecular weight 900,000: Smith, 1966; Wahl *et al.*, 1965; Abramoff and La Via, 1970). Occasionally, biologically active pieces of antibody also may be encountered—for instance, in urine (Remington *et al.*, 1962) or in cattle antiserum (Cowan, 1966b). For immunodiffusion these molecular size distinctions are important, both because of correspondingly different rates of antibody diffusion and because of associated contrasts in reactions with antigen (Paul and Benacerraf, 1966). In recent years the ultracentrifuge has given way to simpler, less expensive ways of estimating antibody molecular size, such as measuring absolute or relative rates of diffusion through agar gels, determining diffusion-limiting pore size in semisolid media, or measuring gel-filtration R_f values (see Chapters 6 and 7).

By definition, all antibodies must be able to complex specifically with antigen. But antibodies differ in effects produced by such complexing and in conditions required for development of these effects. Indeed, they are known by their effects as precipitins (precipitate dissolved antigens), agglutinins (aggregate and sediment suspended antigens), complement-fixing antibodies (on combining with antigen they fix and activate enzymatic serum proteins known collectively as "complement"), opsonins (they combine with particulate antigens to facilitate their phagocytosis), and blocking antibodies (they interfere with manifestations of other kinds of antibodies). Antibody activities need not correspond with antibody immunoglobulin classification, since different classes of antibody may produce similar reactions with antigen. For instance, both γ_M- and γ_G-globulins in an antiserum can be precipitins (Pike, 1967; Tran Van Ky *et al.*, 1966a). On the other hand, a given antiserum will be likely to contain various antibodies with differences in both effect on and avidity for the same antigen (Carter and Harris, 1967; Boyd, 1966; Abramoff and La Via, 1970), and among these, individual antibodies will differ as to the portions (determinants) of the antigen with which they combine (Weiser *et al.*, 1969). These different kinds of antibody in a single antiserum, with their individual variations in relation to one antigen, and their competitive (Fiset, 1962; Christian, 1970) or complementary (Carter and Harris, 1967; Moore, 1961) interplay with each other through combination with the same antigen, define the overall antibody activity of the antiserum (Klinman *et al.*, 1966). As will be seen below, this total activity also is affected importantly by other nonantibody constituents of the antiserum.

Immunodiffusion tests most commonly use precipitins. But in some, antibody complexed with antigen forms clear or "negative" precipitin bands in agar gels, instead of opaque ones (Moore, 1961; Silverstein *et al.*, 1958); and there are immunodiffusion tests that detect blocking antibodies (Patterson *et al.*, 1964a), complement-fixing antibodies (Milgrom and Loza, 1966; Paul and Benacerraf, 1966), agglutinins (Milgrom and Loza, 1967), and antibodies that form no more than primary complexes with antigen (Freeman and Stavitsky, 1966; see Chapter 7 for additional examples). The following discussion centers on precipitins because of their primacy in immunodiffusion. The characteristics and uses of nonprecipitating antibodies in this technique will become evident partly as a by-product of this discussion and partly with later description of specific tests using these antibodies.

PRECIPITINS

Precipitins are antibodies that insolubilize antigen; hence, an antiserum that produces a precipitate when mixed with antigen solution contains precipitins. But this precipitating capacity for an antiserum is the product of complex agents and events including nature of antibodies, interaction between antibodies, interplay with nonantibody serum constituents, physicochemical conditions, and nature of antigen. Consequently, only a functional definition of precipitins is possible, although most frequently these antibodies are 7 S γ-globulins that are divalent and have a high affinity for antigen.

Precipitins can be 30 S (Cowan, 1966b), 19 S (Josephson *et al.*, 1962; Cowan and Trautman, 1965; Pike, 1967), 14 S (Orlans *et al.*, 1961), 7 S (Siskind, 1966), or even 4.5 S globulins (Cowan, 1966b). Their electrophoretic mobility depends on the species of animal making them, on the antigen inducing them, and on the immunization protocol employed (Christian, 1970). Rabbits tend to make γ_2-globulin precipitins (Siskind, 1966); horses more copiously make γ_1-globulin precipitins (Johnston and Allen, 1968); precipitins frequently occur in both electrophoretic classes of globulin in guinea pigs (Wilkerson and White, 1966) and mice (Krøll, 1970) and occasionally also in man and monkeys (Hillyer, 1969). Guinea pigs injected with foot-and-mouth disease virus produced, within 4 days, 19 S γ_1-globulin precipitins which could neutralize virus but not fix complement; but after 15 days they had ceased production of this antibody and instead were manufacturing 7 S γ_2-globulin precipitins which could both fix complement and neutralize virus (Cowan and Trautman, 1965; Graves *et al.*, 1964). Seven days after infection with the same virus, cattle were making precipitins of 19 S and 30 S γ_1-globulin, but later they made predominantly 7 S and 4.5 S γ_1- and γ_2-globulin precipitins (Cowan, 1966b).

Precipitins are called R- or H-type according to how they precipitate antigens (see section on antigen–antibody precipitation, below); and they can be either pseudo- or euglobulins. But production of one or the other of these types is not an exclusive characteristic of just certain species of animals. For example, conventionally immunized rabbits produce pseudo- and euglobulins, and both R- and H-type antibodies (Siskind, 1966). Horses make predominantly R-type precipitins early after immunization with protein antigens; only later do they produce the predominantly H-type precipitins for which they are renowned (Klinman *et al.*, 1964; Johnston and Allen, 1968). Both R- and H-type antibodies in the horse are 7 S globulins (Allen *et al.*, 1965).

Most precipitins are either γ_1- or γ_2-globulins, but α_2-globulin precipitins have been observed in rabbits (Strejan, 1965) and horses (Korngold and van Leeuwen, 1962). Precipitins may (Klinman *et al.*, 1966) or may not fix complement (Dupouey, 1963; Cowan and Trautman, 1965; Cowan, 1966b). Although they tend to have high affinity for antigen, this property alone does not make an antibody a precipitin; nonprecipitins can have equally high association constants (Klinman *et al.*, 1966). Both combining sites on an antibody molecule must be free to complex independently with antigen for it to be a precipitin, since if it is not thus functionally divalent not only will it fail to precipitate antigen, but also it may interfere with other precipitins to the same antigen (Klinman *et al.*, 1964). The ability of an antibody to precipitate antigen sometimes is related to its molecular charge, high isoelectric point favoring precipitating capacity (Carter and Harris, 1967). Since delipified antibodies retain normal affinity for antigen molecules but lose their capacity to precipitate them, antibody-bound lipids probably are required to stabilize the forming lattice of antigen–antibody complexes for visible precipitation (Cline, 1967; Tayeau and Jouzier, 1961b).

Certain antibodies in an antiserum must cooperate to precipitate antigen; others may enhance precipitation but not be necessary; still others interfere with precipitation. No single precipitin can recognize more than one kind of determinant on an antigen molecule. Consequently, different precipitins recognizing two or more antigen determinant sites are required for antiserum to precipitate an antigen (Weiser *et al.*, 1969).[1] Interestingly, this can account for the fact that rabbits immunized with too much human serum albumin produce antibodies but not precipitating antisera to the albumin. Having been made partially tolerant to this antigen, they make precipitins that are reactive with too few antigenic determinants to develop a visible aggregate (Christian, 1970).

Nonprecipitating antibodies can aid precipitins by "coprecipitating" with antigen and thus adding stability and bulk to the antigen–antibody lattice. For instance, certain chicken antisera contain two kinds of antibody, one of molecular weight 600,000 which will precipitate antigen alone, and the other of molecular weight 180,000 which is unable to precipitate antigen without help from the first. Both contribute to antigen precipitation by the whole antiserum (Orlans *et al.*, 1961). Some rabbit antisera, in addition to γ_G-globulin precipitins, contain also γ_A-globulin nonprecipitins which coprecipitate to enhance antigen aggregation by the precipitins. Both antibodies have similar affinities for antigen, but the coprecipitin is more hydrophilic and has a higher negative charge, and alone cannot form large antigen–antibody lattices (Carter and Harris, 1967).

The proportion of contrasting types of precipitin in an antiserum helps to determine its overall precipitating characteristics. Consider horse antiserum to human γ-globulin. Both γ_1 H-type and γ_2 R-type antibodies are present, but the former usually outnumbers the latter. Since the former has a high negative charge and is more hydrophilic, its resultant characteristic of precipitating antigen over a narrow range of proportions is also characteristic of the horse antiserum itself. But since this characteristic is influenced by the presence and quantity of the R-type antibody in the antistrum, in extremes, such as within an early-bleeding antiserum, horse antiserum can have R-type antigen-precipitating characteristics (Johnston and Allen, 1968).

In some antisera, nonprecipitins may compete with precipitins for antigen determinant sites and, instead of aiding, thereby prevent or diminish precipitation. For instance, some canine antisera to bovine serum albumin contain nonprecipitating antibodies which, when mixed with or used adjacent to canine or rabbit precipitating antisera in immunodiffusion tests, prevent these from precipitating the antigen (Patterson *et al.*, 1964a). Early-bleeding horse antisera can exert a similar effect,

---

[1] Most soluble antigens (e.g., albumins) are multivalent but have no more than one of each determinant site; only antigens with large repeating units (e.g., γ-globulins) will have two or more of one kind of determinant site (Pressman, 1967).

but, interestingly, nonprecipitating antibodies prepared by heating guinea pig precipitins do not (Patterson *et al.*, 1964a).

Nonantibody serum constituents usually enhance antigen–antibody precipitation. This is a major reason why antibodies that have been purified sometimes lose much or all of their capacity to precipitate antigen, and why reversed immunoelectrophoresis is more difficult than conventional immunoelectrophoresis (see Chapter 5). In addition to coprecipitins as mentioned above, chicken antiserum contains nonantibody substances that participate in and occasionally are necessary for antigen–antibody precipitation (Orlans and Rose, 1965). One serum factor taking part in this effect has been identified as a macroglobulin resistant to heating for 30 minutes at 56°C. Similar nonspecific "helpers" for antigen–antibody precipitation also are found in rat, mouse, guinea pig, and rabbit antisera (Gengozian *et al.*, 1962), although they may be more essential to antiserum from one species of animal than another. Guinea pig antiserum, for example, is an especially poor subject for reversed immunoelectrophoresis (Cline, 1967). Certain soluble antigen–antibody complexes are insolubilized by the 11 S component of complement (Christian *et al.*, 1963). On the other hand, there may also be constituents of serum that interfere with antigen–antibody precipitation, especially if the precipitins have been weakened somehow (e.g., by delipification: Cline, 1967).

Antibodies may be precipitins in one physical environment, but not in another. This is uniquely illustrated by certain human and horse antibodies which react with antigen in agar gel to develop a negative or clear precipitin band instead of the usual turbid band (Silverstein *et al.*, 1958; Moore, 1961; Fig. 1.1). These antibodies are forming soluble complexes with antigen large enough to be trapped within the agar gel but apparently too hydrophilic to precipitate. The complexes become conventionally turbid, that is, the antibodies become "precipitins," if they are exposed to mild protein denaturants, or if the salt concentration of the gel is increased (Silverstein *et al.*, 1958) or decreased (Crowle, unpublished work). Antibodies unable to precipitate antigen in liquid medium may do so in agar gels (Tayeau and Jouzier, 1961a), presumably because the gel supports the forming antigen–antibody lattice. Delipified antisera without precipitating capacity in liquid may still be able to precipitate antigen in agar gels (Tayeau and Jouzier, 1961b; Cline, 1967). Chicken antisera taken soon after immunization precipitate antigen more efficiently in 1.5 M than in physiologic NaCl solution (Gengozian *et al.*, 1962). Several more examples of environmental effects on antigen-antibody precipitation are described in Chapter 2 as practical means for enhancing immunodiffusion sensitivity.

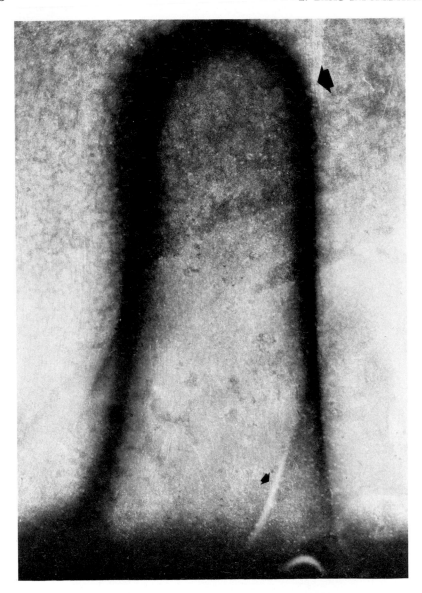

Fig. 1.1. Clear loop of antigen–antibody aggregate (large arrow) in turbid background of agarose gel. This was formed by human serum albumin in two-dimensional electroimmunodiffusion of human serum using a horse antiserum to human serum. One limb of a conventional opaque band of antigen–antibody precipitate is indicated by the smaller arrow. The turbidity of normally nearly transparent agarose gel has been enhanced photographically to accentuate the visibility of the clear loop.

ANTIGEN IN PRECIPITATION

As an essential partner in antigen–antibody precipitation, antigen affects this phenomenon in ways varying from influencing the antibody response made against it to determining manifestations of its reaction with antibodies. Thus, calves injected with whole bovine viral diarrhea virus made only 19 S precipitins, even following booster injections (Fernelius, 1966). But injected with antigen dissolved from this virus they produced 7 S precipitins. Certain Aspergillus antigens induce formation of only γ_G-globulin precipitins in rabbits, whereas others induce production of both γ_G- and γ_M-globulin precipitins (Tran Van Ky *et al.*, 1966). The net electrical charge of rabbit antibodies, both γ_G and γ_M, to various natural and synthetic antigens is reported to be inversely proportional to the net electrical charge of the immunizing antigen (Robbins *et al.*, 1967; see also Nussenzweig and Benacerraf, 1964).

To precipitate with already formed antibody, antigen must be at least divalent; univalent antigens or fragments of antigens can combine with antibodies but cannot bridge them together into a precipitate (Pressman, 1967). In fact, they will compete with multivalent antigens for antibodies and thus can interfere with precipitation. This is the phenomenological basis for precipitation inhibition tests (see Chapter 7). Antigen quantity as well as quality can affect precipitation. Moderate excess of antigen enables both inefficient and efficient antibodies in chicken sera to precipitate at the high salt concentrations often employed for chicken antiserum precipitin tests; the inefficient precipitin–antigen complexes are insolubilized by a salting-out effect (Orlans *et al.*, 1961).

PRECIPITINS OF VARIOUS SPECIES OF ANIMALS

The above discussion shows that the precipitating characteristics of antisera are determined mostly by the collective interaction of their various antibody and nonantibody components. Within moderate limits the antisera from different species of animals have their own predictable antigen-precipitating characteristics. The following discussion will illustrate this while also acquainting the reader with the precipitins of the animals most commonly used to make antisera for immunodiffusion tests.

Rabbits are the most often used producers of precipitins because they respond well to many antigens, yield reasonably large volumes of antiserum, are easy to handle, and are inexpensive. In the classic rabbit antiserum, 7 S γ_2-euglobulin precipitins predominate (Relyveld and Raynaud, 1963). But other kinds of antibody which influence the characteristics of rabbit antisera also are present.

In addition to γ_G-globulin precipitins, rabbits can make a γ_A-globulin nonprecipitin. This coprecipitates with the precipitins rather than inter-fering with them (Carter and Harris, 1967). Against certain antigens they will make both γ_G- and γ_M-globulin precipitins, and within these categories they can produce antibody populations of different electro-phoretic charge (Tran Van Ky *et al.*, 1966a). Against other antigens they will make predominantly γ_1-globulin precipitins (Strannegård, 1962). Sometimes they manufacture precipitins with α_2-globulin mobility as well (Strejan, 1965). The electrophoretic mobility of both IgG and IgM rabbit precipitins may depend on the electrophoretic nature of the inducing antigen, for the net charge of the antibody tends to be in-versely related to the net charge of the antigen (Robbins *et al.*, 1967). Rabbit 19 S γ_M-globulin precipitins are inactivated by reduction and alkylation, or by heating at 65°C for 30 minutes; their 7 S γ_G-globulin precipitins are not (Pike, 1967; Wahl *et al.*, 1965; Josephson *et al.*, 1962).

Rabbit and horse antisera are used as classic examples of R-type and H-type antigen precipitins because of their usually contrasting pre-dominating precipitating characteristics (i.e., 7 S euglobulin, γ_2 anti-bodies precipitating stably with antigen in rabbits; 7 S pseudoglobulin, γ_1 antibodies precipitating unstably with antigen in horses). But rabbits frequently make H-type antibodies. Though present, these antibodies are not usually noticed because they are masked by large quantities of R-type antibodies (Siskind, 1966).

Rabbit antisera usually are employed in physiologic or near-physiologic salt concentrations, and chicken antisera are resorted to when high salt concentrations must be utilized for some technical reason, like main-taining antigen solubility, for reasons given below. But this expedient is unnecessary because rabbit precipitins are effective over a wide range of salt concentrations and may even produce more distinct precipitates with some antigens in 8% NaCl solution than in physiologic saline (i.e., 0.85% solution: Murty and Hanson, 1961). Like precipitating sera of several other species, rabbit antisera lose much or all of their precipi-tating activity, without losing reactivity with antigen, when they are delipified (Tayeau and Jouzier, 1961b; Cline, 1967). This may explain why conditions tending to aggregate lipids enhance antigen precipitation by rabbit antisera, and vice versa.

By volume, horse antisera probably are, next to rabbit antisera, most often used for immunodiffusion. They usually precipitate antigens quite differently from rabbit antisera because their predominating precipitins are 7 S hydrophilic γ_1-pseudoglobulins which form more unstable pre-cipitates with antigen over a much narrower range of antigen–antibody proportions (Sandor and Korach, 1966; see Fig. 1.4). These precipitates dissociate easily in either antigen or antibody excess, whereas rabbit antiserum precipitates dissociate reluctantly in antigen excess and insignificantly in antibody excess. Practically, this means that in immunodiffusion tests rabbit antisera will produce more stable precipitin bands under more adverse conditions than horse antisera, but rabbit antiserum bands will be broader and more diffuse with a consequent possible loss of resolution among closely spaced precipitin bands. Liesegang precipitation (cf.) by horse antiserum is more difficult to identify than Liesegang precipitation by rabbit antiserum.

As in other species, method of immunization, type of antigen, and time of bleeding all affect the precipitating characteristics of horse antiserum (Klinman *et al.*, 1966). Against weak antigens or polysaccharides the horse makes R-type precipitins (Sandor and Korach, 1966). Early in the course of immunization with a protein antigen, horses produce R-type precipitins of γ_2 mobility also, but later they switch to making H-type precipitins of γ_1 mobility[2] (Johnston and Allen, 1968). Both types of precipitin are 7 S antibodies (Allen *et al.*, 1965). Against bacterial antigens and polysaccharides, horse R-type precipitins may be monomers of γ_M-globulin which are unstable and readily polymerize to form the more familiar macroglobulin (Sandor and Korach, 1966). The H-type γ_1-globulin precipitins may be so hydrophilic (Sandor and Korach, 1966) as to cause development of negative precipitin bands (cf. Fig. 1.1) under certain conditions in immunodiffusion tests, especially those of hypotonic salt concentration (Silverstein *et al.*, 1958).

The H-type precipitating characteristics of horse antiserum nevertheless are not entirely attributable to any single kind of antibody among the γ_1-globulins, because more than one electrophoretic class is likely to be present (Johnston and Allen, 1968).[3] But H-type precipitins do seem to have a mutual anatomic characteristic partly accounting for their behavior. Their two antigen combining sites are located on the arm tips of a Y-shaped molecule, and these arms cannot flex apart far enough from each other to achieve strong binding between two antigen molecules (Klinman *et al.*, 1964). Functionally, therefore, they are nearly univalent and must be presented with antigen under nearly optimal conditions to precipitate it. By contrast, comparable arms on R-type precipitins appear to be quite flexible (Dorrington and Tanford, 1970). The H-type antibodies are also more hydrophilic than the R-type (Sandor and Korach, 1966); this attribute sometimes can be countered prac-

---

[2] These are also known as β_2- or γ_A-globulins and, by older terminology, as "T component."

[3] As in rabbits, α_2-globulin precipitins have been observed in horse antisera (Korngold and van Leeuwen, 1962).

tically by salting-out effects, as with chicken antisera (Orlans et al., 1961).

Horses make their classic H-type precipitin responses following customary immunization with aqueous solutions of protein antigen. But if they are immunized instead with antigen in complete Freund adjuvant (see Chapter 2), they may begin and continue to make enough R-type γ_2-globulin antibody to mask the presence of simultaneously produced H-type γ_1-globulin antibodies and so produce R-type instead of H-type antisera (Allen et al., 1965).

Goat antiserum rivals horse antiserum in popularity for immunodiffusion tests because it can be produced in competitive volumes and yet contains the more desirable R-type precipitins (Berrod et al., 1964). Sheep antiserum precipitates antigen only over a narrow optimal proportion ratio with antigen, like horse antiserum, but its precipitates resist solution in antibody excess like those in rabbit antiserum (Relyveld and Raynaud, 1963). Sheep serum contains, in addition to γ_1- and γ_2-globulins, a still more cathodic γ_3-globulin; but its precipitins following immunization with protein antigen in Freund adjuvant and saline are 7 S (Kubo and Benedict, 1969) γ_2-globulins (Cline, 1967).

Most animals seem to respond to strong or persisting antigenic stimulation by producing first 19 S γ_1-, then 7 S γ_1-, and finally 7 S γ_2-globulin precipitins (see Pike, 1967). Thus, 7 days after exposure to foot-and-mouth disease virus cattle are producing macroglobulin γ_1 precipitins, and over the next 3 weeks they graduate to making 7 S precipitins in γ_1- and then γ_2-globulins (Cowan, 1966b). Following "incomplete" antigenic stimulation, antibody production may cease at some intermediate stage. For instance, against certain intact viruses cattle make only 19 S precipitins (Fernelius, 1966). A more mature stage of antibody production may replace an earlier one but progress no further itself: cattle precipitins against Vibrio fetus endotoxin were found to be exclusively 7 S γ_1-globulins (Winter, 1966). Though not often used to make immunodiffusion antisera, swine appear to be satisfactory. Swine antiserum precipitates antigen more in R-type than H-type fashion (Fey et al., 1960). The precipitins are γ_2-globulins, although as in sheep there are also γ_3-globulins (E. Jenkins and D. Lueker, personal communication).

Although rabbits predominate for laboratory production of antiserum, other small animals are frequently used. Among these are guinea pigs, which, like cattle, make γ_1-globulin precipitins following mild immunization with a protein and graduate to making γ_2-globulin precipitins if immunization is stronger (Wilkerson and White, 1966). Their earliest (4 days) precipitins are 19 S γ_1-globulins, and these are replaced in 2 to 4 weeks by 7 S precipitins (Graves et al., 1964; Cowan and Trautman,

1965). Some guinea pig precipitins need complement to precipitate antigen (Paul and Benecerraf, 1966).

Mice make principally 7 S γ_1-globulin precipitins to protein antigens injected in Freund adjuvant (Crowle, unpublished work); against microbial antigens they make both 7 S and 19 S precipitins (Krøll, 1970; Hillyer, 1969), 19 S precipitins sometimes predominating (Krøll, 1970). Mice, which ordinarily provide only very small amounts of antisera, can be made to produce large volumes of precipitin-rich ascitic fluid by intraperitoneal injection with complete Freund adjuvant and antigen (Munoz, 1957). For instance, mice will yield as much as 100 ml in repeated tappings of ascitic fluid precipitins for Australia antigen (Krøll, 1970).

Rats, like mice, tend to make predominantly γ_1-globulin precipitins (Relyveld and Raynaud, 1963). These precipitate antigen in a narrow optimal proportion region like H-type antibodies, but the resulting precipitates are stable to antibody excess, like R-type antibodies (Relyveld and Raynaud, 1963). Monkeys make 7 S precipitins (Sibal *et al.*, 1967). In addition to γ_2-globulin precipitins of R-type, canine antiserum, sometimes contains γ_1-pseudoglobulin nonprecipitins which interfere with antigen precipitation by the γ_2-globulins (Patterson *et al.*, 1964a,c). Consequently, dog antiserum tends to precipitate antigen incompletely in situations of antibody excess. It may contain the nonprecipitating antibodies alone and then will interfere with precipitation of the same antigen by other canine or rabbit precipitating antisera placed, for example, nearby in immunodiffusion tests.

Chickens are excellent alternates for rabbits as laboratory animals, easily producing good volumes of potent precipitating antisera against many different kinds of antigen. But their antisera have puzzled researchers for several years with certain peculiarities. Frequently they precipitate antigen well in liquid medium at high salt concentration (8% NaCl) but little or none at physiologic strength (Orlans *et al.*, 1961), and chicken antisera that do not precipitate well in liquid medium may (Crowle and Lueker, 1961) or may not (Weiner *et al.*, 1964) be effective in agar gels. The following facts may help to solve these puzzling events.

Chickens produce at least three different kinds of precipitin. One, appearing soon after strong immunization and remaining predominant for long periods following weak immunization, is a 7 S globulin which precipitates antigen optimally in 8% NaCl but poorly or not at all in physiologic saline. The second, present only in low concentration, is a 19 S antibody precipitating optimally in physiologic saline. The third, a 7 S antibody with optimal precipitating characteristics in physiologic saline, is produced by hyperimmunization (Benedict *et al.*, 1963). The principal reason that the early 7 S weak antibody precipitates antigen only at high salt concentration is that it is functionally univalent but aggregates spontaneously, though reversibly (Kubo and Benedict, 1969), in salt concentrations of 5.8% or higher to a functionally multivalent trimer or tetramer (Benedict *et al.*, 1963; Hersh and Benedict, 1966; Van Orden and Treffers, 1968a). However, other nonantibody chicken serum components also help it precipitate antigen and contribute to the bulk of the eventual precipitate (Franklin, 1962b; Orlans, 1960; Orlans and Rose, 1965; Hersh and Benedict, 1966; Van Orden and Treffers, 1968b). Complement is one (Orlans, 1960); another is nonantibody 7 S γ-globulin which aggregates with the antibody holding it in divalent complexes (Hersh and Benedict, 1966). Early 7 S antibodies aggregate spontaneously in chicken antiserum aged for 2 to 3 weeks at 4°C or frozen (Gengozian *et al.*, 1962). Spontaneous aggregation probably accounts for reports of efficient precipitins of molecular weight 600,000 mixed with inefficient precipitins of molecular weight 180,000 in some chicken antisera (Van Orden and Treffers, 1968a). Significantly, these 180,000- and 600,000-molecular-weight antibodies are electrophoretically the same (Orlans *et al.*, 1961).

The nature of the antigen itself complicates the situation. Chicken antiserum will precipitate myoglobulin at 8% NaCl but not in physiologic saline, whereas a similar antiserum will precipitate bovine serum albumin 70% as well in physiologic saline as in 8% NaCl (Orlans, 1960). Immunizing method and bleeding time are important factors in comparisons made among different laboratories of chicken antisera against the same antigen. For instance, 7 S inefficient precipitins predominate in sera taken a week or two after intravenous immunization with a protein either in solution or adsorbed on alumina (Weiner *et al.*, 1964; Tenenhouse and Deutsch, 1966);[4] but in hyperimmune sera efficient 7 S precipitins which will precipitate antigen efficiently in physiologic saline predominate (Benedict *et al.*, 1963). The importance of serologic test conditions is underlined by such a finding as inhibition of coprecipitation in chicken antiserum precipitation by the chelator EDTA (Orlans and Rose, 1965). This implicates divalent cations in manifested chicken antiserum activity, but the concentration of these ions is seldom closely monitored or controlled in immunodiffusion tests.

Disagreement over whether chicken antiserum precipitates antigen

---

[4] Tens of milligrams of antigen often are used for "immunization." In rabbits these quantities would produce tolerance to several or all determinants on an antigen. Might some of the inefficiency seen in antisera from chickens so immunized be the unrecognized effect of tolerogenesis such as develops in the rabbit (Christian, 1970)?

well in gels at physiologic salt concentrations surely arises from one or more of the factors indicated above, together with poorly understood additional factors related to gel strength and composition. Presently available information suggests that hyperimmune chicken antisera used at or near antigen equivalence will precipitate as well or better at physiologic salt concentration in immunodiffusion gels than in high salt concentration, but weak antisera may precipitate better in high salt concentration. Nevertheless, trial and error is the wisest course of action in establishing optimal salt concentration for any new antigen–antiserum system; this is also true but not generally recognized for antisera produced by other species, even including rabbits. Although chicken antisera precipitate antigen in R-type fashion (Van Orden and Treffers, 1968b), precipitates formed by their inefficient 7 S precipitins will be less stable at physiologic than at high salt concentrations (Orlans, 1960).

The property of chicken 7 S immunoglobulin to aggregate spontaneously at high salt concentration into 11 to 14 S molecules is shared by pheasant and quail 7 S immunoglobulins (Kubo and Benedict, 1969), which therefore should precipitate antigens similarly. This aggregation is absent from rabbit, porcine, bovine, sheep, or human immunoglobulins, as well as from sera of pigeons, ducks, and geese. Turkey immunoglobulins exhibit intermediate characteristics (Kubo and Benedict, 1969).

Precipitin responses in people resemble in timing and nature those of rabbits. Human antiserum precipitation is predominantly R-type, but as in lower animals the precipitating characteristics of such antiserum depend on the total interaction between several kinds of antibodies which may be present (Pike, 1967). For instance, certain patients with Hashimoto's thyroiditis make 7 S antibodies like the horse antibodies described above which form clear instead of turbid bands in agar gels with thyroid antigens (Anderson *et al.*, 1962a). Moreover, clear-band antibodies appear to be coprecipitated as visible precipitin bands by certain human thyroiditis antisera which do not appear to contain either precipitins or clear-band antibodies themselves (Moore, 1961).

Precipitins also can be obtained from such other animals as the cold-blooded species (Molnár and Berczi, 1965; see Chapter 2).

OTHER KINDS OF ANTIBODY EFFECTIVE IN IMMUNODIFFUSION TESTS

Precipitins are discussed above at some length because they are used in nearly all current immunodiffusion tests. But the few exceptions, with major technological developments that they augur for the future, warrant brief mention also of the nonprecipitating antibodies employed in these tests. Because of their variety, most are even more heterogeneous than precipitins. The reader should refer to sections below on various nonprecipitin serologic reactions, to Chapter 7, and to Weiser *et al.* (1969), Boyd (1966), and Pressman (1967) for more details than are presented in the following paragraphs.

Agglutinating antibodies have the same characteristics as precipitins but react with suspended rather than dissolved antigen and so agglutinate rather than precipitate it. Antibodies that couple with antigens that are either integral parts of or artificially attached to an intact cell, usually an erythrocyte, fix complement thereon, and thus lyse this cell, are called lysins. Complement fixation therefore is their primary characteristic; they may or may not be able also to agglutinate or precipitate antigen. The same kinds of antibody are also called simply complement-fixing antibodies when the antigen with which they react is not one that can be lysed (e.g., a soluble protein). Then they are detected indirectly by a secondary serologic system which recognizes that complement has been fixed and removed from solution.

Many antibodies can combine with antigen without either fixing complement or visibly affecting antigen. Some are detected indirectly because they compete with precipitins for antigen and block precipitation. These blocking antibodies, found frequently in canine antiserum as discussed above, must be competitively avid for antigen but be unable to precipitate it because of functional univalency, unusually strong hydrophilia, or some other such property which both prevents their precipitating antigen and makes them interfere with precipitation by authentic precipitins. Similar antibodies have the opposite effect of coprecipitating antigen with precipitins to add to the total precipitate developed, or cooperating with each other to precipitate antigen. These antibodies probably resemble blocking antibodies but have lower affinity for antigen and so aid rather than suppress precipitation. Or they can be precipitins themselves present in one antiserum to too few determinants on an antigen to precipitate it and therefore requiring help from similar precipitins in another antiserum to different determinants of the same antigen.

Development of radioimmunodiffusion and related techniques which reveal the first stage of antigen–antibody binding (see The Precipitin Reaction, below), infinitely widened the scope of immunodiffusion for revealing antibodies: any antibody capable of binding to antigen theoretically can be detected. A classic example and prototype for future advances with primary antigen–antibody complexing immunodiffusion tests is demonstration of atopic antibodies in human immunoglobulin E (Ishizaka *et al.*, 1966), since previously the only way of detecting these antibodies definitively had been by *in vivo* skin testing. Antibodies that can form only primary complexes with antigen are quite heterogeneous and thus not readily definable. They might even include, for example, the "antibodies" of delayed-type hypersensitivity which may not be conventional immunoglobulins at all.

Antigens

An antigen is any substance that can induce antibody formation in animals and can react with antibodies specific for it (Sela, 1966). These two properties of an antigen—capacity to induce antibody formation (antigenicity) and reactivity with antibodies—are not the same. The first is quite complex because it is determined by intrinsic factors like antigen structure as well as by extrinsic factors like immunization protocol and type of antibody required of the immunization. The second is simpler because in immunodiffusion tests it consists basically of only two events—initial complexing of antibody with antigen determinant groups (ligands), and secondary manifestations of this reaction such as complement fixation or precipitation (Weiser *et al.*, 1969; Pressman, 1967).

Antigenicity

Antigenicity is a meaningless term when used alone because antibody production results not only from properties of the antigen but also from an animal's reaction to immunization with it. But for a given animal and selected immunization procedure, antigens will differ in the type and extent of antibody production which they can elicit and, thereby, in antigenicity (Sela, 1966).

One molecular characteristic determining antigenicity is structure. Antibodies are directed principally against primary structure[5] ligands on a molecule of antigen (Liu *et al.*, 1967; Oudin, 1962; Kaminski, 1965), and so the ligand is the focus of antibody production. But a ligand alone, which may be a few of the amino acids in a peptide chain, a string of sugar molecules, or even a simple chemical like arsanilic acid (Sela, 1966), lacks antigenicity; that is, it lacks an ill-defined biologic characteristic of activating the immunized animal's antibody-making cells. Hence, it is called a hapten. But if the ligand is part of a protein molecule, if it is attached to such a molecule artificially before it is injected, or if it becomes attached to one spontaneously *in vivo* during immunization, then it gains the activating property (sometimes called "adjuvancy") needed

---

[5] Antibodies specific for secondary (Barbu *et al.*, 1963) or even tertiary (Tornabene and Bartel, 1962) antigen structure are reported.

to make it antigenic and stimulate antibody production (Weiser *et al.*, 1969; Sela, 1966; Plescia, 1967; Rapport, 1967). Most proteins and numerous polysaccharides are antigens; several nucleic acids and some lipids are haptens.

Multivalent antigens with many different ligands that stimulate formation of corresponding antibodies potentially are precipitinogens (Oudin, 1962; Kaminski, 1965). But antigens with only one or sometimes two ligands superficially might not be considered precipitinogens because, although they might be able to induce formation of precipitins, their antisera would lack sufficient variety of precipitins to build antigen–antibody lattices large enough to precipitate (Oudin, 1962; see The Precipitin Reaction, below). Practically, then, univalent or, sometimes, divalent antigens are not precipitinogens, though they may be able to stimulate formation of high titers of antibodies.[6] Thus, a substance may be judged antigenic by one criterion but not antigenic by another.

Antigenicity is determined also by poorly defined interdependent quantitative and qualitative factors. As was mentioned in the section on antibodies, animals respond to antigenic stimulation in a temporal and ascending sequence of stimuli beginning with production of nonprecipitating, low-avidity, hydrophilic, γ_1-globulin antibodies, progressing to production of different kinds of antibodies, and eventually making precipitins. Consequently, one exposure to a small quantity of strong antigen could induce precipitin production; for a weaker antigen several larger exposures might be needed; for a very weak antigen, or one available in only small quantity, the aid of a strong artificial adjuvant will be needed. A weak antigen sometimes can be made stronger directly by physical or chemical changes, such as heating it to form aggregates. Then, because of this qualitative change, less quantity will be required to elicit a precipitin response.

The method of immunization determines how the capacity of an antigen to induce antibody formation will be exploited, controlling whether antibodies will be produced and of what type and quantity (see sections on preparation of antisera, Chapter 2). Sera drawn early, after modest immunization, will contain low titers of antibodies, often nonprecipitating, with high specificity; intermediate immunization and later bleedings provide moderate titers of varied antibodies, some of which

[6] Potentially precipitating antisera against a single kind of univalent antigen can exhibit this capacity if two or more molecules of this antigen are coupled to an inert carrier molecule, thus making the necessary divalent or multivalent antigen artificially. Univalent fragments of a multivalent parent antigen, each with a different ligand, can induce formation of an antiserum that cannot precipitate the univalent fragments but can precipitate the whole antigen.

will be precipitins of good specificity; strong immunization followed by bleedings carefully timed for peaking of an animal's precipitin response will produce antisera with very high titers of several antibodies, including potent precipitins of mediocre specificity. In addition to the inherent adjuvancy of an antigen, the "strength" of immunization depends on its schedule and the method of administering the antigen. Within limits, which differ for individual antigens as well as for the animals being immunized, the longer and more repeatedly an animal is stimulated with antigen, the greater variety and quantity of precipitins it will make, and the stronger but less specific will be its antiserum. The limits of stimulation are ill-defined homeostatic controls on antibody production excited by exposure to excess antigen or to antigen in tolerogenic rather than immunogenic form, and resulting in immunologic tolerance with an accompanying undesired suppression of precipitin production.[7]

Options in methods for administering antigen are numerous. The best can be selected from the following general information on antigenicity. The weakest antibody responses develop when the injected antigen is disposed of quickly (e.g., following intravenous injection in water of a soluble, catabolizable antigen); intermediate responses are obtained when the antigen is protected by route of administration (e.g., subcutaneous versus intravenous) or especially by the form in which it is injected (e.g., adsorbed to aluminum hydroxide or insolubilized by heat or chemicals, as opposed to merely being dissolved in saline); strongest responses result from injecting the antigen together with a potent adjuvant which in addition to protecting the antigen also releases small amounts of it repeatedly over a long time for more prolonged immunizing stimulus, distributes the antigen throughout the antibody-producing reticuloendothelial system, and nonspecifically stimulates hyperactivity of this antibody-producing system (e.g., water-in-oil Freund adjuvant).

Much of the type and extent of immunologic response to an antigen depends on the animal being immunized. Generally, the more foreign an antigen is to an animal, the better it will induce precipitin production. In mice, for example, chicken ovalbumin is an excellent antigen, bovine serum albumin is a weak antigen, and native mouse serum albumin is not antigenic. Bacterial polysaccharides elicit production of only R-type

---

[7] For each antigen used in a given way in a given species of animal, there appears to be a wide range of antigen quantities (e.g., from 100- to 1000-fold) over which the induction of precipitin formation can be elicited. Quantities above or below this range will induce instead varying degrees of immunologic tolerance. Because conditions for tolerance induction differ as widely as conditions for immunization, it is impossible to give here any specific advice for avoiding tolerogenesis (cf. Friedman, 1971; Cinader, 1968).

precipitins in horses, whereas against proteins these animals make principally H-type precipitins (Sandor and Korach, 1966). Under equivalent conditions, rabbits make precipitins to proteins more easily than do mice or guinea pigs (Plescia and Braun, 1967; Crowle, unpublished work). Hence, for precipitin production some proteins "are antigenic" in rabbits but not in the smaller animals. On the other hand, purified polysaccharides are not antigenic in rabbits and guinea pigs but are in mice and man (Kabat, 1967).

Antigen Reactivity with Antibodies

The second part of a definition for antigen is that it must be able to combine specifically with antibodies. Every antibody is divalent, but specific for only one kind of antigen ligand (Weiser *et al.*, 1969; Pressman, 1967). For this aspect of antigenicity, then, a ligand alone constitutes reactivity (Paul and Benecerraf, 1966). But only a primary antigen–antibody reaction will develop with a single ligand, and this will be detectable only indirectly (e.g., in blocking tests) or by a primary-type test (e.g., radioimmunodiffusion: Kaminski, 1965). If several ligands are attached simultaneously to separate inert carriers, these, in effect, constitute multivalent antigens, and antibodies to the ligands then can effect a visible reaction. This will be precipitation if the carrier is a dissolved molecule (Paul and Benecerraf, 1966) or agglutination if it is a suspended particle (e.g., erythrocyte).

Most natural antigens are multivalent. If two or more of their ligands elicit corresponding antibodies, then the resulting antiserum will precipitate them. Generally, the more ligands there are on an antigen, the better and faster its antiserum will precipitate it (Kaminski, 1965). But this depends on the corresponding precipitins being present, for too much antigen used in immunization could induce tolerance for a large number of these ligands (Christian, 1970); then, only precipitins to weaker, more inaccessible ligands will be present in an antiserum, and precipitation of what otherwise might have been considered a good antigen will be poor or absent.

Some Practical Examples

The following are specific examples of some of the principles outlined above.

For reactivity with antibodies, simple chemicals frequently are good ligands. Precipitins against dinitrophenyl groups will react invisibly with these alone or, if they have been conjugated to carrier proteins like ovalbumin, will cause precipitation (Paul and Benecerraf, 1966). Small pieces of natural antigens have been studied as ligands in experiments on protein structure using antisera prepared against the whole protein (Lichter, 1967) or against fragments of it (Williams, 1964; see Kaminski, 1965). Protein molecules have themselves been used as "macroligands" by attaching them chemically to carrier erythrocytes which then are passively agglutinated by antibodies linking the erythrocyte-bound protein molecules together (Weiser *et al.*, 1969). Thus, with appropriate antiserum there is practically no limit to what can serve as a ligand in antigen–antibody reactions.

Variation among substances that can induce antibody formation, especially formation of precipitins, is much narrower. Generally, any protein foreign to the immunized animal and of molecular weight $\geq$10,000 can induce antibody formation (Sela, 1966; Weiser *et al.*, 1969). Examples include serum proteins, tissue antigens, microbial constituents, and even synthetic proteins (Paul and Benecerraf, 1966; Maurer, 1962; Sela, 1966). As molecular weights drop below 10,000, or as a protein more closely resembles those in the antibody-producing animal, difficulties in eliciting production of antibody and especially of precipitins increase, and more intense regimens of immunization are needed. For example, insulin is a small molecule and similar to an analogous hormone in the immunized animal. Precipitins are produced to it in mammals only with the help of complete Freund adjuvant (Pope, 1966). This adjuvant also must be employed to elicit production of precipitins to iso- or autoantigens like mouse serum proteins in other strains of mice, or guinea pig aspermatogen in guinea pigs.

Polysaccharides are usually poorer antigens than proteins, possibly because, as simpler molecules than proteins, they have potentially fewer antigenic varieties (Boyd, 1966), or because their physicochemical reactions with other molecules are weaker than those of proteins (Sela, 1966). Nevertheless, a few purified polysaccharides are good antigens in some species of animal. A classic example is pneumococcus polysaccharide which is effective in men and mice but not in horses or rabbits (Haurowitz, 1968). A polysaccharide naturally attached to a protein (e.g., serum glycoproteins: Kabat, 1967) or cruder substance (e.g., yeast cell wall: Hasenclever and Mitchell, 1964) induces antibody formation more easily. Horses will make precipitins to pneumococcus polysaccharide if immunized with the pneumococci themselves (Haurowitz, 1968).

Macromolecules other than proteins and polysaccharides so far have proved to be haptens rather than antigens. Precipitins against nucleic acids (Lacour *et al.*, 1962b; Barbu and Dandeu, 1963; Anderson *et al.*, 1962b; Barbu *et al.*, 1963; Plescia and Braun, 1967) and some lipids (Niedieck *et al.*, 1965; Graf and Rapport, 1965; Rapport and Graf, 1969), for example, have been obtained only when these are complexed to antigenic carriers, usually proteins, and then preferably when injected in adjuvants.

Additional examples of unusual antigens which have been used as precipitinogens are given in Chapter 2 in the section on antiserum production.

The Precipitin Reaction

Serologic precipitation occurs when a clear solution of antigen molecules mixed with a clear solution of corresponding antibody molecules (antiserum) combines with them to turn turbid by precipitation of antigen–antibody complexes. Serologic agglutination results if the antigen is particulate instead of dissolved. Because antibodies are divalent, whereas antigen molecules are generally multivalent, with precipitating antigen molecules (precipitinogens) the same size as precipitins (ca. 180,000 molecular weight) or smaller, most of the bulk of visible precipitate is precipitin. By contrast, an agglutination reaction is signaled by a change in dispersion of an already visible suspension of agglutinogen effected by only a few antibody molecules interconnecting individual particles of agglutinogen. Consequently, much less antibody is needed for agglutination than for precipitation; this is the reason that antisera can be used far more dilute for agglutination tests than for precipitin tests.

In forming, antigen–antibody complexes usually engage other substances nonspecifically, some of which can contribute so materially to these complexes as to determine whether they precipitate. These substances include, for example, serum lipids and complement. In addition, weak antibodies not alone able to precipitate antigen tend to join these complexes as coprecipitins. Antiserum therefore is likely to precipitate antigen better than antibodies purified from it.

Both agglutination and precipitation are employed in immunodiffusion, but because use of the former is rare and the basic principles of the two types of reaction are so similar, only the precipitin reaction will be discussed.

Examples of Antigen–Antibody Precipitation

When a solution of human serum albumin antigen is mixed with rabbit antiserum in a small test tube, within seconds to minutes the previously clear solutions turn turbid. This turbidity coarsens and settles with additional standing, especially at 4°C, and slowly precipitates into a fine layer on the bottom of the tube. This reaction can be quantitated by measuring the degree of turbidity that develops or the amount of antibody precipitated (Fig. 1.2A).

This precipitin test can be miniaturized, while still being performed with liquid medium, by partially filling a capillary tube with undiluted antiserum and then carefully overlaying this with dilute human serum albumin solution. Within a few seconds to minutes a precipitate will develop at the sharp interface between antiserum and antigen as a result of local intermingling of antigen and antiserum by diffusion and convection. Because the reactants form a ring of precipitate, this is known as a ring test (Fig. 1.2B). Historically, it is the direct precedent of immunodiffusion tests.

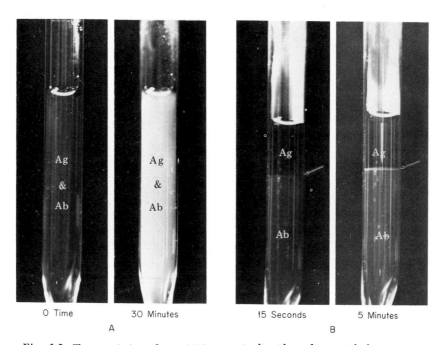

Fig. 1.2. Two varieties of precipitin test in liquid medium with human serum albumin antigen (Ag) and rabbit antiserum (Ab). The "0 time" tube in section A shows a mixture of reactants immediately after it was made. Dense precipitation developing throughout the mixture within 30 minutes is shown in the next photograph. Section B illustrates the classic ring test, forerunner of immunodiffusion tube tests. A faint ring of precipitate already had formed at the interface between layers of antigen and antiserum in the 15 seconds required to layer the antigen over the antiserum and then photograph the tube. The ring (arrow) intensified during the next several minutes at room temperature. Though rapid, versatile, and sensitive, the ring test cannot distinguish different coexisting antigen–antibody systems from each other.

If agar is mixed with the diluted antiserum in this ring test, and after the agar has gelled this is overlaid with antigen solution, the ring test is converted into an immunodiffusion test first popularized by Oudin beginning in 1946 and known as the single diffusion tube test. Antigen molecules diffuse into the antiserum-charged agar gel layer and form a disc of precipitate with their antibodies beginning near the interface and then slowly moving down the antiserum column as antigen, purposely used in excess, continues to feed into and be precipitated within the column of antiserum (see Fig. 3.2).

In precipitin tests conducted in liquid medium, antigen and antiserum form one precipitate; if there are several antigen–antibody systems precipitating at once, they are not distinguishable from each other. But in the semisolid media of immunodiffusion tests each antigen–antibody system of several possibly coexisting can be observed to precipitate in a different plane of the medium. Thus, two precipitin bands might be observed in the single diffusion tube test because two antigens differing in diffusion rate or reactivity with the antiserum employed precipitate in different planes of the antiserum–agar gel (see Fig. 3.2).

This capacity to resolve separate coexisting antigen–antibody systems in a single test is the cardinal value of all varieties of immunodiffusion test. Indeed, these differ from each other principally in means of separating and characterizing antigen–antibody systems. Consequently, additional examples of various antigen–antibody immunodiffusion tests will not be given here; they are found in later chapters.

Events of Antigen–Antibody Precipitation

The discussion that follows is based on general information such as that found in Weiser et al. (1969), Kabat (1967), Pressman (1967), Boyd (1966), and Haurowitz (1968); see also Cinader et al. (1963).

Within a few seconds after antigen and antiserum solutions have been mixed, most antigen molecules will have collided with and attached to antibody molecules (Hughes-Jones, 1963). That is, at least one ligand of the several usually present on each antigen molecule will have complexed with one of the two combining sites[*] of a matching antibody molecule (Oudin, 1962). This constitutes the primary stage of antigen–antibody precipitation. It may progress no further if reactants are

---

[*] The most commonly encountered 7 S antibodies are divalent. The 19 S antibodies and polymers of 7 S antibodies may have more than two effective determinant groups. The 7 S antibodies that polymerize spontaneously (such as in chicken antisera: Van Orden and Treffers, 1968) not only may have more than two determinants but also could have determinants to more than one antigen ligand.

univalent, or if antigen–antibody binding is very weak; it may continue secondary development to multiple antigen–antibody complexes that remain soluble under conditions of antigen excess, or if antigen–antibody binding is not strong; or it may grow visible. Theoretically, the secondary stage of antigen–antibody precipitation begins when the original duo of antigen and antibody are joined by another antigen molecule combining with the second reactive site on the antibody molecule, or by another antibody molecule joining a different receptor on the antigen molecule.

Monopeptide antigen molecules have several ligands, usually all different (e.g., A, B, C, D); antigen molecules consisting of two or more large duplicate units, like a peptide chain, may have two or more of one kind of ligand (e.g., A, A, B, B, etc.: Liu *et al.*, 1967). A precipitin to ligand A will bridge together two molecules of an antigen with this ligand. But if the antigen is a monopeptide, then antibody to other ligands (e.g., B) must also be available for antigen–antibody complexing to progress to the secondary stage and eventually precipitate (Oudin, 1962; see Fig. 1.3). If the antigen is a dipeptide and has two A ligands, then antiserum containing only antibodies to A can precipitate it. Of course, multiple ligands of just one kind can be attached to just one molecule of antigen either as part of its natural structure or artificially (e.g., Siskind, 1966).

Molecules of antigen and antibody originally complex because thermal agitation makes them collide. A primary complex colliding in turn with another antigen or antibody molecule binds it. When these events start, there are myriads of single antigen and antibody molecules. They associate and dissociate by the law of mass action (Hughes-Jones, 1963). Therefore, the higher their concentrations and the greater the attraction or affinity they have for each other, the faster they associate. When the average affinity of antibodies in an antiserum for antigen is high enough, then the tendency for antigen–antibody complexes to dissociate will be outweighed by their tendency to stick together sufficiently for complexes of physically insoluble size to form. Since any factor that suppresses dissociation of the forming complexes (e.g., low temperature, specific or nonspecific coprecipitation, antigen or antibody insolubilization, anti-convection medium) aids antigen–antibody precipitation, and vice versa, the practical affinity for antigen of antiserum antibodies is complicated and environment-dependent (Siskind, 1966). As time passes during development of the antigen–antibody precipitate, the reaction slows because the number of uncomplexed reactants becomes progressively smaller and consequently the likelihood of random fruitful collisions diminishes, and moreover the developing complexes become progressively larger. This, in turn, means that their movement becomes more sluggish and that they themselves become more fragile. Progress in the secondary

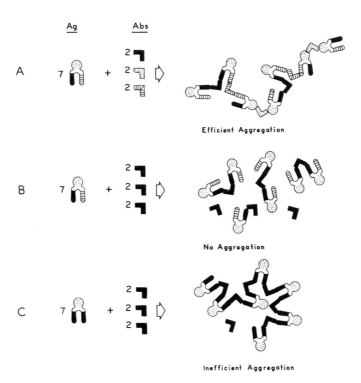

Fig. 1.3. Diagram of primary and secondary antigen–antibody complexing in three different situations. In the first (*A*), trivalent antigen mixed with antiserum containing antibodies to all its three determinant groups develops a good aggregate because the different antibodies cooperate to form the lattice. In the second (*B*), the same antigen is mixed with an antiserum containing antibodies to only one of the antigenic determinant groups. There are plenty of antibodies, but only primary complexing occurs because two of the three determinants on the antigen have no antibodies to combine with; that is, with this antiserum the antigen is functionally monovalent. In the third (*C*), two of the three determinants of the trivalent antigen are the same. Hence, even though the antiserum has antibodies of only one specificity, the antigen is divalent to this antiserum and precipitation develops, although not so well as when antibodies to several determinants are present in the antiserum (as in situation *A*).

stage of antigen–antibody precipitation therefore becomes increasingly affected by environmental factors like temperature, pH, salt concentration, and the physical nature of the test medium, such as whether it is liquid or gel.

THE PRIMARY STAGE OF PRECIPITATION

Primary antigen–antibody combination depends on an antibody combining site recognizing and reacting with a complementary antigen ligand when the two are drawn together by collision. Antigen ligand and antibody determinant sites fit each other by spatial configuration and electrochemical complementarity. They complex by means of weak bonds including, predominantly, attraction between oppositely charged ions, attraction between polar nonionic groups (including hydrogen bonding), and very close-range mutual attraction between atoms, called Van der Waals forces (Hughes-Jones, 1963; Pressman, 1967; Hurwitz *et al.*, 1965). Since none of these bonds is strong, antigen and antibody combining sites must fit together closely to be stable. The closer one fits the other, the faster and stronger is their association and the slower and lesser is their dissociation.

Initial complexing occurs quickly and tentatively. Weak antibodies tend to be "knocked" off their antigen ligands and replaced by stronger antibodies not so easily dislodged (Fiset, 1962). A weak antibody relative to the first stage of antigen–antibody precipitation (said to have low affinity) is one whose combining site either fits the corresponding ligand poorly, perhaps because the ligand is on a cross-reacting antigen and therefore not exactly like that by which the antibody was induced to form, or fits only part of it (e.g., antibody produced early in the immune response). A strong antibody, which is said to have high affinity, is one whose determinant site conforms to the topography of the antigen ligand closely and broadly. An antiserum is likely to have antibodies to an antigen of widely varying affinities (Siskind, 1966); its antigen-precipitating characteristics depend partly on the nature of the distribution of these populations of antibodies and therefore on the way in which antibodies in this antiserum first combine with antigen (Patterson *et al.*, 1964a).

FACTORS AFFECTING PRIMARY ANTIGEN–ANTIBODY COMPLEXING

The rate of this reaction is governed principally by reactant concentrations and only secondarily by environment (Siskind, 1966). It is too fast for convenient measurement when reactants are mixed at concentrations $\geq 10^{-6}\ M$ but slows to measurable rates with reactant concentrations lower by a factor of 1000 (Hughes-Jones, 1963). Practically speaking, at the high reactant concentrations usually employed in immunodiffusion tests, only environmental effects that are unusual enough to interfere directly or indirectly with binding of antigen to antibody will affect their rate of combination. These include, for instance, very high (>9) or very low (<4) pH, very high salt concentrations ($>12\%$ NaCl), electrolyte concentration too low to maintain solubility of euglobulin antibodies, characteristics of a medium that would slow or prevent reactant diffusion (e.g., freezing, use of a dense gelling agent), or reactant-denaturing conditions (e.g., heat $\geq 56°C$). In immunodiffusion tests, then, primary binding of antigen by antibody is essentially instantaneous as the two reactants mix and is unaffected by any but severely nonphysiologic environmental conditions.

THE SECONDARY STAGE OF PRECIPITATION

Theories purporting to explain antigen–antibody precipitation are seldom applicable to more than primary complexing between purified antigens and carefully selected antibodies and the formation of the first few secondary complexes (cf. Webber and Williams, 1963). More advanced secondary stages of antigen–antibody aggregation which lead to visible precipitation are so complicated and so poorly studied as to be understandable today only empirically (Cline, 1967).

The following events are observed to occur in a typical precipitation of antigen by antibody–"typical" referring to use of strong rabbit precipitins reacting with a purified relatively simple antigen like bovine serum albumin (see Weiser et al., 1969; Boyd, 1966; Webber and Williams, 1963; Liu et al., 1967).

Each molecule of antigen has several different ligands; the antiserum has high-affinity bivalent precipitins for each ligand (Oudin, 1962). A combining site for ligand A on antibody molecule a–a will bind the antibody to this ligand in a primary antigen–antibody reaction. Meanwhile, the other free combining site on this a–a antibody molecule has been contacted by and has combined with ligand A on a separate molecule of antigen (Feinstein and Rowe, 1965). Ligands B, C, D, etc., on the two antigen molecules meanwhile have been accumulating antibodies b–b, c–c, d–d, etc., which in turn have trapped additional molecules of antigen with their free sites (see Fig. 1.3). Thus, when proportions of antigen and its various kinds of antibody in an antiserum are balanced, primary complexes develop rapidly into succeedingly extending secondary complexes, and there is maximum precipitation (Blair et al., 1966).

As reactants become complexed and therefore depleted, the growth of what is called a lattice of antigen–antibody molecules slows and eventually ceases (Webber and Williams, 1963). Sometime in its growth, if it is fed by sufficient reactant (mostly antibody), the lattice becomes insoluble (Kleczkowski, 1965), and large enough to have properties of a particle (e.g., $\geqq 100$ nm in smallest diameter), and together with similar lattices forming simultaneously in the same mixture of antigen and antiserum turns the previously clear solution turbid and constitutes a visible precipitate. This precipitate usually requires several days' standing to attain maximum bulk.

The events leading to maximal precipitation in this reaction are altered if antigen and antibody are used out of optimal proportion to each other:

precipitate development is slowed and decreased, and in extremes may not occur at all (Weiser *et al.*, 1969). Inhibition is greatest when antigen is excessive, for the overabundance of antigen ligands on normally multivalent antigen molecules occupies all the divalent antibody molecules in primary or small secondary complexes (see Fig. 1.3). Antigen–antibody complexes have formed, but they are too small to become insoluble (Yagi *et al.*, 1962). Overabundance of antibody molecules is more difficult to achieve because they are only divalent, but if there are enough of them they will crowd available antigen ligands so much as to interfere with bridging by antibody molecules between antigen molecules.

In antigen–antibody precipitation, the central event is primary binding between antibody combining site and antigen ligand (Siskind, 1966). This is especially evident in the specificity of lattice assemblage; it is retained throughout the entire event (Tayeau and Marquevielle, 1958). Since primary antigen-antibody complexing is reversible, antigen–antibody precipitation also should be reversible. But in practice it is usually only partially reversible (Smith *et al.*, 1962b; but see Schmidt and Styk, 1968); and the longer a lattice is allowed to stand, the more resistant it becomes to dissociation. Lattice development can be interrupted or even reversed by any condition that weakens or interferes with antigen–antibody union (e.g., excess antigen, low pH, high salt concentration, presence of certain cations: Hirschfeld, 1963; Grossberg *et al.*, 1962; Edelman and Byran, 1960; Schmidt and Styk, 1968; Hawkins, 1965), but it can also be interrupted or reversed by effects that do not demonstrably diminish antibody affinity for antigen (e.g., antiserum delipification, high temperature: Cline, 1967). Conversely, although antigen–antibody precipitation depends on specific antigen–antibody complexing, it will not occur without the aid of lattice stabilizers (Siskind, 1966; Tempelis and Lofy, 1965; Hellsing and Laurent, 1964; Hurwitz *et al.*, 1965). These are situations not adequately explained by existing theories of antigen–antibody precipitation, and therefore they must be discussed descriptively (Cline, 1967). Empirically they are important in deciding between success or failure of an immunodiffusion test (Lichter, 1967; Tayeau and Jouzier, 1961a,b).

R- AND H-TYPES OF PRECIPITATION

The complexity of antigen–antibody aggregation is illustrated by the classic and important contrast in characteristics of protein antigen precipitation by antisera prepared in rabbits and horses. Test tubes containing a series of antigen concentrations from excessive through optimal to insufficient and charged with equal volumes of antiserum will develop different quantities of precipitate for the two kinds of antisera, as illustrated in Fig. 1.4. Horse antiserum precipitates antigen over a narrow optimal proportions region, and, on either side of this, precipitation may be absent. The optimal proportions region for rabbit antiserum is much broader, and some precipitation is present in all the tubes (Weiser *et al.*, 1969; Boyd 1966).

This contrast between rabbit and horse antisera in precipitating antigen is due to the lesser physical flexibility and greater hydrophilia of horse antibodies and to their coexistence with high-avidity nonprecipitating antibodies which compete with them for the same antigen ligands (Klinman *et al.*, 1964; Patterson *et al.*, 1964a; Siskind, 1966). As was pointed out in the section on antisera, pseudoglobulin precipitins in any species of animal tend to precipitate antigen like horse antiserum, whereas

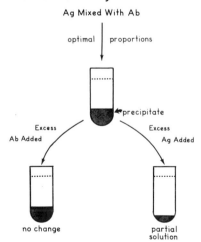

R -type Antibody

1. Horse γ_2-Globulin Antiprotein
2. Horse Antipolysaccharide
3. Rabbit Antibody

Ag Mixed With Ab

optimal | proportions

←precipitate

Excess Ab Added   Excess Ag Added

no change   partial solution

H -type Antibody

1. Horse γ_1-Globulin Antiprotein

Ag Mixed With Ab

optimal | proportions

←precipitate

Excess Ab Added   Excess Ag Added

solution   solution

Fig. 1.4. A contrast of types and properties of the two most often used precipitins. The R-type antibody, typically produced in rabbits against various antigens, forms precipitates with antigen insoluble or poorly so in reactant excesses, particularly in antibody excess. H-type antibody, best exemplified by horse antitoxins, forms a precipitate with its antigen which is readily and usually completely soluble in either antibody or antigen excess. These differences between H and R antibodies control the type of precipitin band formed in immunodiffusion tests and often affect the significance of results.

euglobulin precipitins tend to precipitate antigen like classic rabbit "R" antibodies (Siskind, 1966). The type of antibody that predominates helps to determine the precipitating characteristics of the whole antiserum (Christian, 1970; Patterson *et al.*, 1964).

FACTORS AFFECTING ANTIGEN–ANTIBODY PRECIPITATION

Any factor that stabilizes antigen–antibody lattice growth enhances precipitation, and vice versa. Precipitation also can be enhanced and increased by some substances which become part of and help to stabilize the lattice. Consider the following examples.

Thermal agitation and convection currents in liquid medium limit the ultimate size of lattice growth by weaker antibodies in an antiserum. This is why antigen–antibody precipitation is greater at refrigerator temperature than at room or body temperature (Berg, 1965b) and can occur in a semisolid medium when absent from a liquid one (Tayeau and Jouzier, 1961a,b).

Delipidified precipitating antisera lose their capacity to precipitate antigen without losing antibody reactivity for the antigen (Cline, 1967; Tayeau and Jouzier, 1961b). Sometimes this loss can be restored by "relipidifying" the antiserum (Horsfall and Goodner, 1935), compensated for by reacting the antiserum with antigen in an anticonvection medium (e.g., agar gel: Tayeau and Jouzier, 1961b), or by chemically changing the antibodies to make them more unstable in solution (e.g., with ninhydrin, or by iodination; Marquevielle, 1957; Carter and Harris, 1967). Lipids associated with antibodies probably contribute vitally but nonspecifically to the stability of developing lattices of antigen and antibody by stabilizing nonspecific bonds between reactants and also by displacing water from the lattice (Cline, 1967). Consequently, certain ions such as Cd^{++}, Ni^{++}, and barbital which precipitate lipids enhance antigen–antibody precipitation, and buffers that chelate such ions, like those containing EDTA, tris, or citrate, depress it (Orlans and Rose, 1965; Crowle, 1960a, 1961; cf. Cline, 1967).

Nonprecipitating antibodies can either enhance or inhibit antigen–antibody precipitation. High-avidity functionally univalent or hydrophilic antibodies will interfere with antigen precipitation by precipitins (Patterson *et al.*, 1964a). But low-avidity antibodies will coprecipitate antigen with precipitins, help to stabilize a forming lattice, and add to its bulk (Christian, 1970). Antibodies engaged in a lattice may fix serum complement and less well-defined serum constituents, accomplishing the same effect (Paul and Benacerraf, 1966; Gengozian and Doria, 1964; Gengozian *et al.*, 1962). Additional entraining of immunoglobulins is effected by nonphysiologic electrolyte concentrations which polymerize antibodies, sometimes making univalent ones di- or polyvalent (high salt concentration: Van Orden and Treffers, 1968a), tend to salt out serum proteins onto a lattice (high salt concentration: Orlans *et al.*, 1961), or lower the solubility of antibodies (low salt concentration). Moderate acidity usually produces the same effect (Lichter, 1967). Specific precipitation is enhanced by antibodies to either antibodies or nonantibody serum constituents in the lattice; these auxiliary antibodies may be present naturally or added artificially (Nace, 1963).

In addition to electrolytes, antibodies, and directly involved macromolecules, colloids affect antigen–antibody precipitation, sometimes favorably, sometimes not. High-molecular-weight dextran, polyethylene glycol, and polyvinylpyrrolidone can increase antigen–antibody precipitation in conditions of antigen excess when soluble antigen–antibody complexes are abundant (Hellsing and Laurent, 1964) and presumably also in other conditions that produce large numbers of these complexes. But such colloids, including gelatin and serum albumin, can depress antigen–antibody precipitation in other conditions (Depelchin, 1964), such as when precipitins are weakened by delipidification (Cline, 1967). Indeed, if charged colloids are absent from the reaction solution in which delipidified precipitins are being tested, these will precipitate antigen as effectively as nondelipidified precipitins (Cline, 1967).

Antigen–antibody precipitation usually is studied in solutions of NaCl. Changes in cation or anion composition of the solution, or addition to it of other small molecule solutes, may alter specific precipitation (Grossberg *et al.*, 1962; Hawkins, 1965). For instance, K^+, Cs^+, Mg^{++}, and Ca^{++} mildly reduce the velocity of precipitation; replacing Cl^- with F^- more strongly reduces it. Small polyhydroxy molecules like sucrose, glucose, or glycerol used at $0.3 M$ or more can reduce not only precipitation velocity but also its quantity. Simple amides, like formamide, in concentrations as low as $0.02 M$ will inhibit precipitation. The ions appear to alter ionized portions of antigen and antibody, affecting both primary and secondary reactions, and the polyhydroxy compounds act like detergents and make lattices more hydrophilic. The effect of the amides is puzzling (Hawkins, 1965), but it also may be due to increased lattice hydrophilia (Hurwitz *et al.*, 1965).

In general, antigen–antibody precipitation is enhanced by slightly acid pH (ca. 6.5), moderately high (up to 8% NaCl) or lower-than-physiologic (down to 0.01% NaCl) salt concentration (Molnár and Berczi, 1965; Orlans and Rose, 1965), the presence of normal serum (Orlans and Rose, 1965), refrigerator temperature (Berg, 1965b), the presence of an anticonvection medium that permits easy reactant diffusion (Tayeau and Jouzier, 1961a,b), the presence of colloids (Tayeau and

Jouzier, 1961a), lipid precipitants, and mild protein denaturants. It is inhibited by high pH (above 8.6: Berg, 1965b; Edelman and Bryan, 1960) and low pH (below 5: Edelman and Bryan, 1960), very low (distilled water) or very high (more than 12% NaCl) salt concentration (Edelman and Bryan, 1960), moderate and high temperature, use of an anticonvection medium that inhibits reactant diffusion, and the presence of reactant solubilizers such as lipid solvents and detergents.

ANTIGEN–ANTIBODY PRECIPITATION IN STABILIZED MEDIA

The generalizations made above for antigen–antibody precipitation apply to this phenomenon occurring either in liquid medium or in media stabilized by a gel or similar structure. But important additional factors affect precipitation in stabilized medium (i.e., in immunodiffusion tests). These arise from the basic facts that in immunodiffuson tests antigen and antibody are not mixed together all at once, and that the reaction medium has a semirigid structure. These facts have the following implications.

Mixture of reactants and associated substances in immunodiffusion tests is regulated by their migration by diffusion, electroosmosis, electrophoresis, or hydrodynamic transport into each other. Since each component migrates independently according to its own physicochemical characteristics and, often, concentration, the interaction of several all at once as occurs in liquid medium is rare. For example, liquid antigen added to liquid antiserum in a test tube is exposed immediately to numerous kinds of antibodies, several coprecipitating factors like complement, lipoproteins which may help precipitation, and colloids which can either help or hinder it. But antigen diffusing against antiserum in a double diffusion test encounters successive expanding fronts of antiserum constituents (Orlans and Rose, 1965). Of the more obvious macromolecular substances, albumin would be first (small size, high concentration), followed by transferrin (low molecular weight, high concentration), the predominating 7 S immunoglobulin, some minor 7 S immunoglobulins, immunoglobulins of 11 S or 14 S intermediate size, and finally 19 S immunoglobulins. A 7 S nonprecipitating antibody present in the antiserum in good concentration, by meeting the opposing front of antigen in antigen-saturating concentration before other antibodies arrive in significant numbers, may prevent 7 S precipitins from trailing along behind because of lower concentration from precipitating the antigen, may slow precipitation itself, may slow or stop diffusion of the antigen by engaging it in complexes too large to diffuse readily through the stabilizing medium, or may interfere with reaction between the antigen and the still more laggard fronts of 11 S, 14 S, or 19 S antibodies (Orlans *et al.*, 1961; Fiset, 1962).

If manifestation of an antigen–antibody reaction depends positively or negatively on nonantibody antiserum constituents, then it will be different in immunodiffusion tests than in liquid medium (Orlans and Rose, 1965). Precipitation-inhibiting colloids may be diluted enough by diffusion so that precipitation can occur in immunodiffusion tests when it is absent from parallel liquid medium tests (Tayeau and Jouzier, 1961a); coprecipitins like complement needed for one kind of precipitin to act may cause a single antigen–antiserum system also involving self-sufficient precipitins to develop two separate precipitates (Paul and Benacerraf, 1966); precipitins separated from other serum "helpers," as in reversed immunoelectrophoresis, may not precipitate antigen at all (Cline, 1967).

There are so many varieties of immunodiffusion test that the only generalization one can make from these considerations is that, although antigen–antibody precipitation in immunodiffusion tests is fundamentally the same as it is in liquid media, differences in mixture of principal and accessory reactants and in delivery of influencing factors make secondary stages of antigen–antibody precipitation in a given immunodiffusion test unique to the mixing characteristics of that test alone (Tayeau and Jouzier, 1961a).

Aside from segregating delivery of reactants in immunodiffusion tests, with results that have just been discussed, semisolid media influence antigen–antibody precipitation directly with their semirigid structures. Principally this is in supporting and thus improving lattice formation and thereby enhancing the capacity of weak antibodies to precipitate antigen. Related to this is the ability of these media to prevent diffusion and therefore to localize small antigen–antibody complexes, or larger complexes which are hydrophilic enough to resist precipitation. Visible precipitation therefore need not occur for certain kinds of immunodiffusion to display antigen–antibody reaction, for the complexes, having been fixed in the gel, later can be detected indirectly (see Chapters 2 and 7, and also following section).

Other Serologic Reactions

In most immunodiffusion tests antigen–antibody precipitation is the principal serologic effect observed. But some employ other indicators of antigen–antibody reaction which may be direct (agglutination, complement fixation) or indirect (precipitation inhibition, radioimmunodiffusion). The following paragraphs describe briefly the natures of these other manifestations of antigen–antibody reaction. Their use in actual immunodiffusion tests is detailed and illustrated elsewhere, especially in Chapter 7.

Agglutination

Agglutination is the same as precipitation except that the antigen is particulate rather than molecular (Boyd, 1966; Weiser *et al.*, 1969; Kabat, 1967). In liquid medium tests the evenly dispersed antigen reacting with antiserum is coarsened to become a smaller number of larger particles, which is evident both visibly and by accelerated sedimentation of the antigen. Coarsening is effected by the bridging together or agglutination of individual particles of antigen by antibody molecules into floccules whose characteristics depend mainly on the nature of the antigen. The antibody molecules must be divalent; the antigen particles generally have large numbers of many varieties of ligands. These ligands are the same as the antigen receptor sites of antigen–antibody precipitation, and they complex with corresponding antibodies in the same way and subject to the same influences. Both primary and secondary stages of antigen–antibody combination develop.

The major difference in antigen size between agglutination and precipitation also accounts for a major distinction between the two tests for quantity of antibody necessary to effect visible reaction. So little antibody is needed for agglutination that, practically, when antiserum is diluted to the point of inability to agglutinate antigen, it can be considered devoid of agglutinins. By contrast, an antiserum comparably diluted for precipitation still contains large numbers of precipitins, but these are simply insufficient to produce a visible precipitate. This difference in antigen size also means that in agglutination tests there is no practical range in ratios of antigen to antibody encompassing antigen excess in which agglutination is inhibited, as is easily observed in precipitation; on the other hand and for the same reason, inhibition of agglutination by antibody excess is quite common, whereas inhibition in precipitation is rarely seen.

Any colloid or suspensoid with antigen ligands on it can be used as antigen in agglutination tests. These ligands may be a natural part of the particle of antigen (e.g., structural antigens on viruses, bacteria, erythrocytes; micelles of tissue lipids suspended with surfactants), or they may be placed there artificially (e.g., protein antigen adsorbed on erythrocytes). When they are natural, agglutination is said to be active; when they are artificial, agglutination is said to be passive. Passive agglutination nicely demonstrates the relationships and contrasts between agglutination and precipitation: precipitins for a protein antigen in solution become agglutinins for the protein adsorbed onto such inert particles as latex or kaolin or on erythrocytes, and the quantitative interrelationships between the protein and its antibodies change accordingly.

Immunodiffusion tests utilizing agglutination have been unusual because of the problem of moving antigen through a semisolid medium. But some of these media, like agar and agarose gels, have proved to be more porous than was originally suspected, sufficiently so that they will permit agglutination tests with virus particles (Ragetli and Weintraub, 1965), lipoid antigens (Milgrom and Loza, 1967), and tissue cell fragments (Milgrom and Loza, 1967). A medium stabilizer like agarose can be used in quite dilute form and therefore makes a very porous gel. This together with new ways of employing forces like electrophoresis and rheophoresis (Ragetli and Weintraub, 1964) to forcefully move reactants through gels in immunodiffusion lead us to expect more frequent use of agglutination in future immunodiffusion tests. There are also immunodiffusion tests in which agglutination simply occurs upon rather than within the gel (Angevine *et al.*, 1966; Raunio and Kaarsalo, 1962).

Hemolysis and Complement Fixation

One of the most widely used techniques in serology for detecting antigen–antibody complexing is the complement-fixation test. It has also been adapted for use in immunodiffusion (Milgrom and Millers, 1963). Basically, it is an enzyme-inhibition test in which erythrocytes are the substrate changed by the enzyme system (complement). What makes it uniquely useful in serology is that this enzyme system is directly associated with antigen–antibody interaction in activation tests (hemolysis) or depletion tests (complement-fixation tests: see Weiser *et al.*, 1969).

Complement, which is a constituent of fresh, normal serum, has an affinity for aggregates of certain classes of immunoglobulin and therefore attaches to lattices formed by these, reacting as complement-fixing antibodies with antigen. If the antigen is a constituent of intact erythrocytes, then the fixed complement lyses these cells. Complement-fixing antibodies that react with erythrocyte antigens therefore are called hemolysins. The effect is typically demonstrated in liquid medium by mixing a suspension of sheep erythrocytes with rabbit anti-erythrocyte antiserum known, by effect, as hemolysin, and then adding an appropriate concentration of fresh guinea pig serum as a reliable, measurable source of complement. Within a few minutes the turbid erythrocyte suspension clears to a red solution as the erythrocytes lyse.

In a hemolytic immunodiffusion test, such as for titrating hemolysin, complement and hemolysin are diffused toward each other within agar containing sheep erythrocytes. Where the two meet, they form a band of lysis in the otherwise erythrocyte-turbid gel (Rybak *et al.*, 1963).

Rabbit hemolysin, sheep erythrocytes, and guinea pig serum (complement) have become standard serologic reagents because their interactions are predictable and quantifiable. Typically, one adjusts concentrations of hemolysin and complement to just slightly more than enough to lyse a 2% suspension of erythrocytes and then uses this standardized hemolytic system to detect separate antigen–antibody reactions by their fixing the minimal amount of complement in the system to a level too low for the hemolysin to disrupt the erythrocytes. For instance, protein antigen is mixed in a tube with its antiserum and complement. The consequent antigen–antibody complexes fix this complement. Later, when sheep erythrocytes that have been soaked in rabbit hemolysin to "sensitize" them are added to this tube, they will not lyse because there is no free complement to be fixed to them and the hemolysin. Thus, reaction between the protein antigen and its antibodies is detected by the complement that it fixed.

Complement fixation can be demonstrated similarly in immunodiffusion tests. An antigen is diffused toward its antibodies in a double diffusion plate through agar containing sheep erythrocytes and complement. Later the gel is flooded with hemolysin, and erythrocytes throughout the gel lyse except in the zone where antigen and antibodies have combined and fixed complement (Milgrom and Millers, 1963).

Complement-fixation tests will detect only reactions of antigen with complement-fixing antibodies; on the other hand, since these antibodies need not form large aggregates with antigen to fix complement, these tests are more sensitive for detecting antibodies than precipitin tests and much less affected by antigen-to-antibody imbalances. They require principally the precautions that only complement purposely added to the reaction system be present and that this complement not be inactivated nonspecifically. To satisfy the first precaution one must inactivate complement naturally present in both the hemolysin and the antiserum being tested by heating them a 56°C for 30 minutes. The second precaution is observed by using appropriate controls, such as "reacting" the test antiserum with an antigen unrelated to that for which it has antibodies.

Although complement fixation has not been used much in immunodiffusion tests, one can easily imagine several ways in which it could be (e.g., for a simplified, miniaturized Kolmer test for syphilis) and in which its unique abilities and proved values thereby could be more fully exploited.

Invisible Antigen–Antibody Reactions

Precipitation, agglutination, and hemolysis are visible evidence for antigen–antibody reaction. But complement fixation occurs invisibly during such a reaction, which therefore is detected visibly only with erythrocyte hemolysis as an indicator system. Several other methods have been used in immunodiffusion tests for accomplishing this purpose. The following discussion explains the basic principles of some of them. Examples and applications will be found elsewhere, particularly in Chapter 7.

Invisible antigen–antibody reactions can be detected in three different ways: (1) by changes that they exert on visible antigen–antibody reactions; (2) by means of nonantigen–antibody indicator systems; and (3) by some auxiliary device.

Whenever an antigen–antibody system produces a visible reaction, such as a precipitin band in immunodiffusion, then one can detect antigens and antibodies related to those in the system by tests revealing interference with the visible reaction. The interference can be additive or subtractive. For example, a solution added to a previously standardized solution of antigen might cause more rapid migration of the precipitin band that this antigen forms in a single diffusion tube test. The solution thus is revealed to contain either the same antigen or a related one (see Fig. 3.6). The same solution mixed into the agar–antiserum column of such a test instead will have the same effect for a similar reason (Gussoni, 1964). In the first instance, the quantity of unknown antigen added to that in the standard is greater than that of the standard alone. Hence, net diffusion of the antigen is faster and is also less easily retarded by the antibody in the lower column. In the second instance, mixing the unknown antigen with the antiserum depletes the antibodies available to react with and retard progress of the standard antigen. Consequently, as in the first instance, the precipitin band passes more quickly through the antibody-containing column, not because the antigen source is stronger by addition but rather because the antibody source is weaker by subtraction (Crowle, 1961).

This principle of specifically altering the position, intensity, or shape of a precipitin band formed in immunodiffusion tests by a standardized antigen–antibody system has many variations (Paul and Benacerraf, 1966; Keller, 1966; Casman *et al.*, 1969; Wilson *et al.*, 1962; Goldfarb and Callaghan, 1961). Antigen, or hapten, mixed with antiserum can slow, displace, or prevent formation of a precipitin band, although the antigen–antibody reaction product of this mixture itself is invisible (Paul and Benacerraf, 1966; Malley *et al.*, 1964; Pepys *et al.*, 1962). Antibodies can be detected indirectly in the same way by mixing the unknown antiserum with a minimal concentration of antigen (Keller, 1966; Ray and Kadull, 1964; Patterson *et al.*, 1964; Jameson, 1969; Shivers and Metz, 1962).

Changes in some nonimmunologic characteristic of antigen effected by and indicating invisible antigen–antibody reactions can be either qualitative or quantitative. Classic examples are afforded by immuno-diffusion tests with enzyme antigens. Most prominent is some effect of antibodies on the distribution of the enzyme in a semisolid medium. For instance, one can locate an enzyme in agar by originally including its substrate in the gel, or by placing it on the gel later. Where the enzyme reacts with antibody in the gel its diffusion pattern will be deranged, and this will be detectable by observing the enzyme–substrate reaction whether or not interaction between the enzyme and the antiserum has resulted in visible reaction (Lundbeck and Tirunarayanan, 1970; Thompson and Lachmann, 1970; Hermann and Miescher, 1965). Alternatively, the enzyme may be fixed by antibodies within the gel. Then, when the gel is washed free of uncomplexed enzyme and exposed to the appropriate substrate for the enzyme, a finely localized residual zone of enzyme activity will be evidence of the antigen–antibody reaction that has occurred (Micheli, 1965; Daussant and Grabar, 1966; Kaminski, 1966; Nace, 1963; Beernink *et al.*, 1965; Revis, 1971).

In these reactions, Nature supplies the experimenter with a labeled reactant. Essentially the same principles can be applied to reactants that have no natural label by using an auxiliary technique for detecting the invisible antigen–antibody reaction. Indeed, by this device the experimenter can readily detect the simplest of antigen–antibody reactions—namely, the formation of primary complexes; he can study any kind of antibody and any kind of antigen. There are many ways of accomplishing this, but all can be illustrated by the example of radioimmunodiffusion (Rejnek and Bednarik, 1960; Yagi *et al.*, 1963a). The key to this and similar techniques is to label antigen or antibody directly or indirectly in order to detect its fixation to the opposite specific reactant. Labeling can be radioactive, fluorescent (Nace *et al.*, 1961; Hsu *et al.*, 1963; Ghetie, 1967), enzymatic (Avrameas and Uriel, 1966), heavy metal (Hsu *et al.*, 1963; Bazin, 1967) or visual (Katsh and Matchael, 1962; Bazin, 1967; Castañeda, 1950); and it can be applied as a constituent of a secondary reactant which detects one of the primary reactants (e.g., radioactive antibody to antibody). Consider some illustrations.

If the antigen is made radioactive and reacts with antibody to become fixed as either a visible or an invisible aggregate in agar, and the gel then is washed free of unreacted materials and dried, the aggregate can be detected by laying the dried gel on photosensitive film to detect the resultant region of concentrated radioactivity in the gel. But the antibody reacting with this antigen may not form large enough aggregates with it to resist being washed out of the gel. This problem can be overcome by precipitating this antibody with another antibody to it (e.g., by precipitating human hay fever antibody with rabbit precipitins to the human hay fever antibody) and then diffusing the labeled antigen into the area of this stable aggregate (Onoue *et al.*, 1964; Heiner *et al.*, 1970; Dolovich *et al.*, 1970). The antigen will become fixed to its antibody, even if by no more than a primary stage reaction, which is itself already fixed within the gel by antibody to it. After subsequent washing, the reaction between the labeled antigen and its nonprecipitating antibody will be detectable by radioactivity adhering to the precipitate formed by the nonprecipitating antibody, and antibody to it. The value of this technique cannot be overestimated, for it enables one not only to detect any kind of antibody but also to identify the antibody as belonging to some class of immunoglobulin (Heiner *et al.*, 1970; Yagi *et al.*, 1963a).

Less frequently, antibody is labeled instead of antigen to detect invisible antigen–antibody reactions (Hsu *et al.*, 1963; Ghetie, 1967). Usually, this is done when the antibody can fix antigen in agar but the amount of antibody is too small to produce a visible reaction. As with antigen labeling techniques, labels can be varied; but the most sensitive is that of radioactivity.

Diffusion

In immunodiffusion tests, antigen and antibodies can be mixed in several different ways. The most frequently used and elementary of these is diffusion.

Nature of Diffusion

Random thermal agitation of individual atoms, molecules, and ions is vigorous at the temperatures used for immunodiffusion tests. This agitation is the motive power for diffusion.

As any single molecule of antigen is jostled about, a coincidence of random hits on it by other ions and molecules moves it short distances in one direction or another, and gradually it will diffuse away from its original position. If it had originally been placed in the center of a petri dish of agar gel, given infinite time and unchanging environmental conditions it would eventually diffuse to every other possible position in the gel. The movement of such a molecule is random, so that there is as much chance that it will travel in one direction as another. But if two antigen molecules were placed at one location in the gel instead of one, there would be twice as much chance for this antigen to move in any given direction; and if many were placed in this area this chance would be increased in proportion to their number. Thus, in an immunodiffusion test, the chances for some antigen molecules to diffuse from a well charged with antigen solution into surrounding gel containing no antigen increase in proportion to the total number (i.e., concentration) of all the antigen molecules placed in the well. Consequently, the net rate of antigen diffusion into surrounding gel will be proportional to the difference between the concentration of antigen within the well and the concentration of antigen in surrounding gel. As this difference becomes less by diffusion of antigen molecules away from their original source, the chances for antigen molecules to move in any given direction (e.g., away from the well) become progressively less, and the rate of net diffusion slows progressively. Eventually, when the population of antigen molecules has become distributed evenly throughout the gel it stops.

Factors Affecting Diffusion

The rate of diffusion for any antigen or population of antibody molecules[9] follows rules that make it predictable and mathematically definable (Ouchterlony, 1968; Stiehm, 1967; Meffroy-Biget, 1967b,c,d; Aladjem *et al.*, 1968). The higher the concentration of diffusing molecules at their source, the faster will be their net diffusion away from it. The net rate of diffusion decreases progressively as the antigen becomes more dilute by diffusion. This decrease is much faster when antigen diffuses radially, as from a hole, than when it diffuses linearly, as down a column of gel.

High temperature accelerates diffusion; low temperature slows it. Small molecules diffuse faster than large ones, and round ones faster than those of other shapes. Diffusion varies inversely with medium viscosity, which can be an important factor in concentrated solutions or when some agar in a gel has been partially hydrolyzed during preparation of the gel such as by heating it to remelt it.

---

[9] The characteristics of diffusion as depicted here apply to antibody molecules as much as to antigen molecules, but the latter will be used as an example because they offer a wider variety for discussion of various effects. Many of these characteristics can be demonstrated swiftly, realistically, and cheaply with inorganic chemicals (Young and Brubaker, 1963).

The above rules apply only when reactant diffusion is free; but often it may not be free. For example, localized drying of the gel may attract water and, with it, a flow of antigen superimposed on its diffusion. This effect, sometimes called rheophoresis, can be used purposely to hasten mixing of antigen and antibody (Van Oss and Bronson, 1969). Similar hydrodynamic effects arise from locally high salt concentration, siphoning or percolation (i.e., chromatography), or electroendosmosis (see these subjects, below). These effects may be nuisances, especially if unrecognized and unaccounted for. But trends recently have been to use them to supplement or even supplant diffusion as forces for mixing antigen and antibodies in immunodiffusion tests (see Chapter 7).

Reactant diffusion can be altered in other ways, notably by interaction between medium and reactant. For instance, an antigen may adsorb to or react with the medium (e.g., Hokama *et al.*, 1965), or it may be too large or become too large to pass freely through the network of the supporting medium. The following are some examples.

Agar is negatively charged; consequently antigens with a net positive charge will combine with it. At neutral or alkaline pH, antibodies and most serum proteins are either electroneutral or electronegative and so diffuse unaffected through agar. But in buffers of pH lower than their isoelectric points, protein antigens convert to electropositivity. Some antigens like lysozyme have such a high isoelectric point (pH 11.3) that a buffer with pH high enough to make it electronegative would interfere with antigen–antibody precipitation. Consequently, antigens like these, or antigens converted to high isoelectric point such as by acetylation (Tawde *et al.*, 1963), must be studied in neutral stabilizing media like agarose, cellulose acetate, gelatin, or polyacrylamide, chemically changed to lower their isoelectric points (Weeke, 1968a), or studied in agar chemically electroneutralized (Ragetli and Weintraub, 1966).

Sulfate groups in agar tend to react with lipids and certain antigens like hemoglobin (Wunderly, 1960; Beck and Uzan, 1965). Hence, such antigens as serum lipoproteins move through agar gels more slowly than they would by unimpeded diffusion, and some will be precipitated by the agar.

Problems of reactant–gel interaction like these sometimes can be minimized by changing solvent buffer composition (Wunderly, 1960), but they are circumvented more readily by substituting agarose for agar, because agarose is nearly electroneutral and therefore reacts little or not at all (depending on how it is prepared) with electropositive antigens or with lipids. Cellulose acetate and polyacrylamide are similarly inert. Gelatin is electroneutral (Crowle, 1961), but it reacts with neutral polysaccharides, and also with antibodies to a lesser extent (Dudman, 1965b).

The maximum size of molecules or particles that can move through an immunodiffusion medium depends on the structure of the medium, which, in turn, depends on its nature, concentration, and constitution. The theoretical pore size of 0.67% agar gel is 12 nm, but the structure of agar gels is so heterogeneous that α_{2M}-globulin, for example, which is larger than 12 nm, can diffuse through it (Wunderly, 1960). Large molecules, including viruses (Blair *et al.*, 1966), therefore can diffuse through agar gels, but truly free diffusion of even the smaller antigen molecules probably cannot occur in concentrations of agar exceeding 0.5% (Wunderly, 1960). This explains why one can obtain increased serum antigen resolution in immunoelectrophoresis with 2% as contrasted with 1% agar gels: the movement of several serum antigens is moderately restricted in the gel of higher concentration (Brummerstedt-Hansen, 1967). Changes in the size of a given antigen molecule therefore can affect its diffusion rate even in the most commonly used concentrations of stabilizing medium, and such changes, in the form of spontaneous polymerization for example, are probably frequent (see Preparation of Antigens, Chapter 2).

SHAPE OF REACTANT SOURCE

The shape of the front of the diffusing reactant depends on the shape of its source, on the shape of the container it diffuses in, and on the influences it encounters during diffusion (Wilson, 1964). From a circular source it is radial. From a square source it develops primarily in four planes corresponding to the sides of the square and secondarily in four wedge-shaped areas corresponding to the four corners of the square. A rectangular trough will provide a long, even front of diffusion with acutely curved edges.

Diffusion fronts of reactants from opposing circular wells will meet as oppositely curving arcs, center first, and then with progressing lateral overlap (Fig. 1.5). Diffusion fronts from the sides of square wells or from rectangular troughs will meet each other face-to-face at 180 degrees across nearly the entire face of each front. Only at the ends of these fronts will changes in disposition of encounter develop, but these will be acute. When face-to-face diffusion is confined within a tube, there will be no change of confronting reactant proportions laterally. Elongated troughs positioned at angles to each other of less than 180 degrees (e.g., 90 degrees) cause reactants to diffuse across instead of toward each other (Fig. 1.5).

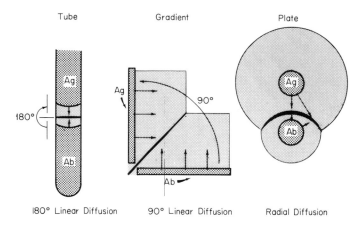

Fig. 1.5. Three basic types of double diffusion test are (1) the tube test, (2) the gradient test, (3) the plate test, which permit antigen and antibody to diffuse face-to-face, across each other at right angles, or both, respectively. The first hypothetically is the most sensitive test, the second is particularly useful for identifying secondary precipitation which may be confusing interpretation of antigen qualitative analyses, and the third because of its convenience is the most often used of double diffusion tests for qualitative comparisons of antigen and antibody mixtures.

A front of diffusion can be changed by anything affecting reactant diffusion locally, such as the presence of the opposing reactant, incompletely dissolved particles of agar, indentations in the gel, a well that is empty or charged with saline, a trough filled with denser or thinner gel, or the edges of the immunodiffusion container. Regarding the last of these, if the quantity of reactant is large, the immunodiffusion container small, and the source of diffusion small, diffusion of the reactant can rebound from the edge of the container, causing some unexpected precipitation in peculiar places (Holm, 1965; Fig. 1.6).

Secondary Precipitation

Generally, a single antigen–antibody system produces only one precipitin band. But there are exceptions, and some are associated with certain characteristics of antigen–antibody diffusion (Lueker and Crowle, 1963).

A forming precipitin band consumes antigen and antibody in its immediate area at a rate established by their relative concentrations and diffusion coefficients. If the two are serologically balanced, the precipitin band remains immobile where it first began to develop, and on either

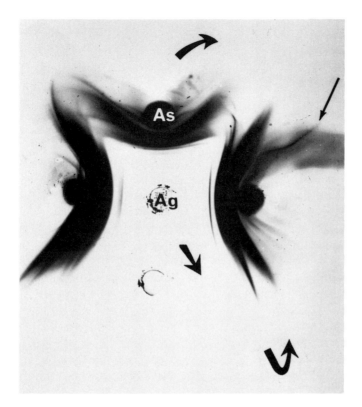

Fig. 1.6. Micro double diffusion plate test in which diffusion of antigen and precipitins "rebounded" from edges of agar gel to precipitate (long, thin arrow) outside the original arena of antigen–antibody interaction. Thicker arrows trace paths of antigen and precipitins.

side of it there is a smoothly rising gradient of free reactant. No secondary precipitation develops. But antigen and antibody frequently are not serologically balanced. If one, antigen for instance, is in slight excess, it will feed into the reaction area faster than the other (antibody) can precipitate it. Some therefore will pass through the forming precipitate and will precipitate on the antibody side. Consequently, the precipitin band will shift slightly toward the antibody source while it is developing.

When antigen and antibody precipitate each other, they create a lack of their respective molecules on either side of the immediate area of precipitation known as a "sink" (Afonso, 1966a; Fig. 1.7). If antigen is in moderate instead of slight excess, the antigen sink will be essentially nonexistent, but the antibody sink will be more prominent than it is in

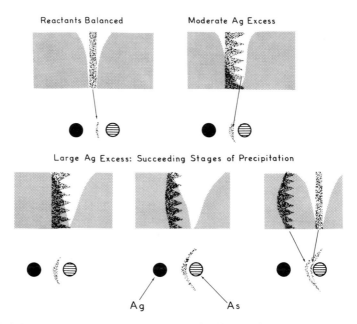

Fig. 1.7. Diagrammatic representation of sink effect and its promotion of Liese-gang precipitation. The shaded areas on either side of the central stippled bar represent concentrations in the gel of antigen (left) and antiserum (right). The stippled bar, or jagged derivatives of it, represents antigen–antibody precipitate. Below each situation (reactants balanced, moderate antigen excess, stages of pre-cipitation in large antigen excess) are diagrams indicating what can be observed in a double diffusion plate test between round wells of antigen and antiserum. Liesegang precipitation occurs only when there is an appropriate excess of reactant, usually antigen, having a diffusion coefficient different from that of its precipitins (cf. Lueker and Crowle, 1963).

balanced conditions, because antibody molecules are not diffusing into the reaction area fast enough to replace those precipitated by excessive antigen. In these conditions free antigen will diffuse not only through the forming precipitate but also some distance beyond it before encountering enough antibody to precipitate, and the result will be development of a second (Liesegang) precipitin band by this single antigen–antibody system (Francois *et al.*, 1956; Crowle, 1963; Crowle *et al.*, 1963; Lueker and Crowle, 1963; Prager, 1956; Gold, 1964; see Fig. 3.8). Liesegang bands develop best when one reactant is moderately excessive and when this reactant has a faster inherent diffusion rate than the other. They are rarely seen when either of these conditions is lacking (Van Regenmortel, 1967). Conditions favoring Liesegang precipitation also can develop when one reactant is mixed forcibly and rapidly with another by electrophoresis in electroimmunodiffusion (Jameson, 1968; Zydeck *et al.*, 1966).

Since moderate excess of one reactant is required for Liesegang precipitation, the phenomenon is self-correcting in immunodiffusion tests with reactants diffusing radially. The stronger reactant dilutes itself faster than the weaker lateral to the original area of precipitation, and so the secondary precipitin band converges with the primary band laterally; the two bands do not cross as they would if formed by different antigen–antibody systems (Fig. 1.8). This hallmark[10] of Liesegang precipitation is absent when there is no change of reactant ratios laterally.

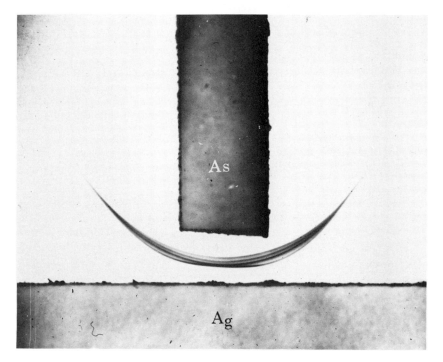

Fig. 1.8. Classic example of Liesegang precipitation between bovine serum albumin antigen and horse antiserum. The importance of the antigen–antiserum ratio is seen directly in formation of four bands of precipitate with this single antigen–antiserum system where antiserum is diffusing from the corners of its source, as opposed to the formation of only three between the antigen source and the middle of the antiserum source. For details of this experiment see Lueker and Crowle (1963).

[10] Multiple bands due to truly different antigen–antibody systems may merge laterally in a resemblance of Liesegang precipitation when local depletion of reactants coincides with the area of band merging (see DeCarvalho *et al.*, 1962, for possible examples).

Consequently, Liesegang precipitation cannot be identified as such directly in tube immunodiffusion tests (see Fig. 3.8).

A different kind of secondary precipitation can appear in immunodiffusion tests with a large excess of antigen. This excess is so great (e.g., as in single diffusion tests) that the antigen sweeps through the atmosphere of antibodies being precipitated as it moves and never establishes an equilibrium. But sudden changes in temperature will alter its speed of diffusion (Lueker and Crowle, 1963; Crowle, 1961). A drop will slow it and give antibody more time to combine efficiently with it at its advancing front and thus form a band of precipitate with increased intensity (stria). A rise will do the opposite, causing its front to move even faster into the already taxed atmosphere of antibody and either not precipitate or precipitate more weakly than before (gap; see Fig. 3.7). Similar secondary precipitates also can develop in electroimmunodiffusion tests (Fig. 1.9).

Gaps and striae form quite easily in single diffusion tests (or in double diffusion tests that inadvertently become single diffusion tests because of large excess of reactant) in which there are sudden, even, small temperature changes, such as are effected by the heating–cooling cycles of a refrigerator. They are more apt to form when the excess reactant also has the higher diffusion coefficient. These artifacts are more readily identified for R-type than for H-type precipitins (see Fig. 3.7), because with the latter the background of weak precipitation marking the progress of antigen diffusion through antiserum tends to dissociate. Unlike Liesegang precipitates, gaps and striae do not tend to converge laterally in plate tests allowing radial diffusion of reactants; they simply fade out. If the distance of diffusion is great enough, or the initial excessiveness of antigen is low enough, a test in which gaps and striae have been developing can convert to producing Liesegang precipitates.

Secondary precipitation can result from a duality characteristic of reactants in addition simply to diffusion-associated factors. For instance, guinea pig antibodies to a hapten–protein complex can form two precipitin bands specific for the same hapten because some of the antibodies precipitate hapten–protein alone, but others form soluble diffusible complexes with it which can precipitate only with the aid of complement. The complement-associated precipitation is likely to develop in a plane of the medium different from that of the complement-independent precipitation (Paul and Benacerraf, 1966). One kind of antigenic determinant can be attached to two different carriers, both of high molecular weight and one higher than the other. A high concentration of antibody diffusing to encounter the determinant on the smaller of the two molecules first precipitates it, but then also bypasses it because diffusion of this

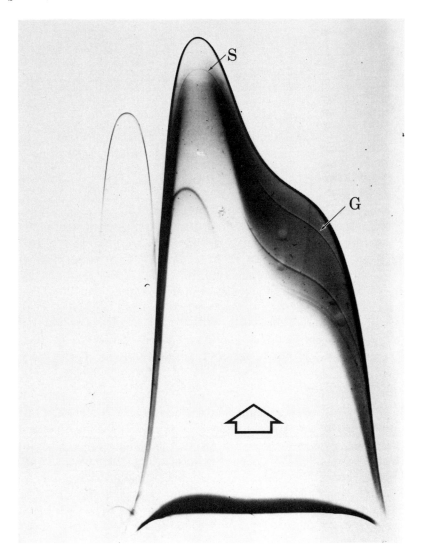

Fig. 1.9. Gaps (G) and striae (S) can be observed in electroimmunodiffusion as shown here in a two-dimensional single electroimmunodiffusion analysis of human serum using rabbit antiserum. The large double loop within which this secondary precipitation was developed was formed by serum albumin. The lower, more anodic loop (cf. Chapter 6) probably was formed by free albumin; the higher, more cathodic loop probably was formed by complexes of albumin and other more basic serum constituents which it carries (G. J. Revis, personal communication). Three partially formed loops were formed by other serum antigens. The very heavy but flat double loop at the base of the electroimmunodiffusogram was formed by albumin prematurely reacting with antiserum before secondary electrophoresis was begun (D. C. Lueker, personal communication).

antigen into the area of precipitation is too slow to keep precipitating the antibodies as fast as they arrive. The bypassing antibodies then encounter the second, slower-diffusing determinant–carrier substance and form a second precipitate. This occurs with antibodies to serum α- and β-lipoproteins (Burtin and Grabar, 1967). Another novel cause of "secondary" precipitation is the presence of precipitins in an antigen solution which precipitate antigen components of the antiserum. This was observed when rabbit antiserum was used to measure IgG in human serum, but the human serum contained precipitins for rabbit immunoglobulins themselves (Ammann and Hong, 1971).

Electrophoresis

Next to diffusion, electrophoresis is the force most frequently used to mix antigen and antibody in immunodiffusion tests, and with recent developments in electroimmunodiffusion techniques may eventually equal it. Since there are several excellent monographs explaining electrophoresis (McDonald, 1955; Wieme, 1959a; Boyack and Giddings, 1963; Wunderly, 1960; Audubert and de Mende, 1960; Bier, 1967), the following discussion is restricted to providing the reader only with practical information for use in immunoelectrophoresis and related techniques.

Nature of Electrophoresis

Electrophoresis can be defined as the movement of particles or ions by direct current through an electrolyte solution. The basic apparatus consists of a power supply for direct current (batteries, direct-current generator, or rectifier for converting alternating line current to direct current), positive and negative preferably nonpolarizing electrodes (platinum, carbon, or some similarly inert conductor), a vessel of buffer for immersing each electrode, and some kind of bridge connecting these two buffer vessels and acting as the support for the material in which electrophoresis will occur. A simple but effective setup is shown in Fig. 1.10 as used with a microscope slide supporting agar gel. Figure 5.9 diagrammatically represents an improvement on this apparatus in which opposite ends of the electropherogram are rested directly on sponges protruding from the buffer vessels.

A simple, visible demonstration of electrophoresis also illustrates its principles. Any of a number of acid dyes, such as thiazine red, can be the substance to be electrophoresed. In preparation for the experiment illustrated in Fig. 1.10, 1% agar was dissolved by boiling in an alkaline buffer such as one of the barbital buffers used for fractionating serum.

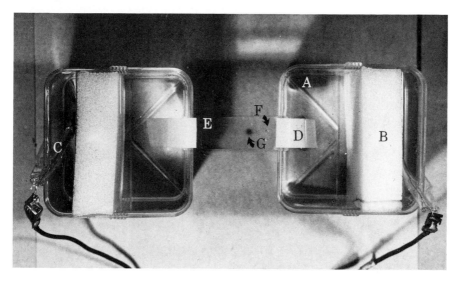

Fig. 1.10. A simple form of agar electrophoresis commonly adapted to immuno-electrophoresis. Buffer vessels (A) contain sponge baffles (B) to prevent electrolysis products from the electrodes (C) changing the pH of buffer in contact with the paper connecting wicks (D). The glass slide (E) has been covered with agar about 2 mm thick; the origin (F) punched in this agar was charged with thiazine red R solution which by electrophoresis at pH 8.2 has moved away from the origin toward the anode and was located at C when this photograph was made.

The hot solution was poured onto a microscope slide and permitted to gel. A hole was punched in the gel at the cathode (negative pole) end of the slide and filled with thiazine red R solution dissolved in buffer, and 100 V of direct current was passed through the gel and its electrolyte, a barbital buffer of pH 8.2 and ionic strength 0.05. The dye migrated away from its origin at a rate directly proportional to the voltage applied and to the dye's electronegativity, and inversely proportional to the buffer's ionic strength, the opposing force of electroosmosis (strong in agar, weak in agarose), and the agar's viscosity. Essentially the same would be observed if a serum protein were used in place of the dye. Factors affecting zone electrophoresis, particularly in semisolid media, include buffer pH, ionic strength and composition, supporting medium charge and physical characteristics, electric current and voltage, temperature, and the concentration and nature of the substances being electrophoresed.

Buffer pH controls chiefly the direction and rate of reactant movement. Since in immunoelectrophoresis and electroimmunodiffusion protein antigens and their derivatives are the most frequent subjects for investigation, pH and other factors will be discussed relative to them. A protein, being composed of amino acids with both acidic (carboxyl) and basic (amino) groups exposed to the environmental solvent, can have a positive charge, a negative charge, or be electrically neutral. The net charge of a protein molecule will vary in kind and intensity with variations in pH of the surrounding medium. At its isoelectric pH, the pH at which the protein is electrically neutral, it may be imagined to have an equal number of carboxyl and amino groups at its surface. As the pH is raised, the positive charge on increasing numbers of amino groups is neutralized by whatever alkali is being used, and the protein molecule becomes increasingly negative as the unaffected carboxyl groups become dominant. Conversely, as the pH is lowered below the isoelectric point, amino groups remain unaffected while increasing numbers of negatively charged carboxyl groups are neutralized, and the protein becomes positively charged. Hence, a serum protein such as γ-globulin with an isoelectric pH of about 7 dissolved in buffer of pH 8.2 will be moderately negative, while another serum protein with a lower isoelectric pH, such as albumin with a value of 4.7, will have a strong net negative charge. A mixture of these two proteins electrophoresed at pH 8.2 therefore will separate because the γ-globulin is less repelled by the cathode than the albumin; they move in the same direction but at different rates. In some media, like agar gel, they will move in opposite directions because of electroosmosis (see below).

BUFFERS

The ionic strength of a buffer affects electrophoretic resolution, apparently because when it is high it will minimize interactions between substances being separated and between them and the supporting medium. But ionic strength also controls the rate of fraction migration, the buffering capacity of the medium, and the amount of current passing through the medium. If ionic strength is low, current carried by the medium will be low, and high voltage can be applied to it without excessive heating. Fraction migration then will be rapid for two reasons. First, at a given ionic strength and pH an increase in voltage or, more precisely, field strength increases the net differences in charge between the substance being electrophoresed and the similarly charged electrode, and consequently their net mutual repulsion. Second, the migrating substance is surrounded by an atmosphere of electrolyte ions of opposite charge so that there is a tendency for fluid around it to move in the opposite direction and against it, thus decreasing its mobility. Since this is proportional to the ionic strength (that is, the electrolyte ions available for forming this atmosphere), the lower this is, the less will this effect influence the migrating antigen. The advantage offered by low ionic strength of rapid fraction movement (and therefore a minimum time during which it can diffuse) in a medium carrying little current may be offset by poor fraction resolution and by reduced buffering capacity, a condition incompatible with obtaining of consistent results. In immunoelectrophoresis and electroimmunodiffusion, the best practice is to use an ionic strength that will permit the most rapid separation (to minimize fraction diffusion) at constant pH with good resolution and lack of trailing. Generally, this is between 0.1 and 0.02.

A formula can be employed to calculate buffer ionic strength, providing that all ions composing the buffer are completely ionized:

$$\mu = \tfrac{1}{2} \sum (i \cdot n^2)$$

in which μ is the symbol for ionic strength, i is the molal concentration of an ion, and n is the valence of the ion. But calculated ionic strength, which is that often stated in tables of buffer formulas, seldom agrees closely with and frequently widely diagrees with what it actually is as determined by electric conductance. For example, the calculated ionic strength of a sodium barbital–hydrochloric acid buffer and of sodium chloride solution will be equal at 0.15, and both usually are presumed to be completely ionized. Yet, the conductivity of the buffer is less than that of the sodium chloride solution. This is illustrated in Fig. 1.11. Fortunately, since this buffer still is the most often used, it does have the same conductance as sodium chloride solution, and the calculated ionic strength for both is the same, in the concentrations employed for immunoelectrophoresis and electroimmunodiffusion.

A trend for greater relative conductance (i.e., degree of ionization) with decreasing salt concentration also is obvious from Fig. 1.11; it shows that eventually the lines drawn for four different electrolyte solutions will converge. Nevertheless, some buffers are made with constituents ionizing so poorly that the calculated ionic strength will never agree with that estimated by conductivity in concentration ranges practical for immunodiffusion tests. This is exemplified by the tris buffer in Fig. 1.11 as well as by barbital buffer made up with acetic rather than hydrochloric acid and occasionally used for immunoelectrophoresis. For example, while calculated and actual ionic strengths of barbital–hydrochloric acid buffer at pH 8.6 and ionic strength 0.05 are equal, for a barbital–acetate buffer to attain equivalent conductivity it must be made up at a calculated 0.079 ionic strength. If it were prepared at a calculated ionic strength of 0.05, its true strength by conductance would be only 0.032. For the very weakly dissociating buffer sodium borate–boric acid

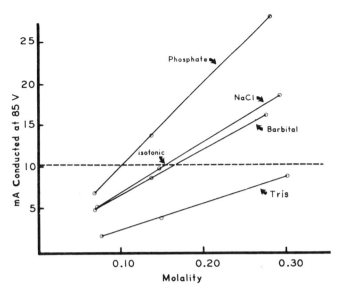

Fig. 1.11. A comparison of the conductivity (mA) under standardized conditions of four different electrolyte solutions at different molalities showing that salts made up at identical calculated ionicities (e.g., 0.15 molal sodium chloride and 0.15 molal sodium barbital–hydrochloric acid) will not necessarily conduct equal quantities of electric current, that as the electrolytes are used in progressively lower concentrations they ionize more completely and therefore conduct more efficiently, and that some buffer constituents ionize so weakly (e.g., tris) that within concentration ranges employed for immunoelectrophoresis their calculated ionicities invariably will be higher than their ionicities determined by actual conductivity studies.

to attain conductivity equivalent to that of completely dissociated sodium chloride at ionic strength 0.05, it would have to be made up at a calculated ionic strength of 0.228 at pH 8.6.

True ionic strength (i.e., current-carrying capacity of dissolved electrolytes) can be calculated only if one takes into account such factors as electrolyte dissociation constants, pH, actual salt concentrations, temperature, and the influence of one kind of ion upon the dissociation of another. This is neither simple nor practical for most users of immunoelectrophoresis and electroimmunodiffusion. Therefore, buffer "strength" should be reported in terms both of quantitative composition, so that someone else can make up the buffer, and of either "equivalent conductance"[11] or

---

[11] This can be determined with a Wheatstone bridge conductance cell, designed for this purpose, and expressed in $\Omega^{-1}cm^2$ for a given temperature. But information obtained in this manner is not available in buffer formularies used for biochemistry, and, since it is meaningless to the average user of immunodiffusion and zone electrophoresis, we prefer reporting buffer conductance as described in the text (cf. Wunderly, 1960; Uriel, 1966).

conductance relative to that of a known and familiar standard solution like sodium chloride. For example, one may determine how much current is conducted by a 0.05 N ($\mu = 0.05$) sodium chloride solution at a given voltage and temperature, make up a barbital buffer at a desired pH somewhat more concentrated than this, measure its conductance at the same voltage and temperature in the same apparatus at three or more different dilutions, and, from values so obtained and graphed, determine exactly what dilution of the original barbital mixture at that particular pH will conduct the same amount of current as the reference sodium chloride solution. Then the electrolyte strength of the barbital could be reported as "conductance equivalent to 0.05 N sodium chloride solution," or it could be reported as some multiple or fraction of this conductance. Satisfactory data of this sort can be obtained with the electrophoresis power supply, beakers, electrodes, and an inverted U tube as illustrated in Fig. 1.12. Note that conductance generally is an exponential function of absolute temperature and therefore that measurements should be made at a standard temperature (Wunderly, 1960).

The importance of a buffer's composition is obvious from what has just been discussed—i.e., that conductivity varies among different buffer salts. But beyond this, certain buffers used under more or less equivalent conditions may provide strikingly different results, some permitting separations not possible with others. Rat serum proteins retain the same relative electrophoretic mobilities in borate buffers of different pH and ionic strength, but they change these mobilities relative to each other with such variations made with other kinds of buffers (Escribano, 1962). Examples of this are given in Chapters 6 and 7. Apparently these differences are due to such effects as complexing between buffer ions and fractions, changes that they effect in fraction dispersion, and their influence on medium-fraction interactions.

CURRENT AND VOLTAGE

Electric current is a villain in immunoelectrophoresis. Other factors such as ionic strength, buffering capacity, pH, and voltage must be regulated so that the separation of components will be as rapid as possible without inducing excessive flow of current, because several complications will arise if this precaution is not taken. One is excessive heating. This leads especially to rapid drying of the electrophoresis medium, which in turn increases the flow of current as electrolytes become more concentrated, and occasionally to development of local "hot spots," such as at the origin if the sample being electrophoresed has not previously been dialyzed against the buffer being used for electrophoresis and exceeds its ionic strength. A heating gel also may shrink and distort the electropherogram (Uriel, 1966). Another product of excessive current

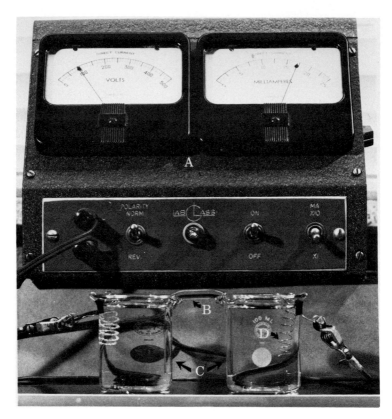

Fig. 1.12. Apparatus required for simplified conductivity measurements on electrolyte solutions employed for immunoelectrophoresis. This consists of a direct current power supply (A), a glass tube bridge (B) filled with electrolyte solution and dipping into two small beaker buffer vessels (C), and a nonpolarizing wire coil electrode (D) in each buffer vessel. The greater the dissociation or actual ionicity of an electrolyte, the greater amount of current will be carried by the bridge (as registered by the milliampere gauge) at a given voltage.

is pH change caused by electrolysis of buffer salts. Normally, this is low enough or baffled well enough to be insignificant, but excessive current together with insufficient baffles, small buffer volume, and poor buffering capacity can cause significant pH change. Current actually passing through the electrophoresis gel can be lowered by lowering the voltage, lowering the ionic strength, or cooling the apparatus and electrolyte.

The term "field strength" has been used somewhat confusingly by various writers describing their zone electrophoretic techniques; it therefore deserves some explanation. A voltage of 100 read on the dial of an electrophoresis power source merely indicates that this is the difference in electric potential between its two electrodes. If all that separated these electrodes were a glass tube 10 cm long filled with electrolyte solution, the field strength would be 100 V per 10 cm, or 10 V/cm. In practice, some types of zone electrophoresis apparatus offer too much resistance to permit realization of full voltage potential across the actual electrophoretic zone. Poor connection between the electrophoresis medium and the cathode and anode buffer vessels is a frequent impediment to application of full voltage. Electrophoretic migration of an antigen depends on how near its origin is to one of the electrodes.[12] Small changes in temperature will cause significant changes in migration; and antigens migrate faster at the beginning of electrophoresis than later, especially at high voltages (Reinskou, 1966b). Because of such practical variations in apparatus, it is more useful to mention in addition to the voltage reading of the power supply, in volts per centimeter of electrophoresis medium, the rate of movement of a tracking dye or a standard antigen like human serum albumin through the gel.

ELECTROPHORESIS MEDIUM

The nature of the supporting medium can profoundly affect results in the electrophoretic separations of immunoelectrophoresis and electroimmunodiffusion. In previous years this was evident as differences among various kinds of agar gel. Today, variations obtainable in electrophoretic separations are potentially much greater as one uses not only different kinds of agar, but chemically altered agars, agarose, media like gelatin or cellulose acetate, and the medium with the greatest potential among its own formulations for variety, polyacrylamide. Examples of these will be given with techniques describing their use in Chapter 2. Here, some generalizations will be made on reasons for their differences.

Agars are negatively charged. Since they form immobile gels, water within them moves toward the cathode to compensate for their tendency to move toward the anode. This effect, called electroosmosis, causes all fractions being electrophoresed to be carried toward the cathode; their progress toward the anode if they are negatively charged is what their progress would be in an indifferent medium minus their electroosmotic movement. Electroosmosis has become an important means for mixing antigens with antibody in such techniques as electroimmunodiffusion (Chapter 6).

---

[12] Human Gc proteins migrate faster as they are placed nearer the anode. This effect is especially troublesome when electrophoresis slides are used in series between electrodes instead of in parallel (Reinskou, 1966b).

Agars also differ in affinities for various antigens such as lipoproteins and therefore may differ in their capacity to resolve these antigens. Some may insolubilize antigens more readily than others and so be ineffective in detecting them. As was mentioned in the Diffusion section, these effects of agar gels are influenced significantly by the nature of the electrolytes mixed with them, and they can be changed radically by chemically altering agars to neutralize their electronegativity or to do the opposite and increase it. A procedure as subtle as adding 0.01% Merthiolate to agar before it is boiled will reduce serum antigen migration rates (Jordan and White, 1965). Increasing the agar concentration from 1% to 2% is reported to decrease serum protein migration in electrophoresis by 40% (Jordan and White, 1965).

Electrophoresis in agarose, a component of agar (see Chapter 2), is nearly the same as that in agar except that a properly prepared agarose has considerably less electroosmosis, no affinity for either acidic or basic antigens, and less tendency than agar to bind with various other substances like lipids. Consequently, antigens that tend to drag and trail during electrophoresis in agar gels migrate more homogeneously and therefore are better resolved in agarose gels.

Electroosmosis is absent from gelatin, cellulose acetate, and polyacrylamide (Crowle, 1961). Electrophoresis through cellulose acetate is like paper electrophoresis except that strips of cellulose acetate are more uniform than paper and do not adsorb antigens as much. Gelatin seldom is used for electrophoresis, principally because it liquefies so easily on heating; hence little is known about its properties as a stabilizer for electrophoresis (Crowle and Hu, 1967). Our experience is that serum proteins separate in it approximately as they do in agarose, but that in immunoelectrophoresis less antigens are detected, perhaps because of gelatin's interactions with various antigens as mentioned in the section on diffusion. Polyacrylamide electrophoresis has become very popular in recent years (disc electrophoresis: cf. Whipple, 1964) because of the inertness and excellent utility of polyacrylamide gels, but especially because their composition can be varied so broadly to prepare gels with sieving characteristics in addition to those of anticonvection medium. Electrophoretic migration of serum proteins appears to be as free in 3% polyacrylamide gels as it is in 1% agarose (Keutel, 1964) and is similar except that the entire pattern in agarose is shifted slightly toward the cathode because of weak electroosmosis. But succeedingly denser polyacrylamide gels can be prepared in several ways, usually by increasing the percentages of acrylamide in them, with corresponding increases in sieving effect—that is, the capacity not only to serve as an inert anticonvection medium but also to act as a filtering gel which can sort antigens from a mixture by molecular size as they are being fractionated at the same time by electrophoretic characteristics (see Chapter 2). Only moderate sieving can be achieved in agar or agarose at the highest concentrations (about 4%) with which they can be worked practically. Starch gels are well known for sieving fractionations and have been used occasionally for immunoelectrophoresis for lack of a better medium of this kind (see Chapters 5 and 6), but it is not likely that they will compete successfully with acrylamide gels, when these are available, because they are not clear, they are more difficult to use, and they cannot be prepared in such great variety.

Gels made with polyacrylamide alone have some properties that make them troublesome to use in conventional immunodiffusion tests, but these can be circumvented by casting them in combination with agarose (Uriel, 1966). Electrophoretically these gels appear to produce essentially the same results as polyacrylamide gels made without agarose.

CHARACTERISTICS OF THE SAMPLE

Electrophoretic fractionation depends partly on the nature of the test sample other than its ionic characteristics. For instance, antigens frequently exist as complexes with each other in native state, and therefore the electrophoretic mobility of a complex and of its component antigens depends on the proportions of one antigen to the other in the original complex, and the degree of complex dissociation occurring during electrophoresis (see Chapter 6). Degree of dissociation in turn depends on such factors as temperature, pH, ionic strength, and electrophoretic voltage.[13] Antigens also may complex with antibodies, each thus altering the other's electrophoretic mobility (Yagi *et al.*, 1962). Some antigens, such as serum α-lipoprotein, are widely recognized to have strongly concentration-dependent electrophoretic mobilities, but there are others for which this effect, though present, is not generally known (e.g., γ-globulin: Russell, 1966). The pattern of serum protein fractionation in agar gel is not the linear sum of the individual patterns that would be obtained by electrophoresing each component separately (Raymond and Nakamichi, 1962b). The presence of albumin, for example, influences the mobility of adjacent serum globulins, apparently by affecting pH, conductivity, field strength, and ionic composition of neighboring gel.

Electrophoretic Mixing of Antigen and Antibody

The function of electrophoresis in immunoelectrophoresis usually has been to separate a mixture of antigens before allowing them to mix with

---

[13] Complexes composed of electrophoretically different components can be dissociated by electrophoresis, this being proportional to the square of the voltage gradient (Ornstein, 1964).

their antibodies by diffusion and thereby to increase both resolving and characterizing capacities of immunodiffusion tests in which there has been no such preliminary fractionation of a reactant mixture.[14] But there is now a rapidly growing interest in using electrophoresis either in place of diffusion to mix antigen and antibody, achieving greater sensitivity and rapidity of antigen–antibody precipitation, or both for preliminary reactant fractionation and for later mixing with an opposing reactant.

The basic aspect of such techniques, collectively called electroimmuno-diffusion (Chapter 6), is to arrange conditions of electrophoresis so that antigen and its antibodies differ somewhat in electrophoretic mobility; then they can be mixed by causing them to migrate into each other or by having one overtake the other. For instance, rabbit precipitins are more cathodic than most serum proteins, so one can detect human serum albumin by charging a cathodic well in agar with this antigen and an anodic well with rabbit antibody to human serum albumin. During electrophoresis the albumin migrates anodally and the rabbit antibodies migrate cathodally (by electroosmosis); the two reactants meet each other between their origins and precipitate (see Fig. 6.20). In this, called "double electroimmunodiffusion," the electroosmotic properties of agar gels obviously are advantageous. Alternatively, human serum albumin can be made to react with rabbit antibodies which are sessile during electrophoresis by arranging conditions for the human serum albumin to migrate into the atmosphere of antibodies (e.g., by using agarose instead of agar and a pH of 8.6 instead of 8.2). The result of this technique, called "single electroimmunodiffusion," will be similar to that of a single diffusion test, a precipitate forming as antigen contacts antibody-containing gel and then growing as electrophoresis is continued and antigen progresses farther into this gel.

Several characteristics of the electrophoresis test can be manipulated to achieve the desired difference in electrophoretic or electroosmotic migration of antigen and its antibodies. Gels can be prepared for no electroosmosis to occur or for this to have either cathodic or anodic direction. Buffer pH can be adjusted to immobilize one reactant but not the other, if they have different isoelectric points. Uncharged antigens can be chemically modified to acquire the charge necessary for them to migrate through antibodies; or, if they are polysaccharides, they can be "activated" electrophoretically by using buffers that contain ions like borate, which combine with polysaccharides. Antibodies or antigens can be "fixed" in an electrophoresis gel by increasing its density, so that dur-

[14] Though less often performed, reversed immunoelectrophoresis effects electrophoretic separation of different classes of antibodies which then react by diffusion with antigen (see Chapter 5).

ing electrophoresis one reactant will be able to migrate but not the other. Specific examples of these various alternatives will be found in Chapter 6.

Other Methods of Reactant Migration

Most immunodiffusion tests employ diffusion or electrophoresis, or both, to move antigen and antibodies through gels for fractionation and interaction. But occasionally the following means are used.

Chromatography

In this procedure, fluid is percolated, siphoned, or drawn by capillary attraction through a porous supporting material so that interactions between solutes, the supporting material (stationary phase), and the solvent (moving phase) cause fractionation of the solutes into physico-chemically different populations (cf. Gordon and Eastoe, 1964). Fractionation develops from differences in affinity for stationary and moving phases of the separating populations. A population with higher affinity for solvent than for solid will move faster through the chromatogram than a population of opposite affinity. The nature of the attractive forces of the stationary phase for solutes being fractionated depends on the characteristics of the chromatographic medium being used. For immuno-chromatography these forces have been adsorption (Přistoupil *et al.,* 1967; Castañeda, 1950), ion exchange (Carnegie and Pacheco, 1964), and molecular sieving (Agostoni *et al.,* 1967; Grant and Everall, 1965).

Adsorption results from solute and stationary phase interacting physically. In immunochromatography this can be the simple and coarse effect of antigen being aggregated by antibody within the meshwork of the stationary phase (e.g., filter paper); but if one of the reactants has a natural affinity for the stationary phase (e.g., bovine serum albumin for cellulose nitrate: Přistoupil *et al.,* 1967), then aggregation need only fix the free reactant onto the specifically modified stationary phase.

Since most antigens have ionized groups, they can be fractionated by ion exchange. For instance, a positively charged stationary phase like DEAE cellulose attracts negatively charged antigen populations, as they percolate by, in proportion to their negativity and thus proportionally retards their progress through the chromatogram.

Some forms of stationary phase, such as Sephadex cross-linked dextran or Bio-Gel polyacrylamide "beads," are constituted of granules which are like microscopic sponges. The holes in these microsponges are of fairly uniform size. As solvent and solute percolate through a bed of these granules, solute molecules tend to diffuse into and out of these holes.

Large molecules nearly the size of the holes will penetrate them infrequently; medium-sized molecules will do so more often; small molecules will spend much of their passage time occupying the holes. Consequently, these molecular populations are sieved apart into large (moving fast), medium (moving slowly), and small (moving very little).

To date only two basic forms of immunochromatography have been described. One is analogous to immunoelectrophoresis in which antigens are fractionated through a chromatogram like thin-layer Sephadex G-200 on a glass slide, and then the fractions are diffused against a trough of antiserum (Grant and Everall, 1965; Hanson *et al.*, 1966a). The other is like a single electroimmunodiffusion test: a spot of antigen in or on paper is overrun with buffer carrying antibody (or vice versa). Antigen-antibody complexes that form become caught within or upon the meshes of the paper and therefore remain at their point of application (Castañeda, 1950; De Banchero, 1962).

Electrofocusing

This is a variety of electrophoresis employing a self-forming and self-maintaining pH gradient in the supporting medium (Longsworth, 1967). An antigen migrates during electrophoresis toward the oppositely charged electrode until it arrives at a zone in the pH gradient where the pH is the same as its isoelectric point. Here, by definition of "isoelectric point," it will have no charge and therefore will migrate no further; it has been electrofocused. As in electrophoresis, antigens separated from each other by electrofocusing next are detected by diffusion against antiserum. Alternatively, they can be detected by electroimmunodiffusion (cf. Svendsen and Rose, 1970).

The pH gradient used in electrofocusing forms from a mixture of low-molecular-weight peptides called "ampholytes" which arrange themselves during electrophoresis by their own isoelectric points into correspondingly different pH zones. Results obtained by immunoelectrofocusing (Catsimpoolas, 1969) resemble those obtained by conventional immunoelectrophoresis, although antigen resolution seems to be poorer.

Hydrodynamics

Reactants can be moved toward or through each other by solvent flow through the supporting medium. Such flow by percolation and siphoning has been mentioned in the section above on chromatography; that of electroosmosis was described in the section on electrophoresis. A similar hydrodynamic phenomenon, perhaps a variety of chromatography, is "rheophoresis" (Van Oss and Bronson, 1969). In rheophoresis, water drawn from an area of the supporting medium by evaporation is replaced by water flowing into it from other regions of the medium. Depots of antigen and antiserum can be arranged so that this water movement aids their mixing. For example, the area midway between antigen- and antibody-charged wells can be exposed to evaporation while the rest of the gel is protected (Van Oss and Bronson, 1969; see Chapter 7). Water moving from protected gel toward exposed gel carries the reactants with it into each other. Precipitation occurs faster and more intensely than it would if resulting from reactant diffusion alone. Rheophoresis frequently occurs in immunodiffusion tests using templates lying on very thin agar gel if they are not adequately humidified. Evaporation at the edges of the templates draws reactant from the central well out toward the satellite wells, accelerating and intensifying precipitation. Capillary attraction by filter paper itself subjected to drying can be used instead of direct evaporation to achieve the same ends, as can partial dehydration of double diffusion plates before wells are charged with reactants.

Ultracentrifugation

Differences in the molecular size of antigen populations are the basis for gel filtration immunochromatography as already discussed. These populations can be separated also by differential sedimentation or centrifugation. The physical bases for this technique, called "immunosedimentation," are that dense molecules sediment faster than light ones, and this can be observed readily in a strong centrifugal field. Antigens will segregate on being centrifuged in an appropriate medium of uniform density or in a medium with density increasing from top to bottom. For instance, in a mixture centrifuged through a sucrose density gradient medium, all molecules will be centrifuged downward. But upon. encountering succeedingly greater medium densities one population after another will find a level that is approximately equivalent to its own density. Here it will "bottom" and not be centrifuged any further, for it will float in the centrifugal field on fluid of greater density below it, after having sunk through fluid of lower density above it.

At present, succeeding levels of the centrifugate are tested for antigens by transferring them to conventional immunodiffusion plates (Córdoba *et al.*, 1965, 1966). But theoretically centrifugation could be performed in a medium containing a gelling agent like acrylamide. Then, following centrifugation this could be gelled by photocatalysis, and the resulting semisolid column could be removed without disturbing the centrifuge-fractionated populations of antigens and analyzed with antiserum as in two-step immunoelectrophoresis (see Chapters 5 and 7).

Chapter 2

General Information

This chapter contains general information useful in several or all varieties of immunodiffusion tests. Nearly all this information was obtained from papers reporting experiments employing immunodiffusion tests; these papers are cited with the double purpose of providing the required basic information and of acquainting the reader with references to numerous applications made of these tests. Only papers published in the last decade are mentioned; reference to earlier, related publications can be obtained from the first edition of this book or from Ouchterlony's reviews (Ouchterlony, 1958, 1962, 1968).

The sequence of this chapter roughly parallels that of an immunodiffusion test: obtaining antiserum, preparing antigen, choosing and using a supporting medium and its solvents, performing the test, observing and recording the results, and transforming the test into a permanent original record of itself.

Antiserum

The analytic reagent of immunodiffusion tests usually is antiserum. It should react with antigen clearly and stably but not with other substances, should be easy to produce in useful volumes, and should store well. Its specificity for antigen may be high, moderate, or low, depending on its intended use. This reagent can be obtained by immunizing animals with appropriate antigens, or by bleeding animals that already have the required antibodies from natural exposure to antigen. Antisera to the more commonly studied antigens usually can be purchased. Occasionally a nonantibody substance which precipitates certain antigens specifically can be substituted for antiserum.

Selecting the Species of Animal To Produce Antibody

Many animal species can produce precipitins useful for immunodiffusion tests. Aside from such traditional producers as rabbits, horses, and goats, these include ducks (Halbert and Ehrlich, 1962; Christian, 1963), chickens (Parlebas and Robert, 1963; Gengozian et al., 1962), turkeys and pheasants (Gengozian et al., 1962), pigs (Ruckerbauer et al., 1965; Boulanger et al., 1961), sheep (Birkinshaw et al., 1962; Thorbecke and Franklin, 1961; Mage and Harrison, 1966), donkeys (Kulberg et al., 1961; Sweet, 1971), guinea pigs (Birkinshaw et al., 1962; Wilkerson and White, 1966), mice (Kubes, 1965; Marbrook and Matthews, 1966), hamsters (Berman and Sarma, 1965), monkeys (Dimmock, 1967; Balayan, 1960), fish (Molnár and Berczi, 1965), and tadpoles (Maniatis et al., 1969).

Chickens are used frequently; they appear to respond better than ducks, pheasants, or turkeys (Gengozian et al., 1962). There are no special problems in eliciting good precipitin production in ungulates, including mules and cattle. Among common laboratory species, we regularly use guinea pigs and mice.

As was indicated in Chapter 1, the characteristics of precipitins produced by different species may differ. But these characteristics depend also on other factors such as immunization protocol and nature of antigen. For instance, calves inoculated with whole bovine viral diarrhea viruses produced only 19 S precipitins; but when inoculated with soluble antigen from the virus they produced only 7 S precipitins (Fernelius, 1966). Guinea pigs injected with ovalbumin in incomplete Freund adjuvant made only γ_1-globulin precipitins, but when injected with the same antigen in complete Freund adjuvant they made both γ_2 and γ_1 precipitins (Stewart-Tull et al., 1965). Horses exposed to protein antigens in saline manufacture first γ_2 R-type precipitins followed shortly thereafter by predominantly γ_1 H-type precipitins. If, instead, they are injected with such an antigen in complete Freund adjuvant, they make both types of antibody at once (Allen et al., 1965). Immunizing extremely young animals may elicit no precipitin response at all, depending partly on the nature of the antigen. Fetal lambs produce antibody to bacteriophage and horse ferritin but not to such otherwise excellent antigens as diphtheria toxoid, or certain entire bacteria (Silverstein et al., 1963b). This indication for the importance of both host and antigen extends further and more generally. Thus, while protein antigens, viruses, bacteriophage, and simple haptens usually stimulate a preponderantly γ_G-globulin response in most mammals after an early phase of γ_M production, enterobacterial lipopolysaccharide somatic antigens stimulate predominantly formation of γ_M antibodies in man and rabbits but γ_G antibodies in guinea pigs (Pike, 1967). Rabbits injected intravenously with hemocyanin produce both types of antibodies, whereas rats produce only γ_M; but if rats are injected with this antigen in Freund adjuvant, then their main response is γ_G-globulin (Pike, 1967).

One species can make a heterogeneous response to antigens from one source. For instance, in patients with aspergillomas, most precipitins to *Aspergillus fumigatus* antigens are γ_G-globulins, but some are of the γ_M class. Rabbits immunized with this mold produce γ_G-globulins against most of the antigens but also produce both types of precipitin against a few (Tran Van Ky *et al.*, 1966a). Gram-negative bacteria tend to induce widely variable antibody responses, making prediction for the outcome of precipitin production difficult (Holme and Edebo, 1965).

SPECIES CHARACTERISTICS

Although the type of precipitin obtained from a species of animal depends partially on the nature of antigen and the immunization protocol, some generalizations about antisera and animal species producing them can be made (see also Chapter 6). Rabbit antiserum is the most popular because rabbits make precipitins readily, and because these precipitins aggregate antigen strongly and over a wide antigen:antibody ratio (Zwaan, 1963). Most rabbit precipitins are γ_2-globulin euglobulins, but rabbit antisera frequently also contain γ_1-pseudoglobulin precipitins (Crowle and Hazeghi, unpublished work; cf. also Siskind, 1966, who describes methods for separating the two types of precipitin). Horses usually make precipitins that form unstable aggregates with antigen and require near-optimal reactant proportions to precipitate (Allen *et al.*, 1965). Goats make R-type rather than H-type antibodies, but they are more difficult to stimulate into precipitin production than rabbits (Ridgway *et al.*, 1962). Sheep are interesting in sometimes having precipitins with electrophoretic mobility slower than γ_2-globulin (Silverstein *et al.*, 1963a), although usually their precipitins are of more conventional mobility (Cline, 1967). Mouse, guinea pig, and rat precipitins are R-type, generally occur in the γ_1-globulins,[1] and may be of either pseudo- or euglobulin solubilities (Anacker and Munoz, 1961; Crowle, unpublished work). Man produces predominantly R-type antibodies of γ_2 mobility.

[1] Experiments with different strains of mice indicate, however, that this characteristic can be strain-dependent. BALB/c mice produce γ_1 precipitins to hemocyanin, but C57BL mice make γ_2 precipitins to it (Fahey *et al.*, 1965).

Chicken antiserum contains a variety of precipitins. In liquid media these generally precipitate antigens more efficiently in salt solutions of ten times physiologic strength than at physiologic strength (Orlans *et al.*, 1961). But if the chicken is hyperimmunized, or if its antiserum is tested in agar gel rather than in liquid medium, its precipitins may aggregate antigen efficiently at physiologic salt concentration (Benedict *et al.*, 1963; Crowle and Lueker, 1961). Dogs are poor producers of precipitating antisera because they make high-avidity nonprecipitating antibodies which compete for antigens with the precipitins (Klinman *et al.*, 1964), although apparently this fault can be overcome partially by immunizing them with antigen in Freund adjuvant (Patterson *et al.*, 1964a).

Antiserum Specificity

In addition to broad considerations determining the choice of animal species in which to make antibody, there are more specific considerations. Perhaps the most important is the purpose for which the antiserum will be used—that is, whether it will be employed to detect differences in antigenic determinants on similar molecules of antigen, to demonstrate taxonomic relationships between different species of animals, or to diagnose a disease. For the first purpose the antiserum should have maximum specificity, for the second maximum cross reactivity, and for the third a combination of high titer and high specificity.

Antisera of highest specificity for animal antigens[2] generally are obtained by auto- or isoimmunizations, because then the immunized animal will be immunologically tolerant of all antigenic determinants except those that distinguish the immunizing antigen from similar antigens in the animal itself (Lichter and Dray, 1964). That is, the immunized animal usually will not produce antibodies to antigenic determinants the same as its own, but can make precipitins to determinants different from its own (Hirschfeld, 1963). For example, if a rabbit is injected with serum from another rabbit which has some γ-globulin determinants different from those on the γ-globulins of the first rabbit, this rabbit will immunologically ignore all the other serum antigens because they are the same as its own but will recognize the slightly different γ-globulin antigen and make antibodies to it (Leskowitz, 1963). Another species of animal (e.g., goat) injected similarly would be so "preoccupied" immunologically with making precipitins to all the other rabbit serum antigens that it

[2] Highest specificity for nonanimal antigens (e.g., bacterial) usually is obtained by immunizing animals lightly. Choice of the antibody-making species becomes relatively unimportant unless the antigens are related to the animal indirectly, such as by symbiosis or parasitism (Dineen, 1963; Olitski and Godinger, 1963).

would tend to "overlook" subtle determinant group differences on a single species of γ-globulin. Even if it were able to detect this distinction, its antiserum would have to be absorbed to remove precipitins of secondary interest and prevent development of a confusingly large number of precipitates in an immunodiffusion test (Leskowitz, 1963).

Isoimmunization has become routine. For instance, isoimmune antisera are used for allotypic classification of rabbits (Dray *et al.*, 1963a) and of mice (Dray *et al.*, 1963b). Rabbits deficient in rabbit serum atropinesterase have been used to make highly specific precipitins by injecting them with rabbit serum containing this enzyme (Margolis and Feigelson, 1964). Guinea pigs have been employed to make precipitins useful for distinguishing between guinea pig tissue culture cell lines (Brand and Chiu, 1966). Isoimmunization nicely detects the presence of a foreign antigen or changed antigen: mice immunized with suckling mouse brain virus produced precipitins only to the virus and not to the mouse tissue antigens (Chan, 1965). But the antigen detected may be neither foreign nor changed. For instance, rabbits will form precipitins to rabbit adrenal gland antigens which are organ-specific, presumably by reacting with antigens that are hidden from the immunologic apparatus within intact organs (Centeno *et al.*, 1964). Isoimmunization avoids the complication in this example of precipitins forming to numerous other rabbit antigens as they would if another species of animal were used to make the antiserum.

If auto- or isoimmunization is not possible, a closely related species should be selected for producing antiserum with maximum discriminatory capacity (Durand and Schneider, 1962a). Monkeys, for instance, produce antisera that recognize more varieties of antigenic groupings on human serum immunoglobulins than do antisera of rabbits, goats, sheep, or horses (Deutsch, 1964; Lichter and Dray, 1964; Lichter, 1964). Buffalo were used to make anti-cattle precipitins, and cattle to make anti-buffalo precipitins, because rabbit antisera against either could not distinguish between buffalo and cow bones in anthropological investigations (Pandey and Pathak, 1966). On the other hand, trial and error have shown that some fine antigenic determinant distinctions can be made without regard to this general rule of taxonomic relationship. In one study sheep, goats, and monkeys were found to respond to only one of two types of human immunoglobulin light chain, and the monkeys made precipitins to human immunoglobulin solely by way of this light chain (Fahey and McLaughlin, 1963). Thus, empirical selection of the antibody-making species may allow some very fine anatomic distinctions to be made among several classes of protein molecule. Pigs make precipitins to "hidden" but not surface determinants of human immunoglobulin λ light chains but often do the opposite for human immunoglobulin κ chains. The reason appears to be chance similarity between human and pig λ chains but not κ chains (Skvaril and co-workers, 1970). Empirically, horse antisera have been found to detect more antigenic variety in human sera than have rabbit antisera (Neuzil and Masseyeff, 1959). Rabbit antisera could not detect antigenic differences between normal and multiple sclerosis cerebrospinal fluid, but horse antisera could (MacPherson and Cosgrove, 1961); horse antiserum detected two IgM antigens in human serum, only one of which was detected by rabbit antiserum (Fessel, 1963b). Unfortunately, differences between individual animals of a species make generalizations difficult. A Pasteur Institute antiserum to human serum lacked precipitins to α_1-antitrypsin (Burtin and Grabar, 1967); similar antiserum from another lacked precipitins to transferrin (Neuzil and Masseyeff, 1959). Both of these are prominent and good antigens.

On the other hand, differences among individual animals in responding to mixtures of antigens, which incidentally makes it necessary to use several antisera for an exhaustive study of a given antigen (Zwaan, 1963), can be a considerable advantage. For instance, analyses of human tissue cell antigens were facilitated by the fact that different guinea pigs do not respond uniformly to these antigens but rather produce antibody specificities in different combinations and in limited numbers. A battery of antisera thus could be employed to differentiate among six established human cell culture strains without the complications of antiserum absorptions (Chiu et al., 1967; cf. also Hirschfeld, 1960b, 1963).

Reasons for different individual antibody responses are many and usually poorly understood, and the differences in response involve quality, quantity, and ultimately individual antigenic determinants. One reason, which extends to species, genus, and higher taxonomic levels, is related to the number of determinant groups on individual types of antigen shared by the species of antigen donor and the species producing the antibodies; the greater this sharing, the more determinant groups will the antibody-producing species tolerate immunologically and therefore not respond to. This distinction, classically demonstrated by the ease with which precipitins are produced in chickens to human but not to duck serum albumins (Ivanyi and Valentova, 1966), can be employed quantitatively to elucidate phylogenetic relationships between animals from the class level (Neuzil and Masseyeff, 1958), through genus and species levels (Durand and Schneider, 1962b), to strain levels as mentioned above. The principle of progressively lesser precipitin response in the progressively closer animal–antigen relationship extends also to adaption of parasites to their hosts: sheep are natural hosts of the parasite *Haemonchus contortus* and make poorer precipitin responses to the antigens of this parasite than do rabbits because of a reduced antigenic disparity between *Haemonchus* and sheep (Dineen, 1963). Consequently, for producing maximum variety of antibody response to a parasite or microorganism one should choose an animal not naturally associated with it. The same precaution holds for a different reason: host animals already may be making precipitins to parasites or symbionts and thus may not respond to immunization well, or they may respond selectively and adversely (Olitski and Godinger, 1963). Of course, "difficulties" like these also can be useful if appropriately exploited.

The fact that different animals can make equivalent titers of precipitins, but these individually can be directed against different antigens in a mixture (Zwaan, 1963) or different determinants on the same antigen (Paul *et al.*, 1970), can cause some confusion. Thus, an antibody producer should not be selected by precipitin titer alone, even against a single antigen. For instance, rabbits and horses may have equivalent titers of precipitins against a given human γ-globulin but react quite differently because the rabbits tend to make antibodies principally against the light chain portions of the immunoglobulins, whereas horses make antibodies well against the heavy chain determinants and often fail to make anti-light chain precipitins at all (Fahey and McLaughlin, 1963). Two antisera with "equivalent" precipitins to IgM can give radically different results with this one kind of antigen because one detects κ IgM better than λ IgM, and the other detects λ IgM better than κ IgM (Reimer *et al.*, 1970).

Other Considerations

For little-studied antigens it is frequently not possible to determine which species of animal is best for precipitin production until several · individuals of several species have been tested. Interpolations of expectations even with well-studied antigens should be made cautiously. But there are considerations other than antiserum specificity that affect choice of the precipitin-producing species. Thus, by general characteristics of antibody production one species may be preferable. For instance, animals producing R-type antibodies are better than H-type antibody producers for making antisera to precipitate low-molecular-weight antigens, because these antigens tend to dissociate from their antibodies so readily (Berrod *et al.*, 1964). R-type precipitins are also preferable for detecting antigens present in an immunodiffusion test in only small quantities, because these antibodies precipitate better than H-type antibodies under conditions of reactant excess (Seligmann, 1961). R-type precipitins appear to be better for quantitative and H-type for qualitative two-dimensional single electroimmunodiffusion tests (see Chapter 6). An antibody producer may have to be chosen for reasons unrelated to the nature of the antibodies themselves. For example, an antigen that is toxic because it acts as a hormone in one species can be used with impunity in another: chickens are preferred to mammals for making precipitins to mammalian insulin for this reason (Patterson *et al.*, 1964b).

Antigen

Successfully preparing antiserum for a given task in immunodiffusion tests depends partly on how the antigen used to stimulate the precipitin-producing animal itself is obtained, prepared, and administered to the animal. Antisera usually have one of three broad tasks to perform in immunodiffusion analyses: detect a maximum number of antigens in a mixture, detect qualitative or quantitative differences in complex mixtures of antigens, or reveal the immunologic anatomy of individual populations of antigens. For these respective purposes one requires antisera with a maximal variety of response, antisera with selective responses, and antisera to single species of antigens or portions of antigens.

Preparing Polyvalent Antisera

Polyvalent antisera are needed, for example, to detect as many antigens as possible in a biological fluid or tissue. The immunizing mixture of antigens should be prepared to contain these antigens in maximal number and best antigenic form, well dispersed, and in concentrations individually that promote antibody formation but do not induce immunologic tolerance or effect antigenic competition. For example, serum is a suitable mixture because it has many separate populations of antigens, most of them appropriate in form and quantity to induce precipitin formation. But even in serum there are problem-producing inequalities among different antigen populations. Some are too weak to induce precipitin formation; others, like albumin and transferrin, are concentrated enough to inhibit formation of homologous precipitins and sometimes also formation of precipitins to weaker antigens.

There are solutions to this type of problem. One can artificially lower the concentration of the stronger antigens while raising the concentration of the weaker antigens. Or, one can use a related mixture (e.g., cerebro-spinal fluid) which lacks or has only traces of the more powerful antigens for initial immunization and later boost precipitin production with the original mixture. This is because antibody production against the weaker antigens has already started, boosting with the stronger antigens can be effected with less fear of antigenic competition, and the concentrations of these stronger antigens can also be kept low without concern that the concentrations of the weaker antigens in a mixture will have been made too low to elicit precipitin formation.

Frequently, antigens may not be soluble in their native state, and when injected in this state they will not induce a comprehensive precipitin response. Extracts must be made to obtain a maximum number of least-denatured antigens. Sometimes this is easy (e.g., aqueous extracts of *Candida albicans:* Biguet *et al.,* 1965a). But one must select the proper object for extraction. Thus, the best source of *Phytophthora* antigens was young, growing tips of the hyphae (Burrell *et al.,* 1966), and *Histoplasma* antigen that was least cross-reactive with antigens from other fungi was obtained from the yeast phase (Sweet, 1971). Sometimes it is difficult and can be done only while risking denaturation, such as in preparing saline-insoluble kidney basement membrane antigens by sodium hydroxide digestion (Myers *et al.,* 1966), or by disrupting influenza virus with sodium dodecyl sulfate to obtain type-specific ribonucleoprotein (Schild and Pereira, 1969). But some denaturation can be advantageous: rabbits are stimulated to form precipitins to their own immunoglobulins by mildly denaturing the immunoglobulins by 18-hour exposure to pH 11.5 (McCluskey *et al.,* 1962). Usually, a variety of insoluble antigens will not induce as wide a spectrum of precipitin responses as the same variety in solution, but it is also true that some antigens become haptens when solubilized, presumably by dissociation from adjuvant carrier molecules; these will not be detected unless injected in native form (e.g., teichoic acid in staphylococci: Singleton and Ross, 1964).

A difficulty in preparing polyvalent antisera against "typical" antigen mixtures is in defining "typical"; an antigen that is not typical of the usual mixture may inadvertently be included in the immunizing mixture. For instance, there is so much variety in the quantity and quality of human serum that one laboratory uses a pool of serum obtained from 1000 different donors to produce antiserum to "normal" serum (Grubb, 1970). Female salmon serum contains an antigen associated with egg production which is absent from male salmon serum; hence, in taxonomic studies using sera from these and related fishes the "typical" serum must be a pool of male sera to avoid confusion from differences attributable to sex rather than strain (Ridgway *et al.,* 1962). Bacterial contamination can convert one Gc type of human serum into another (Nerstrøm *et al.,* 1964).

Some antigens that one might wish to detect with a polyvalent antiserum may be either too weak or absent from the immunizing mixture and thus not induce precipitin formation. If similar mixtures containing these antigens in better proportion can be found, these mixtures can be used legitimately as complementary or substitute antigenic stimulants. For example, cerebrospinal fluid induces better precipitin response to serum α_2- and β_2-globulins than serum itself because there are relatively more of them in the fluid than in the serum (MacPherson and Cosgrove, 1961). But, in employing this practice one must recognize that the substitute mixture may also have antigens of its own not present in the original mixture (MacPherson and Cosgrove, 1961). Such a mixture as tears may not be available in sufficient volume for intense antigenic stimulation called for by some immunization protocols to boost precipitin responses. Then, a mixture sharing antigens but available in larger volume, like serum, can be used for the boosting injections even though it may have several antigens not present in the original mixture. In this circumstance, the boosted animals must be bled within a few days when only anamnestically produced precipitins are present. Sometimes the native antigen to be detected may not be available at all, but precipitins can be made to it with a cross-reacting antigen. Thus, mice produced precipitins that could detect liver antigen in the serum of people with hepatitis or mushroom intoxication when they were injected with mouse liver extract (Bodmer, 1969).

The problem of eliciting production of precipitins not typical of the antigen pool being studied is subtle and must continuously be guarded against in preparing antigens for immunization. Already mentioned is the presence of sex-specific antigen in female salmon serum (Ridgway et al., 1962) and of bacteria-changed Gc serotype (Nerstrøm et al., 1964). Lymph from an injured rabbit paw contains a β_2 antigen not present in lymph from an uninjured paw (Courtice, 1967). Adsorbed antigens are notoriously difficult to remove from tissue; rabbit organs extensively profused remain contaminated with large quantities of serum antigens (Depieds et al., 1962). Unfortunately, this problem often is unsolvable because, although a given antigen may be a contaminant, it may, on the other hand, be a true constituent of the mixture present in sufficient quantity to induce antibody formation but insufficient to be detected by conventional immunodiffusion techniques.

TOXIC ANTIGENS

The problem of producing antisera to toxic antigens is seldom discussed in standard sources of information. The following examples and their solutions suggest general techniques for circumventing it.

Toxins can be detoxified by formalinization (i.e., "toxoiding"). Rabbits injected safely with toxoided Clostridium culture filtrates produced precipitins to the native toxins (Ellner and Green, 1963b). Alternatively, the antibody-producing animal can be exposed to small quantities of toxin and thus build a tolerance to it. Rabbits could withstand immunizations with 2 mg of staphylococcus enterotoxin when their regimen started with 0.9 μg and they received increasing doses weekly. They could be boosted safely 7 days before a final bleeding with 1 mg of enterotoxin (Casman and Bennett, 1964). Similarly, immunization with attenuated bacteria can be followed later by boosting with virulent organisms because of the protective immunity elicited by the attenuated bacteria (Sharon, 1961).

Serum from some animals is toxic for others; both dog and donkey serum can kill rabbits. Injecting such toxic serum in Freund water-in-oil emulsion both avoids this effect and increases antigenic stimulation. Dog serum injected into rabbits in Freund adjuvant elicited local reactions but caused no deaths; later the injected rabbits could withstand boostings with dog serum not incorporated in this adjuvant (Durand and Schneider, 1963).

Preparing Monovalent Antisera

Some of the most remarkable theoretical and technological advances in biology and medicine have been made with immunodiffusion tests employing antisera with precipitins specific for single antigens or portions of antigens. Production of monospecific antisera has become commercially profitable. But, until recently, preparing such an antiserum often has been a difficult task unless, by good fortune, one could find a way empirically of purifying the antigen (e.g., purifying immunoglobulins by precipitating nonimmunoglobulins with caprylic acid: Steinbuch *et al.*, 1970) or a mixture of antigens lacking some antigen and thus useful for selective absorption (e.g., Lambotte and Salmon, 1962; see Antiserum Absorption, below). Fortunately, there are now some relatively simple methods enabling any laboratory to make precipitins to any selected antigen, even if it occurs originally in a very complex mixture.

Moderately selective, simple, and often quite effective is zone electrophoresing the antigen mixture in a gel, cutting out the gel containing the antigen, and then for injection either eluting the antigen or homogenizing the gel together with the antigen (Croisille, 1962; Laron and Assa, 1962a; Weintraub and Raymond, 1963). The electrophoresing medium (e.g., agar, polyacrylamide) thus can serve a second role as adjuvant (Weintraub and Raymond, 1963). Frequently, the resected zone will contain two or three contaminating antigens, but if these are low in concentration relative to the principal antigen, the eluate can be diluted for injection; or it can be injected without adjuvant. Thereby only precipitins to the principal antigen will be produced.

Biophysical characteristics of an antigen can be used to present it selectively to the antibody-producing animal. For instance, certain guinea pig serum constituents adhere strongly to *Escherichia coli*. Therefore, rabbits will produce precipitins selectively to these guinea pig serum components when injected with these bacteria first soaked in guinea pig serum and then washed thoroughly (Beernink and Steward, 1967). This technique also can be used to determine which guinea pig serum antigens do adhere to *E. coli* and participate in its immunologic inactivation. Antiserum to human complement can be made in rabbits by injecting individual rabbits with their own immune precipitates formed in the presence of human complement, because the complement becomes attached to such precipitates (Eyster *et al.*, 1966; Ellis and Gell, 1958). This technique can be used also to produce antibodies to antibodies. For example, various mammals, birds, turtles, and fishes were inoculated with rabbit erythrocytes so that they would make hemagglutinins. The resulting antisera from these various species then were reacted with fresh rabbit erythrocytes, and the agglutinated erythrocytes were washed and injected back into other rabbits (Ambrosius, 1966; Hodgins *et al.*, 1965). The injected rabbits would not produce antibodies to rabbit erythrocytes, of course, but they readily made precipitins to the foreign hemagglutinins (i.e., immunoglobulins) attached to these erythrocytes. Indeed, rabbits of one strain will develop precipitins to antibodies of another strain of rabbits if this latter strain is immunized with some bacteria, and then these bacteria and the resulting antibacterial antibodies are injected as immunological complexes into the first strain (Lerner *et al.*, 1963).

PREPARATORY IMMUNODIFFUSION

The most exquisite and potentially versatile technique for obtaining precipitins against a single antigen among many is to use immunodiffusion itself for purifying it. Although use of this technique was suggested in the first edition of this book, and although it is very powerful, it has not yet often been employed. Essentially, it is to prepare an antiserum against the mixture of antigens, react this with the mixture in some immunodiffusion test, carefully cut out the precipitin band that develops with the antigen of interest, and then immunize an animal of the same species as that used to form the polyvalent antiserum with the resected precipitin band. This animal will make precipitins predominantly to the attached antigen; usually, it will not react to the antibodies forming a large portion of the injected complex. Indeed, these tend to lend adjuvancy to the antigen which they have precipitated. This, together with the use of Freund adjuvant, makes the usually small quantities of antigen obtained by this method sufficient to induce precipitin formation. Once even a low titer of precipitins has become available, they can be used to selectively precipitate larger quantities of the same antigen out of its original mixture in liquid medium or in a scaled-up preparatory immuno-diffusion test, and these can be used for boosting the same animal or for immunizing other animals with the purified antigen. The potentialities of this underexploited but simple technique are awesome if they are considered with some imagination. The following are some examples of its application.

Precipitin arcs from immunoelectropherograms of serum resected carefully from the entire pattern have been used to produce antisera specific for selected serum (Thompson and Lachmann, 1970; Goudie *et al.*, 1966) and saliva (Revis, 1968) antigens. Monospecific precipitins to frog oviductal antigens were obtained similarly by using a double diffusion plate for developing the precipitin bands used for immunization (Shivers and James, 1967). Bands produced in gelatin instead of agar were obtained free of gel by warming the gelatin and centrifuging out the freed precipitate (Smith *et al.*, 1964). With special apparatus utilizing thick gelatin gels, this technique can yield milligram quantities of specific precipitate (see Chapter 4).

Antigen Denaturation

When antigen is removed from its native habitat for any purpose, such as injecting an animal to obtain precipitins, it may be changed to a non-native form. The many ways in which this can occur include dissociating it from native molecular partners, and exposing it to chemical, physical, or biological changes (e.g., oxidation, aggregation, or enzymatic digestion, respectively). These changes are frequently not easy to detect because they are evident only by comparison with what is known to be the native form, and this in turn is uncertain because defining the "nativeness" of antigen usually requires working with the antigen, which may alter the antigen itself during investigation of the problem. A classic example, only recently becoming elucidated, is one of the most frequently studied antigens, serum albumin. Attempts to obtain this in its purest form have led to information artifacts. In water solutions pure serum albumin equilibrates spontaneously into various molecular forms (Ceska, 1969a). The presence of these monomer–polymer transition forms was not widely recognized until they became directly evident in polyacrylamide electrophoresis and more recently by double diffusion tests with dextran-containing agar. These variations are antigenically as well as physically distinguishable from each other (Ceska, 1969a). In whole human serum (native state?) albumin supposedly exists in just the monomeric form.

Purified antigens tend to be denatured more easily than native antigens. Frothing during the preparation of a water-in-oil (w/o) emulsion is sufficient to denature several kinds of antigen (Zwaan, 1963). Purified antigens often are less antigenic than nonpurified (Struck and Heinrich, 1967). "Purification" may even include removing antigen from a parasite to which it has become attached in the host–parasite relationship: rabbit antigens on *Echinococcus* induced precipitin formation when rabbits were injected with the parasite but not when they were injected with just the rabbit antigens alone (Kagan and Norman, 1961). On the other hand, moderate purification can be an advantage by eliminating antigenic competition, for monkeys immunized with whole human serum made no precipitins to ceruloplasmin, but they did when injected with ceruloplasmin alone (Lichter and Dray, 1964).

Success in preparing an appropriate antiserum for an immunodiffusion test therefore calls for carefully selecting and preparing the immunizing antigen. But, given certain minimal precautions in these endeavors, there appears to be no technical obstacle at present to developing monospecific antiserum to any selected antigen to be examined by immunodiffusion or other immunologic tests. Especially encouraging is application of immunodiffusion itself for preparing in native or nearly native form the highly purified antigens needed for immunization.

Immunization Protocols

Laboratories that frequently make antisera have their own favorite protocols for immunizing the animals that they most commonly employ; they vary these empirically to fit changes in the animals, the nature of the antigen, or the purpose of the immunization. The following information is presented as a guide to those who do not already have the benefit of direct experience in antiserum production.

General Considerations

No protocol to fit all precipitin-producing situations can be devised: there are too many variables. Primarily one must decide on the intensity of immunization (Kushner and Kaplan, 1961). Intense immunization (e.g., with Freund adjuvant) will elicit production of large quantities and varieties of precipitins to a maximum number of both antigens in the immunization mixture and antigenic determinant groups on each population of antigen.[3] It tends to provoke development of strong antisera with low specificity. Full response to this type of immunization is slow to develop (weeks or months). Moderate immunization (e.g., repeated injections of antigen in water solution or with weak adjuvants like aluminum hydroxide) tends to provide antisera with increased specificity but only modest content of precipitins, both in variety and in quantity. It is likely to elicit production of precipitins only to the strongest antigens in a mixture. As with intense immunization, moderate immunization may take a long time to mature. Weak immunization (e.g., single injection of an aqueous solution of antigen and/or bleeding early in the immunization schedule) sacrifices strength and variety of antiserum precipitins for maximum specificity. Once this primary decision on immunization intensity has been made, then a protocol can be selected or devised from those available in the literature for similar situations; samples of these are given below.

Most species of animal respond slowly (weeks) to make detectable precipitins after initial (primary) stimulation with antigen; at the same time that they are beginning to make precipitins to the stronger antigens in an immunization mixture, they may also be making some antibodies to the weaker antigens. But these may either not be precipitins or be too weak to detect. On later (secondary) stimulation with the same antigen mixture they will respond much more rapidly (days), making greatly increased titers of precipitins to the stronger antigens, and detectable titers to the weaker antigens against which they had previously shown no detectable response. Immunization protocols take advantage of these contrasting characteristics of primary and secondary antigenic stimulation to tailor the immune response to requirements. For instance, it is a common practice for primary immunization to employ a low concentration of antigens in Freund adjuvant and then 3 to 5 weeks later to utilize a close sequence of secondary stimuli with medium and high concentrations of the antigens in saline. The purpose of this regimen is to initiate antibody formation in the animal to a maximum number of antigens, without risking antigen overloading and thus tolerogenesis, and then to stimulate

[3] Animals can be "overimmunized," whereupon they make much reduced precipitin responses or may even become tolerant and unable to make any precipitin to the immunizing antigen (Christian, 1970; Oehme and Schwick, 1961). Usually, this is the result of injecting an excessive amount of the antigen initially in Freund adjuvant (e.g., >10 mg in a rabbit) or in saline. Unfortunately, animals also can be "underimmunized," which causes them to make nonprecipitating antibodies that can interfere with their production of the desired precipitins. Generally, this is a consequence of injecting small (e.g., ≤ 1 μg) amounts of antigen in saline; it rarely occurs when antigen is injected in Freund adjuvant (Crowle and Terman, unpublished work).

the resulting wide spectrum of antibody production to maximum output. Another reason for only modest primary immunization is to keep antibody production low enough so that a minimum of boosting antigen will be diverted by combining with antibody from its intended function of secondary stimulation. This is accomplished also by waiting for titers of antibodies resulting from primary stimulation to subside somewhat, and by using a series of secondary stimuli such that, although much or all of the first injection of antigen is "consumed" by existing antibodies, antigens injected in the second and third stimuli will not be consumed, because the first injection will have neutralized free antibodies.

Adjuvants

An adjuvant is any substance that intensifies an animal's immunologic response to antigen. It can be native or artificial; and it can be physical, chemical, or biological. As an example of native adjuvancy, most particulate antigens have enough inherent adjuvancy to elicit good precipitin responses by themselves (Fox et al., 1962; Lacour et al., 1962a). This adjuvancy can be mimicked artificially. Haptens acquire adjuvancy when conjugated to appropriate antigenic carriers (Holländer et al., 1966; Brandriss et al., 1965). Aluminum hydroxide and similar insoluble adsorbents (Weiner et al., 1964; Hirschfeld, 1960b) provide adjuvancy by making antigens artificially particulate. Sodium alginate functions similarly (Burrell et al., 1966; Fisher, 1965). Gels like agar, agarose, and polyacrylamide provide some adjuvancy; hency, antigens separated in them by zone electrophoresis are more potent precipitinogens than they would be in their absence (Revis, 1971). Antigen–antibody precipitates, especially when prepared in slight antigen excess, are often better inducers of precipitins against the antigen moiety of the precipitate than antigen alone.

Adjuvants may function by chemical and physiologic effects that they have instead of or in addition to physical effects. Saponin was used to obtain precipitins to trypanosome antigens when other adjuvants had failed (Dupouey and Maréchal, 1966). Guinea pig serum taken some weeks after the animals had been injected with mycobacteria, a component of complete Freund adjuvant, was able to stimulate formation of more precipitins in rabbits than such serum drawn from guinea pigs not pretreated with mycobacteria (Havez et al., 1965). The effect apparently was to increase the quantities of various minor antigens in the immunizing guinea pig serum. Mice infected with lactic dehydrogenase virus showed elevated levels of γ-globulin and produced greatly increased quantities of antibodies to human γ-globulin antigen (Notkins *et al.*, 1966).

Immunology's most popular and effective adjuvant functions by all three effects—chemical, physical, and biological. This is Freund adjuvant, a water-in-oil (w/o) emulsion which may ("complete") or may not ("incomplete") contain mycobacteria (see Appendix I). It is a chemical irritant; it physically distributes antigen piecemeal throughout the body's lymphatic system; and biologically it stimulates the reticuloendothelial system and the associated antibody-making mechanisms of the body. It retains the antigen at the site of injection in effective form for several weeks (Herbert, 1968); a response to antigen some 500 times as great as that seen when antigen is injected in saline is not uncommon. Certain immunization techniques can be employed to obtain nearly the same responses against some antigens without this adjuvant as with it (Parks *et al.*, 1961; Williams, 1962a); but for other antigens (e.g., ethanol-insoluble fractions of porcine brain and adrenal gland) this adjuvant appears to be essential to obtain precipitins (Milgrom *et al.*, 1964a). In addition to serving as an excellent stimulator of antibody production, Freund adjuvant also permits use of otherwise toxic antigens such as scorpion venom for immunization, because these are released slowly enough from the w/o emulsion not to harm the animal injected with them (Irunberry and Pilo-Moron, 1965).

As was indicated above, the difference between incomplete and complete Freund adjuvants is that mycobacteria are added to the latter. This tends to intensify most immunologic responses with mixed blessings. Complete adjuvant may stimulate an animal to make precipitins to antigens closely related to its own (e.g., against rat serum albumin in mice; autoantibodies), but it also can depress production of precipitins to unrelated antigens (e.g., chicken ovalbumin in the mouse) as compared with incomplete adjuvant, presumably because the antibody-producing animal becomes "preoccupied" with making antibodies against antigens of the mycobacteria themselves.[4] Complete Freund adjuvant seldom is used for secondary stimulation because the intense hypersensitivity reaction of the animal being boosted to mycobacteria in the emulsion interferes with reaction of the animal to the other antigens to which it is intended to respond. If large amounts of antigen are used in incomplete adjuvant, the same problem develops. Complete Freund

[4] One should not use complete Freund adjuvant for producing precipitins against microorganisms related to mycobacteria without recognizing that the precipitins obtained may be responses against the mycobacteria rather than against the other microorganisms.

adjuvant tends to change the immune response as well as intensify it; guinea pigs injected with ovalbumin in incomplete adjuvant made only γ_1-globulin precipitins, whereas guinea pigs injected with this antigen in complete adjuvant made precipitins of both γ_1- and γ_2-globulin classes (Stewart-Tull *et al.*, 1965).

Despite the acknowledged effectiveness of Freund adjuvants in eliciting precipitin production, best results sometimes are obtained with other adjuvants or with none at all. For instance, guinea pigs injected with rabbit serum in Freund adjuvant persistently failed to make precipitins to rabbit serum γ-globulins and albumin, whereas both rabbits and chickens injected with similar antigen mixtures in the adjuvant developed full-range responses (Codd *et al.*, 1968). The species of animal chosen to produce the precipitins therefore appears in part to determine the potential utility of this adjuvant. And, as has been mentioned, it is not the best vehicle for eliciting selective antibody responses such as are needed for typing human serum Gc antigen (Reinskou, 1966b).

Variations in Method of Antigenic Stimulation

Most often precipitins are developed in animals by injecting them with antigen subcutaneously or intraperitoneally. But there are exceptions that exemplify technical variations useful for solving special problems of precipitin production. The route of antigen inoculation may, in addition, profoundly affect the type of response obtained.

Rabbits injected intravenously with *Candida albicans* made precipitins against the yeast's polysaccharides, but after intradermal injection they made precipitins preferentially against its proteins (Stallybrass, 1965). Monkeys injected intraperitoneally with Coxsackie virus formed type-specific precipitins, but when infected with the virus orally they made both group- and type-specific precipitins (Schmidt *et al.*, 1965). Allotypic differences among α_2 lipoproteins from different people could be detected with precipitins from rabbits injected intravenously with this antigen (Berg, 1963).

Precipitins have been produced in rabbits by feeding them *Trichinella spiralis* (Tanner and Gregory, 1961). *Herpes simplex* virus rubbed into the scarified cornea of rabbits caused them to produce precipitins to seven or eight different herpes antigens for several weeks (Mäntyjärvi, 1965). Intranasal instillations and intraperitoneal injections were used for inducing mice to produce anti-influenza virus precipitins (Styk and Hána, 1966). Large volumes of precipitins to myxovirus were obtained in the milk of goats by instilling myxovirus into the mammary glands (Pasieka *et al.*, 1970). Very large volumes of precipitins can be obtained from mice, considering their size, by repeatedly injecting them intraperitoneally with antigen (e.g., arbovirus) in complete Freund adjuvant (Ibrahim and Sweet, 1970). Under these conditions the mice produce large volumes of ascitic fluid containing precipitins essentially the same as those found in their serum. Intraperitoneal injection of sarcoma 180/ TG cells enlarges the volume of antibody-rich ascitic fluid produced in mice. Precipitins are readily manufactured as a result either of natural infection or of intentional infection which may be self-limiting (attenuated organism) or chemotherapy-controlled (e.g., *Haemonchus contortus* in sheep: Ozerol and Silverman, 1969; *Stephanurus dentatus* in swine; Tromba and Baisden, 1963, 1964; *Toxoplasma gondii* in rabbits: Strannegåard, 1962; *Histomonas meleagridis* in turkeys: Clarkson, 1963; *Brucella melitensis* in rabbits: Glenchur *et al.*, 1962; Coxsackie virus in man and monkey: Schmidt *et al.*, 1963; the mite *Psoroptes cuniculi* in rabbits: Fox *et al.*, 1967; *Hymenolepis nana* in mice: Coleman and DeSa, 1964; *Plasmodium berghei* in rats: Zuckerman *et al.*, 1969).

Animals can be induced to make precipitins to autologous antigens by effecting appropriate *in vivo* injuries. For instance, rabbits produced precipitins to coagulating gland and seminal vesicle antigens following injury of these tissues by cryosurgery (Yantorno *et al.*, 1967).

Specific Protocols for Immunization

The following data illustrate specific immunization techniques which have been employed to obtain precipitins for different antigens, from different species of animals, and for different situations.

ANTIGENS PURIFIED BY SPECIFIC ADSORPTION OR PRECIPITATION

Rabbit antibodies to trout immunoglobulin were made by immunizing the rabbits with rabbit erythrocytes coated with trout hemagglutins. The erythrocytes were injected into the trout intracoelomically, and the fish were maintained at 15°C. Trout hemagglutinins were harvested 2 months later and mixed with a 10% suspension in saline of freshly prepared rabbit erythrocytes. The agglutinate was centrifuged and washed. Then 1-ml portions of 25% suspensions of these trout antibody (i.e., immunoglobulin)-sensitized cells were injected intraperitoneally three times a week for 2 weeks into rabbits. The rabbits made precipitins to trout immunoglobulins and possibly also to complement (Hodgins *et al.*, 1965).

Mouse serum was electrophoresed in agar at pH 8.2 on a 3¼ × 4-inch glass plate in gel 0.5 cm thick. The area known to contain principally γ_1-globulin (IgF) was cut out, frozen and thawed, and pressed through a fine wire mesh held in the bottom of a 10-ml syringe. The resulting fluid, estimated to contain IgF at approximately 50% of its original concentration in whole mouse serum, was injected subcutaneously into a rabbit at a 1% concentration in the 0.4-ml aqueous phase of a 0.6-ml volume of incomplete Freund adjuvant. The injection was repeated 7 days later. After 21 days the rabbit was producing strong precipitins to IgF but not to three other serum antigens also present in the agar electrophoresis-purified fraction, detected by injecting another rabbit with 10% instead of 1% concentrations of the eluate (Crowle, unpublished work).

Antigen–antibody precipitin arcs were cut directly from immunoelectropherograms of serum developed with polyvalent antiserum, soaked in saline for 48 hours at room temperature to remove diffusible substances, minced with 0.2 ml of saline, emulsified in complete Freund adjuvant, and injected directly into the popliteal lymph nodes of a rabbit.[5] The injection was repeated in 1 month with precipitate homogenized in saline alone (0.4 ml injected subcutaneously to drain into the previously injected popliteal node, 0.4 ml injected similarly into the contralateral leg, and 0.2 ml injected intravenously). Antisera from bleedings, made in 10 to 12 days, were monospecific (Goudie et al., 1966).

TOLEROGENIC SELECTION

Animals can be made tolerant to several antigens in a mixture so that when they are immunized later with this mixture they will produce precipitins only to its weaker antigens for which they have developed no tolerance; or they can be used to make precipitins to one or two antigens in a similar mixture which were absent from the tolerizing mixture (Zwaan, 1963; Berglund, 1963b; Garb et al., 1962; Gold and Freedman, 1965a; Hyde et al., 1965; Antoine and Neveu, 1967). By selective tolerogenesis, then, one can thus make monospecific antisera without purifying an antigen (i.e., without altering its native state) or having to absorb antisera with antigens (see below). One or a few different antigens in similar mixtures of many identical antigens can be detected by this technique of antiserum production. The following are some specific examples.

Rabbits were made tolerant to eye tissue antigens except those of the lens by injecting them daily, beginning at birth, for 15 days sub-

[5] Injection directly into the lymph nodes was meant to enhance precipitin production. But it is not necessary. We have performed similar immunizations with human salivary antigens, injecting precipitin arcs in incomplete Freund adjuvant on days 0 and 7 subcutaneously into rabbits, boosting the rabbits with whole saliva in saline on days 21, 22, and 23, and bleeding the rabbits 1 week later. Good monospecific precipitins were obtained in this manner, for instance, against salivary DC antigen (Revis and Crowle, unpublished work).

cutaneously or intravenously with 10-mg quantities of tolerizing mixture. Two months after the last tolerizing injection and when they had matured, they were immunized routinely with eye antigens but made precipitins only against lens antigens, to which they had not become tolerant (Zwaan, 1963). Precipitins to antihemophilic factor, which is not readily separated from fibrinogen, were made by injecting rabbits neonatally with 5-mg quantities of fibrinogen subcutaneously and repeating this every 5 to 10 days until the rabbits were 8 to 14 weeks old. Then they were immunized intravenously with 5- to 10-mg doses of a mixture of fibrinogen and antihemophilic factor repeated weekly for 4 weeks. At the end of this time they were making precipitins only to the antihemophilic factor (Berglund, 1963b).

Rabbits treated similarly were employed to make precipitins specific for leukemic tissues (Garb *et al.*, 1962; Greenspan *et al.*, 1963), for tumor antigens in carcinomas (Gold and Freedman, 1965a), and for human serum β lipoprotein (Antoine and Neveu, 1967). The use of this technique is discussed more fully in papers by Antoine and Neveu (1967) and Hyde *et al.* (1965).

Protocols for Different Species of Animals

Rabbits are the most often used species (cf. Soothill, 1962; Grabar *et al.*, 1962a; Durand and Schneider, 1962a; Loewi and Muir, 1965). Excellent responses to good protein antigens are obtained by the following protocols. Inject the rabbit subcutaneously on days 0 and 7 with no less than 1 μg and no more than 10 mg of a protein antigen in 0.5-ml volumes of incomplete Freund adjuvant (formula 1, Appendix I). On days 21, 22, and 23, or on any 3 succeeding days over a 5-week period beginning on day 21, inject 0.1, 1.0, and 10 mg of the antigen in saline subcutaneously, intravenously, and intravenously, respectively. Bleed the animal 7 to 10 days later (Crowle, unpublished work).

Human hemoglobulin is a poor antigen. Precipitins to it were obtained from rabbits by injecting them initially with 40 mg of the antigen in Freund adjuvant and then on day 21 injecting them with 20 mg in saline and repeating this at weekly intervals until precipitins appeared in sample antisera (Heller *et al.*, 1962).

Strong multivalent rabbit antisera to ungulate sera can be obtained without using Freund adjuvant by injecting the rabbits three times with 5-ml volumes of ungulate serum at intervals evenly spaced over a 2-week period and following these with two 10-ml injections once a week for 3 weeks. Optimal precipitin titers were attained in 6 to 8 weeks by this technique (Durand and Schneider, 1962a). A protocol for producing good polyvalent antisera to human serum with Freund adjuvant consists of injecting rabbits intramuscularly in opposite thighs with 1 ml each (2 ml total) of complete Freund adjuvant (made of a 1:1 mixture of 1% protein and oil phase containing mycobacteria) on day 0, repeating this in the shoulder muscles on day 14, boosting on days 28, 32, 34, and 36 with 0.5 ml of undiluted serum (intraperitoneally on day 28 and subsequently intravenously), boosting still more with 1-ml volumes intravenously on days 28, 40, and 42, and then bleeding several days later. Boostings can be continued until sample bleedings indicate maximum antibody titer (should reach 5 mg of antibody protein per milliliter; Soothill, 1962; cf. also Ferri and Cossermelli, 1964b; Porter and Dixon, 1966; Bazin, 1966; Grubb, 1970).

Guinea pigs are immunized like rabbits (cf. Loewi and Muir, 1965; Hyslop and Stone, 1969; Patterson et al., 1964b). Injecting the animals' foot-pads has been a common practice, but in our experience is unnecessary; other routes are effective and more humane. For instance, guinea pigs will make precipitins to the notoriously poor antigen bovine insulin if injected subcutaneously with 10 unit quantities in incomplete Freund adjuvant weekly for 4 weeks and then biweekly with 25 unit quantities for 4 months (Patterson et al., 1964b). Against a good antigen like chicken egg albumin, excellent precipitating antisera are obtained by injecting the guinea pigs subcutaneously on days 0 and 7 with 0.1-ml volumes of incomplete Freund adjuvant containing 1 mg of this antigen. The animals are bled 2 to 4 weeks later (Crowle, unpublished work). At this time the animals also can be boosted (e.g., intraperitoneal injection of 1 ml of saline containing 0.1 mg of antigen followed 1 day later by subcutaneous injection with 0.1 ml of saline containing 1 mg and again 1 day later with 1 ml of saline containing 10 mg) and bled still later. Bleedings should be performed some 6 to 10 days after the last boosting injection. The same protocol can be employed to produce multivalent antisera against mixtures of antigens like serum, if appropriate adjustments are made for achieving similar total antigen concentrations. The principal problem in attaining high titers of precipitins in guinea pigs is avoiding acute or protracted anaphylactic shock during the boosting course of injections, and for this reason more than usual care must be taken in boosting guinea pigs than in boosting most other species of animals.

Mice will produce powerful precipitating sera when immunized with antigens in Freund adjuvant and boosted with aqueous solutions as described above for guinea pigs and rabbits (Crowle, unpublished work). Volumes are scaled down to 0.1 ml per injection. Especially interesting is the capacity of some strains of mice to make large quantities of ascitic fluid with high titers of precipitins. For instance, if Swiss

Webster mice are injected intraperitoneally several times, usually at 4- to 7-day intervals, with 0.2- to 0.3-ml volumes of complete Freund adjuvant containing 1 to 1.5 mg of the antigen for the first injection and 0.1-mg quantities for later injections, after several weeks their abdomens become distended with ascitic fluid rich with precipitins to the antigen injected. This fluid can be tapped repeatedly, frequently to yield tens of milliliters per mouse (Anacker and Munoz, 1961). The yield of precipitin-containing ascitic fluid can be increased still more by injecting appropriate strains of mice with sarcoma 180/TG cells late in the immunization schedule (Ibrahim and Sweet, 1970). Up to 100-ml volumes of ascitic fluid with good precipitins to Australia antigen have been obtained in this manner from succeeding tappings of a single mouse (Krøll, 1970).[6] A particular advantage in using mice for making precipitins is that they can be employed in large numbers to provide a much broader variety of potential responses than is commonly available with larger animals; the utilization of mouse ascitic fluid instead of antiserum makes it possible to harvest volumes of "antiserum" approaching in size those obtained from larger animals like guinea pigs.

Rats and hamsters can be immunized well by injecting them subcutaneously with from 10 μg to 1 mg of antigen in 0.1 ml of incomplete Freund adjuvant, boosting them similarly 1 week later, and then at 5 weeks boosting again with a series of daily intraperitoneal injections of antigen in saline beginning with a low dose (e.g., 10 μg) and progressing through medium (0.1 mg) and large (10 mg) doses. These animals should be bled 6 to 10 days after the last boosting (Crowle, unpublished work; cf. also Paul and Benacerraf, 1966).

Horses react well to protein antigens injected in the classic methods of antitoxin production–that is, as alum precipitates; but in our very limited experience with these animals, we did not find them responsive to either ovalbumin or human γ-globulin injected in Freund adjuvant. However, the following protocol is reported to induce production of strong precipitins in the horse to human γ-globulin antigen (Johnston and Allen, 1968). Inject 4 ml of complete Freund adjuvant containing 4 mg of antigen per milliliter subcutaneously, and repeat this 1 month later with the same volume containing 20 mg/ml. Bleedings may be made 5 to 9 weeks after the second immunization. Titers can be raised by a series of booster injections consisting of 1.5 ml of a suspension of alum-precipitated antigen given subcutaneously on 5 consecutive days,

---

[6] Other kinds of body fluids should not be overlooked as sources of precipitins. For example, precipitins in the aqueous humor of eyes from patients with toxoplasmosis are rich in precipitin (O'Connor, 1957).

starting 2 months after the last bleeding, and then bleeding 4 days after the last boosting.

Freund adjuvant appears to be necessary for inducing a comprehensive precipitin response of goats to a mixture of antigens (Ridgway *et al.*, 1962). Goat polyvalent antiserum to human serum has been prepared by mixing a 1:6 dilution of human serum 1:1 with the oil phase of Freund adjuvant, injecting 12-ml volumes of this mixture six times at 7- to 10-day intervals with each dose divided into multiple subcutaneous injections of 1 to 2 ml given at different sites, boosting 2 months after the last injection with a 10-ml volume, and then bleeding several days later (West *et al.*, 1961). Sheep and swine produce good precipitins following immunization by a protocol similar to the first described above for rabbits. Essentially, this is to inject antigen originally in incomplete Freund adjuvant, 3 or more weeks later boost with a series of increasing doses of antigen, in saline, and take bleedings a week or 10 days after the last boosting injection (Crowle *et al.*, unpublished work; cf. also Fireman *et al.*, 1963).

Cattle can be immunized similarly (Hunter, 1969). Like other species of animal, cattle produce weaker but more specific antisera following immunization without Freund adjuvant. Cow anti-buffalo and buffalo anti-cow precipitins were made, for instance, by injecting with alum-precipitated bone antigens in 80-ml volumes twice intramuscularly and following these with three injections of 100 ml each at 4-day intervals by the same route (Pandey and Pathak, 1966). Cattle respond well to bacterial and viral antigens (Nagy, 1967; Myers and Hanson, 1962).

Monkeys and chimpanzees respond like smaller laboratory animals to injections of protein antigens in Freund adjuvant (Lichter and Dray, 1964; Lakin *et al.*, 1967; Hill *et al.*, 1967), and immunization protocols are generally the same. One injects the animals with from 1 to 100 mg of antigen in the adjuvant (complete Freund adjuvant usually has been used) and then boosts later with antigen in incomplete Freund adjuvant, in saline, or as an alum precipitate. Boostings can be made in as few as 3 weeks (Lakin *et al.*, 1967); the animals are bled within 2 months but still will be making useful quantities of precipitins up to 2 years later. Some species of monkey may produce very poor titers of precipitins if stressed during immunization by loud noises, light, or mechanical agitation of their cages (Hill *et al.*, 1967).

Considering their size, convenience of handling, and excellent precipitin production, fowl are used less frequently than they should be. Among the fowl, responses in the chicken have been best characterized. Chickens will manufacture strong precipitins very rapidly to such antigens as mammalian serum proteins; taking advantage of this, experimenters usually have made early bleedings. The precipitins in these early-bleeding chicken antisera are different from precipitins taken later in that they require a high salt concentration for optimal precipitation of antigen, especially in liquid medium precipitin tests (cf. Chapter 1; Van Orden and Treffers, 1968a; Weiner *et al.*, 1964). Chicken precipitins in sera harvested later, especially after boostings, precipitate antigens under more conventional conditions (Benedict *et al.*, 1963). Therefore, there are two contrasting protocols for immunizing chickens: in one, initial injection of a large quantity of antigen in saline is followed by bleedings a few days later to yield precipitins requiring high salt concentration; in the other, initial injection of small quantities of antigen in incomplete Freund adjuvant is followed 2 or 3 weeks later with boostings of antigen in saline and still later with bleedings. In antisera from these bleedings, conventionally reactive precipitins predominate.

As an example of the first variety, roosters were injected intravenously with 30-mg doses of horse ferritin divided over 2 days for a total of 40 mg/kg body weight and then bled after 7 days (Patterson *et al.*, 1965a). Bleedings also were taken 1 week after secondary immunization, performed 4 weeks after the primary. The same schedule elicited good precipitin production in 8 to 10 days against human transferrin (Planas and De Castro, 1961) and was superior, for rabbit γ-globulin and bovine serum albumin, to intramuscular injection of alum-precipitated antigen given eight times over 5 months (Orlans *et al.*, 1961).

As an example of the second variety, chickens were used to produce polyvalent antisera to monkey and human sera by injecting them intramuscularly with 0.5 ml of serum mixed with 0.5 ml of Freund adjuvant followed 1 month later by weekly injections of serum for a period extending up to 15 months (Weiner *et al.*, 1963). We find chickens to respond well to the first immunization protocol for rabbits mentioned above. For instance, chickens were injected subcutaneously on days 0 and 7 with 0.1 ml of Freund adjuvant containing 1 mg of bovine serum albumin antigen and 1 mg of living avirulent tubercle bacilli. They were producing strong precipitins by day 21, and these precipitated better in immunodiffusion tests at physiologic salt concentration than at the higher salt concentrations usually used for chicken antisera (Crowle and Lueker, 1961).

Ducks are reported to make good precipitins to allotype antigens by both types of immunization protocol (Kaminski and Ligouzat, 1964).

Immunizations need not be restricted to warm-blooded animals. For example, *Rana catesbeiana* tadpoles manufactured precipitins to the main hemoglobulin component of the adult frog of the same species when injected subcutaneously into their backs with 5 μg of the dimer

of this antigen emulsified in complete Freund adjuvant, boosted intraperitoneally 1 month later with the same amount of antigen without
adjuvant, and bled by decapitation 1 month after this second injection
(Maniatis *et al.*, 1969).

PROTOCOLS FOR SELECTED ANTIGENS

Frequently, the problem of obtaining appropriate precipitins is less
in the nature of a species' response to a given protocol of immunization
than in the nature of the antigen itself, which does much to govern the
type of response obtained. Some examples of this follow.

Antigens like hemoglobin, enzymes, and hormones usually are poor
precipitinogens because of their nonforeignness and their low molecular
weight. Strong immunization is required for hemoglobin. For instance,
precipitins were obtained in rabbits by injecting them with 5 ml of
foreign hemoglobin solution mixed with 5 ml of Freund adjuvant twice
weekly for 5 consecutive weeks, each injection being divided into two
equal parts with one injected subcutaneously in the inguinal region and
the other similarly in the abdominal area. Precipitins appeared 10 days
after the last injection (Rachmilewitz *et al.*, 1963). In another protocol,
3 to 5% hemoglobin was mixed with an equal volume of complete Freund
adjuvant, and 1 ml of this was injected into the gluteal muscles of an
adult rabbit. Two weeks later, 3 ml of hemoglobin solution were injected
intraperitoneally followed on 3 succeeding days by intravenous injection
of 0.5-, 1.5-, and 2-ml volumes of this solution. This series of boostings
had to be repeated during each of the following 3 weeks, with antisera
collected 1 week after the final injection (Boerma and Huisman, 1964;
cf. also Boerma *et al.*, 1960). Similar schedules of immunization in rabbits produced precipitins to small peptides of human anterior pituitary
gland (Friesen *et al.*, 1962), to human chorionic gonadotropin (Keele
et al., 1962), and against various enzymes (Raunio, 1968).

Despite the general opinion that rabbits are better precipitin producers
than guinea pigs, the latter may be superior in responding to bovine
insulin (Hirata and Blumenthal, 1962). Sixteen milligrams of insulin
dissolved in 10 mg of pH 3.0 hydrochloric acid–saline were emulsified
with an equal volume of complete Freund adjuvant oil phase. Two milliliters of this were used for each injection, three injections being given at
4-week intervals over 8 weeks. Precipitins appeared in sera drawn 4
weeks after the last injection. Similarly immunized rabbits also made
precipitins to insulin, although these did not precipitate as well in double
diffusion tests as the guinea pig precipitins (cf. also Jones and Cunliffe,
1961; Corcos and Ovary, 1965; Ceska, 1969b). Chickens apparently will
manufacture precipitins to bovine insulin quite readily, either following

intravenous–intramuscular injections of the antigen in saline or following its injection in incomplete Freund adjuvant (Patterson *et al.*, 1964b).

Rabbits can manufacture species-specific antiferritin precipitins when immunized with a saturated solution of ferritin in pH 7 phosphate buffer mixed with complete Freund adjuvant and injected subcutaneously into the flanks two or three times a week during 3 weeks (Richter, 1967). They are bled 2 to 3 weeks after the last injection.

There are no unique difficulties to obtaining precipitins to various tissue antigens other than minimizing simultaneous production of precipitins to nontissue antigens adsorbed to the tissues. A typical protocol calls for two subcutaneous injections in rabbits, spaced 1 week apart, of 5 to 10 mg of lyophilized rat bone marrow in complete Freund adjuvant, followed by two intramuscular injections per week of the same extract dissolved in physiologic saline, beginning with 5 mg and increasing by 5 mg each week to end with 20 mg 4 weeks later. After 4 weeks of rest, the rabbits are desensitized by intraperitoneal injection of 5 mg of the extract (to avoid anaphylaxis) and then injected simultaneously with equal quantities of the extract intravenously, intramuscularly, and subcutaneously; they are bled out 8 days later (Beernink *et al.*, 1965; cf. also Boyle *et al.*, 1963). A similar protocol has been used in ducks (Ehrlich *et al.*, 1962) for rabbit eye lens antigens, and in guinea pigs for various rabbit organs (Kasukawa *et al.*, 1966). Other examples include as antigens frog oviduct (Shivers and James, 1967), cultured strains of human-derived cells (Brand, 1965), bovine cortical bone (Kaminski and Gajos, 1962), and salivary gland insoluble lipoprotein (Chrambach and Rodbard, 1971).

Precipitins to isoantigens or alloantigens generally are prepared by immunizing other individuals of the same species as that from which the antigen was derived by the intensive techniques mentioned above for poor antigens (Dray *et al.*, 1963b; Lieberman and Dray, 1964; Skalba, 1964). This is true also for causing animals to make precipitins to their own antigens (i.e., autoantigens). For instance, precipitins were made in rabbits and guinea pigs to their own adrenal tissue by mixing a 20% suspension of organ homogenate with an equal volume of complete Freund adjuvant oil phase for the first three injections (intradermal) given at weekly intervals. These contained 8, 6, and 4 mg of antigen. A similar series of three injections employing incomplete Freund adjuvant was used for boosting, with 1- to 3-week intervals between boostings. The final bleeding was made 1 week after the last inoculation; the immunization period never exceeded 10 weeks (Witebsky and Milgrom, 1962). An alternative, rather interesting technique which can be used to obtain autoprecipitins is to induce mild organ injury *in vivo*, such as by placing a freezing probe against a rabbit's coagulating gland (Yantorno et al., 1967). However, antibody production is likely to be evanescent and weak.

Viruses are good precipitinogens (Styk and Hána, 1968; Bock, 1966; Dimmock, 1969; Ibrahim and Sweet, 1970; Göing and Micke, 1962; Woods et al., 1962; Jordan and Chubb, 1962; Krøll, 1970). Selecting a protocol for them, as for any complex mixture of antigens, depends on whether high specificity (e.g., type-specific antiserum to polio: Woods et al., 1962), strength (Ibrahim and Sweet, 1970; Styk and Hána, 1968), or polyvalency (Dimmock, 1969) is required of the antiserum. Generally, conditions for inducing precipitin formation to bacteria are similar; but because bacteria are larger and more complex than viruses, and because they usually are excellent antigens with their own adjuvancy, using intense immunization may give poorer results than immunizing simply with aqueous suspensions. Better precipitins against streptococcal antigens were produced in rabbits, for example, when heat-killed streptococci were injected intravenously three times a week for several weeks than when they were injected in complete Freund adjuvant (Pierce, 1959; cf. also Whiteside and Baker, 1962; Carlisle et al., 1962; Armstrong and Sword, 1967). If Freund adjuvant is to be used, the incomplete form usually is better because of the possibility that antigens from the mycobacteria included in the complete adjuvant might induce formation of precipitins cross-reacting with the bacterial antigens of primary interest. When homogenates or extracts of microorganisms are being employed for immunization, then one of the immunization protocols using incomplete Freund adjuvant mentioned above for inducing polyvalent responses to complex mixtures of antigens tends to be superior to injections of the antigen mixture in aqueous solution (Cross and Spooner, 1963; Biguet et al., 1965b). Purified microbial polysaccharides frequently are poor precipitinogens because they lack adjuvancy; therefore, precipitins are best produced against them by immunizing with unpurified polysaccharide or with whole microorganisms (Grappel et al., 1967).

Parasites like Shistosoma mansoni (Hillyer and Frick, 1967), Entamoeba histolytica (Lunde and Diamond, 1969), and Toxoplasma gondii (Sherman et al., 1963) readily induce precipitin formation either after infection (Sherman et al., 1963; Hillyer and Frick, 1967) or after injection in Freund adjuvant (Lunde and Diamond, 1969). Insect homogenates in Freund adjuvant also are good precipitinogens in rabbits (mite: Dasgupta and Cunliffe, 1970; bark beetle: Thomas and Krywienczyk, 1966). Precipitins against house flies have been used to discriminate between DDT-resistant and DDT-susceptible strains (Long and Silverman, 1965).

Chickens respond readily to mammal serum antigens partly because there is a big taxonomic gap between them and mammals. For the same reason, rabbits easily make abundant precipitins to serum antigens from such nonmammals as fish; strong immunizations are not required. For example, rabbits made precipitins that could distinguish between male and female salmon serum when they were immunized two times a week for 8 weeks with a mixture of equal parts of salmon serum and 25% poly-vinyl pyrrolidone, 1 ml of this mixture being injected subcutaneously for each injection (Fine and Drilhon, 1963). Intraperitoneal injections of pooled tuna fish serum (Ridgway, 1962a) or of carp serum (Creyssel *et al.*, 1964) elicited formations of similar antisera. The precipitins to carp serum were made with the aid of sodium alginate as an adjuvant, rabbits being injected intraperitoneally first with 1 ml of a mixture of 3 parts of 4% sodium alginate and 1 part of 1% calcium chloride and then, into the same area, with 1 ml of carp serum. Three weeks later each rabbit was injected with 0.5 ml of serum intraperitoneally, and 2 days later with the same volume intravenously. Adequate precipitins usually were obtained within another 15 days; if not, the animals were reimmunized after a 6-week rest (Creyssel *et al.*, 1964).

Rabbits respond well also to plant antigens such as those of wheat or barley (Grabar *et al.*, 1962), potato (Lester, 1965), or various seeds (Vaughan *et al.*, 1966; Lester *et al.*, 1965). Soluble extracts are commonly employed to expedite rapid antigen contact. For instance, dry whole *Brassica* seeds were ground to a fine powder, extracted with petroleum ether to remove lipids, and then air-dried. Protein was extracted from the residue with physiologic sodium chloride at 4°C for 18 hours, precipitated with ammonium sulfate, redissolved in saline, and used for immunization (Vaughan *et al.*, 1966). One part of seed extract containing 10 mg of protein per milliliter was emulsified with 1 part of oil phase of complete Freund adjuvant, and 1 ml of this mixture was injected into each thigh of the rabbit at weekly intervals over a period of 3 weeks. Blood was taken 4 weeks after the last injection.

Simple chemicals which alone are not precipitinogens frequently will induce precipitin formation if attached to antigenic carriers and then used in a routine schedule of immunization. Examples of this for guinea pigs, rabbits, monkeys, and mice are given in the paper of Paul and Benacerraf (1966). Initial exposure to antigen typically is by multiple simultaneous injections with complete Freund adjuvant. The animals are boosted 2 weeks later, and for the succeeding 2 weeks, with antigen in physiologic saline, and then they are bled 1 week after the last booster.

Precipitins can be prepared against lipids also by similar use of carrier substances. Rabbits were immunized with haptenic cerebroside by mixing it with an equal quantity of bovine albumin as carrier and injecting this in complete Freund adjuvant (Niedieck *et al.*, 1965; Niedieck and Palacios, 1965).

CHANGES WITH BLEEDING TIME OF ANTISERUM PRECIPITINS

The importance of the interval between immunization and bleeding in determining precipitating characteristics of antisera used for immunodiffusion has been mentioned several times. Early bleedings generally provide high-specificity, low-activity antisera, and late bleedings provide low-specificity, high-activity antisera (Omland, 1963a; Muraschi *et al.*, 1965; Rodkey and Freeman, 1970). But there are exceptions, variations, and modifying factors to this generalization. For instance, 21-day convalescent bovine serum more readily distinguished between subtypes of foot-and-mouth disease virus than did 7- and 14-day sera (Graves, 1960). Polyvalency and cross-reactivity usually increase with time after immunization (Williams *et al.*, 1964; Biguet *et al.*, 1962a,c,d; Slaterus, 1961); but each antigen–animal relationship is unique and, if previously unstudied, must be observed empirically. For example, there will be large variations among individuals of one species injected by one protocol with the same preparation of antigen (Ferri and Cossermelli, 1964a). A rabbit injected with human serum can make high-titer antialbumin precipitins without forming anti-γ-globulin precipitins early after primary immunization, but later with boostings this relationship is reversed (Ferri and Cossermelli, 1964a). Precipitins to different antigens in a mixture first appear at different times after immunization. Most antigens of *Onchocerca volvulus* had elicited precipitins in rabbits injected with this parasite in Freund adjuvant by the eighth week after immunization, but precipitins to additional antigens occasionally appeared through the twenty-fourth week (Biguet *et al.*, 1962c). Maximum variety of response to *Shistosoma mansoni* took 14 weeks (Biguet *et al.*, 1962a) and to *Aspergillus fumigatus* over 90 days (Biguet *et al.*, 1962d). Unfortunately, the sequence of antibody production to the same antigen frequently differs in two different individuals. For instance, one rabbit produced precipitins to antigens 1, 2, and 3 of *Candida albicans* in 6 weeks; but in another, precipitins to antigens 1 and 3 had appeared within only 3 weeks, while precipitins to antigen 2 were absent until the seventh week (Biguet *et al.*, 1965b).

Boosting injections of antigens usually provoke a rapid rise of precipitin titers, and this rise is partially proportional to the amount of antigen used. But these heightened titers also drop rather quickly afterward, so that bleedings usually should be made a few days after the last boosting

(Godzińska, 1966). They can be made too soon: free antigen or antigen–antibody complexes that act like free antigen can combine with and precipitate antibodies in other antisera (Burstein and Fine, 1964c).

The type of antibody response developed by an animal against a given antigen changes remarkably with time after immunization. Evidence of this for chicken antisera has already been presented above (Orlans *et al.*, 1961); there are many examples of changes in immunoglobulin class and characteristics with passing time and/or changes in antigenic stimulation (Cowan, 1966b; Moore, 1961; Pappaganis *et al.*, 1965; Murray *et al.*, 1965). Animals can pass through a period of good precipitin production and then into equivalent production, instead, of passive hemagglutins (Richter *et al.*, 1962; Rodkey and Freeman, 1970).

The type and sequence of antibody manufacture are associated with the nature of the antigen and how it is administered. Precipitins appear rapidly after antigen has been injected in saline (Orlans *et al.*, 1961; Richter *et al.*, 1962), but they also tend to disappear rapidly. They accumulate more slowly following injection of antigen in Freund adjuvant, rise to higher titers, and persist in bleedings taken over a much longer time. Poor antigens (e.g., RNase, leucine aminopeptidase) eliciting little or no primary response of precipitins may nevertheless elicit good responses following boosting, whereas good antigens (e.g., bovine serum albumin, viruses) provoking strong primary response may elicit little or no secondary rise in precipitin production (Wright and Stace-Smith, 1966; Rodkey and Freeman, 1970). Some investigators find the duration of immunization more important than the dose of antigen (e.g., for precipitin production to bovine parathyroid hormone in rabbits: Williams *et al.*, 1964); others find dose more important (e.g., to produce precipitins to human serum albumin in chickens: Ivanyi *et al.*, 1966). Time is a primary factor when antigenic stimulation consists of infection (Cowan and Trautman, 1965), and apparently if bleedings are obtained frequently enough one can observe cycles of rising and falling precipitin production to a given antigen after just one immunization (Biguet *et al.*, 1965).

Much less is understood about anamnestic precipitin production than about that following initial exposures to antigen. Aside from aiding in the production of maximum-potency antisera, this specific immunologic recall can also be utilized to restore manufacture of precipitins in an animal no longer making any. For example, a rabbit producing no detectable precipitins one year after having been immunized with bee venom sac extract in incomplete Freund adjuvant was boosted with freshly prepared extract in the adjuvant and within 1 to 3 weeks had developed a precipitin response equivalent to its maximum earlier response (Shulman *et al.*, 1966a).

Antisera with "Natural" Antibodies

Occasionally one can avoid preparing antisera by using some from people or animals already exposed naturally to antigen and therefore making antibodies; indeed, this has been an important way in which some allotypic differences between individuals have been discovered. For instance, patients receiving multiple blood transfusions produced precipitins with which polymorphisms in serum lipoprotein were detected (Blumberg, 1963; Blumberg *et al.*, 1962, 1964; cf. Berg, 1964). Infected individuals are a natural source of precipitins for antigens of streptococci and cross-reacting tissue antigens (Kaplan and Svec, 1964), toxoplasma (O'Connor, 1957; Tönjum, 1962), *Paragonimus westermani* (Yogore *et al.*, 1965), *Entamoeba histolytica* (Auernheimer *et al.*, 1966), and *Herpes simplex* virus (Tokumaru, 1965b). People or animals sufficiently exposed to but not necessarily infected with microorganisms also may be producing precipitins (e.g., to staphylococci: Sonea *et al.*, 1962; Cohen *et al.*, 1963; Torii *et al.*, 1964). In response to certain infections they may make precipitins to different but cross-reacting antigens: antisera from patients with infectious mononucleosis precipitate antigens extractable from ox and sheep erythrocytes (Stannegård and Lycke, 1964).

The sera of allergy patients have precipitins to various antigens. The stools of people with gastrointestinal bleeding were found to contain coproantibody precipitin to antigens in cow's milk, and the intestinal secretions of patients with celiac disease contained precipitins to wheat and rye proteins (Katz *et al.*, 1968). Victims of autoimmune disease may be producing precipitins to their own affected tissues (e.g., thyroid, Fahey and Goodman, 1964).

Collection and Care of Antiserum

The production of antiserum to be used in immunodiffusion tests leads to problems of selection, storage, and utilization. Although immunodiffusion tests can be performed with nonprecipitating antibodies, the following data principally concern these, the most often used antibodies.

Selection and Assay

Antisera to be used for immunodiffusion tests should be assayed by immunodiffusion tests, for, although their precipitins can be detected by other techniques (e.g., by the interfacial "ring" test), these techniques neither indicate the variety of antibodies present nor do they necessarily correlate well with titers of precipitins that would be evident from an immunodiffusion test (Cline, 1967). Quantitation adequate for many purposes can be achieved directly by reacting serial dilutions of the antiserum against a given concentration of antigen (Cline, 1967; cf. Fig. 4.14). Indirect tests, such as for capacity of antiserum to neutralize antigen (Klein *et al.*, 1963; cf. Chapter 7), are also useful but detect nonprecipitins as well as precipitins. Qualitatively, a good way to assay the variety of antibodies in an antiserum is by some form of immunoelectrophoresis (Chapter 5); electroimmunodiffusion (Krøll, 1969a; Chapter 6) offers both qualitative and quantitative data simultaneously.

Analyses of antisera obtained from different animals to a given mixture of antigens, or from different bleedings of a given animal, will indicate which is the best for a given use. Often, different antisera will detect different antigens in the same antigen mixture. Then they can be blended appropriately to prepare a versatile polyvalent antiserum (Ridgway *et al.*, 1962). This procedure of blending can be carried back to initial immunization by injecting different animals with different portions of the antigen mixture so as to avoid competition among the many antigens for the immunologic attention of individual animals (Rathbun *et al.*, 1967). A blend of the resultant various antisera is likely to have broader and more even polyvalency than any single antiserum alone.

In assaying precipitins to multiple antigens, the absence of precipitation for a given antigen may not indicate the absence of precipitins for it; each antigen–antibody precipitating system has its own optimal precipitating characteristics, and in a test permitting detection of most of the other systems some may very well not be detected (Hirschfeld, 1963). Therefore, comprehensive analyses require that antigen be matched against antiserum in several different ratios. Moreover, antisera containing what would appear to be equal precipitin titers against a single antigen cannot be assumed to have equal quantities of antibodies to the same antigenic determinants and therefore cannot be expected to behave equally in comparative tests. This is of considerable practical importance in the assay, for example, of human immunoglobulins (Reimer *et al.*, 1970; Stiehm, 1967); commercial antisera against the same immunoglobulin provided different results because they contained different quantities of precipitins against different varieties of the same portion of one antigen (i.e., immunoglobulin light chains).

Antiserum Storage

Problems of storing immunodiffusion antisera with minimal change or loss of activity have attracted less attention than they deserve, and the approach has been principally empirical. Unfortunately, storage characteristics for antiserum from one species may not fit those from another, even against the same antigen. This is also true of antisera obtained within a species or even from just one individual, because there are several kinds of precipitins, and each has different sensitivities to changes that occur within and around it (Van Orden and Treffers, 1968b; Krøll, 1970). Hence, only some general guidelines on antiserum storage can be given here.

The three most common means of storage are by refrigeration at 4°C, by freezing, and by lyophilization. None can be depended upon to prevent changes in precipitin titer. Some antisera can maintain activity for months when stored at 4°C aseptically or with preservatives such as phenol or Merthiolate (guinea pig: De Banchero, 1962; rabbit: Glenn, 1961d). On the other hand, some rabbit precipitins lose activity in 12 days or less at this temperature (Hruby et al., 1969); human precipitins to mycobacterial antigens can lose activity overnight (Morton and Dodge, 1963); and mouse antisera to foreign serum albumins lose precipitating activity rapidly at 4°C (Crowle, unpublished work). By contrast, the antigen-precipitating capacity of chicken antisera may rise during storage at 4°C (Van Orden and Treffers, 1968b).

Freezing seems to be the surest way of preserving precipitins, perhaps because it stops the activity of serum enzymes which often play an important but usually unrecognized role in this deterioration.[7] Freezing prevented most of the deterioration of human precipitins noted above (Morton and Dodge, 1963) and also of the rabbit precipitins (Hruby et al., 1969). But rabbit IgM precipitins have been observed to lose titer while stored frozen (Krøll, 1970), and we have observed diminishing precipitating activity in antisera from several species of animals, including rabbits, stored for several years at −29°C without thawing and refreezing. If the precipitins in an antiserum do not depend for help in precipitating antigen on other nonantibody serum constituents, and if they are themselves relatively stable physically, they can be frozen and thawed repeatedly without apparent harm (Glenn, 1961d; West et al., 1961). But if they do depend on other antiserum cofactors, they can be affected by being frozen and thawed, sometimes even advantageously. For instance, the precipitin titer of frozen–thawed chicken antiserum rose following storage at −20°C for 2 to 3 weeks (Gengozian et al., 1962).

Spontaneous aggregation[8] or changes in solubility probably account

---

[7] Proteolytic degradation of precipitins by plasmin and fibrinolysin probably can be depressed by adding an enzyme inhibitor such as ε-aminocaproic acid to the antiserum (Hruby et al., 1969).

[8] This aggregation, especially of purified immunoglobulins, can be minimized by dialyzing them before storage against 0.1 M glycine.

for most deterioration of antiserum precipitins during lyophilization as well as during freezing (Grubb, 1970). Once the initial damage, if any, to precipitin titer has occurred in the process of lyophilization, there seems to be very little additional deterioration. A strong antiserum stored lyophilized at 4°C for several years retains nearly the same precipitating activity as it had immediately following lyophilization. This observation has practical application for long-term storage of reference antisera, for commercial distribution of antisera, and for such specific purposes as charging paper discs with antiserum and lyophilizing them for later use in field tests (Hamilton, 1965).

Freezing probably is the best general method for storing antisera for immunodiffusion tests for more than a few days and up to a few years; but if a modest loss in activity is acceptable, or if the antiserum can withstand lyophilization, this is probably the better long-range antiserum storage method.

Antiserum Concentration

Some problems of precipitin selection and storage can be minimized by concentrating antiserum or, as will be described later, separating the precipitins from other serum constituents. Usually an antiserum is concentrated because its precipitin titer is low. Frequently, concentrating the whole antiserum is better than concentrating just antibodies separated from it, because antibodies tend to precipitate antigen better in the presence of other serum constituents, and also because the precipitins can be distributed among several immunoglobulin classes, so that several could be lost by selective enrichment of any single class.

Antiserum concentration (i.e., its dehydration) is done in several ways, including lyophilization and reconstitution to two- to five-fold reduced volume (Bednařík, 1966); absorbing water directly from the antiserum with substances like Sephadex G-25 dextran[9] or Bio-gel P-2 polyacrylamide beads, which do not also absorb proteins (Bednařík, 1966); dialysis against a concentrated solution of large inert molecules (e.g., polyvinylpyrrolidone, 50% Ficoll[10]:Bednařík, 1966); dialysis against an inert

[9] Add G-25 to serum at a ratio of 2 gm to 10 ml, mix for 15 minutes, and centrifuge. Concentration is two-fold (Bednařík, 1966).

[10] Dialyze antiserum against 50% Ficoll for 4 hours. Concentration is five-fold (Bednařík, 1966). Similar concentration is obtained by dialysis against 40% polyvinylpyrrolidone (Fey, 1960); polyethylene glycol (molecular weight 20,000) also can be used (Fey and Margadant, 1961). However, these concentrating substances to which dialyzing membranes supposedly are impermeable nevertheless do enter dialyzing bags and may combine with antiserum protein (Crowle, unpublished work). Hence, this concentrating technique should be selected with reservation (Iverius and Laurent, 1967).

powder like sucrose, which draws water out of the dialyzing bag and, although it enters the bag, can later be easily removed (Centeno et al., 1964);[11] ultrafiltration (Lieberman and Dray, 1964); pervaporation; and freezing–thawing. All these methods have the disadvantage of simultaneously concentrating other serum constituents, albumin being particularly troublesome because of its originally high concentration, which raises problems of viscosity, an increased affinity for surrounding water, and increased interaction between serum proteins.

Lyophilization is convenient and effective but should be preceded by dialysis to prevent excessive concentration of salts. But it may directly injure the precipitating capacity of an antiserum (see above). Concentration with Sephadex beads, though convenient and rapid, is not as efficient as lyophilization. These beads also remove salts and thus may alter the physical state of antibody molecules and their solubility. Concentration against a substance like 50% Ficoll is effective and fast, but, as is indicated in the footnote on this substance, macromolecules used for concentrating antiserum tend to enter dialyzing bags to various degrees and may affect antigen–antibody precipitation in later immunodiffusion tests (cf. dextran). Ultrafiltration and pervaporation are effective and simple[12] and would appear to have no disadvantages beyond concentrating all other serum macromolecules simultaneously, but these techniques have not seen much use in immunodiffusion experimentation. Concentrating antiserum by freezing it slowly also is relatively simple but may have the disadvantage of insolubilizing or aggregating serum constituents, including antibodies, important to the precipitin reaction.

Antibody Purification and Concentration

Techniques for purifying and concentrating precipitins differ from those of simply concentrating the whole antiserum: they selectively remove precipitins from other serum constituents. They do so physicochemically or immunochemically. Physicochemical techniques concentrate immunoglobulins without regard to whether they are the antibodies of

---

[11] Enclose the antiserum in the dialyzing bag, and cover the bag with sucrose powder. After 1 to 4 hours, retie the bag to maintain the diminished volume and dialyze it against 0.15 M NaCl to remove excess sucrose and adjust the salt concentration (Centeno et al., 1964). Note, however, that for certain antigen–antibody precipitating systems the presence of even small amounts of sucrose can inhibit precipitation (Hawkins, 1965).

[12] For ultrafiltration one simply vacuum- or pressure-forces fluid through a semipermeable membrane which holds back the macromolecules; for pervaporation, the antiserum is hung in a dialyzing bag in a draft, so that the fluid evaporates as it diffuses through the semipermeable membrane.

interest, whereas immunochemical methods concentrate the antibodies alone by their property of reacting with antigen. The former method is more popular because it is easier, but the latter method is superior for more critical experimentation. Both methods have the disadvantage of removing antibodies from other antiserum constituents which may be necessary cofactors for full activity of the antibodies. Because of this disadvantage, which is important and frequently encountered in practical immunodiffusion, we rarely use purified antibodies (cf. Jochim and Chow, 1969; also see Chapter 6).

Physicochemical methods for purifying immunoglobulins (and therefore antibodies) are broadly divisible into those of selective precipitation and those of fractionation by physical characteristics such as electric charge or molecular size (cf. review of techniques in Steinbuch and Audran, 1965). The method most frequently employed is to mix antiserum with saturated ammonium sulfate (1:1), centrifuge out the resulting immunoglobulin concentrate, and redissolve this in an appropriate volume of a suitable buffer. One composed of 0.05 M sodium phosphate at pH 7.85 and containing 0.3 M glycine both restores physiologic salt and pH conditions and prevents spontaneous aggregation of the immunoglobulins and other macromolecules (Manski *et al.*, 1960). Alternatively, the ammonium sulfate precipitate can be dissolved in a larger volume of buffer which later is reduced by dialysis against polyvinylpyrrolidone (Weiner *et al.*, 1963). Since serum albumin is not precipitated by the ammonium sulfate, this technique reduces considerably the concentration of nonantibody serum protein in its product (De Banchero, 1962); but it does precipitate many other nonantibody serum proteins and therefore may preserve some coprecipitating effects of the whole antiserum.

Lower concentrations of ammonium sulfate, such as one-third instead of one-half saturation in the antiserum (Manski *et al.*, 1960), more selectively precipitate out the euglobulins, but they may not precipitate nonantibody cofactors or pseudoglobulin precipitins (Biguet *et al.*, 1962e). Ammonium sulfate precipitation is practiced most frequently with mammalian antisera. Chicken antisera precipitins can be concentrated similarly by precipitation with sodium sulfate followed by Sephadex G-100 and G-200 gel filtration to remove macroglobulin and transferrin (Tenenhouse and Deutsch, 1966).[13]

---

[13] Antiserum immunoglobulins can be concentrated twenty fold within 30 minutes (Smith, 1968). Desalt the antiserum by filtration through Sephadex G-25 equilibrated with 0.04 M phosphate buffer at pH 7.2, mix with an equal volume of 50% ethanol, precooled to $-19°C$, in an ice bath at $-6°C$, and centrifuge at 12,000 g. Use the resulting pellet of γ-globulins directly for charging the antiserum well of a double diffusion test.

Techniques that precipitate immunoglobulins risk some denaturation of these antibodies (De Banchero, 1962) or chances of degrading them by activating plasmin to plasminogen (Steinbuch et al., 1970). Hence, methods for purifying immunoglobulins by precipitating other serum constituents instead are gaining popularity, including especially methods using the basic acridine dye Rivanol (also known as Ethodin: Zwaan, 1963). For instance, 0.5% Rivanol in distilled water is mixed with rabbit antiserum at 3.5:1, and the resulting precipitate is centrifuged out and discarded. The clear supernatant containing principally immunoglobulins is passed through Sephadex G-50 or G-25, using 0.01 M phosphate buffer, pH 7.2, as eluant, to remove the Rivanol (Zwaan, 1963). But as is true of any batch purification technique, separations are never complete: some nonimmunoglobulins will remain in the solution, and some immuno-globulins will be precipitated (Rejnek, 1964).

The immunoglobulins of human beings, goats, sheep, and cattle can be separated from other serum constituents with caprylic acid because they are soluble in the presence of this acid at pH 5 (Steinbuch et al., 1970). The procedure is as follows: adjust the antiserum to pH 5 with 0.1 N acetic acid, add caprylic acid[14] slowly drop by drop with vigorous stir-ring at room temperature, and continue this stirring for an additional 15 minutes. The supernatant fluid from a subsequent centrifugation will con-tain principally γ_1 and γ_2-globulins. These can be separated from each other, and traces of other serum macromolecules can be removed by additional procedures of purification (Steinbuch et al., 1970).

Electrophoretic or chromatographic techniques may be used instead of batch methods for separating immunoglobulins from nonantibody anti-serum constituents. Agar gel zone electrophoresis, for example, is very simple, quick, and effective, and it minimizes chances of altering or de-naturing the immunoglobulins. Typically, one simply pours 1.5% agar or 1% agarose, made up in one of the conventional immunoelectrophoresis buffers, onto a glass slide (dimensions and gel thickness are selected to suit the size of sample to be electrophoresed; 5 ml can be fractionated on a 3¼ × 4-inch glass plate with 1-cm-thick gel), cuts a trough to receive the sample, mixes antiserum previously dialyzed against the electro-phoresing buffer with an equal volume of double-strength agar or agarose at 56°C, and fills the origin trough with this. The sample is electro-phoresed in a refrigerator for 1 to 4 hours, depending on the dimensions

---

[14] The amount of caprylic acid differs from one animal to another. For 100 ml of serum or plasma adjusted to 5% protein content it is 4, 3, 6, and 6.8 gm, respec-tively, for goat, sheep, cattle, and man (Steinbuch et al., 1970; Steinbuch and Audran, 1969).

of the agar block. Transferrin can be seen as a faint brown band in the gel; it serves both as an indicator for the extent of electrophoretic separation and as a marker for removing the separated immunoglobulins. Most of these will be located cathodic to the transferrin band. Gel containing the immunoglobulins is frozen and thawed, and fluid is expressed from it on a fine wire mesh placed within a syringe of suitable size. The expressed eluate contains immunoglobulins at nearly the same concentrations as the original sample, and only transferrin is likely to be a significant contaminant.[15]

Additional details will not be provided here for electrophoretic and chromatographic fractionation of antiserum, since these can be obtained from handbooks devoted to these techniques in general (cf. Steinbuch and Audran, 1965). A word of caution: note that antibodies belong to different immunoglobulin mobilities and that precipitins to antigens sometimes can be restricted to a narrow region of an electropherogram (Silverstein *et al.*, 1963b; Osterland *et al.*, 1966). Consequently, purifying a specific class of immunoglobulin does not necessarily coincide with purifying the precipitins of a given antiserum.

There are many techniques for purifying antibodies by reacting them with their antigens. Thus, one obtains not only purified immunoglobulins but also only those that have specific antibody activity. However, coprecipitating antiserum constituents like complement also may be present in the product of this type of purification. These methods are described in immunology manuals such as those of Campbell *et al.* (1970) and of Williams and Chase (1967).

The technique mentioned earlier in this chapter for obtaining purified antigen by sectioning a precipitin band from an immunodiffusogram and then dissociating the antigen–antibody complex can also be employed to acquire highly purified specific antibody. In an interesting microvariant of this technique (Nace, 1963), the band is formed by using fluorescent antibody. Then it is cut from the gel, washed in microtubes, minced, and transferred to fixed tissue sections which are to be studied with the fluorescent antibody. The antigen–antibody precipitate is dissociated with mild acid directly on these sections, the liberated fluorescent, now highly

---

[15] Transferrin will not be a contaminant, nor can it be used as a marker for locating immunoglobulins, in agar block separations applied to antisera in which transferrin does not migrate electrophoretically as a β_1-globulin. In guinea pigs, for instance, transferrin has α_2-globulin mobility (Havez *et al.*, 1965). Changing from agar to another semisolid medium also can considerably rearrange the electrophoretic rank of serum constituents; in starch, transferrin migrates with albumin rather than with the immunoglobulins (Korngold, 1963b).

specific antibody is allowed to diffuse into the tissue, and then the pH is neutralized to make it reassociate *in situ* with tissues containing the same kind of antigen from which it was dissociated.

Antiserum or Antibody Modification

Antiserum and/or antibodies can be modified for improved utility in immunodiffusion tests. One of the commonest problems in using antisera in these tests is development of nonspecific precipitates in the gel. This is minimized by using agarose rather than agar. It can also be reduced by removing lipids from the antiserum. This must be done cautiously to avoid denaturing antiserum precipitins. There are several techniques.

One is to achieve spontaneous separation such as occurs with chicken antiserum allowed to stand at 4°C for 2 to 3 weeks (Bornstein and Oudin, 1964). Mouse ascitic fluid "antisera" frequently contain troublesome lipid; this can be removed by ultracentrifuging the fluid in a potassium bromide–sodium chloride aqueous mixture of final solvent density 1.063. This is followed by dialysis against 0.9% sodium chloride, and the clarified fluid then can be concentrated by ultrafiltration (Lieberman and Dray, 1964). Interfering lipids in human antiserum are precipitated with dextran sulfate in the presence of calcium chloride (Burstein and Fine, 1964b). Some workers shake the antiserum with 1% chloroform for 5 minutes, centrifuge, and use the supernatant fluid (Witter, 1962; Talal *et al.*, 1963).

Antiserum lipids can be more carefully and completely removed—for example, to study their effects on antigen–antibody reaction—by slightly more complex methods. For instance, chill the antiserum to 0°C in an ice bath, add it drop by drop to ten times as much 95% ethanol itself chilled to dry ice temperature (-72°C), allow this mixture to stand for 30 minutes at -72°C with frequent agitation, and then centrifuge out the precipitated proteins at -20°C. Extract the resulting sediment three times more with absolute ethanol (1.5 to 2 hours for each extraction) and then three times with anhydrous ether. The ethanol extractions and the first two extractions with ether should be in the cold; the last ether extraction can be performed at room temperature. This procedure yields a dried, lipid-free powder containing antibodies that have undergone little change in capacity to combine with antigen (Cline, 1967). In another technique (Burstein, 1967), one volume of serum is mixed with one of amyl alcohol. The resulting two layers are intermixed for 5 minutes by gentle magnetic stirring, and then the mixture is centrifuged at 10,000 g for 15 minutes. The lower delipified serum layer is withdrawn, clarified by paper filtration, and dialyzed against physiologic saline to remove dissolved amyl alcohol.

Changes can be made in antiserum antibodies themselves. Treating rabbit antiserum with 0.1% ninhydrin for 1 hour at 37°C, or with β-naphthoquinone-4-sulfonate, is said to intensify the capacity of the antiserum to precipitate antigen (Francois *et al.*, 1956; Tayeau and Faure, 1953). Antibodies can be partially digested, such as by pepsin, to produce reactive fragments which may be useful in certain modifications of immunodiffusion tests (Keller, 1966). They can be labeled with fluorescence, radioactivity, heavy metals, or enzymes (Ghetie, 1967). For use in electroimmunodiffusion with certain antigens (e.g., polysaccharides, other γ-globulins, or antigens with the same electrophoretic mobility as the precipitins being used), antibodies can be changed chemically to lower isoelectric pH and thus greater electrophoretic affinity for the anode than they ordinarily have (Weeke, 1968a; Nász *et al.*, 1967; Ragetli and Weintraub, 1965). For instance, precipitins can be carbamylated by mixing 1 volume of antiserum with 2 volumes of 2 *M* potassium cyanate, prepared immediately before use in distilled water, allowing the mixture to stand at room temperature for about 18 hours, and dialyzing out the potassium cyanate against the kind of buffer ultimately to be used for the electroimmunodiffusion test (Weeke, 1968a).

Antiserum Absorption

Obtaining a monospecific antiserum usually is impossible without special immunization or purification techniques. But these may be more complicated than making a polyspecific antiserum monospecific by absorbing out unwanted antibodies. Moreover, specific absorption sometimes also answers immunological questions better than other techniques (Manski *et al.*, 1960; Manski, 1969; Berg and Dencker, 1962; Gomes da Costa *et al.*, 1962; Ver *et al.*, 1962). Specific absorption also is used for quantitations (Mackiewicz and Fenrych, 1961), currently especially so in electroimmunodiffusion (see Chapter 6).[16]

ABSORPTION DIRECTLY IN THE IMMUNODIFFUSION TEST

The principle of this very simple and effective method, first developed by Björklund (1952a), is to incorporate the mixture of absorbing antigens

---

[16] "Reversed absorption," in which antigen is purified by precipitating undesired antigens from a mixture with excess antiserum, can be accomplished. But it is very inefficient, and soluble antigen–antibody complexes are likely to form in the excess antibody and not precipitate (Sandor and Gleye, 1960).

in the reaction gel. As unwanted antibodies diffuse through these antigens, they form complexes in or near their origin of diffusion and thus are delayed or prevented from accompanying the antibodies for which there are no absorbing antigens in the medium as these antibodies diffuse into the reaction area. This technique can be used, for example, to detect a tumor antigen with antiserum to tumor tissue which also contains precipitins to numerous normal tissue antigens: an extract of normal tissue is mixed into the gel, and so only tumor antigen-specific precipitins will be free to diffuse against an extract of tumor tissue which will contain normal antigens as well as the tumor antigen (cf. also Van Regenmortel, 1967; Manski *et al.*, 1960; Gomes da Costa *et al.*, 1962; Berg and Dencker, 1962; Fine *et al.*, 1962).

This technique is very efficient because the antibodies in an antiserum to be absorbed are confronted with a practically inexhaustible source of absorbing antigens (Van Regenmortel, 1967). It can be applied to all varieties of immunodiffusion test (e.g., Schen and Rabinovitz, 1967b; Manski, 1969; Chapters 6 and 7). Absorbing antigen can be incorporated into the gel in several ways: mixing a warm solution of antigen with warm liquid agar before the agar is cast; diffusing the antigen into already cast agar gel either from antigen spread over the entire surface or from the wells subsequently to be charged with the antiserum; electrophoresing the antigens into the gel; or simply mixing antiserum with absorbing antigen before adding the antiserum to a well. Applied locally within a gel to create local specific absorption, the principle of intragel absorption can be employed for both qualitative and quantitative analyses of complex mixtures of antigens. Actually, the principle of intragel absorption is responsible for the reaction of identity in comparative double diffusion tests (Finger, 1964). Specific examples of local absorption will be found in several subsequent chapters.

Reversed immunoabsorption, using antiserum in the gel to absorb antigens, is less efficient than direct immunoabsorption because of the characteristics of antigen–antibody interaction (see Chapter 1). Nevertheless, it can be used effectively in immunodiffusion tests (Sen *et al.*, 1961), presumably because of the consistently large concentration of antibodies through which a rapidly diminishing concentration of antigen molecules would be passing during diffusion (see Fig. 2.1).

BATCH METHOD OF ABSORPTION

The method used most often probably is batch absorption of antiserum with antigen. Antigen is mixed in moderate excess with antiserum, whereupon antibodies to the various antigens added will preciptate and thus be absorbed from the antiserum. For instance, sheep antiserum to human

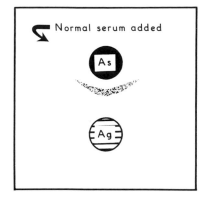

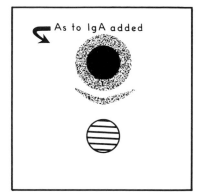

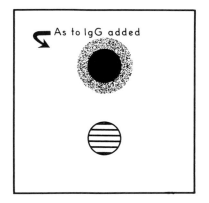

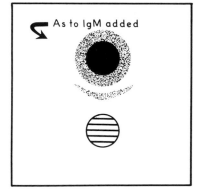

Fig. 2.1. Diagram showing how the class of antibodies precipitating an antigen was identified by using an inhibition double diffusion plate test. These antibodies were mixed with antibodies to different classes of immunoglobulin and then were examined for capacity to precipitate antigen. Antibodies to immunoglobulins A and M (IgA and IgM, respectively) did not inhibit this reaction, but antibodies to IgG did, thus indicating that the precipitins being studied were of the IgG class (adapted from Hanson *et al.*, 1971).

IgA globulin containing precipitins cross-reacting with IgG globulin was made specific for the IgA by absorbing 1 ml with 500 μg of IgG in increments of 100 μg, each being incubated at 37°C for 2 hours and then at 4°C for 18 hours (Fireman *et al.*, 1963). The supernatant resulting from subsequent centrifugation was analyzed for precipitin reactivity to IgG. None was present, and therefore absorption was judged complete (Midgley *et al.*, 1961; Burrell *et al.*, 1966). Dried antigen frequently is used for absorption, both for increased efficiency and to avoid undue dilution of the antiserum (Zwaan, 1963). Using absorbing antigen in small increments is more efficient than adding a large amount all at once (Hochwald and Thorbecke, 1962), partly because there is less chance for weaker antibodies being absorbed to form complexes with antigen in extreme antigen excess. An additional advantage in using modest amounts of absorbing antigen is that the absorbing mixture of antigens may have some quantity also of an antigen for which one does not wish to remove antibodies. Then, employing small amounts of the mixture will remove undesirable antibodies without too greatly diminishing titers of the desired antibody (e.g., antiserum to human growth hormone absorbed with trace amounts of human serum: Hayashida and Grunbaum, 1962). Unfortunately, very large quantities are quite frequently required to absorb all unwanted antibodies in strongly polyspecific antisera. Rabbit antiserum to human gastric mucosa had to be absorbed with 100 to 200 mg of lyophilized plasma per milliliter of antiserum before only antibodies to the mucosal extracts remained (Aronson *et al.*, 1965). This underlines the inefficiency of batch absorption as contrasted with Björklund in-test absorption.

Some precautions in using batch absorption should be mentioned. "Exhaustive" absorption of an antiserum with a mixture of antigens may not have been truly exhaustive because the concentration of minor but significant antigens in the absorbing mixture may have been too low (Laterre and Heremans, 1963). Thus, apparent qualitative differences between partially related mixtures of antigen are hard to rule out as being simply quantitative. Antisera prepared against fragments of an entire antigen molecule may have antibodies that cannot be removed by absorption with the whole molecule itself (Tan and Epstein, 1965). That is, absorption specificity, like immunodiffusion specificity, is against determinants, and these must be properly presented for correct absorption. Determinant specificity is especially evident when one is absorbing antiserum to a single antigen with a cross-reacting antigen and observing the results by the direction and magnitude of spur formation (Finger, 1964; cf. Chapter 4), since in this situation one is consciously removing antibodies to cross-reacting determinants rather than antibodies to whole antigen molecules.

CHROMATOGRAPHIC AND ELECTROPHORETIC ABSORPTION

Antiserum can be percolated through a column of insolubilized antigen, or electrophoresed through a high concentration of antigen molecules for specific absorption. Either technique is much more efficient than batch absorption, and the absorption can be effected without producing an antigen–antibody precipitate.

For chromatographic absorption, a column of antigen is prepared and the antiserum to be absorbed is percolated through it. Antibodies being absorbed become attached to the column, and only antibodies for which there are no corresponding antigens on the column emerge in the eluate. The antigen must either be insoluble or be attached to something that is itself insoluble. The fixed antigen is called an "immunoabsorbent." Techniques for preparing and using immunoabsorbents are described in Volume I of the Williams–Chase series on immunological methods (Williams and Chase, 1967). The following technique is described here both as an illustration and because it is new and widely applicable.

Fifty milligrams of soluble absorbing antigen are added to 200 mg of acrylamide, 120 mg of N,N'-methylenebisacrylamide, 5.6 mg of tetramethylethylenediamine, 0.5 mg of $AlNH_4(SO_4)_2 \cdot 12 \ H_2O$, and 1 ml of $1 \ M$ tris buffer, pH 8.6, all diluted to 11 ml with water; 2.5 mg of potassium persulfate are added. The mixture is kept for 1 hour at 35°C without agitation after addition of the polymerizer (potassium persulfate). The resulting polyacrylamide gel is dispersed with a blender, centrifuged, washed several times, and then used for either batch or column absorption (Bernfeld and Wan, 1963).

This method offers advantages of insolubilizing antigen without denaturing it. In principle, any insoluble particle that will adsorb antigen will serve similarly; therefore, preparation of an absorbing suspension can be quite simple. For example, rabbit antiserum to IgG which contained unwanted antibodies to immunoglobulin κ light chain was absorbed with bentonite particles onto which κ protein had been adsorbed (Claman *et al.*, 1967). Antibodies to IgG were removed from an antiserum to whole human serum by mixing 7.5 ml of 1% IgG solution for 10 minutes with 9 ml of 10% potassium aluminum sulfate adjusted to pH 6.5, centrifuging and washing the sediment which now had the IgG adsorbed to it, and then absorbing 1 ml of the antiserum at 4°C overnight with 0.1 to 0.2 ml of this sediment resuspended in saline to five times its original concentration (Klopstock *et al.*, 1963).

Antiserum Specificity

Although several of the techniques mentioned in the preceding sections concern antiserum specificity, practical aspects of this subject have not been discussed. That is the purpose of this section.

Superficially, defining antiserum specificity is simple: it is the capacity to distinguish one antigen from another immunologically. But complexities associated with varieties of specificity make a single definition impractical. Antiserum specificity depends on the physico-chemical "fit" of the combining site of an antibody molecule for a portion (the ligand: see Chapter 1) of the antigen molecule (Finger, 1964; Maurer *et al.*, 1963b). The specificity of that antibody molecule is relative; it is directly proportional to the ratio of affinity that this antibody molecule has for the homologous ligand that originally induced its production to whatever affinity it may have for physicochemically similar ligands on other molecules of antigen it may encounter (Jennings and Kaplan, 1962). The greater this ratio is, the less likely will the antibody be to combine well with heterologous ligands, and therefore the greater will be its specificity. Hence, immunologic specificity is relative, not absolute.

As was pointed out in Chapter 1, immunodiffusion tests utilize antisera; every antiserum is a collection of individual antibodies, and an immunodiffusion reaction requires cooperation between these antibodies reacting with a population of antigen molecules to develop precipitin bands (cf. Fig. 1.3). The relative specificities of individual antibody molecules for a ligand on one kind of antigen differ over a variable range depending on the characteristics of the antiserum and the nature of the antigen ligand (Dray *et al.*, 1963b; Paul *et al.*, 1970). Ligand specificity of an antiserum therefore is determined by the net reaction of its various antibodies and the antigen ligand (Christian, 1970; Maurer *et al.*, 1963b); this, in turn, may depend greatly on nonspecific characteristics of different populations of antibodies within the antiserum (e.g., relative hydrophilia, spontaneous aggregative potential, capacity to fix complement). Thus, definition of antiserum specificity becomes still more diffuse, having to include even tertiary factors (e.g., temperature, ionic strength, presence of metal ions) which influence expression of the nonspecific characteristics just mentioned.

Interaction between an antiserum and a single population of antigen molecules is not simply the mean interaction between this antigen and the varieties of antibodies in the antiserum (Jennings and Kaplan, 1962). These differ in avidity for antigen ligand, usually in direct proportion to potential cross-reactivity with similar ligands on related antigens (Jennings and Kaplan, 1962). Consequently, antiserum–antigen reaction will be primarily an expression of reaction between antigen and the most strongly combining antibodies (Uriel, 1963) which, though being those most precisely fitting the antigen ligand, are also the most likely to cross-react with similar ligands on other kinds of antigen (Muraschi *et al.*, 1965).

Many antigens have multiple ligands, each differing from the other (exceptions are antigens composed of repeated structures: Seligmann, 1959; cf. Chapter 1). These will be precipitated in immunodiffusion tests only by cooperation between antibodies in an antiserum of different

ligand specificities (Christian, 1970). Since the range of antibody specificities for one ligand on an antigen probably will differ from that for
another ligand on the same antigen, specificity of an antiserum for the
antigen depends not only on the heterogeneity of antibodies to one
ligand but also on the heterogeneities of antibodies to one or more
additional ligands on the same antigen (Dray, 1963). Hence, an antiserum could contain a population of antibodies highly specific for several
ligands, but if it also contained populations of antibodies with low
specificity for two or three other ligands on this antigen, the specificity
of the antiserum in an immunodiffusion test might be very low (Graves,
1960).

This is further complicated by the relative concentrations of antibodies
to various ligands (Dray *et al.*, 1963b; Tremaine and Wright, 1967; Jennings and Kaplan, 1962). Consider the example just given in which
populations of antibodies of low specificity made the antiserum nonspecific even though it might also contain other populations of highly
specific antibodies. If the concentrations of the low-specificity antibodies
were much lower than those of the higher-specificity antibodies, then
the antiserum would appear to have a net high antigenic specificity (cf.
Finger and Heller, 1963; Finger *et al.*, 1963).

Antiserum specificity depends also in part on the nature of the antigen
presented to it (Tan and Epstein, 1965; Dray *et al.*, 1963b; Zelkowitz
and Yakulis, 1970). In one physical form (e.g., molecule opened out,
depolymerized, or partially digested), antigen ligands of "internal" portions of the molecule would be exposed, and interaction between this
form of antigen and a given antiserum would develop according to the
balance of interactions between these internal ligands and their antibodies, and the "external" ligands and their antibodies (Williams, 1964).
The same antigen molecule under slightly different conditions (different
pH, higher or lower salt concentration) might not reveal its internal
ligands, and so its interaction with the same antiserum might be quite
different (Schmidt *et al.*, 1963).

Obviously, then, defining antiserum specificity is exceedingly complex.
One must think on the one hand of individual ligands and their corresponding individually specific but heterogeneous populations of antibodies, and on the other hand of the complex collective interplay of
many different populations of antibodies in an antiserum to their correspondingly different ligands on one population of antigen molecules
(Reimer *et al.*, 1970). Theoretically still more complex are situations,
fairly common in immunodiffusion tests, in which the antiserum contains, in addition to antibodies to various ligands on one antigen, antibodies to various ligands on a number of entirely different populations

of antigens (Dray *et al.*, 1963; Shore *et al.*, 1971).[17] Or, different antigens in a mixture may share common determinants (e.g., IgG and IgM: Nussenzweig and Benacerraf, 1966; Dray *et al.*, 1963b; Reimer *et al.*, 1970).

Fortunately, in practice excellent results can be obtained in preparing and using antisera of tailored specificity employing empirical methods for selectively absorbing unwanted antibodies (Gold and Freedman, 1965a; Middleton *et al.*, 1964; DeCarvalho, 1964; DeCarvalho *et al.*, 1964); varying immunization protocols or bleeding times (Stallybrass, 1965; Korngold and Van Leeuwen, 1961; Berg, 1964; Muraschi *et al.*, 1965; Cooper *et al.*, 1963; Soothill, 1962); using animals that are or have selectively been made tolerant to certain antigens or portions of antigens (Korngold and Van Leeuwen, 1961; Gold and Freedman, 1965a; Henny and Ishizaka, 1969); or arranging test conditions to favor wanted and suppress unwanted reactions (Limbosch *et al.*, 1966; Cooper *et al.*, 1963).

In addition to making the reader aware of the complexities of antiserum specificity, the discussion above also should suggest to him ways in which to use this valuable aspect of immunodiffusion tests to best advantage.

Nonantibody Precipitins

By name, immunodiffusion implies detection of antigen by serum antibodies. Hence the use of nonantibody antigen-precipitating agents in gel diffusion tests is outside of the scope of this book. But the reader should know that this can and has been done, since it may be both cheaper and easier.

"Lectins" are proteins extractable from certain plants which have antibody-like activity (Boyd, 1966). They have been used to precipitate antigens both in liquid media and in immunodiffusion-like tests. Two examples are phytohemagglutinin and concanavalin A, both proteins obtained from certain beans (Goldstein and So, 1965). Concanavalin A is especially effective in precipitating human serum α_{2M}-globulin (Harris and Robson, 1963); phytohemagglutinin precipitates several serum proteins, including albumin, to form diffuse precipitates in "immunoelectrophoresis," but is especially active against α_{2M}, β lipoprotein, and IgM

---

[17] In a mixture of antigens, as with different ligands on a single kind of antigen, one kind of antigen will elicit production of more specific antibodies than another, so that, depending on the purpose of a given immunodiffusion test, one antigen might be better to use than another (Mattern *et al.*, personal communication; Goodman, 1962).

globulins (Morse, 1968; Schmidt *et al.*, 1965). Concanavalin A precipitates with certain glucose- and mannose-containing branched polysaccharides strongly and with rather high specificity (Goldstein and So, 1965); dextrans are strongly precipitated by it (Goldstein and So, 1965; Hazeghi and Crowle, unpublished work).

Any substance that will not react with the supporting medium but will insolubilize or visibly react with antigen can be used in these pseudo-immunodiffusion tests. Basic proteins like lysozyme can be detected in agarose with acid groups attached to large carrier molecules (e.g., dextran sulfate of molecular weight 2,000,000: Kunin and Tupasi, 1970). As was mentioned previously in this chapter, Rivanol (Ethodin) will precipitate serum proteins electrostatically, being especially effective against those most negatively charged. It can be used in increasing concentrations for "immunoelectrophoresis" to precipitate increasing numbers of serum proteins from anode toward cathode. Rivanol was used to detect a weak anodic immunizing antigen of the tubercle bacillus for which no good precipitating antiserum could be obtained (Crowle and Hu, 1965). Acid dyes can be used to detect basic antigens, and vice versa, without having to precipitate them; thiazine red will form a red arc when diffused against lysozyme in agarose (Revis and Crowle, unpublished work). Detergents such as sodium lauryl sulfate precipitate serum proteins and lipoproteins (Palmer *et al.*, 1971).

The potentialities for using these nonantibody precipitins in "immunodiffusion" tests thus seem to be good but, as yet, generally unappreciated.

Preparation of Antigens

Many antigens present no special difficulties in their preparation, storage, or usage in immunodiffusion tests, but others do. For some the difficulties are subtle enough to be overlooked, with consequent misinterpretation of results. Especially difficult are problems of denaturation which may cause such important effects as changes in antigen specificity. Serum immunoglobulin, for instance, can be so changed by holding it at room temperature for 18 hours at pH 11.5, acidifying it, heating it, bubbling it, or freezing and thawing it several times, that it can induce precipitin formation in the animals from which it was obtained (McCluskey *et al.*, 1962).

Source of the Antigen

The best source of antigen is dictated partly by the purpose to which it will be put. Whole serum obviously is a good source for forensic immunodiffusion tests meant to identify blood stains. But certain individual antigens in the serum can be better. IgG, for instance, readily indicates species of origin (Innella *et al.*, 1961). On the other hand, other serum antigens are much hardier and therefore will be identifiable after many years' standing (Milgrom *et al.*, 1964c). Diagnostic antigens may be produced by one form of microorganism of a given species but not by another (Landay *et al.*, 1967; Tormo and Chordi, 1965; Wiggins and Schubert, 1965); antigens of taxonomic or biological utility can be associated with restricted anatomic sites (Lester, 1965; Castro and Fairbairn, 1969). Indeed, the "same" antigens (e.g., albumin) obtained from two different organs of the body are likely to be different (Grieble *et al.*, 1965), perhaps because the antigens are produced differently, or because methods for obtaining them cause changes. For example, unless gastric juice is neutralized immediately there will be extensive proteolysis of its antigens (Hirsch-Marie and Burtin, 1963; Hurlimann, 1963). Serum albumin, transferrin, and IgG normally are absent or very weak in human tears, but the mild trauma of rubbing the eyes will cause all three to be released (Josephson and Lockwood, 1964).

Sometimes there is no ready source of a desired antigen. Then, if proper precautions in interpretation are taken, immunodiffusion tests can be performed with a readily available, related antigen. A classic example: tubercle bacillus antigens can be used to detect precipitins to leprosy bacilli in people with leprosy (Navalkar *et al.*, 1964).

Obtaining the Antigen

Antigens such as serum proteins are readily obtained and used in immunodiffusion tests. Other antigens can be extracted from organs, tissues, microorganisms, etc., simply by allowing these to stand in a suitable solvent (e.g., physiologic saline) for a few hours. Such extractions are largely empirical. Other than sharing the requirement of protection against microbial contamination and denaturation, they are devised to suit expected solubility characteristics of the antigens. The following are some guiding examples of extraction protocols which have been used for special purposes, or to solve difficult problems.

Serum antigens stable to harsh conditions (useful for forensic medicine) can be obtained by boiling the serum in acetate buffer, pH 4.7 (Poortmans, 1962), or boiling and then precipitating the antigens with 71% ethanol (Milgrom *et al.*, 1964c). Complex mixtures of antigens can be simplified by such techniques; organ-specific antigens have been easily prepared by boiling extracts of the organs and precipitating the resulting antigens with ethanol (Milgrom *et al.*, 1965).

Most antigens must be prepared with greater care for their preservation than those just mentioned, for the method of extraction can materially influence the characteristics of the product. For example, the isoelectric point of streptococcus M protein is much higher when it is extracted with acid–alcohol than when it is extracted with water (Wahl *et al.*, 1965). Serum commonly is decomplemented by heating at 56°C for 30 minutes; but, in addition to destroying complement, such heating affects several α and β antigens (Motet, 1964). Simply purifying an antigen can change its electrophoretic mobility: a urinary mucoprotein changed mobility during purification because of concomitant loss of sialic acid (Grieble *et al.*, 1965).

Complications arise also from coexistence of extraneous primary antigen. Some antigens in extracts of an organism like *Entamoeba histolytica,* for instance, are due not to this parasite but rather to bacteria on which it is cultivated, and antisera prepared against the parasite therefore may have antibacterial precipitins (Maddison, 1965). As was mentioned previously, certain proteins extracted from plants precipitate serum constituents spontaneously; unless these constituents are removed from solutions of plant antigens being studied in immunodiffusion tests, they may precipitate with components of the antiserum as though the antibodies in the antiserum were precipitating antigens in the plant extract (Lester, 1965).

Some antigens found empirically in certain sources can become quite important without being either identified biochemically or understood biologically. A typical example is hepatitis-associated antigen found in certain human sera and used as an indicator in double electroimmunodiffusion tests for hepatitis in blood to be used for transfusion (Alter *et al.*, 1971).

Extraction Procedures

The simplest way of obtaining antigen in its native state is to charge an immunodiffusion well with the unaltered source of the antigen. Ideally, the antigen will leach out into the well and thence into the gel to precipitate with antibody. But the technique offers no purification; leaching will be slow and prolonged and so may cause artifact formation; and in fact many antigens will not be released in this manner at all. Nevertheless, this technique is useful. For example, bacteria (antigen source) can be grown on nutrient agar at right angles to antiserum-impregnated filter paper (Liu, 1961a). Wells have been charged with staphylococci (Losnegard and Oeding, 1963), helminth larvae (Sprent *et al.*, 1963), viruses (Mata, 1963), tissues, cells, or blood (Aoki *et al.*,

1963), or cloth, paper, or other materials impregnated with antigen (Innella *et al.*, 1961).

In these tests, antigen is being leached directly from its source to react with antibodies. But much more frequently it is extracted first and then used in immunodiffusion. Difficulty is encountered in this procedure when the native antigen is insoluble. Methods used to solubilize the antigen aim at dissociating it from insolubilizing associations with other substances, or at reducing it to a simpler, more soluble form. Detergents are frequently employed. Viruses have been disrupted with sodium dodecyl sulfate (Schild and Pereira, 1969); mitochondria are dissolved with sodium deoxycholate[18] or other surfactants such as sodium perfluorooctanoate, Lubrol, or Duponol P (D'Amelio *et al.*, 1963a); "insoluble" thyroid lipoproteins have been solubilized with sodium deoxycholate used at 0.2% in the antigen well during the course of the immunodiffusion test itself (Kurata and Okada, 1966). However, antigens solubilized by detergents frequently also combine with these detergents and acquire electrophoretic mobilities determined partly by how they have been solubilized (D'Amelio *et al.*, 1963a). Ultrasonic vibration can, if used carefully, dissolve antigens without changing them excessively (O'Neill, 1964; Sulitzeanu *et al.*, 1963; Anderson *et al.*, 1962b). Enzymes have been employed for many years and are especially useful for separating fractions of antigens from each other (Migita and Putnam, 1963).

Seemingly insoluble tissues like bone and feathers have been studied by immunodiffusion. Solutions of bone antigens were prepared by soaking fragmented, pulverized bone in physiologic saline (Kamaniski and Gajos, 1962; Pandey and Pathak, 1966). Epidermis and feather antigens were extracted from 13-day chick embryos with a 2-hour soaking in 6 *M* guanidine hydrochloride (Ben-Or and Bell, 1965). Extracts of human dermis have been made by lyophilizing trimmed and fat-free skin, grinding it to a fine powder, extracting it with physiologic saline in a high-speed homogenizer, clarifying the extract, and dialyzing it against distilled water (Fleischmajer and Krol, 1967; Aoki and Fujinami, 1967).

The procedure for extracting antigens from plant tissues resembles that for extracting antigens from low-solubility animal tissues. The tissue is defatted and dried. Then it is extracted or pulverized and extracted with a suitable aqueous solvent such as 1% sodium chloride or physiologic phosphate buffer (Jaffe and Hannig, 1965; Lester *et al.*, 1965; Coggins and Heuschele, 1966). Troublesome lipids are removed from dried tissue powder at −15°C (Brown and Bold, 1964). Oxidizing enzymes fre-

---

[18] Suspend mitochondria (e.g., from one rat liver) in 2 to 7 ml of sucrose, and add 0.3 ml of 3% sodium deoxycholate (D'Amelio *et al.*, 1963a).

quently complicate such extractions. They can be neutralized by including a reducing agent like sodium sulfite in the extraction fluid (Lester, 1965). Extracts usually are dialyzed against distilled water and then dried.[19]

Insects are extracted in the same way as smaller organisms. For instance, they can be macerated in physiologic saline containing 0.5% phenol, to preserve sterility, and the clarified extracts can be used for immunodiffusion (Fox *et al.*, 1963).

Certain kinds of lipid antigens can be suspended finely enough in an aqueous solvent for use in immunodiffusion tests. For example, cytolipin K extracted from kidney with a mixture of chloroform and methanol is dried, redissolved in ethanol, and mixed with physiologic saline; or auxiliary lipids like lecithin or cholesterol can be added to the chloroform–methanol extract before it is dried, and the same procedure subsequently followed (Graf and Rapport, 1965). These auxiliary lipids promote specific precipitation of the tissue lipids.

Factors Damaging Antigen during Preparation

To think of purified antigens, even of the hardiest kinds, as truly "native" is probably an illusion, since even small physical changes can alter, remove, or add antigenic determinants. Conformational changes in IgG caused by either heat or treatment with 6 M urea create new ligands (Hirose and Osler, 1967). Formalinization of serum albumin makes it antigenic in the species of animal from which it is obtained (Ruschmann *et al.*, 1962). In the oxidized state, dwarf ragweed allergen has one precipitinogen; this converts to two on reduction (Callaghan and Goldfarb, 1962). Freezing and thawing causes many changes, some as small as a slight shift in electrophoretic mobility (Karlsson, 1965), others as large as insolubilization (Stoffer *et al.*, 1962). Raising the pH of a solution of bovine lens α-crystalline transforms it irreversibly from one antigen into two smaller antigens (Papaconstantinou *et al.*, 1962). Ultrasonication was mentioned above as a technique for solubilizing antigens, but this solubilization tends to cause moderate to extensive changes in many antigens (Norkrans and Wahlström, 1962). Some antigens are especially susceptible: ultrasonication of serum for more than 5 minutes can cause β-lipoprotein to disappear from an immunoelectrophoretic pattern without materially affecting most other serum antigens (Searcy and Bergquist,

[19] Lyophilization is the method used most often. One can also use a "frostless" freezer, which is especially convenient when a small amount of volatile organic solvent is being removed and low temperature must be maintained (Brown and Bold, 1964).

1965). Many antigens are destroyed by heating (Castelnuovo and Morellini, 1962c). Some would appear to be unharmed but if examined carefully enough show subtle but important changes. Milk casein, for instance, retained antigenic specificity but changed its electrophoretic mobility (Aurand et al., 1963). Heating may also promote interactions between different antigens, thus changing them both. Enzymatic changes are common (see below); they can occur as enzymes extracted with an antigen digest the antigen (Simons and Gräsbeck, 1963).

Antigen Purification and Concentration

The objectives of purifying and concentrating antigen are to accomplish this efficiently without unduly denaturing the antigen, and to obtain the antigen in stable form. The techniques are similar to those already described briefly for concentration of antibodies. They include lyophilization (Sinell et al., 1969); ultrafiltration (De Vaux Saint-Cyr and Hermann, 1963); pervaporation (Remington and Finland, 1961); dialysis against a concentrated uncharged ion that is small like sucrose (Mull et al., 1970) or large like dextran (Nielsen et al., 1963), polyvinylpyrrolidone (Rawson, 1962), or polyethylene glycol (Sinell et al., 1969; De Vaux Saint-Cyr and Hermann, 1963); evaporation at reduced pressure (De Vaux Saint-Cyr and Hermann, 1963); and dehydration with dry Sephadex G-25 or G-50 (Shulman et al., 1966b). Of these, techniques that change the physical nature of antigens are the least desirable (e.g., lyophilization: Rawson, 1962; Sinell et al., 1969), and those utilizing other soluble substances such as polyethylene glycol are intermediate.[20] Among the methods remaining one must choose by factors such as convenience, expense, and chances for enzymatic destruction of microbial contamination if the concentration procedure is prolonged or must be performed at higher than refrigerator temperatures. Unfortunately, some antigens are so delicate that they will not remain stable if purified by any technique (Casman et al., 1969).

Antigens can be purified directly from a solution without dehydration by any of several techniques similar to those for purifying antibodies (also mentioned above). Precipitation (e.g., with salts selective for some antigen, such as $MgCl_2$ for serum β lipoproteins: Burstein, 1963) is simple and effective but risks possible irreversible minor to major denaturation. Zone electrophoresis (e.g., in polyacrylamide: DeVillez,

---

[20] These substances tend to mix with the antigen and must later be removed. Carbowax, for instance, is a polyethylene glycol of 20,000 molecular weight. Despite its size, it can diffuse into dialysis sacks, and it has been observed to fix irreversibly to γ-globulins (De Vaux Saint-Cyr and Hermann, 1963).

1964), which is also convenient and efficient, is less likely to cause denaturation, but its yields are small. Immunoglobulins can be cross-linked to prepare an insoluble column of antibodies which will react with antigen specifically. If these are equine antibodies, then antigen later can easily be eluted in highly purified state (DeCarvalho *et al.*, 1964). As has been mentioned previously, antigen can be purified similarly but on a much smaller scale by dissociation from antibody, using complexes obtained directly from an immunodiffusion test.[21]

Antigen Storage

Problems in utilizing antigen for immunodiffusion do not cease when it has been purified and concentrated, for the antigen can change during storage. Antigen may not simply be lost; it may change subtly, even transforming into a "new" antigen. Hence, purported differences observed at different times or in different laboratories in the antigenic composition of some mixture may result from differences developed during storage and therefore reflect differences in storage technique more than differences in composition of the mixture. The following examples will illustrate and forewarn against storage problems.

Immunodiffusion reagents are frequently stored at $-20°C$ and then assumed to change little if any. But changes at this temperature are rather frequent. A weakly cationic protein in cerebrospinal fluid became anionic when stored for several months at this temperature (Dumonde *et al.*, 1963). Certain *Coccidioides immitis* antigens deteriorate at $-20°C$ (Rowe *et al.*, 1965); an α_2-globulin slowly weakens and eventually disappears from human serum (Fessel, 1963a). Beta lipoproteins isolated from human serum and kept for several weeks at $-10°C$ migrate progressively more anodically (Burstein and Fine, 1964b); human serum complement deteriorates at $-18°C$ (Zimmer, 1960). Freezing and storing, or repeated freezing and thawing, cause human IgD to decompose into two components, which might lead one erroneously to "discover" a new variety of immunoglobulin (Škvaril and Rádl, 1967). Similar changes have been observed for IgG.

Probably some of the damage to antigens stored frozen is simply from the freezing and thawing itself (Merrill *et al.*, 1967), and this can also account for many of the damaging effects of lyophilization (De Muralt,

[21] React antigen with antibody at 5° to 6°C for 30 days in a 3- to 4-mm-thick layer of carrageenan (this gels at 28°C and liquefies at 37°C), wash with cold saline, remove the precipitin band with a 15-gauge needle and syringe, warm to liquefy the gel, wash the precipitate with saline, and finally centrifuge out this precipitate (Mohos, 1966). Further manipulation to dissociate antigen from antibody is by standard techniques described in manuals on immunologic methods.

1962). But even when an antigen is not injured by freezing, it can deteriorate during storage in the lyophilized stage: lyophilized *Cryptococcus* polysaccharide, for instance, remained effective for specific precipitin reactions for only a short time (Widra *et al.*, 1968). Ceruloplasmin could be kept from polymerizing following freezing only by storing it at liquid nitrogen temperature (Poulik and Bearn, 1962).

Although some antigens remain unaltered at 4°C while being damaged by storage at −20°C (Rowe *et al.*, 1965), or by repeated freezing and thawing associated with this kind of storage (Merrill *et al.*, 1967), this higher temperature is not any better in general than freezing. The degradation of IgD mentioned above as resulting from freezing and thawing also was seen following 2 months' storage at 4°C (Škvaril and Rádl, 1967). If asepsis is maintained, most problems of storing antigens at 4°C appear to be due to such enzymes as lipases and proteases (Brummerstedt-Hansen, 1967; Nerstrøm, 1964). These enzymes may be natural constituents of the antigen mixture, or they may derive from sources likely to be included in the collected sample, such as blood cells and platelets (Nerstrøm, 1963b, 1964). Of course, without asepsis, microbial enzymes can change various antigens quite rapidly at 4°C (Nerstrøm, 1963b, 1964; Nerstrøm *et al.*, 1964). For instance, proteases from yeasts and bacteria convert human serum Gc_1 into an electrophoretically different substance with the same antigenic identity; Gc_2 is more labile than Gc_1 (Nerstrøm, 1964). Enzymes present in the collected sample can act very quickly: gastric juice antigens are being destroyed even as they are being collected, since there are deteriorative changes evident even when the juice is neutralized immediately after collection as compared with its being neutralized intragastrically before collection (Simons and Gräsbeck, 1963). Storing a sample liquid at higher temperatures (e.g., 37°C), while perhaps appearing to be more physiologic (Kaminski and Gajos, 1965), is simply likely to accelerate enzyme-induced changes (West and Hong, 1962; Brummerstedt-Hansen, 1967).

Antigens vary considerably in stability, which is why suitable storage conditions are difficult to predict. The most susceptible appear to be those associated with lipids (Dencker and Swahn, 1961; Kaminski, 1966; Albutt, 1966; Peetom and Kramer, 1962), those that polymerize easily (Neuzil *et al.*, 1963; Kasper and Deutsch, 1963; Auscher and Guinand, 1964) or change form with small changes in environment (Shulman *et al.*, 1966b; Kaminski and Gajos, 1962; Kasper and Deutsch, 1963; Seligmann *et al.*, 1963), and those that complex readily with other antigens (Perlmutter *et al.*, 1962; Hornung and Arquembourg, 1965; Nerstrøm and Jensen, 1963; Kölsch, 1967; Mannik, 1967).

Certain antigens in some mixtures, like serum or cerebrospinal fluid, are so labile that the "true composition" of these mixtures probably can be determined only on freshly obtained specimens (Hornung and Arquembourg, 1965; Dencker and Swahn, 1961). However, most individual antigens in these and other mixtures are stable enough to be stored for several days or weeks. Despite disadvantages such as those listed above, the best universal antigen storage technique would seem to be to freeze it as soon as possible and then store it at $-20°C$ or lower. Small samples should be used, to avoid repeated freezing and thawing. If the sample cannot be either frozen or analyzed immediately, then it can usually be kept adequately at 4°C provided that it is protected from microbial contamination, and provided also that there are no autolytic endogenous enzymes. Of course, substances added to it as preservatives, such as phenol, Merthiolate, or formaldehyde to preserve sterility, ε-aminocaproic acid to prevent proteolysis (Porath and Ui, 1964), or cysteine to subdue oxidation (Auscher and Guinand, 1964), must not themselves combine with and change the antigen (Ruschmann *et al.*, 1962). One of the least harmful methods for keeping antigen solutions at 4°C aseptically is to filter-sterilize them. But even this can cause loss of antigens by adsorption to the filter, or changes on its surface.

For stable antigens, storage technique can be chosen primarily for convenience. For instance, antigen solution can be dried on a piece of filter paper for later convenient use in an immunodiffusion field test (Cruse, 1966).

Conditions of Analyses

The problems of preparing and storing antigens used in immunodiffusion tests carry over into the tests themselves. Sometimes this is only a matter of preserving antigen integrity; sometimes conditions of a test can be developed to help overcome problems that have haunted preparation and storing of the antigens beforehand.

Immunodiffusion tests should be set up under conditions that best preserve the antigen. This is one reason that most tests are performed at 4°C. At this temperature both spontaneous deterioration of labile antigens and microbial contamination with potentially destructive effects are suppressed. Preservatives like Merthiolate or phenol, which can react with and change certain antigens, are not needed. Micro tests are better than macro tests because they develop rapidly. Even if kept at 4°C, macro tests performed without preservative frequently become grossly contaminated with bacteria in the several days or weeks that they require for full development. Neither the gel nor its solvent should react with the antigen, and ordinarily both should help maintain antigen integrity.

However, sometimes deliberate controlled changes in the antigen are desirable. The following are some examples of effects that varying conditions of analyses can have on antigen and its utilization in immunodiffusion tests.

A colloidal stabilizer like gelatin can be used at 1 mg/ml for preparing antigen solutions (Manski *et al.*, 1961); but, as will be discussed in the section on gels, this may not be wise because gelatin can interfere with antigen–antibody precipitation. Serum albumin is another stabilizer (King *et al.*, 1964), but it also may suppress precipitation (Cline, 1967). Hence, only antigen stabilizers with a specific function should be used. For instance, oxidized and reduced forms of ceruloplasmin differ antigenically. Consequently, a reducing agent like ascorbic acid is used in immunodiffusion analysis of reduced ceruloplasmin to avoid the confusing presence of the oxidized antigen (Kasper and Deutsch, 1963). If both forms are present, only one will be detected in borate-buffered immunoelectrophoresis, whereas both will be evident if a borate–tris–EDTA buffer is used (Kasper and Deutsch, 1963). Keyhole limpet hemocyanin is a physically unstable antigen which varies antigenically and physically at different pH values between 6.5 and 8.5 from a 98 S molecule at the lower pH to an 18 S molecule at the higher pH (Tornabene and Bartel, 1962). For such antigens as these, immunodiffusion solvents should be formulated to preserve antigen in the state which is to be studied.

Certain antigens complex readily with others to change physically and antigenically. Human IgA combines with albumin, haptoglobins, β lipoproteins, and other serum constituents. The resulting complexes sometimes are very difficult to dissociate (Mannik, 1967). In immunoelectrophoresis their formation can be circumvented by raising the voltage of electrophoresis enough to break the complexes; in immunodiffusion, adding cysteine at 0.1 M or thiol compounds can prevent or reverse their formation. Preincubating serum with 0.1 M cysteine hydrochloride is said to prevent spontaneous precipitation of serum macroglobulins within agar, because this is due to oxidation (Seligmann *et al.*, 1963). Interactions of some antigens with agar are partly temperature-dependent; consequently, the occasional practice of mixing warmed antigen with liquid agar cooled to just above its gelling point to form, for instance, a semisolid origin for electrophoresis raises some risks. Some β_1-globulins are sensitive enough to such complexing that they will associate with agar if added to it just after it has been poured and has congealed but has not yet gelled fully (Ferri and Cossmermelli, 1964b).

By physical nature some antigens are incompatible with certain immunodiffusion media, including both gels and buffers. Basic proteins like lysozyme complex with negatively charged agaropectin in agar gels; they are best studied in uncharged media such as agarose, polyacrylamide, or cellulose acetate (Revis, 1971). The "same" media obtained from different sources may give different results: in one batch of agarose the solvent buffer had to be maintained at ionic strength 0.075 and pH 8.6 for studying lysozyme which precipitated spontaneously at lower pH values (Osserman and Lawlor, 1966). Buffer salts themselves can affect antigen directly or indirectly. Barbital tends to precipitate lipids, and so interferes with immunodiffusion analyses of lipoproteins (Berg, 1965b); borate complexes with carbohydrates and can affect analyses of either poly-saccharides or carbohydrate-containing antigens; chelating buffers like tris, EDTA, and citrate, by removing heavy metal ions normally present in agar gels, increase the solubility of lipoproteins (Crowle, 1960a), and they can profoundly affect antigens containing or associated with metals (e.g., transferrin, ceruloplasmin, complement).

Sometimes it is necessary to use special test conditions to detect reactions with certain kinds of antigens. Antigens with predominantly positive charge can be carbamylated to predominantly negative charge without much affecting their antibody-combining capacity (Weeke, 1968a). Univalent antigens can be attached multiply to inert carriers (Batchelor *et al.*, 1966; Brandriss *et al.*, 1965). If the carrier is a small molecule (Batchelor *et al.*, 1966), or if a complete antigen is small, thus having an unusually rapid diffusion rate (Barber *et al.*, 1966a), antiserum can be allowed some preliminary diffusion and antigen is added later. Incubation should be kept short, with such antigen, to avoid dissolving antigen–antibody precipitates with excess antigen. Some antigens will not precipitate under conditions that allow others to precipitate (e.g., a heat-labile mouse tissue antigen used at pH above 8.5: Boyle *et al.*, 1963). Hence, several different test conditions may have to be used to detect most precipitinogens in a mixture. Certain antigens are soluble only at high salt concentration or low pH. By using chicken antiserum which precipitates antigens well at high salt concentration, the first problem can be overcome; the second was surmounted for plasminogen by adding pH 2.0 buffer to the antigen well to acidify the gel immediately surrounding the well before adding the plasminogen itself (Shulman, 1963).

As has been mentioned, lipids in an antigen solution which complicate an immunodiffusion test by precipitating nonspecifically can be removed by pretreating the antigen solution with ether (Chapman, 1961). But occasionally lipids themselves are the antigens. They can be used directly in immunodiffusion tests if they have some hydrophilic groups (Graf and Rapport, 1965), or they can be adsorbed to other lipids with hydrophilic tendencies. For instance, ethanol-soluble cerebroside was prepared for successful use in double diffusion plate tests by mixing 2.9 mg with 2.7

mg of cholesterol and 1.3 mg of lecithin per milliliter of ethanol, and then mixing this solution with distilled water at a proportion of 1:4 (Niedieck *et al.*, 1965).

Purifying antigen before using it in immunodiffusion may or may not be helpful. Usually it is successful for plant antigens, because crude mixtures often contain lectins which precipitate antiserum components nonspecifically (Lester, 1965). However, some enzymes or hormones lose most of their biological activity when purified: prolactin lost 90 to 95% activity without changing precipitinogen activity during purification (Emmart *et al.*, 1963). Hence, a purified antigen may be present and precipitate, but it may have lost its biological activity.

When one cannot use a purified antigen, then appropriate interpretative allowances are necessary. IgM and IgG, for instance, can be quantitated well in radial immunodiffusion because ordinarily they are homogeneous; but IgA has too many molecular varieties for quantitations by this technique to agree well with quantitations by isotopic immune inhibition (Fahey and McKelvey, 1965). There always seems to be a slow component of α_1-antitrypsin in human serum, but this is due not to the presence of another antigen but rather to firm complexing between some of this inhibitor and a more cathodic protein of lower molecular weight (Laurell, 1965b).

If some risk of mild denaturation is acceptable, then immunodiffusion conditions can be arranged to dissociate some antigens either so that particular components can be examined, or because undissociated complexes are too large for diffusion. Detergents are used (e.g., 1% sodium dodecyl sulfate: Schild and Pereira, 1969; 0.1% sodium dibutylnaphthalene sulfonate: Hamilton and Ball, 1966) to fragment viruses to diffusible pieces. One percent Tween 80 was used to aid heart muscle DPNH dehydrogenase diffusion (Mackler *et al.*, 1968). If detergents fail, physical methods can be resorted to: long rod viruses were fragmented to diffusible size by ultrasonic vibration (Hughes and Watson, 1965). This was preferred to their fragmentation with such buffers as ethanolamine or carbonate because these buffers might have introduced changes in antigenicity.

Media for Immunodiffusion

The primary purposes of media within which immunodiffusion tests are performed are to prevent convection currents, to permit intermingling of antigen and antibody either by diffusion or by directed migration (e.g., electrophoresis, rheophoresis), and to entrap forming antigen–antibody complexes so that they can be detected directly or indirectly and be distinguished from each other spatially. The media may have secondary purposes such as participating in antigen fractionation, permitting some reactions to occur while preventing others, or functioning directly in the movement of reactants. To be suitable for immunodiffusion tests, a medium not only must satisfy these purposes but also must be easy to obtain and use, reasonably uniform, and compatible with numerous accessory procedures employed with immunodiffusion to detect, identify, and quantitate antigens and antibodies.

No medium presently available is perfect. Agarose and polyacrylamide are nearly so, but agarose, being a polysaccharide, cannot be used with some stains for polysaccharide antigens, and polyacrylamide is cumbersome to manipulate. The following sections will discuss and compare media that are used for immunodiffusion and then describe their characteristics, preparation, and utilization.

The Media Compared

In decreasing order of popularity, immunodiffusion media include agar, agarose, cellulose acetate, polyacrylamide, and gelatin. Others such as carrageenan, starch, and cross-linked dextrans (Agostoni *et al.*, 1967) occasionally have been used. Although most immunodiffusion tests currently are done in either agar or agarose, it is well to compare all the various media here to indicate reasons for their relative ranks of use and what special advantages one may have over another.

AGAR

Agar is a mixture of two polysaccharides, agarose and agaropectin, extracted by partial hydrolysis of certain seaweeds. It is a familiar laboratory staple—inexpensive, widely obtainable, and easy to use. Inert for most antigens and antibodies that have been studied with it, agar forms nearly transparent gels within which antigen–antibody precipitation can be observed as it occurs. Agar gels are compatible with many different buffer systems and can be prepared at several concentrations. After immunodiffusion reactions have been completed in such a gel, it is easily washed free of most nonreacting constituents of antigen and antibody solutions, and precipitin bands trapped within it then can be subjected to one of many analyses to identify antigens that have been precipitated.

Agar has some disadvantages. Different batches and sources present widely variable characteristics (Masseyeff and Josselin, 1965; Hjertén, 1962). Agar gels have a strong negative charge, which prevents their use with basic dyes and with basic antigens (Masson *et al.*, 1965; Uriel *et al.*,

1963; Brishammar *et al.*, 1961). They may inactivate some antigens (Uriel, 1963; Kunin and Tupasi, 1970), and they cause strong electro-osmosis (Masseyeff and Josselin, 1965; Leise and Evans, 1965; Uriel *et al.*, 1963; Brishammar *et al.*, 1961), although sometimes this is an advantage. Agar has a tendency to complex with some antigens, especially lipoproteins (Elevitch *et al.*, 1966; Beck and Uzan, 1965; Masseyeff and Josselin, 1965; Burstein and Fine, 1964b). Other disadvantages include gel turbidity, especially when the gel is thick and cold (Leise and Evans, 1965), and a tendency to take up polysaccharide stains because it is a polysaccharide. After agar has been dissolved at nearly boiling temperature, to prevent its gelling it must be maintained at a temperature above 45°C; but this promotes its hydrolysis (Uriel *et al.*, 1963) and tends to denature antigens and antibodies which for some immunodiffusion procedures must be mixed with it before it is cast. After it has gelled, it cannot be reliquefied unless it is heated again to near boiling temperature. Although agar gels of 7.5% have been used (Dudman, 1964a), solutions of agar exceeding 4% are viscous and difficult to work with. Hence, except by electrostatic interaction with some antigens (Lawrence and Shean, 1962; Burtin and Grabar, 1967), agar gels are of only minor use for fractionating antigens by molecular sieving (Korngold, 1963a; Raymond and Nakamichi, 1962b; Clausen *et al.*, 1963; Raymond, 1964).

AGAROSE

Agarose is not only agar's strongest competitor for use in immuno-diffusion tests, it is also a component of agar. Agarose is obtained by separating it from agaropectin, the second and undesirable polysaccharide component of agar. It has gained popularity rapidly because it retains nearly all the advantages of agar, and it has some additional ones of its own. Notably, it has practically no charge and so can be used with basic dyes (Hjertén, 1961; Crowle, unpublished work) and basic proteins Brishammar *et al.*, 1961; Revis, 1971; Uriel *et al.*, 1963; Masson *et al.*, 1965); it does not develop much electroosmosis (Uriel *et al.*, 1963; Leise and Evans, 1965; Masseyeff and Josselin, 1965); and it does not inactivate enzymes as readily as agar (Uriel, 1963). Because it has less tendency to complex with antigens (Masseyeff and Josselin, 1965), it produces notably "truer" immunoelectrophoretic characterizations of serum antigens (Burtin and Grabar, 1967; Süllmann, 1964; Burstein and Fine, 1964a), as well as permitting formation of sharper, better-defined precipitin arcs (Brishammar *et al.*, 1961; Styk and Schmidt, 1968; Motet, 1964, 1965; Leise and Evans, 1965; Masseyeff and Josselin, 1965; Styk and Hána, 1966). Its gels are clearer and stronger than agar gels of equal concentration; consequently, it can be used at lower concentration (Leise and Evans, 1965). It can be prepared in a form that does not gel until its temperature drops to about 37°C, so that sensitive antigens are less likely to denature when mixed with it while liquid (Marine Colloids Bulletin AG-LG). It resists hydrolysis better than agar and hence can be used with a wider variety of buffers (Uriel *et al.*, 1963). Because it does not complex with basic molecules, these can be used in agarose gels as agents for precipitating acidic antigens, and acidic molecules can be used to precipitate basic antigens. (Kunin and Tupasi, 1970; Crowle and Hu, 1965). Mammalian cells grow well in agarose, but not in agar gels, which makes agarose the better medium for *in situ* antigen production (Coffino *et al.*, 1970). Agarose gels are somewhat easier to decolorize than agar gels after staining, which is especially important in fluoroimmunoelectrophoresis (Ghetie, 1967).

Agarose would seem to be a nearly perfect gelling agent for immunodiffusion tests, but it does have some disadvantages. Currently it is expensive.[22] Like agar, it is a polysaccharide and therefore useful with only certain polysaccharide stains. It is less useful than agar gels for double electroimmunodiffusion tests because it develops less electroosmosis.

POLYACRYLAMIDE

Although first used for immunodiffusion tests more than a decade ago (Crowle, 1961), polyacrylamide gels only recently have begun to receive the attention that their potentialities warrant for use in these tests. Their slow acceptance is due principally to readier availability and easier utilization of agar and agarose. The superior adaptability of polyacrylamide gels to novel, even extreme, variations in buffer composition and their remarkable capacity for very fine resolution during electrophoresis by molecular sieving have not been especially attractive to users of immunodiffusion because immunodiffusion tests offer very high resolution on their own (Raymond and Nakamichi, 1962b). Only recently have qualitative immunodiffusion analyses matured to a state in which the additional resolution provided by polyacrylamide gels is beginning to invite new interest.

These gels are made by polymerizing acrylamide monomer with methylene bisacrylamide (cf. Chrambach and Rodbard, 1971). They are water-clear, chemically inert, extremely stable, tinctorially inert, and thermostable, and they have no tendency for surface reactions (Antoine, 1962; Mengoli and Watne, 1966; Bloemendal, 1967; Ornstein, 1964).

---

[22] As will be described later, it can now be prepared easily and inexpensively in the laboratory.

Thus, even the faintest precipitin bands are readily visible. Reagents, antigens, antibodies, stains, and indicator reactions can be used in nearly infinite variety (e.g., 8 M urea, pH 1 to 12, 0°C: Poulik, 1966; cf. also Chrambach and Rodbard, 1971). Reactants behave in polyacrylamide gels as though there were no gel, except for molecular sieving (see below). Acrylamide can be polymerized cold (Antoine, 1962). Polyacrylamide gels therefore would appear to be superior to either agar or agarose for immunodiffusion tests because agar and agarose both interact with some antigens, they cannot be used with as many kinds of stains and buffers, they are chemically more delicate, and they must be gelled from warm or hot solutions.

But despite their seemingly ideal characteristics, polyacrylamide gels have not replaced agar and agarose because they are more difficult to work with. The gel is sticky and extremely flexible, and wells consequently are difficult to cut in it (Mengoli and Watne, 1966); it can swell or shrink over wide latitude as water is lost or gained (Antoine, 1962), so that physical conditions within the gel are less automatically consistent than they are in agar or agarose gels; in the porosities that usually have been used, it is very slow to stain and destain, and in these porosities sieving retards or prevents diffusion of many commonly used antigens and antibodies and weakens or prevents their reactions. Polyacrylamide gel is not as easily dried after staining for permanent preservation of the original reactions as are either agar or agarose, and conditions required for polymerization are more complex than conditions required to gel agar or agarose (Mengoli and Watne, 1966). Most of these various disadvantages now can be diminished or overcome as described below. Polyacrylamide may begin to achieve wider usage for immunodiffusion tests as investigators become more familiar with its advantages.

Perhaps the most valuable advantage that polyacrylamides have over any other practical medium for immunodiffusion is that they can be polymerized in many but predictable varieties of pore sizes (Antoine, 1962; Mengoli and Watne, 1966; Weeke, 1969; Raymond and Nakamichi, 1962a; Raymond, 1964).[23] Thus, polyacrylamide can be prepared at 3% to offer no resistance to diffusion by serum macroglobulins, at 4% to selectively retard these proteins (Stobo and Tomasi, 1967), at 5 to 6% to sieve out proteins of intermediate size, at 7 to 9% to stop migration

---

[23] Because of this, deciding upon a "standard, normal" immunoelectrophoretic pattern for something like human serum in polyacrylamide will have to be arbitrary; relatively small changes in technique for polymerizing acrylamide can drastically alter the immunoelectrophoretic pattern obtained under otherwise uniform conditions (Raymond and Nakamichi, 1962b).

of molecules of >20,000 molecular weight, or even at concentrations that impede molecules of <1000 molecular weight (Weeke, 1969; Uriel, 1966). Immunodiffusion tests with too fine a gel porosity to permit diffusion of precipitins nevertheless can be set up by moving antigens, if they are smaller molecules, against the antiserum.

Polyacrylamide gels probably will not displace agar and agarose as primary media for immunodiffusion tests, but they will receive increasing attention and exploitation as they become more practical to use and as their special advantages, especially of variable molecular sieving, are applied to refined qualitative analyses of antigens and antibodies (Morris *et al.*, 1965; Wright *et al.*, 1970).

CELLULOSE ACETATE

The only non-gel medium used more than experimentally for immuno-diffusion tests is cellulose acetate (cf. Kohn, 1970, 1971). This thin, micropore, opaque "paper" originally was a by-product of the development of membrane filters of uniform porosity. Because of its high structural uniformity and physicochemical inertness, it has become favored over filter paper for paper zone electrophoresis and, for similar reasons, it is also useful for various kinds of immunodiffusion tests (Condsen and Kohn, 1959).

Cellulose acetate has the following advantages for immunodiffusion tests (Grunbaum *et al.*, 1963; Kohn, 1967, 1971; Nelson *et al.*, 1964): It requires no preparation for use other than wetting; it can be employed with both acidic and basic antigens; it is compatible with a wider variety of buffers than can be tolerated by agar or agarose; it is economical of reactants (cf. Ringle and Herndon, 1965; Krøll, 1968c); it is easy to handle, especially in washing, staining, and drying (Feinberg *et al.*, 1965); and it provides results rapidly (Kohn, 1961).

The primary disadvantage of cellulose acetate is that, because it is opaque, antigen–antibody precipitation cannot be observed in it until the membrane has been washed and stained (Kohn, 1961, 1971). Because some antigen–antibody precipitates dissociate readily, using cellulose acetate will lead to occasional failure to detect antigen–antibody precipitation which is detected in gel media. In any multiple-antigen immunodiffusion test, to have all antigen–antibody systems reacting at near optimal proportions is unusual. Therefore precipitation bands can develop and then disappear during a cellulose acetate test because of excess reactant and not be detected, whereas in gels one can minimize this problem with periodic observations. Frequent observations during development of a test in gels also provide direct evidence for optimal reaction time, but this information cannot be determined in cellulose acetate without using several tests which are terminated at different times. Other disadvantages to using cellulose acetate are that precise, reproducible application of reactants is diffcult, it is not easy to always achieve the same degree of membrane wetting, and cellulose acetate membranes which have been wet must be carefully protected against even minor dehydration.[24]

Earlier, when most immunodiffusion tests were performed on macro scale in agar gels, cellulose acetate offered some distinct technological advantages. But today miniaturization of gel techniques and utilization of agarose and polyacrylamide have offset these advantages. Hence, cellulose acetate now is used only infrequently.

GELATIN

Gels of gelatin were among the first used in immunodiffusion (Chapter 8). Advantages that they offered in contrast to agar gels included greater clarity, especially at refrigerator temperature; superior protection of labile antigens against denaturation; liquefaction at moderate temperatures; lack of electroosmosis, and utility with either acidic or basic antigens (Crowle and Hu, 1967; Crowle, 1971; McPherson and Carnegie, 1968); and greater opportunity to vary gel density, and therefore molecular sieving (Naylor and Adair, 1962). Of these only the characteristic of liquefying at moderate temperature remains to recommend gelatin in preference to any other medium for some immunodiffusion methods, for this characteristic permits easy harvesting of antigen–antibody precipitates which have been formed in a gelatin gel and thus the production of small to moderate amounts of highly purified antigen or antibodies (see Preparatory Linear Double Diffusion, Chapter 4). All the other advantages now can be obtained by using one or another of the alternative media (e.g., polyacrylamide for gel clarity; either polyacrylamide or agarose for use with basic antigens and for minimal electroosmosis; polyacrylamide for molecular sieving; agarose with antigen stabilizing additives).

Gelatin has some very decided disadvantages: its low liquefaction temperature makes refrigeration during a test essential except for very short periods or when the gel is quite concentrated; practically none of the antigen-identifying stain and indicator techniques used with other media can be applied to gelatin; and its physical structure interferes directly with both reactant migration and antigen–antibody precipitation

---

[24] The membrane can be immersed in mineral oil for complete protection against dehydration during the reaction period, but this is said to affect lipid-associated antigens and therefore to be unsuitable for some tests (Grunbaum et al., 1963).

(Dudman, 1964a; 1965b), which results in low sensitivity, prolonged reaction periods (weeks may be necessary: Naylor and Adair, 1962; Dudman, 1964a), and suppressed antigen–antibody precipitation.

Interestingly, as with the disadvantage of easy liquefaction, which can be turned to an advantage in preparatory immunodiffusion, the disadvantage of interfering with antigen-antibody precipitation by gelatin also has become something of a unique advantage (Dudman, 1965b). This effect appears to be especially strong against neutral polysaccharide antigens, so that precipitin bands due to polysaccharide antigens or determinants in an immunodiffusion pattern developed in one of the other media can be identified by including gelatin in that medium, or by preparing a two-medium test using gelatin gel for half of it and agarose, for example, for the other.[25] At present, then, the only indications for using gelatin gels in immunodiffusion tests are when an easily liquefied gel is required, and when one wishes to identify antigen–antibody precipitation involving polysaccharide antigens.

OTHER MEDIA

Carrageenan is an agar-like gel which has the advantage of gelatin: it can be liquefied at a moderate temperature (37°C) (Mohos, 1966). Cross-linked dextran (Sephadex) has been used for immunochromatography; so has filter paper (Chapter 7). Sodium alginate is gelled by Ca^{++} and can be liquefied by chelation (Ouchterlony, 1968). Starch has been employed because of its notable capacity for molecular sieving (Poulik, 1966; Korngold, 1963a; Brummerstedt-Hansen, 1962), but polyacrylamide appears to be better and "cleaner" and can be used in onestep immunodiffusion. These and a few other media with special purposes also will be discussed briefly below along with the more common media, and relative to their special uses.

Selected Techniques for Preparing Media

Since immunodiffusion media can be prepared in more ways than there is space here to discuss, the following sections relate only a few methods selected for universality of application or particular utility. Special features of the methods or media, and problems that may be encountered with them, also are mentioned.

---

[25] However, the absence of a precipitin band in gelatin gel does not prove that the antigen involved is a polysaccharide, because gelatin gel also can prevent precipitation of some protein antigens, like tobacco mosaic virus protein (Dudman, 1965b).

NATURE OF AGAR GELS

Agar is extracted from the outer layers of red algae seaweeds by holding the layers overnight at 80°C in 0.2% sulfuric acid. The liquid extract, with sodium hydrosulfite added for bleaching, is filtered and cooled, and the resulting gel of agar is cut into suitable pieces. These are frozen and thawed, and the liberated water, with various impurities, is discarded. Then the residual agar is sun-dried (Mori, 1953). This crude commercial agar is further purified, before sale for more critical applications, by washing with water or alcohol, filtration, freezing–thawing, electrodialysis, and precipitation by alcohol (Hjertén, 1961). Because there are so many ways to purify agars, those available from different sources may have distinctly different properties (Karlsson, 1965).

Agar dissolves in water at 95° to 100°C. At concentrations of 1 to 2% usually employed in immunodiffusion tests, a hot agar solution, on being cooled to 45° to 50°C, congeals to form a dimensionally stable gel with fibrillar or meshlike structure and irregular pore size (Crowle, 1961). The average pore size of agar gel is inversely proportional to the concentration of the agar (Jordan and White, 1965; Ackers and Steere, 1962). The size, shape, and type of particle or molecule that can migrate through agar gels depends partly on this pore size, but it also depends on other direct factors such as frictional forces between the agar micelle and the migrating molecule, the affinity of the molecule for water, the affinity of the molecule for agarose or agaropectin in the agar, and the molecule's flexibility as well as the flexibility of the gel's meshes. Other less direct factors include movement of water through the gel, such as by syphoning or electroosmosis, and electrophoretic migration of the molecule through the gel (Clausen et al., 1963; Wunderly, 1960; Ragetli and Weintraub, 1964; John, 1965; Zwaan, 1963). The structure of agar gels may differ according to the nature of their solvents and the presence of various solutes (Wunderly, 1960).[26]

Irregularity of pore size in agar gels, together with the fact that at given concentrations pore size can vary among agars of different manufacture (Ackers and Steere, 1962), explains the diverse estimates that have been made for maximum sizes of molecules or particles that can or cannot migrate through agar gels. For example, the effective pore diameter of 2% agar once was estimated to be 3 nm (see Crowle, 1961). This estimate clashed with observed diffusion of antigen and antibody,

[26] These various considerations also apply to the other semisolid media used in immunodiffusion but appear to be best understood for agar because it has been the most extensively used.

since the dimensions of human serum albumin and of IgG, respectively, are 15×3.8 nm and 23.5×4.4 nm. This paradox was avoided by postulating a highly heteroporous structure for agar gels. A newer estimate of pore size in 2% agar gel then became 12 nm (Wunderly, 1960). In an empirical study the pore radius in 2% agar has been measured at 45 nm, and in 1% essentially no pores were detectable (Fig. 2.2). Thus, whatever will diffuse through water should diffuse through 1% agar gel (Ackers and Steere, 1962). According to this study, the pore radius decreases quickly at concentrations above 2%, narrowing down to 12 to 15 nm at 6%. Agar (and presumably also agarose) gels therefore can be made into sieving media;[27] but at commonly used concentrations of

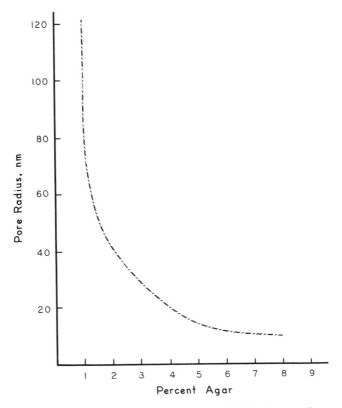

Fig. 2.2. Graph adapted from Ackers and Steere (1962), showing decrease in pore radius of gels made with increasing quantities of agar.

[27] A small area of agar cast at 4% in surrounding 1% agar was used as a local sieve to help identify macroglobulin in immunoelectrophoresis of pathologic sera (Kořínek, 1964).

about 1% they should not much affect migration of even small suspensoids. This explains recent observations in apparent conflict with earlier expectations that such antigens as clover yellow mosaic virus with a length of 539 nm can diffuse through agar gels (Ford, 1964). These particles themselves, and not just portions of them, are migrating to be precipitated (agglutinated?) by antibodies, for electron microscopy showed the antigen–antibody aggregates to consist largely of intact virions (John, 1965; Ragetli and Weintraub, 1964).

But to assume that, because mean pore size in a given agar gel is large enough, free migration of an antigen molecule smaller than such pores will occur, is erroneous both empirically and theoretically: the proportion of relatively smaller pores rises with the increase in concentration of the agar, and one observes empirically that only at concentrations of 0.5% (Meffroy-Biget, 1966) to 1.0% (Ackers and Steere, 1962) is migration truly free. At higher concentrations the effects of impeded migration of antigens and antibodies which are not known to interact with agar itself are seen as changing electrophoretic migration rates, slower diffusion, and slower but stronger precipitation (Zwaan, 1963; Van Oss and Heck, 1963; Brummerstedt-Hansen, 1967; Clausen et al., 1963).

Agar, usually because of its constituent agaropectin, is not an inert medium. Consequently, certain antigens like basic proteins and lipoproteins which are small enough to migrate freely through agar gels actually do so poorly or not at all (Zwaan, 1963). The effective permeability of agar gels also is affected by accompanying solutes. For instance, sucrose at 3.33% increased diffusion of antigen in agar; both dextran and carrageenan at 0.025% decreased diffusion rates fivefold (Wunderly, 1960). Since only a small amount of appropriate solute can drastically affect reactant migration in agar gels, the technique for dissolving agar in preparing for immunodiffusion tests should be kept consistent from test to test. Differences in the proportion of agar hydrolyzed by heating in preparation of a gel can affect the results (Crowle, 1961; Murty and Hanson, 1961).

AGAR PURIFICATION

Most of the gelling effect of agar is due to its agarose (see below), whereas most of its usually undesirable effects (turbidity, reactivity with basic proteins and with lipoproteins, electroosmosis) are due to its agaropectin (Burstein and Fine, 1964b). One might, therefore, question the utility of agar at all, now that agarose can be purchased or prepared so readily. But the phenomenon of electroosmosis is helpful for electroimmunodiffusion, and the interaction between certain antigens and agaropectin in agar gels sometimes improves their resolution (Wunderly, 1960). Moreover, agar still is easier and cheaper to obtain.[28]

Before convenient techniques were developed to prepare agarose several, often elaborate, methods were devised to "clear" agars. Their purposes ranged from simply ridding the gel of lint and dust (filter hot agar solution through paper or other coarse material), through reducing electroosmosis (lower the sulfate content), to deionizing the agar (Crowle, 1961). Today, most of these purposes are accomplished automatically in deriving agarose from agar. Therefore, for most immunodiffusion tests originally requiring highly purified agar it is better now to use agarose (Miller and Feeney, 1964).

Nevertheless, agar is an excellent medium for nearly all currently used immunodiffusion tests. Laboratory-grade agars, such as are used in bacteriologic media, usually are better and cheaper than agars specially purified and sold for use in immunodiffusion tests, and they are generally satisfactory without additional purification (Glenn, 1961; Jameson, 1968, 1969a; David-West, 1966; Alexander and Moncrief, 1966). When these are not available, cruder agars can be substituted after some simple purifications such as the following.[29]

Soak the agar shreds or granules in several changes of distilled water before using them. Make a 4% concentration of gel, dice it, dialyze or electrodialyze it, and then either use this gel to make more dilute gel by reheating and appropriate dilution, or dry it and later dissolve the resulting flakes as needed. Dissolve the agar in the solvent to be employed, and filter[30] it while hot through several layers of lintless gauze, coarse filter paper, shredded paper, or diatomaceous earth; or centrifuge it at high speed (e.g., 5000 g) for 10 minutes in a centrifuge rotor preheated to 80°C. Make agar gel and then chill, freeze, and thaw it to

[28] Heavy metal impurities like Cd^{++} and Ni^{++}, found more often in various agars than in agaroses, frequently contribute significantly to increased sensitivity of immunodiffusion tests (Crowle, 1960a, 1961; Alexander and Moncrief, 1966).

[29] Agars to be used for immunoelectrophoresis or electrophoresis should be deionized to reduce their contribution to heating during electrophoresis (Wieme, 1959). Electrodialysis of agar gel (Wieme, 1959) is the quickest and most effective technique, but dialyzing small cubes of gel against distilled water, or making agar gel and disrupting it through several freeze–thaw cycles, are adequate, rapid, large-yield methods. Large quantities of agar granules also can be deionized efficiently with chelating agents (Crowle, 1961).

[30] Convenient small-volume filtration: draw hot agar solution into a 10-ml pipet tipped with a loose cotton plug. Remove the plug and apply the filtered agar to the immunodiffusion plate or slide (Afonso, 1964a).

disrupt the gel and express the water and dissolved impurities (Crowle, 1961; see this reference also for more complex methods of physico-chemical purification).

Before the advent of agarose many attempts were made to reduce the often marked electroosmosis of agar by washings, deionizations, or empirical changes in calcium or sulfate composition. In geographic areas where agarose may not be readily available, may be too expensive, or cannot be prepared conveniently for lack of reagents or equipment, it is simpler to change the agar chemically to an electroneutral gel. Indeed, agar gel charge can be tailored to fit special purposes (Ragetli and Weintraub, 1966). Results obtained by these techniques of alteration depend partly on the source of agar employed, on the type of chemical group attached to the agar, and on the number of groups introduced (Ragetli and Weintraub, 1966). Davis (New Zealand) agar charged with tri-methylaminoacethydrazide showed 30% less electroosmosis than agarose; diethylaminoethyl-altered Difco Bacto (United States) agar actually developed anodic electroosmotic flow.

PREPARING AGAR GELS

Most agars[31] make gels that are structurally too weak for convenient handling at concentrations below 1%; cutting wells and punching holes neatly becomes difficult (Omland, 1963a; Kunter, 1963; Vanegas Alvarado, 1961). Hence, unless the gel is not to be manipulated after it has been cast (e.g., in tube diffusion tests, in which concentrations of 0.6% generally are employed to decrease background turbidity), agar should be used at concentrations between 1.0 and 1.5% (Jordan and White, 1965).[32] At 2%, agar gel is still easier to manipulate; but moderate sieving effects begin to appear at this concentration, diffusion is slower, and sensitivity begins to drop (Darcy, 1961; Vanegas Alvarado, 1961; Brummerstedt-Hansen, 1967). Higher concentrations can be used for special purposes (Nelken and Nelken, 1962; Kořínek, 1964), but because agar solutions above 4% are too viscous to work with easily, if the purpose of using a higher concentration is to increase sieving then it is better instead to "thicken" 1% agar gel with acrylamide (Uriel, 1966), since this not only is a better molecular sieve but also is more easily regulated (see section below on polyacrylamide).

---

[31] One batch or source of agar may provide better immunodiffusion results than another, so that if a problem in resolution or sensitivity has been encountered several agars might profitably be tested (Karlsson, 1965).

[32] Equivalent "hardness" was obtained for gels made with 1% Difco Nobel agar, 0.7% Oxoid Ionagar No. 2, 1.5% Difco purified agar, and 0.8% agarose (Jordan and White, 1965).

Agar gels are made by adding dried agar to buffered water (exotic buffers, very high or very low pH values, or high salt concentrations will affect solution and gelling of agar:[33] Lachmann, 1962), and then heating this to boiling temperature. The agar granules will dissolve in a few minutes. The solution must be swirled or mixed well to distribute the dissolved agar evenly; there should be no agar granules visible as high-refraction particles if solution is complete. In high altitude laboratories the agar is best dissolved in a screw-capped tube, or in an autoclave or pressure cooker. Avoid excessive heating to minimize hydrolysis of the agar (Witter, 1962).

The solution of agar can be cast boiling hot or at lower temperatures down to just above 45°C, at which it congeals, depending on the nature of the test. For instance, it should be used hot for casting easily and evenly in thin layers on unwarmed surfaces.[34] On the other hand, for single diffusion tests and some kinds of electroimmunodiffusion, antiserum is mixed with the agar before casting. Then it must be cooled to 56°C or less to prevent denaturing antiserum precipitins. For this procedure, the antiserum is warmed to this temperature[35] and mixed with agar pre-cooled to 56°C, and the mixture is cast. If the casting procedure is delicate, as in a micro single diffusion tube, then all components that are to come into contact with the agar–antiserum mixture must be warmed also.

For doing several tests a week, one can prepare several tubes of agar solution all at one time, maintain them liquid at 64°C, and use them during that week as required (Mansi, 1958). Alternatively, one can make several tubes of agar gel in one-use volumes, store these gelled, and then reliquefy one or more as needed. Problems associated with these conveniences include principally agar hydrolysis and microbial contamination and, if storage is prolonged, dehydration (Murty and Hanson, 1961).

Agar can be used immediately after it has gelled. However, letting·

---

[33] If an "exotic" solvent must be used, the gel can be made and cast in distilled water and then soaked for 24 hours in the solvent desired (Paul and Benacerraf, 1966). An unsatisfactory solvent in a purchased gel can be replaced similarly.

[34] Although thin gels are best for most immunodiffusion tests because they provide optimal resolution and sensitivity, for some, like a single radial diffusion in which resolution is not so important, a thicker gel gives better sensitivity (Rumke and Breekveldt-Kielich, 1969).

[35] Even at 56°C, antiserum components may be denatured. Complement is rapidly inactivated, and lipoproteins react quickly with agar. To avoid this problem, one can use other gelling agents such as carrageenan, special agarose, or acrylamide, which gel at lower temperature, or one can cast the agar and then charge it with reactant by preliminary diffusion (see Chapter 6).

the gel harden fully for several minutes to an hour, depending on gel thickness, makes later manipulation and especially cutting easier. Gel "ripening" for several days, recommended by some for accelerating immunodiffusion reactions (DeCarvalho, 1960), probably is simply a partial dehydration, which speeds absorption of reactants and therefore development of the reactions themselves. It seems to have no other merit (David-West, 1966).

AGAROSE GELS

Agarose, one of the two component polysaccharides of agar, is a neutral galactose polymer composed of alternating residues of 3,6-anhydro-α-L-galactopyranose and β-D-galactopyranose (Hjertén, 1961; Beck and Uzan, 1965). Although originally purified by Araki in 1937 (Russell et al., 1964), it did not begin to achieve its present, rapidly do not precipitate lipoprotein. They permit free diffusion of basic as well as acidic molecules (cf. Miller and Feeney, 1964: Hjertén, 1961; growing popularity for use in immunodiffusion tests until Hjertén described a simplified method for its preparation (Hjertén, 1961).

Agarose gels resemble agar gels but are clearer and purer, are more rigid at equivalent concentrations, exhibit no adsorption phenomena, and Hegenauer and Nace, 1965). Although agarose gels exhibit very little electroosmosis (Jordan and White, 1965; Ragetli and Weintraub, 1966), they do show some. This may be due to carboxyl groups of pyruvic acid (Ragetli and Weintraub, 1966).

PREPARATION OF AGAROSE

Although marketed agarose is expensive, until recently preparing agarose from agar in a laboratory was difficult enough (cf. Hjertén, 1961, 1962; Uriel et al., 1963) to justify purchase of the commercial product. But today it can be prepared quickly, economically, and easily by precipitation from hot agar with polyethylene glycol of 6000 molecular weight (Russell et al., 1964; see Fig. 2.3).

Make a solution of 4% agar (e.g., Ionagar No. 2, Difco Bacto agar) in boiling distilled water. Prepare a 40% w/v solution of 6000-molecular-weight polyethylene glycol (Carbowax 6000). Warm this to 80°C, cool the agar solution to the same temperature, and mix them 1:1. Agarose that precipitates is collected by centrifuging the mixture for 10 minutes at 4000 to 5000 rpm in an angle rotor head, such as the Servall GSA, preheated with hot water.[36] The still-liquid supernate, containing

---

[36] Alternatively, collect it by filtration through 110-mesh nylon cloth (Russell et al., 1964).

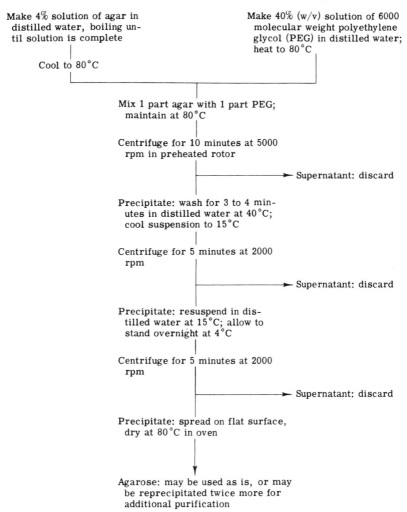

PREPARATION OF AGAROSE FROM LABORATORY AGAR*

Make 4% solution of agar in distilled water, boiling until solution is complete

Cool to 80°C

Make 40% (w/v) solution of 6000 molecular weight polyethylene glycol (PEG) in distilled water; heat to 80°C

Mix 1 part agar with 1 part PEG; maintain at 80°C

Centrifuge for 10 minutes at 5000 rpm in preheated rotor

→ Supernatant: discard

Precipitate: wash for 3 to 4 minutes in distilled water at 40°C; cool suspension to 15°C

Centrifuge for 5 minutes at 2000 rpm

→ Supernatant: discard

Precipitate: resuspend in distilled water at 15°C; allow to stand overnight at 4°C

Centrifuge for 5 minutes at 2000 rpm

→ Supernatant: discard

Precipitate: spread on flat surface, dry at 80°C in oven

Agarose: may be used as is, or may be reprecipitated twice more for additional purification

*Adapted from Russell *et al.* (1964).

Fig. 2.3. Flow diagram for preparing agarose from laboratory-grade agar. The technique shown follows that described by Russell *et al.* (1964).

principally agaropectin, is discarded. Wash the precipitate for 3 to 4 minutes with strong agitation (e.g., in a blender) using distilled water at 40°C, and cool the suspension to room temperature. Centrifuge out the agarose, and discard the supernatant fluid. Wash the precipitate again with vigorous agitation, and let it soak overnight in distilled water at room temperature. Collect the washed precipitate by centrifugation, wash it with acetone, and finally dry it at 80°C. The product, already a high-quality agarose, can be improved somewhat for ultimate quality by one or two more precipitations from hot solution with polyethylene glycol. Up to a 40% yield of the original weight of agar is obtained. The gel strength of agarose prepared by this technique is greater than that prepared by older methods (Tsuchiya and Hong, 1965).

A modification of this technique has been described employing polyethylene glycol of molecular weight 4000 (Hegenauer and Nace, 1965). It is said to facilitate washing of the precipitated agarose. A larger quantity of this lower-molecular-weight polyethylene glycol is required than of the 6000-molecular-weight chemical. In this modification ionic surfactants also are used for dispersing the precipitated agarose more finely for washing and for retarding gelation of the agaropectin. Precipitation temperature appears to be important: there is a higher yield at 80° to 100°C, but more agaropectin is coprecipitated; at 40° to 60°C agaropectin contamination is diminished, but flocculation of agarose is poor and its recovery consequently is low.

The above procedures can be used successfully with Difco Bacto agar and Ionagar No. 2; but with other agars, results may differ, sometimes being better and sometimes worse. For instance, crude agar shreds are poor starting materials (Hegenauer and Nace, 1965). Agar usually is derived from the seaweed *Gelidium amansii* because this agar has high gel strength (Tsuchiya and Hong, 1965). But if agar extracted from *Gelidium pristoides* is used instead, only 7% w/v polyethylene glycol of molecular weight 6000 is necessary to precipitate agarose (Russell *et al.*, 1964). In the future, high-quality commercial agarose probably will become available at prices competitive with those of agar, because source agars will be selected for agarose content rather than for qualities as agars. For instance, alkali-pretreated *Gracilaria verrucosa* yields an agar some thirteen times as rich in agarose, relative to agaropectin, as conventional agars (20:1 versus 1.5:1 ratios, respectively; Tsuchiya and Hong, 1965).

PREPARATION OF AGAROSE GELS

Because agarose is relatively new to the field of immunodiffusion, there are only modest data on its use. However, it is similar enough to agar that the information given above for agar is generally applicable to agarose.

This polysaccharide forms a stronger gel than agar and so can be used at 1% with improved physical qualities but with no more molecular sieving than an equivalent concentration of agar; or it can be used at

a lower concentration (0.8%) for gels of about the same physical consistency as a 1% agar gel but with greater clarity. We have obtained
gels that would be adequate for many varieties of immunodiffusion test
using only 0.2% SeaKem (Marine Colloids, Inc.) agarose in distilled
water.[37] Microbial contamination on agarose gels is usually less than that
of agar gels under equivalent conditions.

Agarose solutions are made like agar solutions, although some currently
available batches require more vigorous heating to dissolve. For instance,
agarose from Mann Research Laboratories required heating at 120°C
(autoclaving) for 10 minutes to dissolve; by contrast, SeaKem agarose
dissolved easily at 100°C (Leise and Evans, 1965). As agarose becomes
more popular, readers will find varieties with useful properties that can
only partly be anticipated here. For example, one recently offered commercially can be cooled to 37.5°C before it begins to gel,[38] which is very
convenient if it is to be mixed with labile antiserum or antigen. Another
variety now is supplied as a dried film on a plastic base. It has a pattern
of wells punched in it and is prepared for use by rehydration in hot
water (Marine Colloids, Inc.).

POLYACRYLAMIDE GELS

Polyacrylamide gels are synthetic linear polymers of acrylamide cross-
linked at intervals by N,N'-methylenebisacrylamide (Chrambach and
Rodbard, 1971). Their formation is aided and accelerated by initiators
chosen for optimal effect and fastest polymerization under given environmental conditions, such as buffer composition, temperature, and nature
of the immunodiffusion apparatus.

Polyacrylamide gels are soft, moist, very flexible, sticky, water-clear,
and dimensionally rather unstable because they swell or contract readily
on gaining or losing water (Murray, 1962; Frederick, 1964; Chrambach
and Rodbard, 1971; Keutel, 1964; Hermans *et al.*, 1960). Some of these
characteristics as well as their porosity depend on the concentrations of
both acrylamide and bisacrylamide and on their proportions to each
other (Bloemendal, 1967; Poulik, 1966; Davis, 1964). Increases in the
concentrations of both tend to increase the stiffness and friability of the
resulting gel, whereas if concentrations of both are decreased, the gel
becomes more elastic and softer (Davis, 1964). Holding the acrylamide
concentration constant and raising that of the bisacrylamide tends to

[37] Bio-Rad Laboratories (Richmond, California, 94804) reports the same for the
agarose they sell (Bull. EP-1, 1970).

[38] Available as Sea Plaque Agarose, Marine Colloids, Inc. A 1% solution of this
substance liquefies at 70°C and gels at less than 32°C (Tech. Data Sheet AG-LG,
Marine Colloids, Inc., Rockland, Maine 04841).

increase gel stiffness; doing the opposite decreases its effective median pore radius. The proportions of these two chemicals to each other and their absolute concentrations can be adjusted to prepare gels with any of many different porosities ranging from 0.5 to 3 nm (Chrambach and Rodbard, 1971) median pore radius.[39] However, the pores are not rigid; if a molecule or particle larger than the putative median pore is subjected to electrophoresis, it may or may not migrate through the gel, depending on the voltage applied to it (Raymond and Nakamichi, 1962a). One of the most important attributes that polyacrylamide gels offer immunodiffusion users, not found in any other medium now being used, is easily and widely variable distinction between molecules by size—that is, a form of gel filtration. One can fractionate molecules ranging from molecular weights of less than 1000 to greater than 10^6 (Chrambach and Rodbard, 1971); one can also prepare polyacrylamide gels with pore size varying across the gel from large, through medium, to small (Wright et al., 1970). Mixing polyacrylamide with other gelling agents like agarose combines some of the advantages of both (e.g., sieving by the polyacrylamide, easy handling and drying after staining by the agarose: Uriel, 1966). Pore size in polyacrylamide gels diminishes as the gel sets (Davis, 1964); therefore, unlike agarose gels, polyacrylamide gels may be significantly affected by "aging" in immunodiffusion, especially if a slow polymerizing catalyst like riboflavin is used.

Large-pore gels are prepared by using the lowest possible concentrations of acrylamide and bisacrylamide (Davis, 1964). At concentrations below 2% acrylamide and 0.5% bisacrylamide a gel usually will not set, but slight increases in one or both chemicals will result in formation of usable gels. Certain substances added to the mixture (e.g., 20% sucrose) facilitate gelling and improve the mechanical properties of the gel (Davis, 1964).

The characteristics of polyacrylamide gels, and the conditions under which the gels will form, depend on the condition of each ingredient used, especially of the primary ingredients and the catalysts (Davis, 1964). Acrylamide must be stored in a cool, dark, dry place to reduce spontaneous polymerization and hydrolysis; under these conditions its average shelf life is several years. Since bisacrylamide also will polymerize spontaneously, it should be stored similarly, and it has a similar shelf life. Catalysts, buffers, and other ingredients of these gels may contain or acquire impurities which make gel structures irreproducible

---

[39] Like agar gels, polyacrylamide gels consist of a meshwork of fibers, and pore size is not uniform but rather is distributed in slightly skewed, non-Gaussian manner (Chrambach and Rodbard, 1971). The length and thickness of the fibers in this gel depend on the degree of cross-linking.

(Chrambach and Rodbard, 1971); for maximum reliability these ingredients should all be fresh and, if purity is suspect, they should be recrystallized, redistilled, or otherwise repurified.

Because polyacrylamide "disc" electrophoresis has become popular for analyzing complex mixtures of macromolecules (cf. Frederick, 1964), the ingredients for making polyacrylamide gels now are readily available. They can be obtained in various premixed forms in kits from which one can prepare gels that are reproducibly uniform for disc electrophoresis. But these have not been designed for use in immunodiffusion tests, and until such mixtures are available primarily for this purpose, it is better to work with the separate components according to formulas devised for immunodiffusion. These ingredients are available, for instance, from Distillation Products Industries, Division of Eastman Kodak Co., Rochester, New York.[40]

PREPARING POLYACRYLAMIDE GELS FOR IMMUNODIFFUSION

Unpolymerized acrylamide and some of the catalysts used in its polymerization are insidiously neurotoxic by inhalation or contact and must be handled carefully (Bloemendal, 1967; Ferris *et al.*, 1962b).

There are some general principles to the various techniques employed for preparing polyacrylamide gels. Concentrations and proportions of acrylamide and bisacrylamide are chosen empirically to form gels that permit full or selective movement of antigens and, during development of antigen–antibody precipitates, permit movement of at least one reactant toward the other. Choosing a concentration partially is governed by the natures of buffers, additives, and immunodiffusion containers, or of the reactants themselves (cf. Chrambach and Rodbard, 1971). One should aim for as complete and rapid a polymerization as possible for uniformity of results; polymerization should be at least 95% complete, and it should occur within 5 to 15 minutes. Polymerization inhibitors, especially oxygen, should be avoided or eliminated; and conditions that aggravate inhibition of polymerization such as low temperature, acid pH, acetate buffers, glycine buffers, and amino compounds should be avoided (Poulik, 1966; Murray, 1962; Radhakrishnamurthy *et al.*, 1963). If the gel is to be used for electrophoresis, the temperature of polymerization ideally should be the same as the temperature of electrophoresis to minimize thermal contraction or expansion of the gel. Once

---

[40] Acrylamide = Eastman 5521; *N,N'*-methylenebisacrylamide = Eastman 8383; *N,N,N',N'*-tetramethylethylenediamine (TEMED) = Eastman 8178; riboflavin = Eastman 5181. Bio-Rad (Richmond, California) offers a kit of purified but separate components that the user can employ in the proportions in which he wishes to make polyacrylamide gels.

formed, polyacrylamide gels do not deteriorate; consequently, there is no restriction to using ideal polymerizing agents for most types of immunodiffusion test (Uriel, 1966). If these are not compatible with antigen or antibody or with antigen–antibody reaction, they can be removed readily by dialysis or electrodialysis in a compatible solvent which thus replaces the incompatible one. This raises no time problem, for polyacrylamide gels can be prepared weeks or months before they will be needed and then stored indefinitely in the solvent to be used. However, if the gel is to be used without removing its catalysts, then a polymerizing technique like photopolymerization, which will minimize the catalysts to both reduce ionic strength and avoid catalyst reaction with antigen or antibody (Brewer, 1967), is desirable (Antoine, 1962). Polyacrylamide at 2.5 to 3.5% will permit diffusion of antibodies and most antigens (Uriel, 1966); at 4%, diffusion of 19 S antibodies is restricted (Stobo and Tomasi, 1967); at 3 to 6%, the diffusion of low- and medium-molecular-weight antigens is repressed; 7 to 9% gels affect the diffusion of molecules in the 10,000- to 20,000-molecular-weight range (Uriel, 1966). Below 3%, polyacrylamide is said to have almost no sieving effect on such mixtures as antigens and antiserum. Stock filtered solutions of acrylamide and bisacrylamide can be kept for several weeks, but solutions of some of the catalysts are not stable and should be freshly prepared (Raymond and Nakamichi, 1962a). As in agar or agarose immunoelectrophoresis, choosing an appropriate buffer for polyacrylamide immunoelectrophoresis is important (Frederick, 1964).

The following are some techniques for preparing polyacrylamide gels useful for immunodiffusion tests.

Mix 20 parts of acrylamide powder with 1 part of bisacrylamide (Poulik, 1966), and dissolve this in enough distilled water or physiologic phosphate buffer at pH 7.4 to make a 3%, 4%, or 5% solution (according to pore size required). Filter the solution through Whatman #1 paper. Add 1.2 ml of 10% β-dimethylaminopropionitrile and 1.2 ml of 10% ammonium persulfate to 300 ml of the acrylamide solution. The volumes can be adjusted to the task, but the proportions are important (Crowle, 1961). Transfer 15 ml to a 9-cm petri dish, and cover with a layer of heptane, mineral oil, or some other inert nonaqueous fluid. Heat the petri dish over steam. The acrylamide will gel within 3 to 5 minutes. Pour off the heptane or mineral oil, and use the gel for any of several kinds of immunodiffusion test. If a nonvolatile fluid like mineral oil is used, it can be washed off the gel with one that is volatile (e.g., ether).

We have used this technique for several years because it is reliable and easy, and it requires no special equipment. Oxygen is easily excluded during polymerization with the protective overlay of organic solvent.

Containers other than a petri dish can be employed to suit special purposes, or supports such as a glass microscope slide can be placed within the petri dish and the gel polymerized upon them. Later they are cut free of surrounding gel and used independently. Polymerization is greatly accelerated by heating the petri dish with steam, but it will occur readily though more slowly at room temperature. Hence, a labile substance like antiserum can be incorporated in the polymer without heat denaturation. The most important characteristic of this technique is exclusion of oxygen by organic solvent. Other characteristics, such as concentrations and proportions of acrylamide and bisacrylamide and the nature of catalysts,[41] can be varied to suit formulations developed for use in immunodiffusion by other investigators.

Some of the disadvantages of handling polyacrylamide gels can be circumvented by preparing them in mixture with agar or agarose (Uriel, 1966). The procedure is as follows.

The slab of gel is formed by pouring acrylamide–agarose mixture at 50°C between two glass plates prewarmed to 55° to 60°C, held apart by thin 3-mm spacers, and resting on a level surface. In separate beakers prepare 50 ml of 1.6% agarose solution (dissolved by boiling) and 50 ml of acrylamide–bisacrylamide mixture (e.g., containing 3 gm of acrylamide and 0.08 gm of bisacrylamide), and then bring them both to 50°C in a water bath. To the warm agarose solution add 0.06 gm of ammonium persulfate and 0.06 ml of TEMED (polymerizing catalysts[41]). Mix this solution vigorously to dissolve the ammonium persulfate. Then mix the agarose and acrylamide solutions together energetically and rapidly (10 to 15 seconds), and pour the mixture between the two glass slides used for casting the polyacrylamide–agarose slab. Let this stand for 35 minutes at 55° to 60°C to promote polymerization, and then transfer it to a 4°C refrigerator to accelerate agarose gelling (complete in 20 to 40 minutes). Disassemble the casting apparatus, and immerse the gel in the buffer required for the immunodiffusion or immunoelectrophoresis test; keep the gel refrigerated in this solution until it is used. Subsequent procedures are essentially the same as operations for agarose gels themselves.

Agar can be employed for the above procedure instead of agarose. The proportions of agarose (0.8%), agar (1.2%) and TEMED (0.06%) remain the same regardless of changes in proportions or concentrations of the acrylamides and of the ammonium persulfate (Uriel, 1966). The propor-

[41] Our use of dimethylaminopropionitrile is obsolescent; *N,N,N',N'*-tetramethylethylenediamine (TEMED) is more efficient (Davis, 1964). Proportions of components then would be, for instance, 98 ml of acrylamide solution:1 ml of 5.0% ammonium persulfate:1 ml of 5.0% TEMED. This mixture will gel in about 1.5 hours at room temperature.

tion of acrylamide to bisacrylamide also is kept constant at 37.5 parts of acrylamide to 1 part of bisacrylamide. As the concentrations of the acrylamides are raised, the quantities of ammonium persulfate can be lowered: for 3%, 5%, 7%, and 9% final concentrations of acrylamides, use 0.06%, 0.05%, 0.03%, and 0.015% ammonium persulfate, respectively. The gel should be washed free of catalysts by soaking it with repeated changes in the immunodiffusion buffer for several hours or overnight. Polyacrylamide–agarose gels are best prepared in distilled water, but they can be made also in buffers commonly used in immunodiffusion and immunoelectrophoresis except, as mentioned above, some like acetate or glycine which inhibit polymerization. Although the gel being cast is left in the oven for several minutes, polymerization usually is complete in 3 minutes or less.

Perhaps the gentlest technique, biochemically, for polymerizing acrylamide is with light. Photopolymerized polyacrylamide gels seldom need washing to remove catalysts because the low molarity of added salts (less than $0.0002\,M$) will not materially affect conduction of electricity in electrophoresis (Antoine, 1962). The end concentration of polyacrylamide in the following technique is 4.25%. The gel is stiff enough so that it can be cast with a relief mold embedded in it. When this is removed after polymerization, it leaves a pattern of wells to receive reactants. As was discussed above, some sieving and impediment of diffusion occur at this concentration of polyacrylamide, but not enough to be objectionable for most immunodiffusion tests.

Dissolve 30 gm of a 20:1 mixture of acrylamide and bisacrylamide in 100 ml of distilled water. Mix 13.98 ml of this stock solution with 73.6 ml of distilled water or of the buffer to be used in the immunodiffusion test, observing precautions on buffer composition mentioned above, 0.74 ml of 0.64% $Na_2S_2O_3$, and 11.68 ml of 0.005% riboflavin. Transfer this mixture to the vessel within which polymerization is to take place (e.g., a petri dish), place the vessel in the bottom of a large beaker,[42] fill the beaker with carbon dioxide gas to exclude atmospheric oxygen and promote polymerization, and expose the solution to intense light, such as two 500-watt photographic flood lights aimed down on the solution from 40 cm directly overhead. Polymerization should occur within about 6 minutes.

Even though the acrylamide has gelled within a few minutes, with this weak polymerizing system gelling may not be complete until some time afterward (see above). Since exclusion of atmospheric oxygen is especially important, best results are obtained by degassing the acrylamide solution *in vacuo* immediately before it is used. Other gases cannot be

---

[42] The gel should be level. Either a flat-bottomed beaker that has been leveled can be used, or the bottom of the beaker can be covered with mercury on which the petri dish containing the acrylamide solution is floated (Antoine, 1962).

substituted for carbon dioxide to exclude oxygen: under nitrogen, for instance, polymerization did not occur satisfactorily (Antoine, 1962). Polymerization can be hastened by performing it at 50°C or warming the acrylamide–catalyst solution to this temperature before illuminating it; then illumination can also be less intense. Although riboflavin is present in only small concentration, it is not biochemically inert and may affect some immuodiffusion reactions by photooxidation (Antoine, 1962). Therefore, immunodiffusion tests using polyacrylamide made by this technique should be developed in the dark. In casting the gel by this method, one can include molds for making wells, or submerged support slides later to be cut free of surrounding gel. With care one can cut wells in polyacrylamide of this concentration using a sharp corkborer (Stobo and Tomasi, 1967), especially if the borer is silicoated.

Polyacrylamide has been used in tube immunodiffusion tests (Mengoli and Watne, 1966) with essentially the same riboflavin-mediated polymerization. Tube enclosure greatly facilitates polymerization. Plates of glass separated with appropriate spacers serve well (see the agarose–polyacrylamide procedure, above). Specially prepared templates for immuno-electrophoresis in polyacrylamide have been used partly to take advantage of this and partly for technical conveniences of reactant placement (Keutel, 1964; Van Orden, 1968). One of these templates (Keutel, 1964) was designed to rest on a 3¼ by 4-inch glass slide and to have projections that serve both to support it at proper distance above the glass slide and to cast a series of troughs and origin wells. It was used with 2.8% acrylamide and with riboflavin for polymerization. Even at this low concentration, polyacrylamide was observed to retard development of immunodiffusion reactions: they were complete in 24 hours in a comparable agar gel test but required 72 hours for full development in the polyacrylamide. Use of a template with chemically polymerized acrylamide has also been described (Van Orden, 1968).[43]

Cellulose Acetate

Cellulose acetate is a thin "paper" of uniform dimensions and structure for a given type, several types differing principally in average pore size.

---

[43] Polymer is made from solutions *a*, *b*, and *c*. Solution *a* is a mixture of 48 ml of 1 N HCl, 36.6 gm of tris, 0.23 ml of TEMED, and 100 ml of water. Solution *b* consists of 9.5 gm of acrylamide, 0.5 gm of bisacrylamide, and 100 ml of water. Solution *c* is 0.15 gm of ammonium persulfate dissolved in 100 ml of water. Stock solutions *a* and *b* can be kept for several months at 4°C but should be warmed before use; solution *c* must not be kept for more than 1 week. Mix *a*:*b*:*c* = 1:3:4, enclose in the templates described in this paper, and polymerize at 56°C for 20 minutes (Van Orden, 1968). The final concentration of polyacrylamide will be 3.75%.

Although cellulose acetate manufactured for membrane filtration can be used for immunodiffusion, that made for electrophoresis tends to give better results. This can be purchased in different sizes and shapes from distributors of filtering apparatus, electrophoresis equipment, and immunodiffusion supplies. For use it needs only to be saturated with buffer, charged with reactants, and then held for a few hours or overnight under very humid conditions for immunodiffusion reactions to develop. Any of several porosities can be used. In a comparison of 47-mm discs made for filtration, membranes with porosities of 0.45, 0.64, 0.80, 1, 2, or 3 microns all developed satisfactory immunodiffusion patterns. Those with the smallest porosities developed very fine precipitin bands and required three to four times as long for reactions to consummate as the same bands developing in the membranes with larger porosity (Monier, 1963).

PREPARING CELLULOSE ACETATE FOR USE (cf. Smith, 1960)

The membrane is floated on buffer solution until it is thoroughly saturated. Then it is blotted lightly between filter papers; no sheen of moisture should be on its surface. Reactants are applied, and the membrane subsequently is incubated by any of various methods described in the apparatus section of this chapter. The aim in reactant application is to soak a small volume into the surface of the membrane without having much spread. During sample application and later incubation the membrane must be rigorously protected against drying by keeping it in a very humid chamber or, for incubation, by submerging it in oil.

GELATIN

Gelatin is a protein extracted from skin, tendons, ligaments, and similar tissues by boiling them. It can be used for immunodiffusion and immunoelectrophoresis at concentrations from 1.5% to as much as 30%; the usual range is 1.5 to 4.0% (Smith et al., 1962b; Dudman, 1965b; Eiguer and Staub, 1966; Crowle and Hu, 1967; Crowle, 1971). The concentration selected depends on the characteristics of the batch being used,[44] the temperature at which it will be employed (gels of 2% or less liquefy at room temperature), and the "pore" density required for restricting diffusion of antigens (such as in molecular weight determinations: Twade et al., 1963).

Gelatin gels are prepared like agar gels. Mix the dried granules into

---

[44] Food gelatins (e.g., Knox) and those used in bacteriologic media (e.g., Difco Bacto gelatin) are satisfactory. Since gelatin is rarely used for immunodiffusion tests, there is little direct information on factors in its preparation or purification which might affect its utility in these tests.

the required volume of buffer or distilled water, heat to boiling but avoid excessive or prolonged heating, distribute the dissolved gelatin well by vigorous mixing, transfer the gelatin solution to the immunodiffusion vessel, and finally allow the gelatin to set at 4°C. Gelatin gels of 2% or less are soft and delicate; those of 3% or more physically resemble agar gels commonly used in immunodiffusion, although they are more elastic and are stickier. With proper care they can be cut to form troughs or wells. Gelatin, like polyacrylamide, can be used in mixture with agar (e.g., 0.75%: Dudman, 1965b; or 1%: Eiguer and Staub, 1966) to form better-quality gels (cf. also Smith *et al.*, 1962a).

Even in low-concentration gelatin gels, immunodiffusion reactants diffuse so slowly that reactions that are completed in agar gels within 1 or 2 days may require days or weeks in gelatin. The sensitivity of immunodiffusion tests in gelatin is low, partly because gelatin interacts with antibodies and various kinds of antigens. This interaction can be intense enough for several antigens, notably neutral polysaccharides (Dudman, 1965b), to prevent precipitation. Gelatin gels once were recommended for immunodiffusion of basic antigens because the antigens could not be studied in agar gels (Crowle and Hu, 1967), but the ready availability now of agarose makes this recommendation obsolete. Polyacrylamide is better than gelatin for molecular sieving (Naylor and Adair, 1962; Tawde *et al.*, 1963). Therefore, except for special purposes, like the selective interference with polysaccharide mentioned above, gelatin today has little to recommend its use in immunodiffusion. When gelatin is added to agar gels as an antigen stabilizer and to minimize nonspecific precipitation (Kagen, 1965), its potential for interfering with immunodiffusion reactions should not be overlooked.

CARRAGEENAN GELS

These are prepared with an agar-like galactose polymer extracted, also like agar, from seaweeds. One variety suitable for immunodiffusion was described in the first edition of this book (Crowle, 1961) as K-agar (Baltimore Biological Laboratory, Inc.), used at 1.5% in a solution containing 0.5% KCl, or at twice that concentration if NaCl is used. It dissolved at 66°C and gelled at 55°C in the presence of KCl; in the presence of NaCl these temperatures were 59°C and 40°C, respectively. It formed a turbid gel unless filtered while hot through filter paper. K-agar still is available from the same supplier.

Marine Colloids, Inc., markets a carrageenan as Gelcarin GS-30 which, because it liquefies at 37°C and gels at 28°C, has been used for preparatory immunodiffusion—that is, to harvest the antibody of antigen–antibody precipitin bands directly from the gel without having to heat the gel enough to denature the precipitins (Mohos, 1966). An agar-like gel was obtained as follows: dissolve 12 gm of GS-30 in 1 liter of 0.9% NaCl and autoclave it for 20 minutes at 120°C. Add 3 ml of $1 M$ KH_2PO_4 and 7.5 ml of $1 M$ K_2HPO_4, potassium salts being used to increase gel strength, and 100 mg of Merthiolate to prevent microbial growth. Filter the mixture through four layers of cheesecloth. Pour the filtered mixture into immunodiffusion containers, allow it to gel, and use it like agar. Reactions should be developed at 4°C. After they have developed, individual precipitin bands can be cut out and released from the carrageenan gel by warming it to body temperature. Carrageenan may be a good source of low-melting point agarose.

STARCH GEL

The most important characteristic of starch gels for immunodiffusion tests is their capacity for molecular sieving. Because polyacrylamide gels have equal or better capacity, are more convenient to use than starch gels, and make clear gels whereas starch does not, starch alone probably will be little used for immunodiffusion tests in the future. Starch has been used in combination with agar (Hase, 1964). Its application to special immunoelectrophoresis and electroimmunodiffusion tests is described later (Chapters 5 and 6).

Composition of Immunodiffusion Test Solvents

The most common solvent for immunodiffusion tests is physiologic sodium chloride, usually buffered to near neutral or slightly alkaline pH.[45] Although this is a good general-purpose solvent for these tests, frequently results can be improved for a given antigen–antiserum system by using another. Because the mechanisms of antigen–antibody precipitation are still only poorly understood, such alterations usually have been empirical. Some illustrative examples are given here to help the reader select an optimal solvent for his particular system.

A general principle is that test conditions that tend to insolubilize antigen or, especially, antibody (e.g., low salt concentration, high salt concentration, the presence of ions like barbital or cadmium which tend to precipitate lipids attached to antibody molecules) also tend to increase

---

[45] Immunoelectrophoresis tests generally are performed in weaker, more alkaline buffers to minimize heating during electrophoresis and to improve electrophoretic separation of antigens.

test sensitivity; of course, they also increase risks of nonspecific precipitation.

Salts Lower Than Physiologic

Rabbit antiserum precipitates most commonly used antigens more strongly and faster at below-physiologic than at physiologic salt concentrations, probably because of coprecipitation by α_{2M}-globulin (Halpern *et al.*, 1961). Human IgM antibody against denatured DNA was found to precipitate this antigen in 1% agarose made in 0.06 M phosphate or 0.06 M barbital but not in phosphate-buffered physiologic saline (Hannestad, 1969). Bacterial antigens are precipitated more distinctly in agar at NaCl concentrations of 0.01 M than at physiologic 0.15 M (Omland, 1963a); the same appears to be true of egg antigens reacting with mouse or rat antisera (McDonald and Duhig, 1965). Antisera from hay fever patients have been reported to precipitate ragweed antigens at low but not at physiologic salt concentration (Perelmutter *et al.*, 1962).

The helpful effects of low salt concentration in immunodiffusion tests are not restricted to antibodies: plant viruses apparently are better dispersed and react less with agar in 0.01 M phosphate than in 0.14 M NaCl (Wetter, 1967a,b). With antigens such as these, as salt concentration in the gel is increased, precipitin band curvature bends progressively more acutely toward the antigen source of diffusion (see Chapter 4). Some basic proteins like deoxyribonucleoprotein react spontaneously with agar gels and precipitate at NaCl concentrations ranging from 0.15 to 0.01. This problem has been circumvented to reveal specific precipitation of these antigens by using NaCl at only 0.007 M (Messineo, 1964). Precipitation of DNA by antibodies could be demonstrated in agar double diffusion tests using either distilled water or 0.15 M NaCl but not 1.0 M NaCl (Anderson *et al.*, 1962b). These various observations of the effectiveness of antigen–antibody precipitation in low-ionic-strength solvents or even in distilled water (Abbood Al-Hilly, 1969) explain the good precipitation ordinarily seen in immunoelectrophoresis, which puzzled earlier workers by not fitting traditional ideas that precipitation cannot develop well in weak electrolyte solutions.

Salts Higher Than Physiologic

As salt concentrations are raised, salting-out effects should cause antigen–antibody precipitation to become progressively stronger until precipitation nonspecificity becomes an overriding problem. Hence, moderate increases in salt concentration on the whole should be beneficial to immunodiffusion tests. But this expectation is countered by competing effects like decreasing attraction between antigen and antibody with rising salt concentrations (cf. Chapter 1), changes in antigen character-istics (Messineo, 1964), and actual diminution of specific precipitation (Anderson *et al.*, 1962b; Perelmutter *et al.*, 1962). Upward changes in salt concentration therefore should not be made without due consideration.

Salt concentrations several times as high as physiologic enhance pre-cipitation of antigens by chicken antisera, especially those of early bleed-ings (cf. below, and Chapter 1). This can be true also of antisera from other animal species like ungulates and rabbits. For instance, rabbit antiserum reacted with duck hepatitis virus antigen in several salt con-centrations from 0.85% (physiologic) to 12% (a concentration commonly used for chicken antisera) produced the most distinct precipitin bands at 8% NaCl (Murty and Hanson, 1961). For the same antigen both bovine and chicken antisera also reacted best at 8% NaCl. Rabbit antiserum pre-cipitated human serum antigens better at 8% NaCl in agarose than at 0.85%; faint bands especially became stronger (Motet, 1965). Both human and rabbit antisera precipitated rubella virus antigens well at 0.45% NaCl (Schmidt and Styk, 1968). Bovine antisera reacted optimally with myco-bacterial antigens in NaCl concentrations of 18%, but precipitation was nearly invisible with these antisera at 0.85% NaCl and did not become readily visible until a concentration of 4% was used (Wedman *et al.*, 1964, 1965; Richards *et al.*, 1966b). A lower concentration of $CaCl_2$ (0.85% to 2.0%) could be substituted in this system, but not without some non-specific precipitation.

That antisera can precipitate antigen in higher-than-physiologic salt concentrations is useful for certain antigens which are poorly soluble in moderate or low salt concentrations. Rabbit antiserum was effective, for instance, in precipitating chicken muscle myosin at the 4% NaCl required to maintain myosin in solution (Winnick and Goldwasser, 1961). Potas-sium chloride has been used at 0.5 M with this antigen and rabbit anti-serum (Finck, 1965); NaCl could be substituted if employed at 1.5 M. Wheat flour gliadin antigen will not migrate through agar at physiologic salt concentrations, but it will do so readily in a conventional buffer for either immunodiffusion or immunoelectrophoresis if urea is added to make a concentration of 3 M (Escribano and Grabar, 1966). Weak anti-sera usually precipitate antigen better in increased salt concentrations provided that antigen is present (Orlans *et al.*, 1961). But there are notable exceptions: increasing the salt concentration of 0.85% up through 12% was detrimental to mouse antisera precipitating chicken ovalbumin, progressively less antigen precipitating as the salt concentration was increased (Anacker and Munoz, 1961).

Some antisera (e.g., from mice and rats) precipitate antigens best at physiologic or lower concentrations of NaCl; others (e.g., rabbit antiserum) precipitate antigen well over a wide range. Still others seem to precipitate antigen better at high than at physiologic concentrations. As has been mentioned, this is especially true of early-bleeding chicken antisera (Orlans *et al.*, 1961; Murty and Hanson, 1961; Aoki *et al.*, 1963; Gengozian *et al.*, 1962; Witter, 1962; Goodman, 1962).[46] Bovine, ovine, and equine antisera are reported to function somewhat better at high salt concentrations (Orlans *et al.*, 1961; Ozerol and Silverman, 1969; Tempelis and Lofy, 1965), and so are turkey antisera (Clarkson, 1963).

Salt concentration changes may affect the immunodiffusion medium as well as either antigen or antibody. For example, one laboratory found that using more than 6% NaCl caused agar gel to become too soft for convenient cutting of reactant wells (Aoki *et al.*, 1963). Consequently, 4% NaCl was used instead, because this promoted good precipitation with the chicken antiserum being tested without unduly softening the gel.

Buffer Salt Composition

This is especially important for immunoelectrophoresis and related techniques using electrophoresis. Distinguishing between various buffers by capacity to resolve separate antigens in mixtures is complex and specialized and so will be done in the chapters dealing with electrophoresis (cf. also Escribano, 1962; Fine *et al.*, 1962b; Cleve and Bearn, 1961; Wehmeyer, 1965; Bednařík, 1966; Lyster *et al.*, 1966; McNeill and Meyer, 1965; John, 1965; Burtin and Grabar, 1967). The following information therefore deals only with effects that different buffers have on antigen–antibody reaction in semisolid media.

Two factors are involved: pH and solute composition. Most immunodiffusion tests use buffers of neutral or slightly alkaline pH (pH 7.2 to 7.4). But occasionally higher or lower pH is preferable. For instance, sheep antiserum to an allotypic determinant on the Fd fragment of rabbit Ig could precipitate it at pH 5 but not at pH 7 (Lichter, 1967); bovine antisera precipitated mycobacterial antigens better at pH 5.0 than at neutrality (Wedman *et al.*, 1965). Borate buffer was used at pH 9.2 to detect swine fever virus antigens optimally with swine antiserum (Hantschel and Bergmann, 1965). Even small pH differences have been reported to be important: an antiserum that detected only one precipi-

---

[46] Just as mammalian antisera can precipitate antigens well at high salt concentrations, so can chicken antisera precipitate efficiently (especially when hyperimmune and used in gels) in physiologic or lower salt concentrations (Weiner *et al.*, 1963; Planas and De Castro, 1961; Lueker and Crowle, 1963).

tinogen from different species of *Brucella* in double diffusion plates at pH 7.4 detected two at pH 7.0 (Gargani and Guerra, 1962).

However, unless variations in pH are extreme, other aspects of the solvent composition will usually be more important than pH. The following generalizations can be made from known characteristics of various salts. Chelators which remove divalent ions decrease immunodiffusion test sensitivity by neutralizing precipitation-enhancing effects of such metals as Cd^{++} and Ni^{++} frequently found naturally in agar, or cofactor effects of Ca^{++} such as in fixation of complement. Chelators include such pH buffers as citrate, acetate, tris, and EDTA. Acetate or borate buffers can interfere with antigen–antibody precipitation by combining directly with reactants, for acetate complexes with proteins, and borate complexes with polysaccharides and with agar itself.

Solutes may have unanticipated and still unexplained effects. Some uncharged ingredients like sucrose, which may be included in a buffer to decrease gel dehydration, can suppress antigen–antibody precipitation. But other neutral solutes can enhance it (see below). Barbital buffers tend to enhance precipitation, probably by precipitating lipids attached to antibodies (Crowle, 1961; Cross and Spooner, 1963; McCormick, 1963). Nevertheless, some varieties of antigen–antibody precipitation in immunodiffusion are better in phosphate-buffered gels or simply in saline than in barbital-buffered gels (Paniker and Kalra, 1962; Hannestad, 1969), especially those involving polysaccharide antigen (Widra *et al.*, 1968). Buffer composition can affect immunodiffusion tests indirectly by regulating natural protein–protein binding. For instance, barbital buffer reduces thyroxin binding to prealbumin, whereas a tris–maleate buffer enhances it (West and Hong, 1962). Attempting to maintain "natural" conditions by using serum as a diluent of antigen for immunodiffusion tests, instead of some nonserum solvent, may not provide results any less confusing. Thus, enzymes in serum used as a diluent for bacterial endotoxin cleaved this into several components, so that a number of precipitin bands appeared when simpler diluents revealed only one (Rudbach and Johnson, 1962). "Inert" polyhydroxy compounds like sucrose or glucose used at $0.03\,M$ or higher can inhibit antigen–antibody precipitation (Hawkins, 1965). Sodium chloride itself can be troublesome, for in concentrations somewhat below physiologic it was observed to cause dissociation and destruction of a ribosomal antigen, an effect that could be avoided by using a tris and magnesium acetate buffer (Quash *et al.*, 1962). On the other hand, the presence of magnesium ions ($0.13\,M$ $MgCl_2$) in immunodiffusion agar analyses of tobacco mosaic virus caused nonspecific precipitation of this virus by its colloidal interaction with the agar in the presence of Mg^{++} (Wetter, 1967b). Since ions like Mg^{++} and

Ca^{++} are prominent contaminants of agar, any constituent of an electrolyte solution affecting these indirectly can also influence the immunodiffusion test. Chelators like EDTA, for instance, diminish complement fixation to antigen–antibody complexes by binding calcium (Lachmann, 1962) and thus depress the enhancing effects on precipitation that complement can have (see also Mardiney and Müller-Eberhard, 1965). This is one particular reason (another is explained below) for the lower sensitivity (see Dudman, 1964b) of immunodiffusion tests set up with chelating electrolytes like EDTA, tris, or citrate.

Some attractive attributes of borate as a buffer in immunodiffusion and immunoelectrophoresis tests include its buffering range, its capacity to effect separations of antigens during electrophoresis which are not possible with other buffers, and its antiseptic properties which eliminate any need for separate preservatives. However, it is especially reactive with certain arrangements of hydroxyl groups on polysaccharides, whether free or constituents of predominantly protein antigens. This affects both the electrophoretic mobilities of such antigens, sometimes advantageously, and their reactions with antibodies (Heiner and Rose, 1970a). Borate reacts so much with agar gel itself that the conductivity of a borate buffer drops fivefold when it is mixed with agar (Escribano, 1962).

The various data above indicate that there are many considerations in selecting an ideal buffer for a given antigen–antibody system. Most prominently, the buffer should maintain antigen integrity and permit its precipitation by antiserum. Its pH and ionic composition should be adjusted empirically to optimize results, and its overall composition supplemented if necessary with appropriate additives (see below). The experimenter should be flexible in choosing and preparing buffers for immunodiffusion and not be overly bound by tradition.

Solvent Additives

Aside from basic ingredients such as electrolytes and buffering salts, solutes used in immunodiffusion tests include various special additives with miscellaneous purposes such as preventing microbial contamination, enhancing precipitin reactions, and modifying one or the other of the reactants to facilitate its diffusion and/or precipitation.

The use of antibacterial preservatives is becoming progressively less common as a need for them is diminished by the increased rapidity with which immunodiffusion reactions are completed, and as realization spreads of the deleterious effects that they may have on antigen–antibody precipitation (Alexander and Moncrief, 1966). Merthiolate (thimerosal) is commonly used at a final concentration of 0.01%, although it has been used at 0.5% (Nelken and Nelken, 1962). At these concentrations it can reduce and delay bacterial contamination but not stop it. It has been observed to prevent antiserum precipitation of three different antigens from bean pod mottle virus (Bancroft, 1962), to alter polio and foot-and-mouth disease virus antigens (Cowan, 1966a), to interfere with immuno-diffusion tests on isometric plant viruses (Koenig, 1970), and to reduce precipitation of tetanus toxoid by human precipitins (Alexander and Moncrief, 1966). Merthiolate may exert these changes by reacting with sulfhydryl groups (Cowan, 1966a), or it could act by adsorption–denaturation (Koenig, 1970). It can dissociate precipitates that already have formed, and it can change antigen electrophoretic mobility (Koenig, 1970). The effects of this preservative depend partly on how it is used. For example, it reduced electrophoretic migration rates when added to agar before the agar was dissolved but did not when added to the already liquefied agar (Jordan and White, 1965). However, for most antigen–antibody systems its effects have been negligible (David-West, 1966).

Sodium azide is another popular preservative which also serves as both electrolyte and pH buffer (Gooding, 1966; Chaparas and Baer, 1964).[47] It is generally used at 0.5%, but has been employed at 0.01 through 2.0% (David-West, 1966). At 2% it delayed precipitation of bovine and sheep serum antigens by rabbit antiserum (David-West, 1966), but it did not otherwise inhibit this system, nor did it affect pre-cipitation of polio or foot-and-mouth disease virus antigens as did Merthiolate (Cowan, 1966a). It has been found to inhibit precipitation of some *Rhizobium melilote* antigens when used at 1% and therefore had to be used at 0.025% for tests with these antigens (Dudman, 1964b). It can interfere with some indicator reactions used to identify antigens in precipitin bands after they have formed (e.g., ceruloplasmin: Weiner *et al.*, 1963).

Other preservatives used in immunodiffusion tests include phenol (add 0.25 ml of melted phenol to 100 ml of agar made with sodium citrate to the desired pH: Schubert *et al.*, 1961), thymol (5 ml of 5% thymol in isopropanol in 1 liter of buffer or agar solution is especially useful to preserve immunoelectrophoresis buffers: Nelson *et al.*, 1964; Kohn, 1961), 0.02% Zephiran (Sarcione and Aungst, 1962), and chloroform (Augustin and Hayward, 1961). Phenol can discolor agar when used with some antigens (Gooding, 1966), can precipitate antiserum lipids (Witter, 1962) and thus obscure specific precipitates or mimic specific precipita-

[47] Another preservative electrolyte is borate (e.g., 0.025 M borax in 0.5% NaCl: Sandor *et al.*, 1967), but borate presents the problem already mentioned above of complexing with polysaccharides.

tion (Wachendörfer, 1965), and can decrease the number of precipitin bands developed by some complex antigen–antibody systems (Ver *et al.*, 1962). The effects of the various other preservatives have not been much investigated, but one may expect that by their nature as preservatives they will affect the integrity of some antigens and interfere occasionally with immunodiffusion tests.

Of the preservatives commonly used, 0.5% sodium azide would appear to be the most innocuous and yet effective, but preservatives should be avoided altogether by performing rapid immunodiffusion tests at 4°C.

Reaction-Enhancing Additives

Antigen–antibody aggregation may be insufficient in an immunodiffusion gel to be visible. Frequently this invisible aggregation can be reinforced to visibility by adding substances to the electrolyte solution which aid in the accumulation and coarsening of antigen–antibody lattices.

At one time certain acid dyes added to agar were thought to have such an enhancing effect, but their activity proved to be due to contamination with Cd^{++} (Crowle, 1960a). Recent tests with purer dyes detected no enhancing effect (Murty and Hanson, 1961); on the other hand, the enhancing effectiveness of cadmium salts used in low concentrations (e.g., 0.05% $CdCl_2$ or 0.03% $CdSO_4$) is now well established (David-West, 1966; Kaminski and Ligouzat, 1964). The potential effectiveness of these ions depends on conditions of the test. Little effect is seen in agar gels naturally contaminated with Cd^{++} or Ni^{++} (Crowle, 1960a), but it will be evident in purified agars and in agaroses. It is more effective with weak antisera than with strong, and with antisera from some animal species (e.g., guinea pigs) more than others (e.g., rabbits: Crowle, 1960a). Useful concentrations are determined partly by the nature of the other electrolytes composing the immunodiffusion buffer. Less will be needed in distilled water, for example, than in barbital buffer (David-West, 1966).

Fewer precipitin bands tend to develop in highly purified, carefully prepared agar gels or in polyacrylamide gels than in gels made from cruder agar. This is due partially in crude agar gels to the presence of dissolved polysaccharides produced by moderate hydrolysis of the agar during its preparation. This natural benefit can be exploited artificially by including appropriate additives in the cleaner gels (Hellsing and Laurent, 1964). Thus, adding such substances as dextran and polyethylene glycol to agar gels greatly increases specific precipitation in some immunodiffusion tests. Dextran of molecular weight 80,000 was used at 4% to enhance precipitation of antigen in antigen excess by rabbit antiserum (Hellsing and Laurent, 1964). Diffusing an 8% solution of 250,000-molecular-weight dextran from the antiserum trough in a developing immunoelectrophero-gram increased precipitin arc resolution and intensity, and it permitted distinguishing antigen isomers from each other (Ceska, 1969a). Poly-ethylene glycol of 20,000 molecular weight was used at 8% as a "chaser" in the antiserum trough following diffusion of the antiserum in immuno-electrophoresis to increase from one to four the precipitin bands formed between a guinea pig antiserum and a pork insulin solution (Ceska, 1969b). Using 0.2% proteose–peptone as a diluent for enterotoxin in-creased the sensitivity of a microimmunodiffusion test for this antigen thirtyfold (Casman et al., 1969).

Additives like dextran are thought to enhance antigen–antibody pre-cipitation by steric exclusion phenomena which depress protein (i.e., antibody) solubility (Ceska, 1969a; Hellsing, 1969). Proteins reacting specifically with antibody can accomplish the same effect. These include coprecipitins and complement (see Chapter 1). They can be added as supplements artificially to an immunodiffusion test, or they may already be present in the reagents being used. Paradoxically, adding complement has been observed also to depress precipitation (Schmidt and Styk, 1968), and the possibility that added coprecipitating antibodies might compete with precipitins must be entertained as well. Detergents like sodium dibutyl naphthalene sulfonate (Leonil SA) used at 0.5% increase the sensitivity of immunodiffusion tests when certain viruses are used as antigens (Hamilton, 1965). Probably they act, as explained below, by dissociating antigens or by preventing them from aggregating spontane-ously during immunodiffusion.

Reactant Modifiers

These are additives that can modify a reactant to facilitate its function-ing in immunodiffusion tests. They may dissociate aggregates of antigen into soluble pieces, prevent spontaneous aggregation of dissolved antigens or of antibodies, or suppress denaturing conformational changes in a re-actant. For instance, deoxyribonucleoproteins which are insoluble in or are precipitated by 0.15 M NaCl can be prepared and tested in 0.1 M glycine using an agar washed to remove potentially precipitating con-taminants (Messineo, 1964). Since antiserum electrolytes also can cause nonspecific precipitation of deoxyribonucleoproteins, an antiserum should be dialyzed against 50 volumes of 0.1 M glycine before being used (Messineo, 1964). Nonspecific precipitation around antiserum and anti-gen wells has been suppressed by using 1 M glycine in agar gels (Casman and Bennett, 1965). This additive probably prevents protein–protein interactions, inhibits spontaneous polymerization (e.g., of immunoglobulins), and stabilizes macromolecules which might otherwise precipitate during an immunodiffusion test (Ragetli and Weintraub, 1964). But since it decreases electrostatic interaction, it also can reduce specific precipitation for some antigen–antibody systems. ϵ-Aminocaproic acid has been used like glycine at 0.1 M during electrophoresis (Taylor and Staprans, 1966), but it too has been observed to inhibit antigen–antibody precipitation from a little at 0.1 M to completely at 1.0 M (Atchley and Bhagavan, 1962). Urea has been added at 3 M to immunodiffusion tests employing conventional buffers to facilitate diffusion of wheat gliadin antigen (Escribano and Grabar, 1966).

Ribosomes can be stabilized for immunodiffusion analyses with a solution of 0.01 M magnesium acetate in 0.01 M tris at pH 7.5 (Quash *et al.*, 1962). Detergents like sodium dodecyl sulfate (0.02%) or sodium dibutyl naphthalene sulfonate (0.5%) promote diffusion of some virus antigens (Hamilton, 1965) and inhibit spontaneous aggregation of immunoglobulins (Wilheim and Lamm, 1966). However, sodium decylsulfate used at 0.04 M to reduce reaggregation of IgG fragments formed a diffuse arc of precipitate close to the antiserum well (Helms and Allen, 1970). Unlike antigen–antibody precipitates, this precipitate was soluble in 0.15 M NaCl and thus could be distinguished in immunodiffusion slides from true antigen–antibody precipitates by washing the slides with saline before final observation.

Miscellaneous Additives

Problems associated with adding chelating agents to immunodiffusion electrolyte solutions have been mentioned above. But there are also advantages. Reactions can be "decomplemented" with minimal risk of denaturing reactants by including 0.01 N EDTA in the solvent (Wollheim and Williams, 1965). Antigens like C-reactive protein which interact with divalent cations like Ca^{++} naturally present in most agars can be protected from such interaction by adding a chelator like citrate (Hokama *et al.*, 1965). These agents are also used (e.g., 0.4% citrate) to reduce nonspecific precipitation of antiserum lipoproteins in agar (Goldin and Glenn, 1964a).

Environmental Conditions for Immunodiffusion Tests

Best results usually are obtained in high humidity and at refrigerator temperature with gels buffered to near-neutral pH (David-West, 1966). But there are exceptions. A controlled drop in humidity can accelerate antigen and antibody diffusion and interaction (cf. Chapter 7), and so can a rise in temperature; carefully regulated lowering of pH can increase immunodiffusion test sensitivity, and high pH values may reveal more antigenic determinants than neutral pH (David-West, 1966).

With rabbit antiserum to bovine and sheep serum antigens, precipitation between pH values of 6.2 and 7.2 did not vary much; at lower values of 4.2 and 5.2 there was no precipitation (David-West, 1966). At a pH of from 8.2 up to 11.2 the number of precipitin bands increased, and they developed more quickly. These are exceptions to the usual observations that optimal precipitation occurs at pH levels between 6.5 and 8.2 (Wedman et al., 1964).

Although risk of nonspecific precipitation is high at a pH of less than 6.5, it is worth taking for some antigen–antibody systems. For example, gastric antigens like pepsin and pepsinogen denature at alkaline pH; hence, they have been studied in double diffusion tests at pH 5.8 (Varandani, 1963).[48] Human gastric mucosal pepsinogens were immunoelectrophoresed at pH 5.6 in a citrate buffer to preserve pepsinogen biological activity (Kushner et al., 1964). Some antibodies, such as heated guinea pig precipitins (Pruzansky and Feinberg, 1962) and sheep precipitins (Lichter, 1967), tend to form soluble precipitates with their antigens at neutral or alkaline pH. Their precipitation of antigen can be detected at pH 5.0 in acetate buffer.

Low temperatures generally increase immunodiffusion test sensitivity because of diminished thermal agitation tending to disrupt antigen–antibody aggregates that are forming. They also diminish chances for undesirable changes either in the test (microbial contamination) or in the reactants (denaturation; enzymatic digestion). A disadvantage to using lower temperatures is slower reaction development, but modern immunodiffusion techniques are rapid enough for this to be an insignificant objection.

For most antigen–antibody systems, precipitin bands will be stronger and better defined, and there will be more of them in multiple systems, when the test is held at 4°C instead of at room or body temperatures (Maurer, 1962; Berg and Egeberg, 1965; McDonald and Duhig, 1965; Wedman et al., 1964; David-West, 1966; Jochim and Chow, 1969; Abbood Al-Hilly, 1969). Some advantages of moderate and low temperature development can be obtained by permitting reactions to develop nearly completely at room temperature and then finishing incubation at 4°C (Damian, 1966), but this maneuver invites development of temperature

[48] At low pH, immunoglobulins tend to aggregate, and they diffuse sluggishly. Consequently, molecular weight estimates for antigens made by precipitin band curvature (see Chapter 4) at low pH tend to be spuriously low.

artifacts. Apparently there are some exceptional antigen–antibody systems which precipitate at room temperature as well as (Dudman, 1964b; Hirschfeld, 1963) or better (Lemcke, 1965) than in the refrigerator.

Reactions developed at different temperatures may be qualitatively or quantitatively different. This is because antigenic specificity is determined partly by the tertiary (three-dimensional) structure of a protein, and this can alter with changes in its environment, including temperature. The antigenic configurations of tobacco mosaic virus thus were found to differ at 2°C, 37°C, and 50°C (Rappaport *et al.*, 1965). By analyzing at different temperatures then, one may be working with antigenically different forms of a single substance. Similar effects are exerted in immunodiffusion tests also by changes in pH, ionic strength, and protein concentration (Rappaport *et al.*, 1965).

Tests with any antigen tending to interact with the immunodiffusion medium or its constituents are especially sensitive to environmental changes. For example, C-reactive protein seems to increase its diffusion rate with rising temperature in saline-constituted agar (Hokama *et al.*, 1965). Because it interacts with Ca^{++}, it diffuses faster also in the presence of a chelating agent like citrate. On the other hand, temperaure-induced changes in its rate of diffusion are less in agar made with citrate than in agar made with glutamate salts.

The incubation time for immunodiffusion tests varies over wide extremes from a few minutes in micro tests at body temperature or in electroimmunodiffusion to several weeks in double or single diffusion tube tests held at 4°C and employing a diffusion-impeding medium like gelatin. It also varies with the intention of a test, for in one instance only a single definite precipitin band need be detected, but in another, development of a maximum number or maximum intensity of bands may be required. Optimal development for maximum number will tend to differ from that for maximum intensity, since resolution begins to decrease as closely situated bands begin to thicken (Omland, 1963a).

Apparatus

Some basic varieties of apparatus are commonly used in several kinds of immunodiffusion test. These will be described here to avoid repetition in later chapters.

Containers and Supports for the Medium

Immunodiffusion media are fragile and delicate; they must be protected from dust and dehydration. Various supports and containers have been devised to satisfy these functions. Gels are cast in glass or plastic tubes ranging from capillary size to large test tubes for single aud double diffusion tube tests, and in various kinds of dishes (e.g., petri dishes),[49] or in specially designed containers for single or double diffusion plate tests. More commonly in recent years, the medium is cast on glass, plastic (e.g., Plexiglas: Jensen, 1965; polystyrene: Goldin and Glenn, 1964a), or film (e.g., cellophane: Correni, 1964; Mylar and Cronar[50]) plates or sheets of various sizes, because plate tests offer improved sensitivity, resolving power, and rapidity. These flat supports are used for electrophoresis, immunoelectrophoresis, and various forms of electroimmunodiffusion. Size variations in these plate supports are large, ranging from microscope slide cover slips to large glass plates several centimeters to the side; usually they are single- or double-width microscope slides or glass photographic projection plates (e.g., 3¼ by 4 inches, or 9 × 9 cm). Cellulose acetate, being a somewhat different medium, can be supported between water-repellent sheets of plastic, suspended in midair by tension at each end of the strip, or laid upon a bed of pins such as the bristles of a nylon hair brush.

All supports or containers for immunodiffusion tests should be inert. Glass vessels to receive a preliminary coating of agar or agarose to promote later adherence to gels of these materials must have oil-free, clean surfaces. Typically, the glass tube or slide is boiled in weak detergent, rinsed several times in distilled water, and finally rinsed in methanol, ethanol, or acetone (Casman et al., 1969). Other cleansing techniques include soaking the slide in dichromate–sulfuric acid cleaning solution, rinsing it in tap water and then in distilled water, and air-drying (Hirschfeld, 1960b); soaking it overnight in 90% ethanol (Murty and Hanson, 1961); or washing it manually with an efficient window cleaner, and then polishing it with lintless cloth. Vigorous methods usually are required, even on so-called "precleaned" microscope slides which have stood in an opened box in laboratory atmosphere for several days. Sometimes these

[49] Convenient little boxes with hinged lids that snap shut and are made of polystyrene are readily available in some countries. They make excellent disposable containers for immunodiffusion tests (Goldin and Glenn, 1964a).

[50] Mylar and Cronar are thin celluloid-like polyester films originally developed for photographic film and magnetic tape. They are sometimes used in place of glass to support immunodiffusion gels because of advantages in handling and storing (Cawley et al., 1965b) and particularly in flexibility (Cawley et al., 1965a; Cawley, 1969). These films satisfy requirements for inertness, and for resistance to staining likely to be used later on an immunodiffusion test, and they can be treated to adhere efficiently to immunodiffusion media (Cawley, 1969). Agarose gels can be cast on such a film, well patterns cut, and the film dried and kept until some later time when it can be rehydrated for use (Marine Colloids Bulletin AG-8-T).

can be freed of their grease film by a 30-second flaming (Hutchison, 1962). A test for adequate cleanliness is to drop some water on the glass. The water should form an even film and not a bead, if the glass is clean.

Agar Coating

This procedure prepares the surface of a glass support or container to adhere firmly to agar gel and prevent capillary leakage of reactants between glass and agar surfaces. When used on a plate or slide, it also serves to hold the gel to the support through washing and staining procedures. Polyester films can be coated like glass (Cawley, 1969), but plastics like polystyrene and Plexiglas cannot because they are hydrophobic. This is an inconvenience in washing and staining, but because of their hydrophobic properties these plastics usually present no problem of reactants seeping between them and agar surfaces during an immunodiffusion test.

The coating is applied by dipping the warmed, clean glassware in hot 0.2% agar or agarose solution in distilled water (concentrations as high as 2.0% have been used: Potter and Kuff, 1961), or filling and emptying the tube or other container with hot agar solution, draining, and air-drying, drying in a hot-air oven (Adamson and Cozad, 1966; Morton and Dodge, 1963), or drying on a hot plate (Potter and Kuff, 1961). Alternatively, one can brush hot agar solution onto the surface of a slide with a brush, piece of cotton, gauze, or similar material (Casman *et al.*, 1969). Excellent, even, and effective coating is obtained by spraying the surface of the slide with boiling hot agar solution using an atomizer, and then drying it at 60° to 80°C (Adamson and Cozad, 1966; Crowle, unpublished work). The substance used for coating should be the same as that used to make the gel; that is, agarose should be used for agarose, and the same kind of agar should be used for both coating and casting.[51]

Casting the Gel

Agar and agarose gels are cast in many shapes and forms. Space would be wasted in describing these here (see the first edition of this book for illustration of the many varieties). Instead, some basic generalities will be discussed.

For best results the agar solution should be boiling hot when it is poured. If it must be cooled, in order to add a labile ingredient like antiserum, then the casting container or support should be warmed to a

[51] Acrylamide gels do not appear to require precoating of their containers or supports (cf. Frederick, 1964).

temperature above that of the gelling point of the type of gel being used. The pipet or syringe to be used for transferring the agar solution should also be warmed by pumping hot water, or the hot agar solution itself, up and down in it several times.

For some varieties of casting, leveling the container or support is not necessary because a flat, uniformly thick slab will be produced automatically by the apparatus, or because a level surface is unimportant. But leveling is important in casting agar in a petri dish, or on an uncovered microscope slide. This is effected in one of three convenient ways. One is to support the solidifying gel on a platform leveled with adjustable screws. A second is to pour agar into a pan, let this gel into a level surface, and then use this as a support for the casting vessel. Of course, the pan of agar must not be moved away from its original location on the workbench. A third way is to use mercury as a support, floating the casting vessel or a platform for it (a wooden platform can be floated on less dense and dangerous fluids like water) on the surface of the mercury.

When agar is being cast in a tube there will be a curved meniscus between it and a second layer which one may wish to cast on top of the first. Practically, this is rarely of any consequence because of the thinness of the ascending edges of the meniscus relative to the width of the rest of the interface. However, if a flat interface is required, it can be prepared with specially designed casting apparatus (Polson, 1958).

In today's increasingly frequent use of glass plates and slides for all varieties of immunodiffusion test, a premium is placed on obtaining a flat, thin, uniform casting of the gel. An easy way to do this, regardless of the size of the plate to be used, is as follows (see Fig. 2.4; Crowle, 1972).

Prepare two plates, one cleaned rigorously and agar-coated as mentioned above, and the other coated thinly with a silicone (e.g., polished with a silicone-containing grease).[52] The agar-coated slide is laid upon supports, such as applicator sticks, to raise it a little from the workbench; no leveling is needed. At each corner of this slide is placed a small spacer (e.g., a 3 × 3-mm square of 0.5-mm-thick polyethylene). The siliconized plate is laid upon these spacers slightly offset from the edge of the lower slide, and hot agar is pipetted between the two along this offset edge. Before the agar gels, the top slide is nudged back square with the lower slide. The agar gels quickly. After it has gelled, the sandwich of the two slides with agar gel between them is transferred to a refrigerator for 5 minutes or more to harden the gel. Then it is removed, and the siliconized

---

[52] A rigid plate of water-repellent plastic (e.g., Plexiglas) can be substituted, but it should have an unscratched surface.

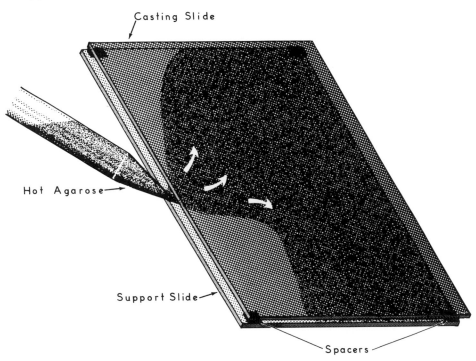

Casting Slide

Hot Agarose

Support Slide

Spacers

Fig. 2.4. Sandwich method of casting a thin, uniform layer of agarose on a glass plate, usually a single- or double-width microscope slide. Four corner spacers govern the thickness of the gel. The lower support slide previousy has been agarose-coated (see text) so that the cast gel will adhere to it well; the upper casting slide has not been pretreated. After the cast agarose solution has gelled and has been cooled, preferably at 4°C, the casting slide can be slid off its surface and the gel used for whatever kind of immunodiffusion test it has been prepared for.

slide is carefully lifted or slid from the surface of the gel. The resulting very uniform slab of agar subsequently can be used for conventional immunodiffusion tests with holes punched in it, with Plexiglas templates laid upon it for highly sensitive microimmunodiffusion tests, for electrophoresis and immunoelectrophoresis, or for various forms of electroimmunodiffusion. Its use for these various techniques will be described more fully in later chapters. Similar uniformly flat slabs can be cast with a three-sided spacer clamped between glass slides (James *et al.*, 1966), and essentially the same technique is used for agar–acrylamide castings (Uriel, 1966) and for sufficiently stiff gels of polyacrylamide alone.

As was mentioned earlier, a nearly infinite array of reactant arrangements is possible for immunodiffusion tests. Molds, cutters, cutting templates, and gels preformed in several useful patterns are available commercially. Sometimes it is not possible to find one that satisfies some special purpose, or one may wish to prepare his own test patterns. There is an increasing tendency to use reactant-holding or reactant-placing templates because of the uniformity of results that these offer, because of the generally greater sensitivity of tests employing them, because in their use the surface of the gel is not broken, and because they both feed reactants into the gel and also prevent its dehydration. Many of the simpler varieties can be made from sheets of Plexiglas or similar plastic with a small saw and drills (Crowle, 1958), but more complex templates, especially those with troughs in addition to holes, are more difficult to make by machining. The reader therefore is referred to the paper of Van Orden (1968) which describes a simple and inexpensive technique for casting templates themselves with dental acrylic resin using 4% agar gel as a casting pattern and laundry soap as a casting form.

Applying Reactants

There are three principal ways in which reactants can be applied to immunodiffusion medium: by migration from wells cut or cast in thicker medium, by migration from deposits on the surface of thin medium, or by mixing with the medium before it is cast.

WELLS AND TROUGHS

The first method—charging wells or troughs formed in the gel—has been the most popular. If the well is to be cut, then its bottom should be sealed with a drop of the same medium (e.g., hot agar solution) to prevent reactant from seeping between gelled medium and its container or support. This precaution may not be necessary for wells 2 mm or less in diameter. If holes are to be cast, then a primary layer of gel should be poured both to support the hole-making forms evenly and to provide the cast holes with sealed bottoms. Holes to be cut in the agar can be made with many different kinds of cutters. Empty .22-caliber firearm cartridges have been used (Wright and Stace-Smith, 1966). Corkborers, and hypodermic needles cut and sharpened like a corkborer, are frequently employed. For small holes a capillary tube with squared-off tip will do. Maximum pattern reproducibility and convenience are obtained with a cutting guide (Mansi, 1958; Sandor et al., 1967), or one of the several mechanical improvements on such devices, either purchased from a commercial supplier or specially prepared (cf. Hackl, 1962; Neuzil and Masseyeff, 1959; Piazzi, 1969; Weeke and Thomsen, 1968). Troughs, such as are needed for immunoelectrophoresis, can be cut along a straightedge or similar guide using two razor blades taped on either side of a spacer the width of the trough required, but better placement and more uniformity are attained by using a "punch" made to cut an entire trough length in one motion. One can be made by embedding two razor blades with an appropriate spacer between them in a holder of cork. Cutters marketed for this purpose by several suppliers provide excellent uniformity and, though expensive, are usually worth purchasing if large numbers of one kind of test are to be performed. Holes cut or cast in immunodiffusion medium should be charged evenly (e.g., level with the surface). A large well can be charged level with the surface using a reduced volume of reactant by placing a space-occupier (e.g., glass or aluminum plug) in it (Feinberg, 1956).

Casting wells and troughs has lost much of the popularity that it enjoyed when macro immunodiffusion tests were the most commonly employed because it is slow and difficult, and because gel around the casting forms is not flat. Wells and troughs therefore currently are nearly always cut.

SURFACE CHARGING

The simplest and most efficient technique for delivering reactants into immunodiffusion media is to deposit them on the surface and let them diffuse in. For example, a square of Plexiglas with a pattern of wells drilled through it is slid or laid on a flat, thin slab of agar gel or polyacrylamide, and the wells are charged with volumes of reactant that are quite large relative to the thickness of the agar gel (Fig. 2.5). Alternatively, the gel is covered with a template of water-impermeable plastic, like Saran Wrap, with holes punched in it, and a droplet of reactant is placed on the gel over each of these. Still more simply, droplets can be laid directly on the bare surface of the medium (cellulose acetate: Grabner *et al.*, 1968; Rabinowitz, 1964; Feinberg *et al.*, 1965; Vergani *et al.*, 1967; gelatin: Crowle and Hu, 1967), or pieces of paper impregnated with reactant can be distributed to appropriate positions on the gel (Hamilton, 1965) or inserted into slits cut in the gel (Hermans *et al.*, 1960). For all these methods of surface application, the gel surface should

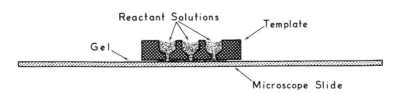

Fig. 2.5. Cross-sectional diagram showing how a Plexiglas template feeds large volumes of reactant into the relatively very thin layer of reaction gel on a microscope slide in a micro double diffusion plate test.

be free of excess moisture. A convenient way to remove moisture is by gentle wiping with a razor blade (Hermans *et al.*, 1960), or the gel can be exposed to room atmosphere to evaporate excess water. Cellulose acetate strips can be impregnated with antiserum by spraying the antiserum onto the strip and then rubbing the surface gently with a glass rod to ensure even distribution (Vergani *et al.*, 1967). Agar and agarose can be charged similarly, or by applying suitable volume to the surface as a drop of fluid and rubbing it in with a glass rod (Afonso, 1966b) or rolling it in with a glass tube (Firestone and Aronson, 1969). Such a drop also can be spread evenly by capillary attraction under the cover of a glass plate or sheet of plastic (Crowle, 1972; Fig. 2.6; cf. also single electroimmunodiffusion, Chapter 6).

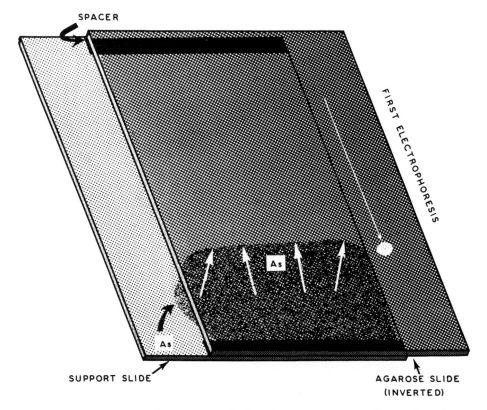

Fig. 2.6. Diagram indicating method of applying antiserum evenly to gels such as are used for single diffusion or electroimmunodiffusion tests. Here antiserum is being applied to a portion of agarose on a double-width microscope slide into which a mixture of antigens already separated in first electrophoresis will be electrophoresed in the second step of two-dimensional single electroimmunodiffusion (cf. Chapter 6).

Direct Mixing

This technique is self-explanatory. Reactant is mixed with liquid medium, and the mixture is cast into or on a suitable container, gelling the reactant within the medium. Agar or agarose must first be dissolved with heat, and then their solutions cooled and the reactant solution warmed to a temperature low enough to minimize reactant denaturation but warm enough to prevent gelling. Polyacrylamide and gelatin can be mixed with reactants and gelled at room temperature or lower.

Delivering Reactants

For the several micro techniques now commonly used, reactants are delivered most conveniently with a small glass syringe and attached 26-gauge needle that has been bent and had its tip filed square, with a Pasteur pipet and rubber bulb, or with a short length of capillary tubing alone. The latter is dipped into reactant which is drawn into it by capillary attraction; then its tip is touched to the well which is to receive the reactant, which in turn draws the fluid out of the tube in proportion to the angle at which the tube is held. Small volumes of reactant can be applied uniformly to the surface of a thin medium by touching the surface with the tip of a bacteriologic inoculating needle which has been dipped into the reactant solution.

Developing the Reactions

Immunodiffusion reactions may take from a few minutes to several weeks to develop. The principal problems to avoid during this time are dehydration, contamination with bacterial growth, and development of temperature artifacts. The second and third problems already have been discussed. The first, dehydration, ranges from being insignificant in short-term reaction development within thick gels, to being severe in prolonged reaction development within thin gels or cellulose acetate. Dehydration also can be considerable in immunodiffusion tests involving electrophoresis (e.g., electroimmunodiffusion) because of heat developed by the electric current.

Drying during electrophoresis, which may be prolonged overnight for some tests, is sometimes avoided by immersing the developing electropherogram in an inert fluid like petroleum ether which both prevents dehydration and, by its own evaporation, keeps the electropherogram cool (Wieme, 1959). However, this procedure is both troublesome and potentially dangerous because of the explosion hazard of the petroleum ether. Another somewhat safer though less efficient technique is to enclose the electropherogram within a humidified chamber during electrophoresis, and also to turn it upside down (cf. Fig. 5.9). This method suffices for nearly all occasions not involving high-voltage electrophoresis. Additional protection against dehydration can be obtained by laying a sheet of Saran Wrap upon the surface of the gel.

For immunodiffusion tests that develop simply by diffusion, dehydration is adequately suppressed by keeping the gel in humid atmosphere. For example, microscope slide immunodiffusion tests can be enclosed in a petri dish containing a disc of filter paper, a piece of gauze, or sponges saturated with water. Incubating the immunodiffusion test upside down provides added protection against drying. Incidentally, dehydration occurring during a test can influence both the speed of its development and the sensitivity, for partially dehydrated gel draws the reactants into it faster than they would enter by diffusion alone (cf. immunorheophoresis, Chapter 7).

Occasionally, such as for time-lapse photography, it is not practical to humidify the immunodiffusion chamber in an ordinary manner or to keep it cool to encourage maintaining its moist state; or the medium may be so sensitive to dehydration (e.g., cellulose acetate) that the methods described above are inadequate. Then it can be submerged in an inert liquid like mineral oil.[53] A preservative like cresol (0.2 ml of 5% solution dissolved in ether added to 100 ml of oil: Agostoni et al., 1967) or toluene (0.1%) should be added as an antiseptic. Although glycerin has been recommended for preventing dehydration in place of mineral oil (James et al., 1966), it may not be inert toward antigen–antibody precipitation. After a test, mineral oil can be removed from the surface of gels easily with a volatile solvent like petroleum ether, heptane, toluene, or ether. For cellulose acetate, only solvents that do not affect the membrane should be used, or the membrane can be washed briefly with detergent (Kohn, 1971).

Reaction Enhancement

There are many ways to enhance immunodiffusion reactions and make them easier to read and, frequently, to obtain data from what otherwise might seem to be reactionless tests. The following are some examples.

---

[53] Some workers object to immersing cellulose acetate in mineral oil because it may interfere with later washing and staining (Rabinowitz, 1964). There are devices especially made to maintain adequate cellulose acetate humidity without mineral oil (Monier, 1963).

Antiserum Modification

This was mentioned earlier relative to preparing and concentrating antibodies. Certain antisera (e.g., rabbit but not horse) precipitate antigen better when treated with ninhydrin or sodium β-naphthoquinone-4-sulfonate (Tayeau and Jouzier, 1961a). One percent ninhydrin in physiologic saline is mixed with an equal volume of antiserum and allowed to stand for 0.5 hour at 37°C.

Application of the Reactants

The way in which reactants, especially antiserum, are used in an immunodiffusion test considerably affects sensitivity. Maximum sensitivity results when enough antigen and antibody mix to form a visible precipitate (see Chapter 1). Using templates with funnel-like feeding of much reactant into a thin gel is very effective (Crowle and Lueker, 1961; cf. Fig. 2.5). Moving reactants against each other rapidly and wholly by electrophoresis, as in two-dimensional electroimmunodiffusion, accomplishes the same end by preventing loss of reactant by diffusion (see Chapter 6). Special containers have been invented to do the same (Crowle, 1961; Smith, 1960). Taking care to recognize possible development of concentration artifacts, one can charge reactant sources repeatedly to "build" visible precipitates when none previously were evident. For instance, in macro double diffusion, wells were charged once daily for three consecutive days, filter paper being used to remove residual fluid from wells before each recharging (Schenberg, 1963). Micro tests were recharged similarly, but at intervals of only 2 hours. Alternatively, antiserum wells can be charged with concentrated antibody, such as a pellet of ethanol-precipitated immunoglobulin, for a twenty-fold increase in sensitivity (Smith, 1967), or with a thick paste of concentrated immunoglobulin (Castro and Fairbairn, 1969).

Steric Exclusion

Already mentioned as a problem in composing electrolytes used for immunodiffusion, this effect also can be helpful: using 2% dextran of 10,000 molecular weight in agar produced a "dramatic sharpening of all immunoprecipitin lines" in immunoelectropherograms (Ceska and Grossmüller, 1968). Infusing 20,000-molecular-weight polyethylene glycol into a developed reaction area from the trough of an immunoelectropherogram (Ceska, 1969b) causes similar enhancement and presumably would do the same if used in wells of a double diffusion test, or if employed to flood the surface of any immunodiffusogram. Sensitivity of the double diffusion test has been increased significantly by using 6000-molecular-weight polyethylene glycol at concentrations up to 4% in agar gel (Harrington *et al.*, 1971).

Protein Denaturants

Used carefully, any condition or chemical that will precipitate proteins also can enhance specific antigen–antibody precipitation without causing undue nonspecific precipitation. This enhancement need be no more than antigen–antibody aggregate fixation within an immunodiffusion medium, so that, although the aggregate may remain invisible, it nevertheless can be detected later by staining. Hence, staining procedures themselves can be considered as enhancers of immunodiffusion reactions (Crowle, 1961; Rümke and Breekveldt-Kielich, 1969).

The discs of radial single diffusion tests can be intensified for better reading by flooding them with 5% acetic acid for 1 to 3 minutes, pouring off the excess, and blotting up the residue; table vinegar can be used as a readily available substitute (Kaufman, 1970). If the plate is to be processed for staining, it should be washed as soon as possible with a strong neutral buffer (e.g., physiologic phosphate buffer of pH 7.4) to reverse generalized nonspecific protein precipitation which also has begun. One percent tannic acid has been used similarly (Alpert *et al.*, 1970). Two- to tenfold enhancement is achieved in 10 to 15 minutes after flooding the single diffusion plates with this acid; longer treatment makes the agar opaque. Double diffusion plates (Wallraff *et al.*, 1965) and immunoelectropherograms (Afonso, 1964a) have been enhanced by washing them first with saline to remove nonprecipitated serum proteins and then soaking them in 1 to 2% acetic acid until a faint cloudiness begins to appear around the antiserum source. Residual acetic acid should be washed away with water. To photograph a faint precipitate, one can intensify it with acid alcohol (3% HCl in 95% ethanol) and photograph the band when nonspecific precipitation just begins to appear (Cuadrado, 1966).

Antigen–antibody precipitation can be intensified by soaking the gel in 10% formalin in physiologic saline (Nász *et al.*, 1967). Washing away nonprecipitated proteins and subsequently fixing aggregates with 5% mercuric chloride in 2% acetic acid both enhances sensitivity and prepares precipitin bands for better staining (Radola, 1960a,b). Soaking an immunodiffusogram in 1% cadmium acetate or mercuric chloride can enhance developing reactions and can shorten incubation time from 3 days to 24 hours (Casman *et al.*, 1969). Immunoelectropherograms can be intensified by first washing them and then exposing them to 1% tannic acid for 24 hours (Cawley, 1969).

Using any of these denaturants may preclude later use of certain analytic tests on the nature of antigen being precipitated, if such tests depend on a biological activity which is injured by the denaturant (Cawley, 1969).

Semispecific Precipitation Enhancement

Some chemicals have particular affinity for portions of antibody molecules and react with these to stabilize and intensify antigen–antibody precipitation. Cadmium and nickel, for example, react with antibody lipids (Crowle, 1960a, 1961). Soluble salts of these cations incorporated in the medium often enhance a reaction during its development. More often, they are applied as weak solutions after antigen and antibody have reacted (David-West, 1966; Kristoffersen, 1969; Balayan, 1960; Fink *et al.*, 1969; Long and Top, 1964; Smith and Shattock, 1964; Romanovsky, 1964; Steigerwald *et al.*, 1960). Typically, immunodiffusograms are flooded at the end of incubation with a solution of 0.03% cadmium sulfate (David-West, 1966), 0.0125% cadmium chloride (Smith and Shattock, 1964), 0.0125% cadmium acetate (Kristoffersen, 1969), or 0.025% cadmium nitrate (Long and Top, 1964). Barbital ions resemble Cd^{++} and Ni^{++} in precipitating proteins by way of attached lipids. This probably is why tests in barbital buffers tend to be more sensitive than similar tests performed in other buffers (Crowle, 1961). Barbital enhancement also can be used after reaction development: monkey antiserum and Rauscher leukemia virus precipitates were enhanced by soaking immunodiffusograms initially developed with physiologic saline in a barbital buffer for 10 minutes (Fink and Cowles, 1965). As indicated in the section above, using an immunodiffusion buffer that decreases reactant solubility will intensify antigen–antibody precipitation. For example, guinea pig precipitating antisera converted to inability to precipitate by heating at 56°C for 30 minutes could be made to precipitate antigen in immunodiffusion tests by utilizing pH 5.0 low ionic strength buffer (Pruzansky and Feinberg, 1962).

Specific Enhancement

Since much of a precipitin band is antibody (see Chapter 1), it should be possible to make a faint or invisible band stronger and readily visible by increasing the bulk of antigen–antibody aggregate using antibody against the antibody in the aggregate. Radial single diffusion precipitation tests were enhanced two- to fourfold by diffusing sheep antibody to rabbit γ-globulin into the surface of agar in which reactions between antigen and rabbit antiserum had taken place (Rümke and Breekveldt-Kielich, 1969). Some slight additional enhancement was obtained by following this in turn with an infusion of guinea pig antiserum to sheep immunoglobulin (cf. also Rümke and Breekveldt-Kielich, 1969). Double diffusion tests also have been enhanced in this manner (Nace, 1963).

Use of Special Immunodiffusion Techniques

Several methods of arranging reactants in immunodiffusion tests or of moving them about in the medium provide enhanced sensitivity. Most of these will be discussed in connection with the major varieties of technique in later chapters, but an illustrative example is that of placing a solution of antigen too weak to precipitate with antiserum near the tip of a reference precipitin band forming between the same antigen in higher concentration and its antiserum. This causes the tip of the forming precipitin band to bend, an effect readily visible but exerted by a quantity of reactant which is insufficient alone to produce a visible precipitate (Deckers, 1967).

Nonspecific Precipitation in Immunodiffusion Tests

This frequent problem of interpretation has no ready solution. It arises whenever precipitation develops that is not due directly to aggregation of antigen by antibody. Some nonspecific precipitates are readily identified, but even yet are not adequately explained. The following are some examples of nonspecific precipitation.

Protein–Protein Interactions

Reactions like those of antigen with antibody have been observed between other components of antiserum and antigen, as follows: erythrocyte constituents and nerve tissue extracts (Kubes, 1965); histones and DNA (Seligmann, 1959); albumin and hemoglobin (Anderson et al., 1962b; Wilson and Warren, 1962; Kagen, 1965; Harris and Fairley, 1962); unknown and prostatic fluid (Barnes et al., 1963), basic proteins (lysozyme?), acidic Bacillus anthracis polypeptide (Leonard and Thorne, 1961); α-globulin and trypsin or chymotrypsin in intestinal secretions (Brown, 1971); α_1-lipoprotein in sera from tuberculosis or lung carcinoma patients and constituent of Old Tuberculin (Murray and Blumberg, 1965); γ_1-globulin and pancreas extract (Fodor et al., 1962) as well as a β-globulin from erythrocyte lysates (Jenkins and Pepys, 1965); a substance in hen's serum associated with egg laying and a normal component of cock or nonlaying hen serum (Petrovský and Slavíková, 1970); acid proteins and histones from cell nuclei (Black *et al.*, 1962) and other basic tissue antigens (Berenbaum *et al.*, 1962); haptoglobin and hemoglobin (Seligmann, 1961); a γ_2 rat serum globulin and unknown components of some normal rat sera and rat tissue, either normal or tumor (Deckers and Maisin, 1963); and proteins and detergents in tissue extracts (D'Amelio *et al.*, 1963a).

The reaction between human serum albumin and hemoglobin is both interesting and typical of the vexing problems associated with understanding of nonspecific precipitation. The albumin displaces globin from methemoglobin and forms methemalbumin; the globin is denatured in the presence of agar and precipitates (Harris and Fairley, 1962). This may occur quite unexpectedly, such as in reacting a rabbit antiserum to human serum with human serum when the antiserum has previously been absorbed with a suspension of cells to make it more specific, and these have included erythrocytes. Globin precipitation occurs in agar gel but not in liquid medium or gelatin gels, and it does not occur in agar gels at 4°C (Wilson and Warren, 1962; Kagen, 1965; Seligmann, 1961). A reaction such as is seen between normal nonlaying chicken sera and a component of laying hen's serum (Petrovský and Slavíková, 1970) is likely to be confusing in allotyping experiments. Reactions between the mostly acid proteins of antisera and basic proteins of various antigen preparations, or even between such basic proteins of antiserum as lysozyme and acid proteins of antigen solutions, probably have been relatively rare in most immunodiffusion tests as performed in the past, since they generally have employed agar. This is because agar itself is acidic and restricts diffusion of molecules with net positive charges (i.e., basic). But with agarose and polyacrylamide growing in popularity as media for these immunodiffusion tests, encounters with nonspecific precipitation due to protein–protein (or acid–base) interactions will undoubtedly become more frequent, as demonstrated by the precipitation of antiserum α-globulin by intestinal secretion trypsin or chymotrypsin (Brown, 1971). Special awareness of this problem also will be necessary when, for instance, detergent-dissociated tissue extracts are to be studied; either detergent (D'Amelio *et al.*, 1963a) or tissue protein (Black *et al.*, 1962) can precipitate nonantibody acidic proteins of the antiserum. Special buffer components may create the same problem (Quash *et al.*, 1962).

Unfortunately, arbitrary tests for distinguishing between nonspecific precipitations and specific antigen–antibody precipitation are not always reliable. For example, the serum lysozyme–acid protein reaction mentioned above (Leonard and Thorne, 1961) is strongest in medium made with distilled water and decreases with increasing salt concentration; but as was pointed out previously, certain antigen–antibody systems exhibit the same property. The reaction between human serum and hemoglobin occurs in agar but not in aqueous medium or gelatin and does not develop at 4°C; but the same is true of some antigen–antibody systems (e.g., those involving polysaccharide antigens). Additional criteria for distinguishing specific from nonspecific precipitation therefore are helpful. They will be discussed below.

Other Forms of Nonspecific Precipitations

Serum, antiserum, and tissue lipids, immunoglobulins, and lipoproteins tend to precipitate spontaneously in agar gels (less in agarose: Burstein and Fine, 1964b; Teichmann and Vogt, 1964; Burtin and Gendron, 1971) and sometimes also with normal serum constituents (Niedieck, 1967). Some of these precipitations are pH-dependent (i.e., electrostatic reactions: Niedieck, 1967), and agar gels contain a factor which precipitates serum proteins at acid pH with maximal precipitation at pH 5 (Zwaan, 1963; cf. also Brishammar et al., 1961). Agaropectin in agar was implicated in precipitation of human immunoglobin (Burtin and Gendron, 1971). Antigens prepared in phosphate buffers may develop precipitates owing to complexing of calcium in agar with phosphate in the buffer (Feinberg and Temple, 1962). The presence or absence of calcium in immunodiffusion medium also more specifically affects certain antigens: C-reactive protein may be precipitated, or its diffusion rate may be depressed (Hokama et al., 1965).[54] Bee venom phospholipase diffusing against antiserum lipoproteins may cleave these into soluble proteins and precipitating lipids (Barker et al., 1966). A similar effect occurs between an antiserum and serum from patients with acanthocystosis who suffer β-lipoprotein deficiency; apparently like bee venom their sera contain a phospholipase, too (Murray and Blumberg, 1965). Gamma-globulin complexes that are present in a reactant, whether the result of aggregation by antigen or not, may combine with and precipitate complement diffusing from another reactant source (Winchester et al., 1969). Antigen can be bound to certain constituents of stomach fluids, thus leading erroneously to the conclusion that these fluids contain antibodies (Kraft et al., 1970).

---

[54] Protein–protein interactions which occur naturally (e.g., between serum albumin, as a carrier, and various other substances) may affect electrophoretic mobility, enzyme reactions, diffusion coefficient measurements, and similar aspects of tests (Jacotot et al., 1965; Priolisi and Giuffré, 1965; Raymond and Nakamichi, 1962b; Lang and Hoeffgen, 1963). Protein–protein complexes can dissociate during electrophoresis and later produce perplexing results because of new reassociations.

Because many sera contain C-reactive protein, especially after some "stress" to the donor of the sera, and C substance is found widely in nature, this nonimmunologic precipitating system is a frequent source of confusion. C polysaccharide occurs, for instance, in various helminths, several species of *Aspergillus* mold, some of the dermatophytes, and several bacteria (Biguet *et al.*, 1965a). Antiserum from patients infected with microorganisms making C substance therefore cannot be considered, on reacting with extracts of these microorganisms, necessarily to be making specific antibodies to them.

False "Nonspecific Precipitation"

Although the usual error is to misinterpret nonspecific precipitation as specific precipitation, the opposite important mistake also can be made. For example, isoprecipitins in human sera which react to precipitate antigens like those of the Ag and Lp serum-type systems have been detected by serum–serum interactions and would have been overlooked if simply attributed to nonspecific precipitation (Berg, 1965a). Precipitation of a single band with two kinds of enzymatic activity might be thought of by this apparent nonspecificity not to involve antibodies, when in reality antibody can be precipitating a common carrier antigen with two different kinds of enzyme attached to it (Lang and Hoeffgen, 1963).

Tests for Nonspecific Precipitation

No one test is foolproof; several should be used. Perhaps the best combination is to show that the precipitate contains a large proportion of immunoglobulin, that this will precipitate "antigen" only when derived from an animal or man previously exposed to the antigen, and that its titer in the "antiserum" waxes and wanes according to the antiserum-maker's intensity and frequency of exposure to the antigen. The presence of immunoglobulin in the precipitate does not alone identify specific precipitation, since some substances have natural affinity for immunoglobulins. *Staphylococcus aureus* protein A, for instance, has a high affinity for γ-globulin and precipitates this regardless of whether it is an antibody to the A protein (Forsgren and Sjöquist, 1966). A normal human sweat prealbumin precipitates normal human serum γ-globulin (Page and Remington, 1967).

Although the presence of γ-globulin in a precipitate therefore does not necessarily prove that it is an antigen–antibody precipitate, its absence probably proves that it is not an antigen–antibody precipitate. A sensitive test for this is to observe whether the precipitate will take up a heterologous antibody to the antibody which it is supposed to contain (labeled with radioactivity, fluorescence, or in some other obvious way: Okubo, 1965); whether the presence of such an antibody can interfere with development of the precipitate (by complexing with the immunoglobulin: Murray and Blumberg, 1965); whether the precipitating substance in the "antiserum" has a γ-globulin electrophoretic mobility (e.g., by reversed immunoelectrophoresis: Dufour and Tremblay, 1964; Barker *et al.*, 1966; see Chapter 5); or, for some systems in which the precipitate is primarily lipid (e.g., phospholipase–lipoprotein interaction), whether the precipitin band has any protein in it at all (Murray and Blumberg, 1965).

Other arbitrary tests have been useful for certain systems. Hemoglobin–serum albumin reactions fail to develop at pH values above 8.2, whereas antigen–antibody precipitation is not inhibited until higher pH values are reached (Seligmann, 1963). Precipitates of C-reactive protein and C substance generally dissolve in 5% trisodium citrate, but antigen–antibody precipitates do not (Biguet *et al.*, 1965b). Calcium phosphate precipitates dissolve in 5% sodium citrate (Feinberg and Temple, 1962). Nonspecific precipitates like those between serum and hemoglobin (Kagen, 1965), between basic tissue constituents and acidic serum proteins (Berenbaum *et al.*, 1962), between histones and DNA (Seligmann, 1961), and between chicken antiserum and agar gel (Orlans *et al.*, 1961) tend to form better at 0.01 to 0.10 M NaCl concentrations and either do not form or are unstable in higher concentrations of NaCl. Precipitation between basic tissue components and acidic serum proteins was absent at 2% NaCl; the hemoglobin–serum precipitate did not form at 5 M NaCl; chicken antiserum ceased to form a ring of nonspecific precipitate in agar gel at 3% NaCl. These concentrations usually do not interfere with antigen–antibody precipitation in agar gels; but sometimes they can, as has been discussed before, and so these arbitrary tests can only be considered as suggestive. Nonspecific precipitation developing between prostatic fluid and normal human or rabbit serum could be washed from double diffusion plates by a soaking with pH 7.2 phosphate buffer followed by prolonged soaking in unbuffered physiologic saline (Barnes *et al.*, 1963).

If a precipitate has been observed to form between antiserum and a tissue extract and there is question as to whether it is due to antibodies in the antiserum, the antiserum can be boiled and then should no longer precipitate the tissue extract. Any antiserum "precipitin" surviving this test probably is not antibody (Deckers and Maisin, 1963). Occasionally nonspecific precipitation can be avoided fortuitously: the use of 0.1% sodium azide in agar gel prevented hemoglobin–serum precipitation (Anderson *et al.*, 1962b).

A somewhat more specific test for distinguishing antigen–antibody precipitation from nonspecific precipitate is especially useful when one is testing miscellaneous substances for the antigen, and when these miscellaneous substances are likely to contain nonspecific precipitins (e.g., testing for staphylococcal enterotoxin: Casman and Bennett, 1965). The unknown should be placed in a well adjacent to a well charged with known antigen; any precipitation occurring between the unknown and antiserum is likely to be specific if the precipitin band coalesces with the band forming simultaneously between the antiserum and the known antigen (see reaction of identity, discussed in Chapter 4). Of course, comparable methods for determining the antigenic specificity of a precipitin band, such as absorption of antibodies by antigen, would have comparable meaning.

Washing and Staining Immunodiffusion Patterns

After antigen–antibody precipitation has taken place in an immunodiffusion test, techniques more or less akin to, and often developed from, histochemical procedures can be used for such purposes as preserving an original record of the test, facilitating examination of the results, and increasing information output (Uriel, 1958). Now that immunodiffusion tests are performed more often on small glass slides than in petri dishes or tubes, it is a common practice to wash the slide, and then stain, dry, and preserve it like a histological specimen. The staining procedure can be selected to enhance distinction of precipitin bands from their background, making both observation and photography simpler and better. Any of many indicator tests can be applied to analyze a precipitin band for the kind of antigen it contains. Formulas for the most generally useful stains and indicators are given in Appendixes V through IX. The following paragraphs provide descriptions of general washing and staining techniques and references to the literature for less frequently used stains and indicators.

Preparation for Staining

The purpose of washing an immunodiffusogram nearly always is to prepare it for applying a stain or indicator.[55] Its primary intention is to remove nonprecipitated constituents of antigen and antiserum solutions without either dissociating antigen–antibody precipitates or deleteriously altering such constituents as enzymes to be detected by their activity with some substrate. Washing may have the secondary purposes of enhancing

[55] An exception would be preparative immunodiffusion in which the antigen–antibody precipitate is to be used for some supplemental purpose after the washing.

or accentuating either antigen–antibody precipitation itself or reaction of antigen–antibody precipitates with indicator substances.

Washing may be followed directly by staining, or the washed immuno-diffusogram may be dried and then stained. The former is preferable when the immunodiffusion medium is no more than 0.5 mm thick, or when drying may injure the activity (e.g., enzymatic) of an antigen that is necessary for its detection (Uriel, 1958). The latter is better for a thicker medium, when the indicator procedure requires placing the im-munodiffusogram in contact with another object like a photographic emulsion in radioautography, or when a wet medium is incompatible with an indicator procedure such as coloration for lipids (Uriel, 1958). If washing is to be followed immediately by staining, then the first opera-tion of the staining should be preceded by soaking the immunodiffuso-gram in the staining solvent (e.g., 2% acetic acid if one is to use acid dye dissolved in 2% acetic acid). If the slide or plate is to be dried first (Cawley et al., 1965b), then salts of the washing buffer must be removed before or during the drying procedure.

Washing Procedures

Wash baths must be capable of leaching nonprecipitated constituents of antiserum and antigen solutions from the reaction gel. Since some constituents of antiserum, such as the euglobulins, are insoluble in dis-tilled water, the wash bath usually is physiologic saline, and frequently it is buffered to a slightly alkaline pH of from 7.4 to 8.2. This is because most antiserum constituents have isoelectric pH of 7 or lower and will be more soluble in such a buffer than in unbuffered saline, which tends to be acid because of atmospheric carbon dioxide. Occasionally, wash baths of different composition may be required. For instance, baths of high NaCl concentration tend to remove nonspecific precipitation while not much disturbing specific precipitation (see section above on nonspecific pre-cipitation). They also may be needed to prevent dissociation of specific precipitates formed by some chicken (Weiner et al., 1964) and rabbit (Motet, 1965) antisera. Baths of moderately acid pH (e.g., pH 5.0: Lichter, 1967; pH 6: Raunio, 1968) may be used to enhance or preserve otherwise weak specific precipitation or maintain antigen integrity. Tap water in some areas may contain enough dissolved salts to wash unreacted antiserum components from an agar gel adequately and so greatly in-crease both the rapidity and the convenience of washing (Hutchison, 1962). The wash bath must also be compatible with unreacted antigen solubility. If washing is prolonged and at room or higher temperature, the wash bath should contain an antiseptic such as 1.0% sodium azide

(Auernheimer and Atchley, 1962). Such additives as chloroform, toluene, thymol, phenol, and Merthiolate also can be used with due recognition that they may injure labile antigens.

The composition of succeeding wash baths can be changed empirically and to suit special purposes. For instance, the first few rinses can be composed of salts needed to leach out most antigen and antiserum constituents;[56] these can be followed by tap water to leach out remaining constituents and the salts of the original buffer, and this in turn can be succeeded with distilled water to remove all salts before drying, or by the solvent for the stain to prepare the gel for staining (Uriel, 1958; Albutt, 1966).

The length of washing and the number of solvent changes depend on such factors as density and thickness of the gel, wash fluid volume, temperature, agitation, nature and quantity of reactants in the gel, and extent of leaching required. Thick gels of a given kind need much more leaching than the thin gels currently most popular in microimmunodiffusion tests; and these, which are usually about 1 mm thick, in turn must be washed longer (e.g., 48 hours in saline followed by distilled water rinse for 4 to 5 hours: Brummerstedt-Hansen, 1967) than gels as thin as 200 μm. A general rule is one day's washing for each millimeter of gel thickness (Uriel, 1963). Dense gels are harder to wash adequately: polyacrylamide, for instance, is several times as resistant to leaching as a comparably thick agar gel, because macromolecules diffuse more slowly through polyacrylamides than through agar (Van Orden, 1968).[57] The efficiency of washing rises with increases in wash fluid volume, in temperature, and in vigor of agitation. Washing techniques include replacing the wash bath occasionally and rocking the wash container frequently (e.g., 3 days of washing an immunoelectropherogram in physiologic

---

[56] These first rinses themselves can be preceded for immunoelectropherograms by a 30-minute fixation in 5% formalin in pH 7.4 phosphate buffer to help stabilize marginal antigen–antibody precipitation (Albutt, 1966). However, the advisability of fixing immunoelectropherograms before staining is debated (Yokoyama and Tsuchiya, 1963).

[57] Although practiced only infrequently, electrophoretic "washing" (see electrodialysis, below) is very quick and effective, especially for thick and dense gels. It can be quite simple. For instance, one can lay the agar-covered slide in the bottom of a petri dish filled with suitable washing buffer and having electrodes at opposite sides. The slide is laid across the path of the electric field, current is turned on, and unreacted antigen and antiserum components migrate out of the gel. All those with isoelectric pH different from the pH of the buffer will be removed within a few minutes. Electrophoresis should be performed again for a few minutes at a different pH to remove components not efficiently extracted during the first electrophoresis. Using low ionic strength and high voltage accelerates this washing, but the possibility of thereby dissociating weak antigen–antibody complexes must not be overlooked.

saline changed once or twice a day: Uriel, 1958), using a large volume of bath and continual rocking or stirring (Yokoyama and Tsuchiya, 1963; Mancini *et al.*, 1965), using special circulating or cycling devices (Sassen, 1965), mixing and periodically but automatically replacing the bath, or using a continuous flow of lukewarm tap water. When part of the antigen is insoluble (e.g., bacterial suspension), it can be rinsed from the surface or wells of the gel with a gentle spray of water (Slaterus, 1961). The presence of antiserum constituents like lipoproteins which are difficult to wash from agar gels can be avoided altogether by using purified antiserum immunoglobulin in place of whole antiserum (Talal *et al.*, 1963), or by using a delipified antiserum (see section on antiserum preparation).

Washing is completed when a protein stain applied to the immunodiffusogram colors only precipitin bands. But "complete" washing by this criterion may not be possible if reactants have complexed with the gel. It may not be necessary, however, if the precipitin bands are easily seen; consequently, a light or moderate background of color is frequently acceptable. Some additional removal of reactants can be achieved during the drying procedure, if this precedes staining, and washing can be shortened if the gel is dried under filter paper. This is accomplished by laying a distilled water-soaked filter paper upon the surface of the gel, itself horizontal and flooded with distilled water (Jouannet, 1968), without trapping any air bubbles, and then letting this paper–gel combination dry at room temperature, in a warm-air oven (Uriel, 1958, 1963), or for least distortion at 4°C (Jouannet, 1968).[58] During this drying, water evaporating through the filter paper carries reactants with it into the paper and out of the gel. Thick filter paper with strong, smooth, fiber-free surface structure, such as Eaton-Dikeman #652, should be used. Even better is cellulose acetate (Uriel, 1966) or cellulose acetate with any kind of filter paper resting on it. After the slide has been dried, the paper is readily removed. Any fibers remaining on the agar can be rubbed off gently with a little distilled water or solvent that is to be used for staining. If only a paper with loose fibers, like Whatman #1, is available, this can be removed from the gel before it has dried completely, and drying then is completed without the paper (Rybák *et al.*, 1963). Since Whatman #1 paper is thin, it should be used in three or more layers. A slide can be dried under filter paper before washing; then washing itself may either be unnecessary or be shortened considerably (Hirschfeld, 1960b).

Most of the information above applies to agar and agarose gels. Polyacrylamide, as mentioned before, is difficult to wash; therefore, unless it

[58] If the gel is moderately thick and has wells or troughs, these should first be filled with the same kind of gel. This minimizes distortion and possible cracking originating from these gel discontinuities during drying (Proctor, 1966).

is quite thin, it is best washed electrophoretically.[59] Cellulose acetate films are washed in the same way as thin layers of agar gel (e.g., 4 hours or more in saline and 10 minutes in distilled water: Johnson *et al.,* 1964). Often these films have been kept under mineral oil during reaction development (Vergani *et al.,* 1967). Then, the oil must be removed first by rinsing with an inert volatile solvent like petroleum ether or benzene; this is followed by washing in saline (Rabinowitz, 1964). Oil also can be washed off cellulose acetate with a detergent.[60] Agar gels that have been incubated under oil should be rinsed with a solvent like petroleum ether before washing.

Staining

Precipitin bands can be intensified, made more visible and easier to photograph, and analyzed for type of antigen or antibody that they contain by reacting them with various indicators (Salvaggio *et al.,* 1970; Uriel, 1965; Cawley *et al.,* 1965b; Casman *et al.,* 1969).[61] This usually is called "staining," because most often it results in coloring a precipitin band; but it also includes many procedures that should not properly be considered staining and some that involve no color at all. The general procedure is to apply indicator (stain) and then differentiate. Indicators include dyes, enzyme substrates, substances that detect changes in enzyme substrates, and indicators that are coupled as labels to substances that react specifically with a constituent of an antigen–antibody precipitate. Examples of these include acid dyes for proteins, hydrogen peroxide for catalase (Uriel, 1963), starch–iodide for amylase (Daussant and Grabar, 1966; Revis, 1968), and radioactivity- or fluorescence-labeled antigen to detect specific antibody activity (Uriel, 1958).

Indicator reactions can be general or specific (Uriel, 1963, 1965). General reactions detect a type of antigen, for instance, on the basis of broad chemical properties (e.g., proteins, polysaccharides, lipids).

---

[59] Microimmunoelectropherograms with thin polyacrylamide gels of only 2.8% can be washed adequately like agar gels with 0.9% NaCl followed by distilled water (Keutel *et al.,* 1964).

[60] Submerge the strip for 30 seconds in a weak solution of detergent, rinse in a strong jet of tap water, soak in 0.2% Haemo-sol for 5 minutes with gentle agitation, rinse in distilled water, and air-dry on a sheet of filter paper (Vergani *et al.,* 1967; Ringle and Herndon, 1965).

[61] Although most immunodiffusion patterns are improved by washing and staining, occasionally these procedures cause precipitin band dissociation (Crowle and Hu, 1965; Cawley *et al.,* 1965; Cawley, 1969). Hence, a pattern should be observed both before and after staining. This seems especially true of precipitates developed with rabbit antiserum if their immunodiffusograms are stained after drying rather than before (Cawley, 1969; Crowle, unpublished work).

Specific reactions identify specific antigen by unique characteristics (e.g., its content of some metal like iron or copper, its enzymatic activity for a selected substrate, or its immunochemical constitution).

STAINS FOR PROTEINS

These are the most frequently used because of their nonselectivity: since they stain the antibodies or precipitin bands, they will color nearly all of them (Nace and Alley, 1961). The basis for using these stains is to lower the pH to about 3 to transform antibody proteins and most protein antigens into positive molecules, and then to expose them to an acid (negatively charged) dye. Agar gel, for which most of these stains originally were developed, retains its net negative charge at this pH and therefore is not stained by acid dyes. Hence, these subsequently can be removed by leaching with a mildly acidified water which can be essentially the same as that used for the staining itself.[62] Variations in formulas and techniques for immunodiffusion protein stains have been developed for such reasons as differences in affinity between different stains and different kinds of antibody, the relatively greater capacity of one dye over another to stain a precipitin band in one medium than in another, the greater efficiency with which precipitin bands of one color can be photographed than those of another, and personal preference or stain availability. Nearly any of the acid stains used in histochemistry will suffice, but some are better than others because of the greater intensity with which they can color a precipitin band.[63] Red or green dyes photograph best (see section on photography). Several formulas and protocols for these stains are given in Appendixes V through IX. The following are some general considerations which affect the choice and use of a given stain.

Precipitin bands of equivalent density may not stain equally well because of differences in antigen–antibody ratio, the presence of nonprotein antigen, or different affinities of a given stain for different kinds of antibody (Nace and Alley, 1961; Cawley, 1969). Occasionally we have observed bands that would not take up any of the commonly used protein

---

[62] Basic dyes like methylene blue, crystal violet, and fuchsin can be used to stain precipitin bands in agarose and polyacrylamide (Crowle, unpublished work).

[63] Favorites are buffalo black (also commonly known as amido black and amido schwartz 10 B), nigrosin, light green SF, thiazine red R, and azocarmine A or B; others include ponceau S (Ringle and Herndon, 1965), thioflavine S (Alexander and Moncrief, 1966), Biebrich scarlet (Dimmock, 1967), crocein scarlet MOO, bromphenol blue, bromthymol blue, indigo carmine, ponceau fuchsin (Crowle, 1961), aniline blue, and Coomasie brilliant blue (Kronman, 1965). Of the various dyes, coloring capacity for proteins is said to decrease roughly as follows: Coomasie brilliant blue R > nigrosin ≫ others (Uriel, 1966; Kronman, 1965).

stains. Since there appears to be no consistently "best" protein stain (cf. Crowle, 1961; Yokoyama and Tsuchiya, 1963; Jochim and Chow, 1969), it is wise to have different kinds of stain available, to use such aids as mordants in stain solutions, to employ multiple stains (Crowle, 1961; Rabinowitz, 1964), and to observe immunodiffusograms by dark-field lighting before staining (Nace and Alley, 1961). Dyes of one name can vary enough to perform quite differently in the same protocol (e.g., buffalo black: Pastewka *et al.*, 1966).

Protein stains are used on both undried and dried gels, but results are not parallel. Staining is fast, and destaining is simple and efficient with dried gels, but in our experience, and in that of some others (Hutchison, 1962), it is also distinctly inferior to staining gels not yet dried. Many precipitin bands in an immunoelectropherogram dried before staining may stain poorly or not at all. To a certain extent this problem can be circumvented by thoroughly moistening the dried gel before staining (Hutchison, 1962), but the better practice is to stain the gel before it is dried. If precipitin bands have been inadequately stained by one protocol, another with a second kind of stain can be superimposed on the first; or, the first stain can be removed by washing the slide in mildly alkaline solution, rinsing it in weak acid, and then restaining it. Bands that were once stained but have faded on prolonged storing can be reintensified somewhat by a brief dipping in distilled water; or they can be restained (Casman *et al.*, 1969).

The procedures used for staining thick agar gels, thin gels, cellulose acetate, or polyacrylamide are basically the same, changes in protocol being made only to suit the medium. For instance, agar gels more than 1 mm thick are better stained if detached from their original support, so that staining and washing solutions can diffuse into the gel simultaneously from above and below. Considerable time can be saved for thick gels if they are dried before staining. For thin gels on glass or polyester (Cawley *et al.*, 1965a) supports, staining can be reduced from the hours required for thicker gels to minutes (e.g., 10 minutes for gels 200 to 400 μ thick), and there is no need to dry them first. Precipitates on cellulose acetate, which should not be dried before staining (Grunbaum *et al.*, 1963; Rabinowitz, 1964), can be stained with a very weak dye solution like 0.001% nigrosin. Color is absorbed from the solution by the precipitates but not by the membrane, so that there is no need for differentiation (Bideau and Masseyeff, 1964). This way of staining also has been used with 0.03% nigrosin for agar (Lange *et al.*, 1966). Cellulose acetate is stained most uniformly by laying the film on the staining solution, allowing this to permeate the film, and then submerging the strip in the stain for several minutes (Rabinowitz, 1964). Polyacrylamide in thicknesses currently most often used is dense enough to require several hours for the stain to penetrate; it is best destained by electrodialysis.[64] However, thin 2.8% gels used in micro tests can be stained and destained by the same protocols as are used for thin agar layers (Keutel et al., 1964). Polyacrylamide–agarose combination gel immunodiffusograms are stained like those of agarose alone (Uriel, 1966).

OTHER GENERAL STAINS

Polysaccharides and glycoproteins in precipitin bands always have been rather difficult to stain in agar or agar-like gels because these gels themselves are polysaccharides. Alcian blue and Mayer's mucicarmine were once recommended for this purpose (Crowle, 1961), but they stain these gels too much to be very useful (Terando and Feir, 1967; Hazeghi and Crowle, unpublished work). They might be useful for polyacrylamide or cellulose acetate but apparently have not been utilized with these media. Schiff's reagent and the paraphenylenediamine reaction are reliable and effective. The former has been improved somewhat by changing reagents and protocol to produce an insoluble and strongly colored formazan derivative with glycoproteins or polysaccharides (Uriel and Grabar, 1961). This eliminates a need for cumbersome auxiliary techniques such as covering the stained gel immediately after staining with a vinyl protective coating or storing it in a weak solution of sulfur dioxide (Stewart-Tull, 1965). Polyacrylamide gel patterns are stained by the same techniques as are used for agar or agarose gels, allowing for differences in their thickness and density (Stewart-Tull, 1965).

Lipid or lipid-associated antigens in precipitin bands usually are "stained" by soaking them in a saturated solution of a lipid-soluble colored chemical like Sudan black or Oil red O (e.g., Brummerstedt-Hansen, 1967; Burtin and Grabar, 1967). Some of this chemical dissolves in the lipid and colors it. Since these stains are insoluble in water, usually they must be used on previously dried immunodiffusograms. However, if this is inconvenient, as with polyacrylamide, the gel can be soaked before staining in the stain solvent (e.g., 40% ethanol: Hermans et al., 1960) and then transferred to the stain itself. There are also some water-soluble lipid stains (e.g., Nile blue A: Crowle, 1961), although they are seldom used. One, reported recently, depends on the characteristic of tetracyclines to precipitate serum lipoproteins (Rabinowitz and Schen, 1965). Thus, when a washed immunoelectropherogram is exposed to tetracycline solution, subsequently washed, and then viewed under ultraviolet

[64] It could probably also be stained rapidly by electrophoresing dye into it, since precipitin bands would not be affected by the electrophoresis.

light, lipoprotein-containing precipitin bands will fluoresce brightly. Thioflavin T has been employed in the same kind of test (Gombert, 1969).

Nucleic acids or antigens containing them can be stained specifically with acridine orange (Cowan and Graves, 1968; Forsgren, 1966; Ohlson, 1963) or with a mixture of methyl green and pyronin Y (Zwaan, 1963; Kurnick, 1955). Immunodiffusograms exposed to acridine orange can be examined and photographed under a high-intensity ultraviolet light: single-stranded RNA or DNA will be flame red, whereas double-stranded RNA or DNA looks yellow-green (Cowan and Graves, 1968). Low concentrations of dye should be used to minimize background fluorescence— 0.01% to differentiate between nucleic acids, and 0.001% to detect them. In immunodiffusion slides stained with the methyl green–pyronin Y mixture, polymerized DNA is green, whereas depolymerized nucleic acids are red (Kurnick, 1955).

Specific Indicators

In the past decade, identifying antigens in immunodiffusion precipitates by histochemical tests has become quite common (Uriel, 1958). This is especially so for enzymes, because their substrate reactions are so specific. The advantages of using specific indicators are more than just identifying antigen in a given precipitin arc. For instance, some arcs which are blurred or even invisible when viewed directly become clearly evident when tested for enzyme activity (Uriel, 1963). Complexes of antibody with carbonic anhydrase from human red cell lysates were detected in this manner when there was no evidence of their presence either directly or after staining with amido black (Micheli, 1965). Tissue glycosidase aggregates similarly were revealed only by their enzymatic reaction (Raunio, 1968), as was lactic dehydrogenase (Nace, 1963). Since the capacity of a stain or indicator to detect an antigen depends on the sensitivity and visibility of its interaction with the antigen, specific enzymatic reactions tend to be very sensitive because they are self-amplifying (Zwaan, 1963). Indeed, suitable enzymes can be used to label antigen or antibody for effects similar to and comparable with radio-autography (see Chapter 1). Indicators for a given enzyme can reveal its presence in more than one precipitin band (i.e., in isozymes: Uriel, 1963) or in separation of enzyme from carrier–enzyme complexes (Revis, 1971).

Retention of biochemical activity by an enzyme that has reacted with antibody might seem paradoxical, since the antibody might be expected to neutralize the enzyme as antitoxin neutralizes toxin. But usually this does not occur, partly because in immunodiffusion tests complexes are not formed in antibody excess, and partly because most of an enzyme's antigenic determinants are not the same as its determinants of enzymatic activity, and enough of the latter will remain free to react visibly with the enzyme's substrate (Uriel, 1965; Arnon and Schechter, 1966). In fact, enzymes complexed with their antibodies appear to be more stable than free enzymes (Raunio, 1968). The surrounding gel also helps to stabilize enzymes, so that those that might be expected to lose activity during drying of the gel before staining instead retain their activity (Raunio, 1968; Uriel, 1963). However, enzyme antigens occasionally will indeed be affected by reaction with antibody. Some antisera are more likely to change them than others (Kaminski, 1966), and in reacting with an enzyme an antibody may alter its structure or mask important portions of it, making it appear physically or chemically different from its native form and thus possibly providing misleading information on its nature (Uriel, 1958).

Although reactions to detect enzymes are the most common specific indicators in immunodiffusion tests, other tests detecting any peculiar characteristic of an antigen also fit this category. These include, for instance, identification of ceruloplasmin by its copper (Uriel, 1963), of transferrin and ferritin by their iron (Uriel, 1965; Ślopek et al., 1966; Richter, 1967), of certain lipoproteins by their capacities to oxidize ferrous iron to ferric iron (Schen and Rabinowitz, 1967a), and of haptoglobin by its affinity for hemoglobin which itself is readily detected by peroxidase activity (Uriel, 1963; Schneider and Arat, 1964).

A larger number of specific indicator reactions for antigens in immunodiffusion and gel electrophoresis probably have been devised or improved by José Uriel than by anyone else. Two of his more recent publications (Uriel, 1963, 1971) therefore should be consulted by the reader for techniques or references to descriptions of techniques for revealing antigens by these means. See also Uriel, 1965; Uriel et al., 1963; Cinader et al., 1963; Lawrence and Melnick, 1961; Tran Van Ky et al. (1966b, 1967) (several different indicator systems); Cawley et al. (1966); Bao-Linh et al. (1964); Shulman et al. (1964b, 1965) (acid phosphatase); Cabello et al. (1965) (arginase); Daussant and Grabar (1966); Hirsch-Marie and Burtin (1964); Uriel and Avrameas (1964); Hersh and Benedict (1966); Revis (1968) (amylase); Micheli (1965) (carbonic anhydrase); Uriel (1961) (carboxylic esterases); Howe et al. (1963); Laterre and Heremans (1963) (catalase); Talal and Tomkins (1964); Bao-Linh et al. (1964) (glutamic dehydrogenase); Cawley et al. (1966); De Vaux Saint-Cyr et al. (1963); Dony and Muyldermans (1970); Terando and Feir (1967); Bao-Linh et al. (1964) (esterases); Raunio (1968); Dony and Muyldermans (1970) (lipase); Dony and Muyldermans (1970) (mucopolysaccharides); Vanha-Perttula *et al.* (1965) (amino peptidase); Cawley *et al.* (1966) (peroxidase); Cawley *et al.* (1966); Bao-Linh *et al.* (1964) (proteases); and Terando and Feir (1967) (tyrosinase). Enzyme–antibody precipitates sometimes can be identified directly during an immunodiffusion test by incorporating substrate in the gel (e.g., elastin for elastase: Uriel and Avrameas, 1964; fibrin for trypsin, and thus also for serum α_1-trypsin inhibitor: Kueppers *et al.*, 1964).

PREREACTION STAINS

A reactant or medium can be labeled before its use in an immunodiffusion test. Coloring serum albumin with Evans blue dye so that migration of the albumin can be observed in monitoring serum electrophoresis is a common example.[65]

Reactants can be labeled with radioactivity, fluorescence, or enzymes, in addition to color. The labeling procedure ideally should not impair the activity of the reactants. Occasionally, a substance will have its own "label" (e.g., iron in transferrin or ferritin); sometimes it will have a natural affinity for some indicator. Serum lipoproteins, for instance, combine with tetracycline, which, in turn, can be detected by fluorescence under ultraviolet light (Schen and Rabinowitz, 1966a).

An indicator need not be attached to either reactant; it has only to indicate the presence of a reactant. Some examples were given above. For instance, elastase is detected by elastin, and protealytic enzymes are detected by fibrin incorporated in the gel. *Clostridium perfringens* α toxin was identified in immunoelectropherograms by its lecithinase activity in egg yolk–agar gel mixture, because it causes the egg yolk to become turbid (Stephen, 1961).

CODING STAINS

Some stains are used for coding marks in the medium before it is used. Cutting or notching may suffice. Cellulose acetate membranes are marked with ball-point pens. Agar gels can be marked with any basic dye, or with one like Alcian blue with an affinity for polysaccharides. A grid marking with Alcian blue has been used, for instance, for preparative agar zone electrophoresis (Micheli, 1963). Alcian blue should be useful on agarose, which basic dyes will not stain. Colloidal marker can be employed: India ink was used to mark agar gels for reactant positions when there were no wells for orientation (May and Rawlins, 1962).

[65] Add Evans blue dye at ≤ 1 mg/ml of serum to be electrophoresed. Serum albumin marked with Evans blue has become a standard reference substance both for assessing progress of an electrophoretic run and for measuring the relative electrophoretic migration of other serum constituents.

Differentiating, Drying, and Preserving Immunodiffusograms

After the chromogenic reaction between antigen and indicator has occurred, or precipitin bands have been stained, excess reagents or stain should be removed from the medium to facilitate observation and to prepare a permanent original record of the test. For many indicator reactions there are special differentiating procedures, but some generalizations can be made.

To be dried clear an immunodiffusion medium must be free of salts; final rinsings should be either in distilled water or in water with volatile solutes (e.g., acetic acid) that leave no residue. Alternatively, if non-volatile solutes must be included in the final rinsings, the medium can be dried under or between filter papers, which draw off both solvent and most of the solutes. No trouble should be encountered in washing and drying agar, agarose, and cellulose acetate; the technique is the same as that used in washing out unreacted antigen and antiserum as mentioned above except that it is much faster, because most chromogen molecules are small, and destaining or differentiation solutions are formulated to correspond specifically to the staining procedure. The art of these procedures for polyacrylamide gels is less well developed. Either they must be submitted to prolonged leaching, or they can be electrodialyzed (cf. Pun and Lombrozo, 1964; Ferris *et al.*, 1962a, 1963);[66] methods for drying them are mentioned below. Agarose–polyacrylamide also is best electrodialyzed (Uriel, 1966).

Agar and agarose gels are easily dried and preserved if they are 1 mm thick or less and are supported on agar- or agarose-coated glass slides or similarly coated polyester films (see above). Undue distortion around wells or troughs cut in the gel should be avoided, and the gel should be protected from dust while drying. Gels that are less than 0.5 mm thick and are dried at temperatures of 37°C or less rarely develop significant distortion; they can be protected from dust by being dried upside down, or under a cover or in a cabinet.

If the gel is thick enough for objectionable distortion to develop during drying, this distortion can be reduced to negligible by drying the gel in contact with filter paper as described above, by filling its wells and troughs with the same gel before it is dried, or by filling these discontinuities and covering the entire surface with an additional thin layer of gel (Longbottom and Pepys, 1964). Gels thicker than 1 mm should be soaked

---

[66] These may be electrodialyzed as described above for electrophoretic washing of gels, except that the wash buffer usually is simpler, of weaker ionic strength, and likely to have lower pH. For example, to destain polyacrylamide that has been stained with amido schwartz, the destaining solution can be 0.5% acetic acid.

in water containing 1 to 2% glycerol, or in 10% glycerol in 60% ethanol (Longbottom and Pepys, 1964), just before drying, both to minimize distortion and to prevent cracking of the gel or its peeling from its support; thinner gels do not require this glycerol rinse (Auernheimer and Atchley, 1962; Alexander and Moncrief, 1966).[67]

Thick agar gels dry into films sturdy enough to be handled without supplementary support. However, the thinner gels of most immunodiffusion tests must be dried onto a suitable support like glass or flexible polyester film if they are to be kept and handled. The hard, durable film that results can be stored for at least a decade without deteriorating. Therefore, unless the immunodiffusogram is to be handled repeatedly and roughly, nothing further need be done.

More positive protection for the dried immunodiffusogram can be achieved by covering it with mounting medium and a suitable cover slip as for mounting histologic sections (Bennett and Boursnell, 1962); or it can be covered with a dipping, painting, or spraying of clear lacquer, varnish, or similar finish. A shellac finish described specifically for such use consists of 2 ml of shellac, 2 ml of glycerol, and 96 ml of ethanol. The immunoelectropherogram is dried at 60°C and then brushed with this mixture while still hot (Salvaggio *et al.*, 1970).

Dried cellulose acetate membranes can be preserved indefinitely. But because they are fragile, and stained precipitin bands are more readily seen in them if they are made transparent, they are best preserved like a histologic section. Place a few drops of mounting medium on a microscope slide, lay the dried membrane on this without trapping air bubbles, place a little more medium on the membrane, and finally lay a cover slip or second microscope slide upon this. If the membrane is to be made transparent but not kept permanently, it can simply be soaked in mineral oil (Kohn, 1960; Nelson *et al.*, 1964). Later, the oil can be washed out with xylene and replaced with mounting fluid if preliminary observation suggests that it should be kept more permanently. Alternatively, excess oil can be blotted away, the membrane can be mounted between a cover slip and glass slide, and the mounting sealed with nail enamel applied along the edges of the cover slip (Johnson *et al.*, 1964).

For the membrane to be cleared with either mineral oil or mounting fluid, it must be completely dry. Cellulose acetate also can be cleared and preserved clear by washing it in 10% acetic acid in methanol, laying it on a glass plate, immersing it in dioxane:isobutanol (7:3), and, when

---

[67] In our experience, using a glycerol rinse actually has interfered with preservation of uncovered microimmunodiffusograms. The color of the stain may fade or change, the dried agar may soften and become tacky, and a peculiar channeling detachment of the gel from its glass support may develop.

it has become completely transparent, drying it in a hot air oven at 80°C (Vergani *et al.*, 1967). Alternatively, the membrane that has just been destained with acetic acid solution (e.g., following protein staining) can be placed on an inclined glass plate and sprayed with glacial acetic acid containing glycerol at 1%. Then it is dried at 80°C, cooled, and removed from the plate (Agostoni *et al.*, 1967). Or it can be soaked in 30% glacial acetic acid in 95% ethanol and dried on a glass plate at 70°C for 20 minutes (Grunbaum *et al.*, 1963; cf. also Grabner *et al.*, 1968).

Polyacrylamide gels in thicknesses currently most often employed have been difficult enough to dry so that most experimenters have resorted to preserving the stained and differentiated gel in the differentiating medium (e.g., 2% acetic acid) without drying. However, some techniques have been devised for drying relatively thin films successfully. Since recent reports indicate that thin films of dimensions such as are commonly used with agar in microelectrophoresis can be dried on a microscope slide just like agar gels (Keutel *et al.*, 1964; Jensen, 1965; Van Orden, 1968),[68] these special methods may be more of historical than of practical interest (see Antoine, 1962; Hermans *et al.*, 1960; Herrick and Lawrence, 1965, for details).

Polyacrylamide–agarose gels have several of the desirable physical properties of pure agarose gels, one of the most useful being that they can be dried by the same techniques as are used for agar or agarose (Uriel, 1966).

Special problems in drying other kinds of less-used media (e.g., Sephadex G-200 for immunofiltration: Grant and Everall, 1966) will be explained where they arise in discussions on the application of these media (cf. Chapter 7).

Observing, Recording, and Photographing Immunodiffusion Reactions

Although most immunodiffusion tests are easy to set up, the results of even the simplest frequently require careful study for correct interpretation. The careful observation needed for such interpretation is aided

[68] The polyacrylamide must be dried slowly to prevent its becoming brittle and cracking. The dried gel can be protected with a clear plastic spray (Van Orden, 1968), as suggested above for agar gels. This drying can be performed as well before staining and destaining, thus facilitating these procedures in polyacrylamide gels (Keutel *et al.*, 1964). If the supporting slide is covered with 1% agar gel before the polyacrylamide is laid on it to dry, somewhat thicker gels can be dried without special techniques (Jensen, 1965).

by selection of appropriate methods for studying the immunodiffuso-grams. Some of these are described in the following pages.

Observing

One observes an immunodiffusion test to detect all real precipitin bands (as distinguished from nonspecific precipitates or secondary pre-cipitates); to note their shape, curvature, length, breadth, boundary sharpness, and position; and to determine whether and how the precipitin bands interact. As succeeding chapters will show, these data identify antigens, reveal important characteristics of both antigens and their antibodies, and elucidate their specific interactions as determined by the kind of antigen–antibody reaction developing, the relative quantities of reactants present, the involvement of specific and nonspecific reactants, and the relationships between antigens and antibodies. Immunodiffusion tests are studied, and records of them are made, both during their development and afterward, when they have been subjected to auxiliary revelatory procedures.

Gel immunodiffusion tests are best observed by indirect illumination against a dark background (i.e., dark-field lighting). Shining a bright light obliquely up through the bottom of the pattern while holding it over a black bench top or cardboard is simple and very effective. Lighting devices for photographing immunodiffusion patterns by dark-field light-ing, as described below, also can be used; and special illuminating systems for both purposes can be purchased from suppliers of immunology equip-ment. Sometimes precipitin bands are observed by transmitted light by means of photometric scanning devices which can detect small differences in light transmission through the medium, but to the human eye and the camera precipitin bands are much more readily evident by indirect lighting. If the observations are being made while the reactions are still developing, induction of temperature artifacts should be avoided by cir-cumventing sudden, extreme changes in temperature, such as occur, for instance, in removing an immunodiffusion test from a refrigerator, warm-ing it with illuminating lamps, and then returning it to the refrigerator (see Chapters 1 and 3). Because cellulose acetate is opaque, reactions developing in this medium cannot be observed until they are revealed either by clarifying the membrane (following washing and drying) or by staining the antigen–antibody precipitates.

Patterns of precipitin bands perceived after revelatory techniques such as staining are likely to differ from those seen before, because some bands can dissociate during washing and staining, invisible aggregates may become visible precipitates, and preciptin bands may become thinner, thicker, shorter, longer, or otherwise change directly or indirectly because of the operations applied to them. Therefore, readings made both before and after staining provide the most complete information.

Stained immunodiffusograms are studied informally by transmitted diffuse white light (e.g., x-ray viewbox) and low-power magnification (e.g., up to 10×; higher magnification begins to reveal the internal structure of precipitin bands, which is usually useless and confusing information). Detailed observations can be made by or before a group of people by projecting the image of the stained pattern with either a photographic enlarger or a slide projector on a white surface in a darkened room.

Recording

The kind of observation made from a test depends principally on the purpose of the test. One may record the number of precipitin bands and perhaps also their relative positions and intensities in simply qualitative analyses of an antigen solution (e.g., by arbitrary numerical notations). On the other hand, the presence of a certain band may have particular significance, and so coalescence of a band among several formed between an antiserum and a mixture of antigens with one formed between the same antiserum and a reference antigen will suffice (e.g., "+" or "−" notation; free-hand drawing). Examining relationships between antigens requires notations, drawings, and photographs of the interaction between their respective precipitin bands in double diffusion plate tests, of changes in relative position (Russell, 1965), of intensity, and of apparent migration of a band in the presence of test antigens. Band curvature may be important, as in estimating relative molecular weight of an antigen; then, one should note not only the direction of curvature, but also signs of whether the test was set up appropriately (e.g., sharpness of the band, movement or stability in the gel with time, curvature when formed by different ratios of antigen to antibody, or in different buffer systems; see Chapter 4). Valuable data can be obtained from immunoelectropherograms by observing whether a precipitin arc is symmetrical, double-humped, or skewed (Chapter 5); and in electro-immunodiffusograms additional information is available from such data as the height of a precipitin loop, whether it is sharp and where, the distance between its "legs," and its relationship to other antigens present (Chapter 6).

For all these observations it is always safest, because of unanticipated questions or data that might arise sometime in the future, to employ an immunodiffusion technique that provides either the original patterns themselves for permanent preservation or patterns that can be photographed readily and efficiently (Nace and Alley, 1961). Printing or drawing a projected immunodiffusogram on gridded paper is useful in nearly all these analyses. As photometric scanning devices of increasing sophistication are applied to making records of immunodiffusion tests (Smibert *et al.*, 1961; El-Marsafy and Abdel-Gawad, 1962; Glenn, 1961a, 1963, 1968; Glenn *et al.*, 1963, 1965) they may replace printing and drawing techniques to some extent and may also eventually be programmed to select and identify certain characteristics of special importance in a given test.

Photographing

All important varieties of immunodiffusion test can be performed in thin or very thin media on supports like microscope slides. Hence, original records of nearly all such tests can be preserved. The best photographs of an immunodiffusion test are prepared from these; they can also be analyzed by photometric scanning (Von Der Decken, 1967). However, both photographs and scannings can be made on the raw test, even as it is developing. Many varieties of photographic technique have been described for recording immunodiffusion results, but major differences among these are few. Essentially, the photograph is produced either by shadowgraphy (light passing through the immunodiffusion medium is barred by precipitin bands) or by dark-field illumination (light passing obliquely through the transparent medium is reflected onto photosensitive material by the precipitin bands; Hirschfeld, 1960b; Almeida *et al.*, 1965). Shadowgraphs are the cleanest and clearest and should be used, whenever possible, for publication. Dark-field photographs can show more detail than shadowgraphs, but this is why they often make mediocre illustrations for publication: the smallest dust particles, pieces of lint, or changes in the continuity of the medium show up starkly. Technically, dark-field photographs are also more difficult to make, and usually they require intermediary photographic steps, like having to make a final print from a photographic negative, which tend to lessen the quality of the final reproduction (Almeida *et al.*, 1965).

SHADOWGRAPHS

The easiest way to make a shadowgraph is to place the fresh, unstained immunodiffusion test[69] into tap water directly upon photosensitive

---

[69] This may be a microscope slide on which antigen–antibody precipitation has taken place in a relatively thin layer of agar gel. Other supports and containers can be used but should not if they have generally poorer optical characteristics (curvature, irregular surface, varying thickness).

material in the dark, expose this to light for a suitable length of time, and then develop the photosensitive material by conventional techniques (cf. Németh, 1964). Water immersion secures good contact between the photosensitive material and the slide, and prevents unnecessary reflections and refractions at well or trough edges (Jones and Marshall, 1960). Well and trough discontinuities also can be avoided by filling these with 1% agar saturated with charcoal (Myers and Hanson, 1962). Photographic contact printing paper is the cheapest photosensitive material to use in shadowgraphy; projection paper is more sensitive but more expensive. Since copies or enlargements of the images obtained on photographic paper are not readily made because it is opaque, a photographic negative material (film, projection slides) should be employed for this purpose (Jones and Marshall, 1960). This material also offers better resolution and latitude, is available in a greater variety of photographic characteristics, and allows much greater control over the quality of the shadowgraph eventually produced. However, it is more expensive than photosensitive papers.

The light used for producing a shadowgraph is important: either it should be a point source, or it should be focused (Jones and Marshall, 1960).[70] If it is diffuse (e.g., from a broad overhead light), the edges of the precipitin band images will be indistinct, weak bands will not register, and resolution will be poor. Exposure time depends on the type of photosensitive material employed (cf. Gilder, 1963) and is determined initially by trial and error. Methods for developing the photograph have too many variations to detail here. They are described in manuals on photography.

Shadowgraphs of excellent and colorful (nine different colors are available) quality can be prepared easily, inexpensively, and rapidly with Technifax Diazochrome color film (Scott Graphics, Inc., subsidiary of Scott Paper Company, Holyoke, Massachusetts: Cawley, 1969). This film can be handled in ordinary room light, and it is capable of reproducing immunodiffusion patterns with good sensitivity and resolution. Development is simple and requires only ammonium hydroxide; and the product is a durable, nonbreakable sheet of plastic which can be stored in a laboratory notebook, used as a projection slide, or attached to a case-history record. We use the following procedure (Crowle and Jarrett, unpublished work; see Fig. 2.7).

Lay a sheet of Diazochrome on the workbench with its emulsion side up, and place the dried, stained immunodiffusogram upon this film face

---

[70] Ultraviolet lighting is said to be superior to lighting with visible light for recording unstained immunodiffusion precipitates of viral antigens (i.e., nucleic acids: Thomson, 1964).

down. Lay a glass plate on top of the immunodiffusogram and film to bring the two into flat, close contact. Hold a photographic flood lamp 1 inch above the glass plate, and expose the film to this light for 40 seconds. Develop the Diazochrome film for 1 minute in 10% ammonium hydroxide in distilled water or tap water. Wash the film briefly in tap water, and blot it dry with a paper towel.

Light for exposing Diazochrome must be intense; optimal exposure depends not only on the intensity of this light but also on the amount of background stain in the immunodiffusogram. The film can be developed by simply dipping it in ammonium hydroxide solution, but a discarded Dippit container, originally used for stabilizing Polaroid 3¼ × 4-inch projection slides but cleaned out and refilled with ammonium hydroxide solution, is very convenient for this purpose. Diazochrome copies of immunodiffusograms show nearly the same detail as the original pattern itself, and they are convenient to use as negatives to prepare enlarged prints for publication.

Shadowgraphs also can be produced inexpensively and easily with some kinds of office copying machines (Cawley *et al.*, 1965a; Cawley, 1969), although their quality is comparatively poor.

Shadowgraphs produced from dried, stained immunodiffusograms are of higher quality than those from wet, unstained patterns, for several reasons. In the dried gel there is no depth to precipitin bands and thus no problem of appropriately lighting two adjacent ribbons of precipitate. The dried gel can be placed upside down and directly in contact with the photosensitive material, as was already mentioned for Diazochrome copying, so that reproduced bands will be quite sharp. Impurities in a gel stain poorly and so are not recorded on a shadowgraph from a stained slide, whereas they tend to be recorded on one from an unstained slide. The color of the stain used on the immunodiffusogram can be selected to enchance recording of the precipitin band,[71] and, as was discussed previously, poorly visible precipitates can be enhanced by adding a mordant to the stain. Since precipitin bands are thinner in dried patterns, resolution is better (Hirschfeld, 1960b). There are some disadvantages to using a dried, stained pattern, the two most obvious being that some precipitin bands will disappear during washing and staining procedures, and that others stain so poorly that they will not register photographically.

Shadowgraphs made by projecting the image of the unstained (wet)

[71] Red and green stains record excellently on conventional photographic material sensitive only to blue light (e.g., photographic paper, certain photographic film, lantern slides), and red-stained bands produce excellent results on orthochromatic films sensitive to green and blue light (Wadsworth, 1963). Blue-stained bands record poorly on these materials, although they record quite well on Diazochrome film.

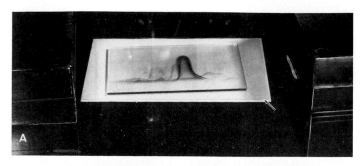

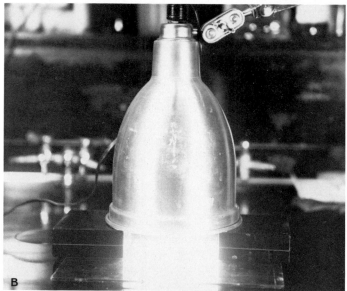

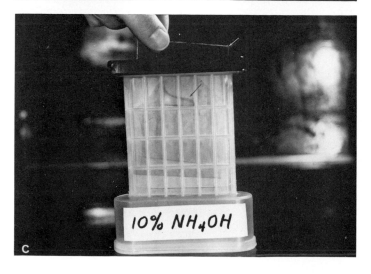

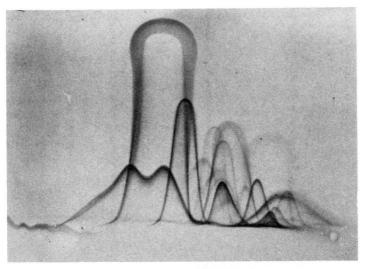

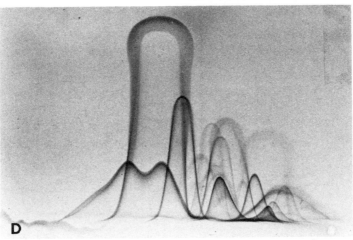

D

Fig. 2.7. Steps in preparing a Diazochrome copy of a stained immunodiffusion pattern. In *A* the pattern has been laid face down on Diazochrome film which, in turn, rests on white protective paper. In *B* the film is being exposed to a photographic floodlight resting on two microscope slide boxes which themselves rest upon a thick glass plate weighing down the pattern to hold it flat against the Diazochrome film. Typically, exposure is for 45 seconds. Next (*C*), the film is developed in a Polaroid Dippit tank (used only for convenience; any other container will suffice) whose original solution has been replaced with ammonium hydroxide solution as indicated. The black arrow shows part of the pattern which has begun to appear; the white arrow indicates the top edge of the film being inserted into the developing solution. Development is complete in a few seconds. After being rinsed briefly in tap water and blotted dry, the Diazochrome copy is almost indistinguishable from the original pattern itself (upper versus lower patterns, *D*). All procedures indicated can be performed in normal room light.

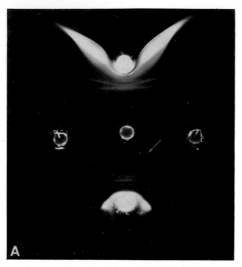

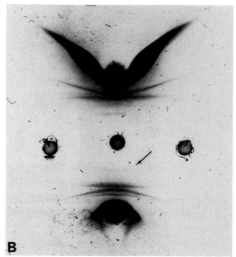

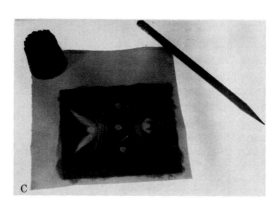

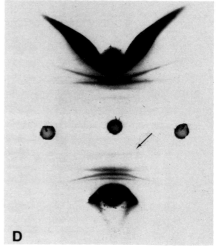

Fig. 2.8. Steps in the preparation of a black-on-white photograph of an immuno-diffusion pattern. Photograph *A* is a projection print made directly from the stained slide onto photographic paper. Photograph *B* is a contact print made from unre-touched photograph *A*. Note many specks of dust; arrow indicates faint precipitate which must not be lost during the various procedures employed. Photograph *C* shows retouching on back of photograph *A* using pencil, burned cork, and illuminating box. Photograph *D* shows final product made by contact printing from retouched photo-graph. Dust specks are gone, but precipitin bands including the faint one indicated by the arrow are all evident. Indeed, this faint band is easier to see in this black-on-white reproduction than in the white-on-black photograph *A*.

or stained pattern from a photographic enlarger or projector onto photosensitive material tend to be better than those made by contact printing (Nace and Alley, 1961; Goodman, 1962). Since light values are reversed in making a shadowgraph (except with Diazochrome, which produces a positive image), this will result in a print in which precipitin bands appear white on a dark background; that is, they have the same appearance as if the immunodiffusogram were being lit by dark-field lighting and photographed. Although esthetically this is a pleasing effect, prints in which precipitin bands appear black on a white background are more easily reproduced for publication, and precipitin bands tend to be more obvious while dust and lint specks tend to be less noticed. Therefore, in preparing a photograph for publication or illustration, it is usually preferable to make the final illustration from the shadowgraph, using the latter as a negative (see Fig. 2.8). For example, the shadowgraph can be made on photographic negative material (e.g., sheet film, lantern slide plate), and then this can be used to make a final contact or projection print on photographic paper. Aside from changing light values back to those of the original stained slide (i.e., dark bands on a light background), this intermediate shadowgraph can be retouched to remove blemishes, spots, specks, or other distracting artifacts for a cleaner final print (Fig. 2.8).[72] Alternatively, the shadowgraph can be made by projection printing of its final size on photographic paper, and this, after such retouching as may be necessary, can be used face-down on similar paper to make the final contact print (Fig. 2.8D).

Projection slides usually are made in the same way. But they can also be the stained immunodiffusograms themselves if blank projection plates were used either as the original support for the immunodiffusion test, or to support the gel of the test after it has been stained and dried onto the photographic plate.

Shadowgraphs usually are made directly from the immunodiffusogram. However, they can also be prepared from photographs of stained transilluminated immunodiffusograms.

PHOTOGRAPHS

There are basically two different ways of making photographs of unstained immunodiffusograms: photographing them with dark-field illumi-

---

[72] To materially change the precipitin bands themselves by retouching is neither ethical nor wise unless this is clearly noted in the accompanying legend (cf. Fig. 1.1). For instance, a weak band that has been enhanced by retouching will erroneously impress the viewer as a strong antigen–antibody reaction, unless he knows that it has been retouched. Moreover, retouching imparts a subjective interpretation to immunodiffusion patterns which may actually be incorrect.

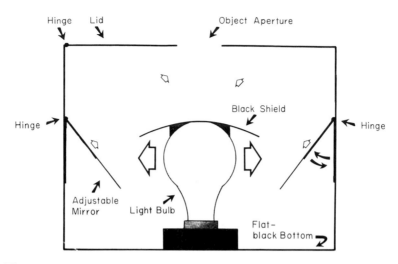

Fig. 2.9. Diagram of a simple and inexpensive viewing box for immunodiffusion reactions which also serves as an excellent dark-field illuminator for immunodiffusion photography. The object aperture is made to fit the size of the most often used cell. Preferably, the bottom of the box and the shield resting upon the light bulb should be covered with black velvet cloth, although a nearly comparable nonreflecting black background is obtained if both are painted with a "flat" black paint. The inside of the box also should be so painted.

nation, or projecting a dark-field image from a photographic enlarger which has been modified to illuminate the immunodiffusogram, which is placed in the negative carrier, only with indirect light.

Many lighting arrangements have been devised for the former technique (see Jensh and Brent, 1969; Nace and Alley, 1961; Murchio, 1960; Schubert *et al.*, 1961). They all attempt to obtain maximum and uniform light reflection from precipitin bands extending across the immunodiffusogram with minimum reflection from the background gel (Nace and Alley, 1961). A simple way of achieving this end is to project light up into the gel at a small angle from the side while it is held over a black, nonreflective background (Wadsworth, 1963). The simple illuminating box illustrated in Fig. 2.9 gives excellent results with petri dish-sized immunodiffusograms (see also Gilder, 1963). Even illumination of smaller immunodiffusograms, such as those currently employed in micro tests, is easier and makes less "formal" lighting arrangements quite adequate (Murchio, 1960; Smith, 1968). Thus, light sources may include anything that will illuminate the slide evenly while not scattering light excessively either on the background or into the camera lens (e.g., microscope lamp, small slide projector, appropriately shrouded incandescent lamp, or stroboscopic light). Some precipitin bands will dissociate when heated by conventional illuminating sources, and a medium such as gelatin may liquefy from lamp heat or room heat. To solve this problem, photographs can then be made with stroboscopic or flash bulb lighting (Maurer, 1962).

Dark-field photography probably is the easiest and most convenient way of recording large numbers of immunodiffusion patterns. A camera with its own built-in lighting system and using Polaroid film is commercially available principally for this purpose. Once an adequate light source has been devised and proper photographic exposure determined, good records can be made with a conventional 35-mm camera and roll film (Nace and Alley, 1961; Murchio, 1960). Normal contrast is better than high contrast film for most purposes (Wadsworth, 1963; Jensh and Brent, 1969; Jackson, 1964). Polaroid film is more expensive than conventional roll film, but it produces immediate results. If it is a film like 55N/P, it will produce both a print for the data book and a negative which can be used later in conventional fashion to make additional prints (Jordan and White, 1965; Wadsworth, 1963).

Occasionally, a precipitin pattern that has been stained will have some bands that have not taken up enough stain to register by shadowgraphing, or a selective stain picking out only one of several bands is employed (Gilder, 1963). Then, dark-field photography should be used (Nace and Alley, 1961). Stained gels which are dry when they are to be photographed in this manner should be soaked for a few minutes in the same solution as that used originally for destaining to restore to the unstained bands a capacity for light reflection (Nace and Alley, 1961).

Dark-field photographs of immunodiffusion tests are best when reflections from objects other than the precipitin bands themselves are avoided. Thus, use gels at low concentration. Warm them to room temperature to decrease their turbidity, use clear gels like polyacrylamide or gelatin, and filter the gels during their preparation to remove lint. Use immunodiffusion techniques in which the gel surface is unmarred and flat, or if there must be wells or troughs, fill them with gel, water, or mineral oil before photographing them. Submerge the slide in lint- and bubble-free water in a clear, unscratched, optically suitable container (e.g., new flat-bottomed glass petri dish: Nace and Alley, 1961).

Making projection prints with an enlarger modified for dark-field lighting is convenient and avoids some of the difficulties of photographing immunodiffusograms by dark-field lighting (Almeida *et al.*, 1965; Stuart, 1970). A big advantage to this technique is that the reaction image can be printed on large negatives which can be retouched easily and then can be used for contact printing of final photographs to produce black precipitin bands on a white background. However, this method is less versatile and generally less convenient than simple dark-field photography.

OTHER TYPES OF PHOTOGRAPHIC AND SEMIPHOTOGRAPHIC RECORDING

Radio-labeled constituents of bands make their own "light" for radioautography. Their radioactivity, just like visible light, reduces silver salts in photographic emulsions to silver. The basic technique is to place the dried immunodiffusogram with its gel in direct and tight contact with photosensitive material like x-ray film, Contrast Process Ortho, Royal Ortho, Royal Pan, or even Contrast Lantern Plates (Kodak products). Wrap this in a light-tight container, or place it in a dark box, allow the exposure to continue (hours, days, sometimes weeks, depending on the strength of the radioactivity in the label, and the amount of labeled reactant in the precipitate) until from previous experience adequate exposure is known to have occurred, and then develop the photosensitive material according to standard photographic techniques (cf. Minden et al., 1966; Van Furth et al., 1966; Silverstein et al., 1963a; Patterson, 1961; Hochwald et al., 1961; Clausen et al., 1963). Since the result will be a contact print of radioactive precipitin arcs, these arcs can be identified by direct comparison with stained precipitin bands in the original immunodiffusogram.

Fluoroimmunoelectropherograms, in which one of the reactants is fluorescence-labeled or in which a fluorescent stain has been used, are photographed under ultraviolet light illumination using a medium sensitivity photographic film and a filter on the camera lens to suppress stray ultraviolet light (Ghetie, 1967). The photographed immunodiffusogram later can be stained more conventionally for comparison of fluorescent (as photographed) and nonfluorescent precipitin bands.

There are several reasons for occasionally recording precipitin band patterns by drawing. For example, reproductions of line drawings are easier and cheaper to make for publication than continuous tone photographs. No matter how good a photograph may be, some faint bands in a pattern simply may not be evident in printed reproductions. The presence of one particular band among many may need to be accentuated.

Perhaps the simplest technique available to the average laboratory for making a drawn reproduction of the pattern is to project the stained image of the immunodiffusogram from a photographic enlarger or slide projector onto paper in a semidarkened room and then trace precipitin bands of interest, and markers such as well outlines, onto the paper with a hard pencil. Later this pencil drawing can be embellished to whatever artistic extent one desires. A simple technique for depicting precipitin bands outlined in pencil in this manner, but destined for line drawing reproduction, is to use a prepared pattern of random dots (e.g., Artype, Zip-A-Tone; see Fig. 2.1) which can be cut to the shape of the penciled pattern and pressed with its own adhesive to the paper. Similar results can be obtained by tracing an immunodiffusion pattern from an enlarged photograph onto transparent film (e.g., cellophane) and then photographing this on a white background (Bonilla-Soto *et al.*, 1961). Some such films are coated on one side with a ground glass-like surface which accepts pencil marks readily. These can be used for excellent tracings by projecting the immunodiffusion pattern onto the sheet from behind while making the tracing.

A semiphotographic method of making such reproductions is to print the immunodiffusion pattern on photographic paper, wash, fix, and dry the paper, use India ink to indicate bands of interest by outline and pattern, and then reduce and remove the silver image from the photographic print leaving only the India ink markings intact.

DENSITOMETRY

Photographs are objective records of immunodiffusion patterns, but like the patterns themselves they usually are interpreted subjectively. Semiobjective measurements made from these or the original patterns, such as the number of precipitin bands, their positioning relative to each other or to reactant sources, and their intensities or density profiles, can be made fully objectively and more accurately by densitometric scanning. Although in some special applications this method of recording immunodiffusion results has been highly developed (Glenn, 1961a, 1963, 1968), in general it is not yet much used. The future probably will witness development of instrumentation for sophisticated qualitative and quantitative as well as comparative analyses of immunodiffusograms by densitometry. Present immunodiffusion techniques are good enough so that, coupled with current technology of densitometric scanning and computerized analysis, they probably could provide routine clinical tests yielding simultaneously data on thirty or forty different serum antigens which would indicate which are quantitatively or qualitatively abnormal.[73] From electroimmunodiffusion tests such results could be available within as little as 5 hours (see Chapter 6).

The basic principle of densitometric scanning is simple (cf. El-Sharkaway and Huisingh, 1971; Butler and Leone, 1968; Smibert *et al.*, 1961). As a beam of light is moved across an immunodiffusion pattern, a light-sensitive detector into which this beam is aimed detects changes in the

---

[73] Results from such an analysis made anywhere could be radiotransmitted to a central computer for interpretation (Glenn, 1963).

intensity of the light beam caused by its interruption in varying degrees by stained or unstained precipitin bands in the immunodiffusion medium. Sometimes the densitometer is used to scan a photographic transparency of the immunodiffusion pattern instead of the pattern itself (Ceska, 1969a), but this is only an expedient required by the use of an immuno-diffusion technique and a scanning device that are not compatible. Except for special purposes, it should be avoided because photography introduces unnecessary variables into the analyses. The scanning can be as simple as moving the immunodiffusion pattern across the beam of light on a calibrated microscope stage and measuring changes in light intensity emanating from the microscope objective (Crowle, 1961); or it can range in automated sophistication through various intermediate levels (Smibert *et al.*, 1961; El-Marsafy and Abdel-Gawad, 1962) to the still unrealized potentials mentioned above.

Chapter 3

Single Diffusion Tests

In single diffusion tests one of the two reactants, either antigen or antiserum, remains stationary (the internal reactant) while the other (the external reactant) diffuses into and complexes with it. Broadly, there are two types of single diffusion test. In one, the external reactant diffuses linearly into an elongated column or strip of medium charged with the internal reactant. In the other, the external reactant diffuses radially into the internal reactant-charged medium surrounding it. Radial single diffusion tests are more commonly used, but linear single diffusion tests have greater historical and theoretical importance.

Mechanisms of Single Diffusion Tests

Linear Tests

One of the oldest (Oudin, 1946) and best characterized of immuno-diffusion techniques, the classic linear single diffusion test (Glenn, 1961c,d; Couffer-Kaltenbach and Perlmann, 1961), is performed by partially filling a small tube with agar gel mixed with a small amount of antiserum as the internal reactant and then, after this has gelled, over-laying it with antigen solution as the external reactant. Antigen is used in large immunologic excess relative to antibody. Hence, immediately after the antigen is layered upon the antiserum column, the tendency for antibody to diffuse upward into the antigen is suppressed, and the antigen instead diffuses downward into the antiserum.

Downward diffusion of the antigen quickly dilutes it at its advancing

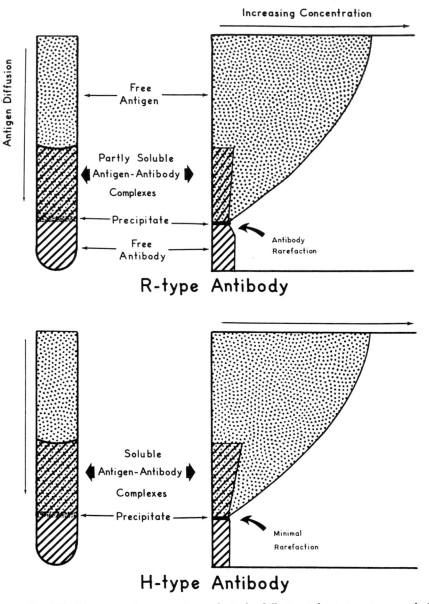

Fig. 3.1. Diagrammatic comparison of single diffusion tube tests set up with R-type and H-type antibodies. In the tubes, antigen, by virtue of an intended original excess over antibody below it, diffuses downward across the interface meniscus, diluting itself by this diffusion until it forms a visible precipitate with antibody. This precipitate, a band with a flat front, appears to move slowly down the antibody-

front from initially too great an excess to be precipitated by the antiserum to what later becomes a precipitating ratio with the antiserum. Consequently, a short distance below the interface of the two reactants a faint precipitate begins to appear. More antigen feeds into and passes through this area, diluting itself by diffusion while encountering essentially unchanging concentrations of antibody in succeedingly lower planes of the antiserum-charged agar. This intensifies the developing band of precipitate but also makes it appear to move into the internal reactant column in the following manner (see Fig. 3.1).

While antigen diluted by its diffusion precipitates with antibodies at the antigen diffusion front, it is being followed by continued diffusion of more antigen in higher concentration behind it, higher because it is closer to the original source of the antigen and because it is not being precipitated by antibodies which already are occupied by the antigen molecules that preceded those passing through this area behind the antigen diffusion front. As was explained in Chapter 1, secondary stages of antigen–antibody precipitation occur; they stabilize rather slowly and are susceptible before stabilization to interference with further development from the presence of one or the other reactant in excess, especially if this happens to be antigen. Consequently, as free antigen feeds into the back of the antigen diffusion front where unstabilized precipitation is developing, it tends to dissolve the developing precipitin band from behind. Thus, there is precipitation at the diffusion front and partial reversal of this behind the front, so that the precipitin band is more truly a wave of precipitation moving through the internal reactant with a sharp front and a trailing edge which is ragged in R-type antiserum and fairly sharp in H-type antiserum (Fig. 3.2).

---

charged column. It leaves behind it a trail of specific precipitate when R-type antibody is used but little or none if H-type antibody is used. In a single diffusion tube are found (1) free antibody, (2) forming, relatively stable, and dissolving specific precipitate, and (3) free antigen. The state of these constituents can be imagined as depicted in the diagrams to the right of their respective tubes. There are two points of particular interest. One is that large quantities of soluble antigen–antibody complexes will exist above the moving precipitin band front and below the interface when H-type antiserum is utilized. What the proportion of these is to free antigen in the same area is not known. A much smaller quantity of soluble complexes will be found in this area when R-type antibody is used. The second point is that, immediately ahead of the advancing precipitin band front, the concentration of antibody is less than further on down the tube for reasons explained in the text. This will be more marked for R-type than for H-type antibody.

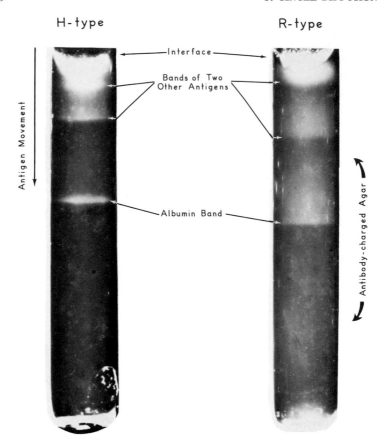

Fig. 3.2. Photographs contrasting and comparing precipitin zones in single diffusion tube tests set up with H-type (horse) and R-type (goat) antisera, respectively. These were antisera against whole human serum, and Cohn Fraction V from human serum was used as antigen in both tubes.

So long as the rate of antigen diffusion at its front is great enough to prohibit significant back-diffusion of antibodies from antiserum-containing gel lying ahead, the migrating wave of precipitate corresponds to the front of the diffusing antigen (Glenn, 1961d). Therefore it is an indicator of the rate of antigen diffusion and, accordingly, of antigen concentration and/or the diffusion coefficient (Read *et al.*, 1965; Glenn, 1961d; Couffer-Kaltenbach and Perlmann, 1961).

If external and internal reactants are balanced serologically at the beginning of the test, the band forms and remains at or near the interface (Fig. 3.3).

Ag Added to Tubes in Decreasing Concentrations, Left to Right

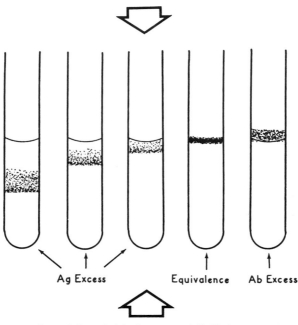

Ag Excess   Equivalence   Ab Excess

Quantity of Ab Same in All Tubes

Fig. 3.3. Antigen–antibody equivalence in the single diffusion test is determined by adding decreasing concentrations of antigen solution, under otherwise standardized conditions, to equal concentrations of antibody, and observing which in the series of tubes so formed shows development of a precipitin band at the antigen–antibody interface which is compact and does not tend to move into either antigen or antibody layers. In this tube, antigen and antibody are feeding into the precipitation area at rates that are serologically equivalent for the single diffusion tube, the diffusion and reaction of each exactly counterbalancing that of the other.

THEORETICAL CONSIDERATIONS

The rate of precipitin band front movement is directly proportional to the external reactant concentration and inversely proportional to the concentration of the internal reactant (Becker *et al.*, 1951; Glenn, 1961b,c). When conditions provide a large excess of antigen reacting with a low concentration of antibody, measurements over a period of time of precipitin band movement and plotted against the square root of that time ($\sqrt{t}$) will fall along a straight line with a certain slope, k (Fig. 3.4; Glenn, 1962b). The steepness of this slope at any single antigen

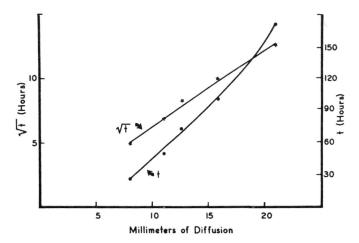

Fig. 3.4. Data obtained from the experiments of Augustin and co-workers (1958) with the bovine serum abumin-rabbit antiserum system in single diffusion tube tests have been plotted here to illustrate the linear relationship between millimeters of diffusion of a protein antigen (as detected by movement of its precipitin band front) and the square root of the time ($\sqrt{t}$) at which measurements were made. For comparison and to illustrate that this relationship means that with increasing time the antigen front moves progressively more slowly, a plot also has been made from the same data of distance versus time (t).

concentration varies with the quantity of antibody[1] in the gel (Perlmann *et al.*, 1960). Thus, if k is plotted along the ordinate of a graph and antibody concentration is plotted along the abscissa, k increases in a straight-line relationship with increases in antibody concentration. On the other hand, if the antibody concentration is held constant in a series of tubes in which various antigen concentrations are employed, then the steepness of the slope k is inversely proportional to antigen concentration, although k is not a very sensitive indicator of changes in antigen concentration or of diffusion coefficient (Couffer-Kaltenbach and Perlmann, 1961). The value k, then, is a potential index of the concentration of either reactant (Preer and Telfer, 1957). However, a linear relationship between k and log antigen concentration at the beginning of diffusion holds only for quantities of antigen that are not too high, while a similar relationship between k and log antibody concentration exists only at antibody concentrations that are not too low (Becker *et al.*, 1951; Glenn, 1961b). Differing k values obtained for varying concentrations of

---

[1] The "quantity of antibody" actually is "quantity of antibodies against all exposed determinants on an antigen." Consequently, the quality of an antiserum partly determines its effective quantitative strength. With IgG as antigen, for instance, one antiserum might react with heavy chain determinants, another with light chain determinants, and still another with both (Oudin, 1961).

antigen used against one antibody concentration, plotted against log concentration of the varied reactant, yield a straight line whose slope, m, is proportional to the square root of the true diffusion coefficient of the varied reactant, under ideal experimental conditions (Neff and Becker, 1956). But even ideal conditions may not permit demonstration of this constant relationship with some antigens (e.g., thyroglobulin) which tend to react with agar or to dissociate or associate during an experiment (Neff and Becker, 1956).

With an otherwise satisfactory system for demonstrating the linear relationship between $\sqrt{t}$ and apparent precipitin band movement, the relationship will not be linear at the beginning of measurements when diffusion distances are very small, because k actually equals $x/(\sqrt{t} + t_0)$ rather than $x/\sqrt{t}$ (Neff and Becker, 1957). Neither will it be linear when one of the reactants nears exhaustion so that its diffusion becomes discontinuous (Glenn, 1961d). For example, if the rate of band movement is measured in the lower reaches of the antibody column where antibody concentration remains constant but antigen concentration has become very low, both by dilution through diffusion and because its source is becoming exhausted, antibody just ahead of the precipitin front has time to diffuse significantly toward the zone of precipitation causing this to decelerate more rapidly than is compatible with linearity (Spiers and Augustin, 1958; see Fig. 3.1). The higher the ratio of antigen to its equivalence quantity with the concentration of antibody used, the further antigen can advance into the antibody column without deviating from this linear relationship between the time it takes to travel a given distance and that distance (Spiers and Augustin, 1958). It is obvious that such deviation will occur closer to the interface as antibody concentration is increased; the distance over which linear movement of the precipitin zone (i.e., antigen) will take place will be shorter (Becker and Neff, 1958). Hence, only when antibody concentration is very low can the "back-diffusion" of this reactant with its retarding effect on antigen diffusion be ignored in determining the diffusion coefficient of an antigen. Since linearity of band movement depends on maintenance of relatively constant antigen concentration at the interface, if the antibody concentration below it is high, an insufficiently long antigen column will speed the onset of the nonlinear phase of precipitin band movement. Obviously, when low antibody concentrations are used, the length of the antigen layer can be varied over wide limits without such inconsistencies (Becker *et al.*, 1951).

SOME FACTORS AFFECTING MOVEMENT OF THE PRECIPITIN BAND

Precipitin band movement will be affected by any physical characteristics of a test that alter reactant diffusion rates. Results may differ in two otherwise identical tests if in one the antigen is liquid and in the other it has been gelled. At a high antigen-to-antibody ratio, for example, penetration of the antigen into the antibody column can be significantly more rapid when it diffuses from a solution rather than a gel unless the antibody concentration is very low (Augustin *et al.*, 1958). Over a wide range of antigen-to-antibody ratios, measurements of antigen diffusion rates are more likely to scatter when a solution rather than a gel of antigen is utilized. These difficulties seem to be due primarily to whether or not convection currents develop in the antigen layer (Augustin *et al.*, 1958; Preer and Telfer, 1957). A liquid antigen solution with a higher specific gravity than the antibody layer on which it rests will develop convection currents, for as antigen diffuses across the interface into the antibody layer locally and at the bottom of its column, its concentration drops, causing also a drop in its density. Then, as the denser upper solution descends to replace the lighter interface layer which rises, a convection current is initiated which tends by its mixing of antigen solution to maintain a constant antigen concentration at the interface. On the other hand, if the specific gravity of the antigen column is less than that of the antibody column, no convection mixing will occur, and antigen in the interface region, becoming less concentrated than that above it, will be replenished only by diffusion from above. In either situation, linearity between time and the diffusion rate of the antigen will hold, but the slope (k) of the linear relationship for the two will differ. The change in slope occurs rather abruptly in a transition from one condition to the other if the specific gravity of the antigen solution is varied experimentally (Preer and Telfer, 1957; Fig. 3.3).

The nature of both antigen and antiserum solutes (sometimes called "nonspecific substances" or *nss*) can affect results (Becker *et al.*, 1951; Oudin, 1952, 1954). For example, if the same antigen used at equal concentrations is allowed to react with the same antibody in two different tubes, the antibody being diluted with saline in one tube and with normal serum in the other, the apparent antigen diffusion rate will be greater in the first tube than in the second (Oudin, 1954). Practically, this makes it imperative that equivalent solute conditions be maintained among several tubes in which, for example, comparisons of various antigen concentrations are being made. Generally, an *nss* in the antigen solution tends to increase the apparent rate of diffusion of antigen. An *nss* in high concentration in the antibody layer usually exerts the opposite effect (Oudin, 1952). These effects may be due partly to specific gravity differences between the two reactant layers (Oudin, 1954). Mathematical compensations for some of the effects are available (Becker *et al.*, 1951).

Unfortunately, an entire explanation for the effects of *nss* on antigen diffusion rates is not available. The value k for an antigen is very sensitive to variations in the viscosity of the antibody layer (Preer and Telfer, 1957). One might expect, therefore, that increasing this layer's viscosity to a given extent by adding to it any of various *nss* uniformly would decrease the antigen diffusion rate. However, some additives such as sucrose reduce k out of proportion to their viscosity-increasing effects. Moreover, when sucrose is added to the antigen solution to increase its viscosity, the rate of antigen diffusion does not drop as would be expected but actually rises. These unforeseen results have been explained tentatively as due to some ordering effect that the sucrose molecules might have upon the random motion of antigen molecules, causing them to move more readily down a sucrose gradient rather than against it, regardless of the factor of viscosity (Preer and Telfer, 1957). The potential error of this effect is not small. The k value for bovine γ-globulin dissolved at 2.5 mg/ml in 0.63 M sucrose has been found to equal that of a globulin concentration of 4.2 mg/ml made up in solution without added sucrose (Preer and Telfer, 1957).

The marked effects of viscosity on k have just been mentioned. If the diffusion rate of an antigen is being compared in some way among several single diffusion tubes, for reliability these comparisons should be in tubes having antibody columns of equal viscosity. Although viscosity is not difficult to control by addition of *nss*, as has been explained, this remedy may create new problems in place of the one it removes, and so it must be used cautiously. Varying the viscosity by changing either the type of agar (or other gel) employed or its concentration is another remedy, but it also invites interference of unpredictable factors (Augustin *et al.*, 1958; Becker *et al.*, 1951). Differences in batches of agar may explain divergent results obtained on similar problems in different laboratories (Augustin *et al.*, 1958). Thus, the viscosity of washed agar is less than that of crude agar. Diffusion rates can differ as determined in the same batch of agar, depending on how many times it is melted and gelled. For example, the diffusion rate for chicken ovalbumin in reheated agar was found to be lower than it was in agar heated only once (Neff and Becker, 1956, 1957a,b). Although minor variations in agar concentration usually do not affect diffusion rates much, they can if the diffusing antigen molecules are large enough for the agar gel to impede their diffusion (Becker *et al.*, 1951). Measurement of diffusion coefficients for quantitation of antigens like lysozyme which tend to combine with agar is, of course, not practical in agar; another type of gelling agent like agarose or polyacrylamide with no charge and perhaps with different chemical properties would have to be utilized.

Antigen does not diffuse into antibody-charged gel as freely as it does into gel with no antibody. Ideally, its leading edge at the front of the moving precipitin zone should be maintained at a constant concentration corresponding serologically to an equivalent quantity of antibody which it meets in the gel (Spiers and Augustin, 1958). Hence, there should be no free antigen below the precipitin zone and no free antibody above it (Spiers and Augustin, 1958). The precipitating time for the serological system being studied must be reasonably short for this condition to hold (Ouchterlony, 1958). The extent of retardation of antigen by reaction at this front depends on how quickly it can react with and "neutralize" each new plane of antibody exposed to it. Only when antigen is used in large serological excess, then, can it be thought to migrate under conditions approaching free diffusion in the agar gel (Oudin, 1952). This also suggests that the least concentration of antibody compatible with visible precipitin band formation should be used in single diffusion tests (Oudin, 1952). Using a low antibody concentration also circumvents a tendency for it to diffuse significantly toward the advancing precipitin zone front. If the concentration happens to be high enough, it forms a gradient ahead of the front, for, as the precipitate forms, antibody is removed locally from solution, creating a regional rarefaction (Fig. 3.1) into which antibody further ahead of this band tends to diffuse; results will depend partially on the steepness of this antibody gradient and the diffusion coefficient of antibody (Crowle, 1960b,c). This condition probably always exists, but it becomes insignificant when it is suppressed by certain experimental conditions. Thus, it is minimal when antibody concentration is very low and its molecular weight is high (e.g., macroglobulin antibody), or when a large excess of low-molecular-weight antigen is used against it (Fig. 3.1).

Antibody not only affects diffusion of antigen at the front of and within the precipitin zone; it also may affect it some distance behind the front, as fresh antigen tends to react with already formed but not necessarily stable antigen–antibody complexes left behind the advancing precipitin zone. This is especially likely when H-type antibody is being employed. No way of measuring this very complex interaction or of handling it mathematically has yet been devised (Augustin et al., 1958; Spiers and Augustin, 1958). The problem is particularly thorny because individual sera vary in how readily their precipitates redissolve in reactant excess or in how susceptible they are to rearrangement of reactant proportions. The final composition of antigen–antibody aggregate will be reached on levels well above the precipitin zone with H-type antibody (Spiers and Augustin, 1958). Under certain circumstances, such rearrangement of complexes formed with this type of antibody may result in production of multiple precipitin bands by a single antigen–antibody system (Crowle, 1960c, 1963; Lueker and Crowle, 1963). Although the linearity of diffusion rates is not affected by this antigen–antibody interaction, an apparent diffusion coefficient is likely to be spuriously low.

Incubation temperature significantly affects the results, as has already been partially explained in Chapter 2. Of special interest for single diffusion tube tests is the observation that changes in apparent migration of antigen into antiserum are not always consistent enough with changes in temperature between 20° and 35°C to permit use of a mathematical constant for adjusting data obtained at one temperature to equivalence with data obtained for the same antigen–antibody system at another temperature (Glenn, 1961d).

INTERPLAY OF MULTIPLE ANTIGEN–ANTIBODY SYSTEMS IN ONE TEST

Antiserum in a single diffusion tube may have antibodies to several antigens constituting the antigen mixture being analyzed. Each antigen–antibody system will react independently of the other because the biophysical and immunologic characteristics of each system are unlikely to be identical with those of any other. Hence, two different systems usually precipitate in different planes of the reaction column and continue to do so during most of the test period. Thus, if a mixture of antigens A and B is diffused into gel containing antiserum with antibodies to both, the two may at first precipitate in a single broad band immediately below the antigen–antibody interface. But as time passes they will be distinguished from each other by a progressive separation of their two respective bands. Each of these will migrate through the antiserum gel independently of the other and at its own characteristic rate, as determined by such factors as concentration of the antigen forming it, this antigen's diffusion rate, the concentration of antibodies forming it, and miscellaneous properties of the immunologic reactions between the antigen and its various antibodies, because theoretically it is very unlikely that for any two antigen–antibody systems all these factors will be exactly the same.

But practically, the distinction between two different systems tends to blur in single diffusion tubes, especially when R-type antibody is being employed, because the trail of the leading wave of precipitation tends to extend back over the front of the following wave of precipitate (cf. Fig. 3.2). This is why various double diffusion or immunoelectrophoresis tests are preferred for qualitative analyses. Nevertheless, because of the distance over which waves of antigen–antibody precipitate travel in single diffusion tubes, these tubes have yielded some of the most detailed information obtained from any kind of immunodiffusion test on interactions of cross-reacting precipitating systems. This information, sum-

marized in the following paragraphs, is general; although it was obtained
from and applies principally to single diffusion tube tests, it applies also
with slight modifications to all varieties of immunodiffusion.

Although two entirely independent antigen–antibody systems will not
interfere with each other, cross-reacting systems will. This may be either
troublesome or helpful, depending on the test situation. It would be
useful, for example, in determining whether a solution contains antigen
A or antigen B. One can mix a sample of this solution with some of each
of the two antigens and then compare this mixture in single diffusion
tubes with control tubes charged with antigen A or antigen B alone,
and with the unaltered solution itself. If antigen A is present in this
solution, then its concentration in the solution will be added to that of
the supplementary antigen, and the rate of migration for the band in
the tube receiving antigen A will be accelerated. By contrast, its migration rate in the tube receiving antigen B will remain unchanged (Fig.
3.5). The degree of change effected by this admixture of known and
unknown also would indicate the concentration of antigen A in the test
solution.

This additive effect of identical antigens being mixed together is immunologically equivalent to Ouchterlony's familiar "reaction of identity"
as classically seen in double diffusion plate tests (see Chapter 4); the
independent development of precipitin bands by different antigens A
and B in a single diffusion tube is the immunologic equivalent of Ouchter-

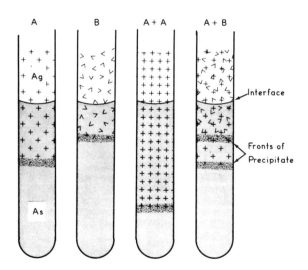

Fig. 3.5. Diagram showing effects on precipitin band formation and location in
single diffusion tube tests of mixing together identical or different antigens.

lony's "reaction of nonidentity." The analog of a "reaction of partial identity" also can be observed in single diffusion tubes.

Consider an antigen with determinants x and y and another with only determinant x. Antigen xy diffused into gel containing antiserum to determinants x and y (i.e., antiserum to antigen xy) would form one precipitin band. Antigen x diffused into this antiserum similarly would form one precipitin band. But suppose that antigens xy and x were mixed for testing in three different proportions to each other: xy predominating, xy and x at equivalent concentrations, and x predominating. With xy predominating only one band would form, consisting of mixed aggregates of xy and antibodies to determinants x and y. No uncomplexed antibodies to either determinant would remain to react with antigen x, trailing behind. With equivalent concentrations of each there would still be only one precipitin band formed, consisting of a mixture of antibodies to both determinants complexed with both antigens. But the apparent diffusion rates of antigen xy would be increased (as they would also for x, though proportionally less) because x, by "aiding" antigen xy in complexing with antibodies to shared determinant x, would be decreasing the number of antibodies through which antigen xy must diffuse. This additive effect would be less than that which would result from adding antigen xy, instead of x, to xy because only the one determinant is shared between antigens xy and x. With x predominating, two precipitin bands most likely[2] would form—that developed by x at the front and migrating as though no xy antigen were present, and that constituted by xy trailing behind and composed of antigen xy and antibodies only to its y determinant, since all antibodies to x would have been consumed by reaction in the more advanced front of antigen x (see Fig. 3.6).

These examples of related antigens affecting each other's precipitation in single diffusion tubes is an oversimplification of actual fact in several ways, most importantly in referring to the determinants involved. "Determinant x" should be understood to represent a series of determinants common to the two antigens, and "determinant y" a series of determinants present on antigen xy but absent from antigen x (see Chapter 1 for expansion on this subject). As a corollary to this, antiserum against both x and y would have antibodies to all the determinants represented by these two letters, while antiserum to x alone would have antibodies only to determinants represented by "x." But no two antisera, even if taken

---

[2] Only one precipitin band still might form if the concentration of antibodies to y relative to that of antibodies to x were very low in the antiserum being used. Then, even at increased relative proportion to antigen xy, antigen x still could not advance far enough ahead of it to form a detectably independent band.

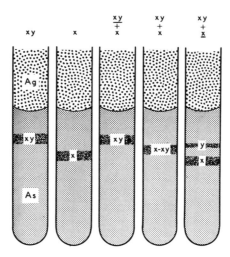

Fig. 3.6. Diagram depicting various possibilities for precipitin band formation in single diffusion tube tests with cross-reacting antigens x and xy and antiserum containing corresponding antibodies, when the two antigens are used singly or mixed in different proportions. Labels on the precipitin bands indicate the antigen(s) forming them. Underlining for antigens in the third and fifth tubes from the left indicate that these antigens are being used in predominating concentration.

from the same animal on successive bleedings separated by only a relatively short time, would be likely to have identical spectra of precipitins to each of the many individual determinants collectively constituting either "determinant x" or "determinant y" (see section on antiserum, Chapter 1). Moreover, antigens being compared may be cross-reactive in two directions rather than just one.

Suppose that one antigen has determinants x and y, and a second has determinants x and z. Because both antigens have determinant x, an antiserum against determinant x alone will not distinguish between the two: they will precipitate in single diffusion tests, as well as other immunodiffusion tests, as though they were antigenically identical. An antiserum containing antibodies to determinant y alone could detect only antigen xy, and an antiserum containing antibodies against determinant z alone would detect only antigen xz. An antiserum containing antibodies to determinants y and z but not to x would detect both antigens as though they were unrelated. This explains the importance of antiserum in immunodiffusion tests.

The truer relationship between antigens xy and xz would be revealed by an antiserum with antibodies against all three determinants x, y, and

z.[3] This would react with both antigens to form two precipitin bands in the single diffusion tube test. But because determinant x is shared by the two antigens, the two precipitin reactions will not form independently of each other. For example, the apparent migration rates of each antigen would be higher if the two were used mixed rather than independently against this antiserum because of mutual aiding against antibodies to the shared determinant x.

If the concentration of one of the cross-reacting antigens is considerably lower than that of the other, the nature of their cross-reactivity will not be revealed by one test alone. With antigen xy in higher concentration and diffusing ahead of antigen xz, the precipitin band formed by antigen xy would propagate through the antiserum at the same rate as it would if it were diffusing by itself. But progression of the precipitate formed by antigen xz to the rear of the xy precipitate would be faster than predicted on the basis of its absolute concentration, because cross-reacting antigen xy will have lowered the concentration in the antiserum column of antibodies reacting with x. This would indicate cross-reactivity between the trailing antigen and the leading antigen, but it would not indicate cross-reactivity in the other direction. Such would be revealed only by reversing the proportions of the two antigens and noting an accelerating effect on migration of antigen xy behind the xz precipitate.

The interplay of related antigen–antibody systems in single diffusion tubes has been discussed rather extensively here because this type of test reveals in greatest detail the events of such interplay which account for the three basic distinctions for compared antigen–antibody systems in all immunodiffusion tests—identity, nonidentity, and partial identity. Therefore only the somewhat different manifestations of these distinctions and associations will need discussion for plate tests, below, and for the immunodiffusion tests described in Chapters 4 through 7.

SECONDARY PRECIPITATION

The movement and position of a precipitin band contribute information not only on the nature and quantity of the antigen but also on whether the band is primary or secondary. One antigen–antibody system which forms only a single (primary) band under carefully controlled

---

[3] Such antiserum would be obtained from an animal immunized with both antigens, or it could be made by mixing antisera from different animals immunized with the separate antigens. A practical aspect to this is often overlooked: in comparing two species of bacteria by an immunodiffusion test, for instance, one should use an antiserum containing antibodies to both and not an antiserum against just one of the two.

conditions may form more (secondary) bands under such influences as sudden temperature changes. The differences between these two types of band can be illustrated best by discussing how they, particularly the secondary bands, are formed (cf. Crowle *et al.*, 1963; Crowle, 1960c, 1963; Lueker and Crowle, 1963).

Highly purified human serum albumin allowed to diffuse in high concentration against very dilute antibody to it at constant temperature will form only one precipitin band which moves down the antibody-charged column in the predictable fashion described above. This is the primary precipitate. However, if, during this test, the environmental temperature suddenly is decreased by a few degrees, the rate of movement of the precipitin band front will decrease. Then, this front appears to split into two precipitin bands, one continuing to move forward, but the other, for most antibody systems (see below), remaining at its plane of formation. This is a secondary band, or *stria* (Fig. 3.7), and its immobility is characteristic (Wilson, 1958). A stria also can be induced to form if the antigen concentration overlying the antibody column suddenly is lowered (Wilson, 1958). A sudden rise in temperature or an increase in antigen concentration usually causes an opposite effect—the appearance of a clear area or *gap* (Fig. 3.7), also usually immobile, in the ragged trail of precipitate most types of antibody leave when the advancing precipitate band does not completely dissolve immediately to its rear in antigen excess. If only one observation of a single diffusion tube is made after several hours of incubation and the temperature has varied several times, even though only a few degrees, the several secondary precipitin bands which may have been developed by the one antigen–antibody system will be misinterpreted as indicating the presence of several antigen–antibody systems. Hence, definitive single diffusion experiments require both rigidly controlled temperature and multiple observations of the number of precipitin bands and their movement.

As postulated on the basis of experimental evidence by Wilson (1958) and supported by experiments in the author's laboratory (Crowle *et al.*, 1963; Crowle, 1960c, 1963; Lueker and Crowle, 1963), a gap probably is formed in the single diffusion test when at the precipitin band front there is a sudden rise in the diffusion rate of antigen (due either to increased temperature or to an artificial change in the antigen concentration at its origin), and temporarily the concentration of antigen in this area exceeds the quantity with which antibody can combine to form a visible precipitate. Beyond this gap antigen again becomes dilute enough, by diffusion and by encountering increasingly greater quantities of antibody, to resume forming visible precipitate. If conditions remain stable thereafter, this "new" precipitin band continues to migrate down-

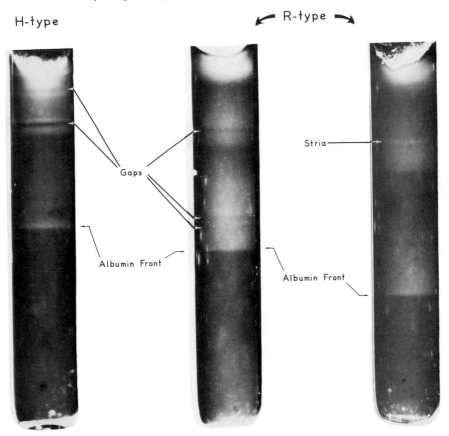

Fig. 3.7. Photographs of single diffusion tubes set up with H-type and R-type antisera showing the temperature artifacts, gaps, and striae. Gaps formed when the temperature of incubation of the first two tubes suddenly was raised, while stria in the third tube resulted when the temperature suddenly was lowered.

ward in the usual way while the gap in its trail remains stationary. A stria, on the other hand, seems to develop when a momentary slackening of antigen diffusion rate occurs, whereupon, also momentarily, antibody at the front of the precipitin zone has a chance to arrange itself with antigen with which it already has begun to react into a more stable lattice under conditions closer to equivalence with the antigen than is ordinarily possible in the single diffusion test. This momentary respite for the antibody results in a precipitate which, because of its increased stability, may be heavier, and is less soluble in antigen than the primary precipitate, so that it remains conspicuously and virtually unaltered in the trail of poorly dissolving antigen–antibody complex left by the moving primary zone. It tends, therefore, to remain sharply defined and heavy.

The characteristic immobility of striae and gaps is not without exception. These artifacts, temperature-induced with H-type antiserum, have been observed to migrate (Lueker and Crowle, 1963). However, they also usually disappear after a short while, the stria dissolving and the gap merging into a background of equal clarity as precipitate trailing the primary band is completely dissolved. The formation of temperature-induced artifacts is more likely with low- than with high-molecular-weight antigens (Wilson, 1958).

Another kind of secondary precipitate, resembling the classic Liesegang precipitation of inorganic chemistry (Stern, 1954; Van Oss, 1959; Crowle *et al.*, 1963), has been reported several times to occur in double diffusion tests (e.g., Burtin, 1954) and has been detected in single diffusion tests employing H-type antiserum (Fig. 3.8; Crowle, 1963; Lueker and Crowle, 1963). Under the usual conditions in which it is employed, the single diffusion test is said not to develop this type of precipitate (Oudin, 1952). These "usual" conditions entail maintaining a very high antigen-to-antibody ratio (Lueker and Crowle, 1963). As this ratio falls with increasing distance that an antigen has to diffuse with time in a single diffusion tube, the susceptibility of the system to Liesegang ("periodic") precipitation increases, and so after prolonged incubation one may observe a band to split into two or more. If there are two

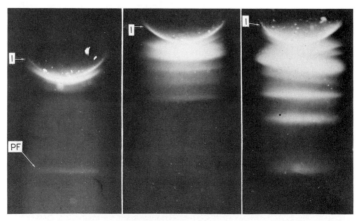

Fig. 3.8. Three photographs taken at different intervals to demonstrate formation of secondary (Liesegang) precipitates in a single diffusion tube above the primary front band (PF, seen only in the first photograph) and originating from the interface (I), and to show that in this instance, when horse antiserum was employed against crystallized human serum albumin, none of these secondary bands remained stationary.

antigens in a solution and one is rather weak, this antigen may begin
Liesegang precipitation well before the stronger antigen, and as a result
the experimenter may conclude wrongly that the solution contains more
than two antigens. Liesegang precipitation is readily identified in plate
tests by lateral convergence of primary and secondary precipitin bands
(cf. Chapter 1, Chapter 4; Lueker and Crowle, 1963; Crowle, 1963), but
in tube tests such convergence cannot develop; consequently, secondary
precipitation is especially deceptive in tubes.

PRECIPITIN BAND CHARACTERISTICS

   The form that a precipitin zone assumes in single diffusion tests can
be instructive (Oudin, 1955). For example, the breadth of such a zone
depends on the nature of both reactants constituting it (Fig. 3.2). A
sharply defined band with a short trailing edge is formed by H-type
antibody because its precipitates dissolve so readily in antigen excess
(Augustin, 1957; Ouchterlony, 1958). On the other hand, R-type antibodies yield broad precipitin zones, rather than bands, whose leading
edges may or may not be sharp but whose trailing edges tend to be long
and ragged, extending into the upper reaches of the antibody-charged
agar column where finally they may fade into the slight background
turbidity of the agar gel. This is, of course, because these antibodies
form precipitates only sparingly soluble in excess antigen.

   The influence of antigens upon zone shape is illustrated by photometric comparison of zones formed by human serum components with
rabbit antiserum (Glenn, 1958; Glenn and Garner, 1957). Human serum
albumin forms a zone with a sharp leading edge in which the degree
of opacity of the precipitin band rises very abruptly; its trailing edge,
although not so compressed as it would be if horse antiserum were being
used, drops off in density fairly sharply. Human serum β- and γ-globulins,
on the other hand, produce a zone more symmetrical in its density distribution, the density rising gradually at its front and fading off slowly
at its rear to merge with other precipitin zones behind or into the background turbidity of the agar. Precipitin bands as they are first formed
are their sharpest and, with time, tend to broaden, for as a precipitin
zone moves down the antibody column, its trailing edge, originally
exposed to the precipitate-dissolving effect of high antigen concentration,
is subject to progressively lower and less effective antigen concentrations
as the gradient for this reactant broadens behind the zone (Glenn and
Garner, 1957). The steepness of the optical density gradient trailing
after a zone measured photometrically at different intervals during a
test thus is a measure of a constantly changing antigen gradient, and
potentially it is an identifying characteristic for a given antigen, since

this gradient should change equally against one antiserum over a period of time.

Most protein antigens which have been studied in single diffusion tests have been observed to precipitate with either R or H antisera in bands with sharp leading edges, while polysaccharide antigens tend to form bands whose leading edges tend to be fuzzy (Becker, 1953; Oudin, 1952). However, this general difference probably is not particularly reliable because, as more proteins are studied, several are being found that resemble polysaccharides in their precipitin band characteristics. Moreover, as Oudin has observed, antiserum from one rabbit against a protein antigen may yield a sharp band front, while antiserum from another rabbit against the same protein produces a band with a fuzzy front (Becker, 1953). This latter observation is interesting in itself as probably helping to characterize the antibodies constituting an antiserum. Thus, whether an antiserum produces a fuzzy-edged or a sharp-edged zone could depend on whether it contains a high proportion of nonprecipitating antibodies; or the nature of the antibody may be such that antigen and antibody combine in a relatively narrow range of ratios to form a sharply defined front (Becker, 1953).

RESOLUTION

The value of a single diffusion test depends, in the final analysis, on the distinguishability of its precipitin bands, which with complex antigen–antibody systems often is not very good. A band must be dense enough to be visible; that is, sufficient antibody for it must be present (Oudin, 1952). Yet, to achieve this for a minor antibody by using less diluted antiserum may be impractical because coexisting stronger antibodies will form precipitin bands broad enough and dense enough to obscure the appearance of the much fainter minor system band. Concentration artifacts also may be invited by such adjustments (Crowle, 1960c, 1963; Lueker and Crowle, 1963). Another form of this problem is that two precipitin bands which should be resolved are not, because physical conditions cause them to precipitate and so to migrate together (Munoz and Becker, 1950; Wilson, 1958). They may do so during an entire test (Munoz and Becker, 1950), or they may first form a single band which later splits into two and still later merges again into one (Wilson, 1958). Hence, double diffusion tests are superior to single diffusion tests for studying complex antigen–antibody systems.

Radial Single Diffusion Tests

In a radial single diffusion test, the external reactant in serologic excess to the immediately surrounding internal reactant is deposited in a well cut in, or at a point on, a thin flat plane of internal reactant-containing medium. From this it diffuses radially into, and combines with, the internal reactant to form a disc of precipitate that expands out into the surrounding medium until at maximum size the front of the diffusing external reactant has reached serologic equilibrium with the surrounding internal reactant, and the disc stops growing (Mancini *et al.*, 1965). Radial single diffusion tests have become much more popular in recent years than they were when the first edition of this book was written because of their unique utility in quantitating antigens and antisera more easily than most other immunodiffusion tests (Becker *et al.*, 1969). Ironically, their attainment of first-rank importance among immunodiffusion tests probably will soon be lost as they are replaced by the much faster and more efficient technique of electroimmunodiffusion.

THEORETICAL CONSIDERATIONS

The rate of movement of the wave of precipitation in radial single diffusion tests is not proportional to $\sqrt{t}$, as it is in linear single diffusion tests, except in the earliest stages of the test (Mancini *et al.*, 1965; cf. Hill, 1968, for mathematical considerations and references thereto). This is because in a radial test the ratio of the volumes of external reactant to internal reactant is very small, and because dilution of the external reactant is very fast.[4] Hence, although the rate of precipitate expansion can be used to quantitate a reactant in these tests, it is too variable and difficult to measure accurately to provide precise data (Hill, 1968). On the other hand, these characteristics of the radial test make the external reactant reach serologic equilibrium with the internal reactant reasonably quickly and quite reproducibly, so that the terminal size of the disc of precipitate, measured as area or diameter, accurately indicates the amounts of both reactants and their proportions to each other (Fig. 3.9). The final size of the disc of precipitate has a straight-line relationship to the initial concentration of the external reactant and is similarly but inversely related to the internal reactant concentration (Mancini *et al.*, 1965; Vergani *et al.*, 1967).

The internal reactant functions in the linear test primarily as an indicator for the progress of external reactant diffusion; it is usually not expected to precipitate the external reactant enough to slow its diffusion. The linear test therefore provides primarily physical data from which are derived qualitative and quantitative characteristics of the external reactant.

[4] Dilution of other solutes accompanying the external reactant is equally accelerated. This, together with the use of a serologic end point (Mancini *et al.*, 1965) rather than measurement of diffusion rates, makes radial tests less susceptible than linear tests to foreign influences like *nss*.

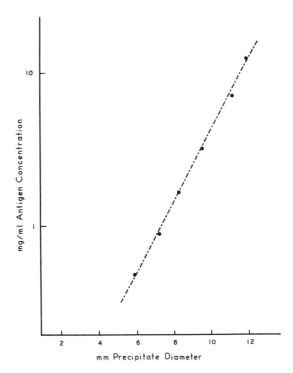

Fig. 3.9. Graph adapted from Fahey and McKelvey (1965), showing the linear relationship between antigen concentration and the diameter of discs of precipitate in single diffusion plate tests. The data were obtained with human IgG as test antigen.

By contrast, in the radial test migration of the external reactant is inhibited significantly and progressively by the internal reactant until it is stopped when, by the dilution and attrition of its preceding migration through the internal reactant and medium, its concentration comes sharply to equilibrium with that of the internal reactant. The higher the relative concentration of external reactant, the farther its disc of precipitate will expand before being arrested; and the lower the concentration, the less the precipitate disc will expand. Reciprocally, the weaker the internal reactant (e.g., antiserum), the farther the external reactant (i.e., antigen) can migrate before reaching equilibrium. A basic difference between linear and radial tests is, then, that the first provides primarily physical and the second primarily serologic data (Colover et al., 1963).

As a result of this difference, the radial test is more independent of physicochemical influences. For instance, the incubation temperature profoundly affects results in the linear test, but the final size of a precipitate disc in a radial test is temperature-independent (Mancini *et al.*, 1965). Indeed, radial tests often are performed at body temperature to shorten the time required for precipitation to reach maximum size. Another important result of this difference between linear and radial tests is that the internal reactant plays only a small role in results obtained from linear tests, whereas it has a major role in shaping results produced by the radial test (Hill, 1968). Consequently, results in a radial test depend directly upon the balance of reaction between available determinant groups on a population of antigen molecules and the concentration, variety, and specificity of antibodies to these several determinant groups in the opposing antiserum. This is a cause both for certain "failures" and for certain advantages in radial tests.

The straight-line relationship between the concentration of antigen, as the external reactant, and the size of the precipitate that it forms in a radial test will fail if the antigen population is physically heterogeneous so that it occurs in different proportions of subpopulations from sample to sample; if there are concentration-dependent interactions between antigen molecules, antigen and accompanying solutes, or antigen and immunodiffusion medium; or if the antiserum is not monospecific for the antigen but contains antibodies which also can react with contaminating antigens (Braun and Aly, 1969; Fahey and McKelvey, 1965). Since data from radial tests are serologically defined, they must be related to serologic standards; either the standard must be serologically identical to the unknown, or differences between them must be recognized and compensated for to obtain accurate quantitations. For example, antiserum to IgA standardized for serum IgA will give falsely low absolute values of salivary IgA because the latter is a larger molecule (Vaerman and Heremans, 1969; South *et al.*, 1966). Or among several antisera standardized against a predominantly k-type IgG there could be major differences in quantitations of IgG in general, due to possibly different proportions among these antisera of precipitins with λ specificity (Fahey and McKelvey, 1965; South *et al.*, 1966; Reimer *et al.*, 1970). Erroneously high values for IgM were traced to the presence in the patient's sera of low-molecular-weight varieties of IgM (Jones, 1970). Standards must be prepared for each antigen–antibody system; one cannot confidently interpolate data from one system to another (Fahey and McKelvey, 1965).

Although the straight-line correlation between antigen–antibody concentrations and area of precipitate holds over a wide range of reactant concentrations (Vergani *et al.*, 1967), it can fail in extremes. When antigen concentration is too high, for instance, failure may result because of indefinite equilibration of the antigen with the antibody due to such factors as partial reversibility of antigen–antibody precipitation within the disc of precipitate from the large excesses of antigen therein, or because the excess of antigen has been sufficient to deplete the antibody concentration in the surrounding gel which, for optimal results, should be uniformly available (Fahey and McKelvey, 1965; Hill, 1968; Massey-eff and Zisswiller, 1969). This will depend partly on the nature of the antigen, excesses of fast-diffusing antigen with relatively few determinants presumably being more likely to produce irregular results than slow-diffusing antigens with larger numbers of determinants; it can also depend partly on the geometry of the test setup and placement of sample wells. Apart from technical difficulties of obtaining accurate measurements for the disc of precipitate, when antigen concentration is too low, back-diffusion of antibodies may account for deviation from the straight-line relationship.

There is a tendency to read results from radial diffusion plates before final disc size has been attained because disc growth may continue for several days. Such premature reading accentuates these problems of extremes in external reactant concentration (McCracken et al., 1969). It should be avoided or compensated for by use of adequate standards for each individual test from day to day (Patnode et al., 1969). It decreases the accuracy of these tests in inverse proportion to the diffusion coefficient of the antigen being quantitated, because the disc of precipitate formed by a slow-diffusing antigen will be smaller than that formed in the same time by a fast-diffusion antigen; hence, distinctions between comparably different concentrations of antigen (i.e., between the sizes of their discs of precipitate) will be harder to measure for the slow antigen than for the fast antigen.

The apparent effective diffusion rate of external reactant in a radial diffusion test can be determined indirectly by measuring either the diameter of its precipitate at a set time during its active expansion or the time that it takes to reach equilibrium with the internal reactant and for the disc of precipitate to cease growing (Mancini et al., 1965). Since values obtained in this manner will depend (as they do in the linear test) on the initial concentration of the external reactant and (as they do not in the linear test) also on the concentration of the internal reactant, they will be relative and thus require the experimenter to use proper control standards for both antigen and antiserum. It is possible, in this manner, to estimate the approximate diffusion coefficient and molecular weight of a homogeneous population of antigen molecules (Fahey and McKelvey, 1965).

As is indicated above, the radial test is relatively insensitive to several extraneous influences affecting linear tests. On the other hand, radial tests have their own peculiar sensitivities. For instance, although within reasonable limits the size of the external reactant well has little effect on the linear relationship between reactant concentration and precipitate disc size, the volume of the external reactant is very important (Becker, 1969). For quantitatively reproducible results this must be the same from test to test. Apparently this is because, relative to the large surrounding volume of medium, the volume of the external reactant is small, but relative to the final disc size, it is fairly large. Hence, small changes in this volume mechanically affect initial movement of the external reactant into the surrounding medium ("wash" it in), thus, in effect, changing the diameter of the starting circle of diffusion and ultimately the final disc size (Mancini *et al.*, 1965). The linear test is insensitive to this factor because in it the volume of the external reactant usually is as large as that of the internal reactant.

In most radial tests the volume of the internal reactant is massive relative to that of the external reactant. But when by design (Masseyeff and Zisswiller, 1969) or by accident (Fahey and McKelvey, 1965) it is not, then the internal reactant can become depleted, with a resulting breakdown in linearity of reactant and precipitate disc proportions. This may not be disadvantageous (actually, it is the basis for demonstrating the "sink effect" discussed below, and for showing reactions of identity in comparative radial single diffusion tests), but it must not be overlooked. Another factor of moderate (Mancini *et al.*, 1965) to prominent (Hill, 1968) importance, depending on how results are being measured, is that the thickness of the reaction medium should be uniform. Small changes in thickness cause disproportionally large changes in total volume of the internal reactant into which the constant volume of the external reactant is meant to diffuse.

The best quantitative results are obtained in radial tests when a monospecific antiserum is used against a homogeneous antigen and hence only one precipitating system is present. Only one disc of precipitate should develop; however, extreme and sudden variations of temperature can cause temperature artifacts, and so they should be avoided (Mancini *et al.*, 1965). When multiple rings of precipitate develop at constant temperature in a test supposedly involving only a single precipitating system and with antigen as the external reactant, they may be the periodic precipitates of Liesegang (Lueker and Crowle, 1963), or the precipitating system may not be serologically as pure as was originally thought. Qualitative radial double diffusion analyses should be performed to determine which answer is true, for the lack of any opportunity for lateral precipitin band convergence in radial single diffusion tests precludes ready identification of Liesegang precipitation. An unusual cause of spurious precipitation is for antibody in the sample of antigen to precipitate antigen in the antiserum—that is, an unintentional superimposition of a reversed test (see below) on the conventional test (Ammann and Hong, 1971). For instance, human serum as the external reactant being analyzed for an immunoglobulin may contain precipitins that can precipitate goat serum albumin present in the goat antiserum to human immunoglobulin being used as the internal reactant.

COMPARATIVE TESTS

Radial single diffusion tests can be used to compare antigens and antisera directly (Mancini *et al.*, 1970), although mostly as a matter of curiosity, since several other kinds of immunodiffusion tests are better for this purpose. Figure 3.10 illustrates reactions of nonidentity, partial identity, and identity as seen in such tests (cf. also Fig. 8.1).

Radial single diffusion plates are especially well suited to demonstrating one of the most interesting phenomena in immunodiffusion, the sink effect (Fig. 1.7, Chapter 1). When identical antigens are deposited fairly close to each other in antiserum-charged gel, they will influence the growth of each others' discs of precipitation (Crowle, 1960b; Mancini

Single Diffusion Reactions

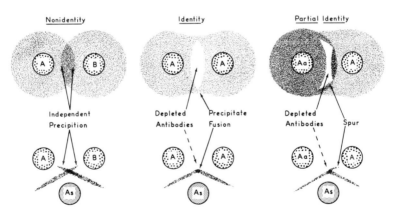

Comparable Double Diffusion Reactions

Fig. 3.10. Diagrams showing the appearance of reactions of nonidentity, identity, and partial identity, in single diffusion plate tests, and comparing them with the appearances of analogous reactions as they occur in double diffusion plate tests. (Drawn from photographs in Mancini *et al.*, 1970.)

et al., 1970; Benaš, 1963). If they are barely within each others' spheres of influence, the disc of precipitate for each will bulge toward the other; if they are closer together, their discs will be flattened across the plane between them (see Fig. 3.11). The reason for these effects is that in single diffusion tests the internal reactant is not as static as the name of these tests implies, for it diffuses toward the advancing front of antigen (sometimes called "back-diffusion") to replace that which is being precipitated by the antigen in the sink effect (Nordin *et al.*, 1970; Crowle, 1960b). Under appropriate conditions this back-diffusion can be large; then it shapes precipitation to the extent to which it occurs. The sink effect and the resulting alterations in the diffusion rate of serologically related reactants in immunodiffusion tests account for some of the more notable characteristics of these tests, including merging rather than overlapping of discs (single diffusion) or of precipitin arcs (double diffusion) in reactions of identity, the growth of related reactions toward each other and especially the bending of precipitin arc tips in Ouchter-

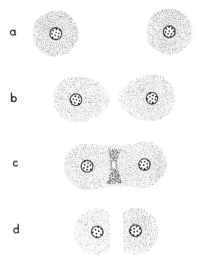

Fig. 3.11. Diagram showing interaction of identical antigens placed in wells at different distances from each other in antiserum-charged agar. When the wells are far apart (*a*), no interaction is evident. As they are placed progressively closer together the growing discs of precipitate bulge toward each other (*b*), coalesce in a reaction of identity (*c*), or interfere with each other's development (*d*). The effects seen in *b*, *c*, and *d* are due to different degrees of antibody depletion by the sink effect between the two converging identical antigens. Examples of these effects can be seen between the discs of albumin precipitate in Fig. 6.11. (Drawn from photographs in Benaš, 1963.)

lony's reaction of identity, and Liesegang precipitation (Lueker and Crowle, 1963; Crowle, 1963).[5] On the other hand, the approach and overlapping without geometric disturbance of two unrelated precipitating systems in a radial single diffusion plate illustrates more dramatically than perhaps any other immunodiffusion reaction the serologic indifference unrelated systems have for each other and reveals clearly the gross physical nature of nonidentity reactions in immunodiffusion (see Fig. 8.1 for examples).

REVERSED TESTS

Usually antigen is the external reactant in single diffusion tests. But these tests can be reversed, antiserum playing this role (Stiehm, 1967; Nariuchi et al., 1970; Becker, 1969; Döhner, 1970). Reversed tests are seldom used because obtaining a persisting antibody excess needed to produce a usefully visible and measurable precipitate is difficult, and because most analyses for which reversal of procedures might be contemplated (e.g., titration of the antiserum, identification and characterization of its antibodies)[6] are better accomplished by conventional use of antigen as the external reactant, or by employing other kinds of immunodiffusion test. Moreover, the edges of precipitate discs in these tests are poorly defined.

The interpretations of these tests appear superficially to be similar to those of conventional tests. Thus, the final size of the reaction disc is directly proportional to the concentration of antibodies and inversely proportional to the concentration of antigen (Nariuchi et al., 1970; Becker, 1969). But these tests are complicated by the usual heterogeneity of antibodies against one antigen as contrasted with the usual homogeneity of antigen reacting with an antiserum.[7] Thus, the wave of precipitation in a reversed test is effected by the cumulative influence of different classes

[5] Because of the geometrical sensitivity of precipitate disc formation to the type of interaction between related antigen–antibody systems, the comparative radial diffusion test might be especially useful for directly quantitating degrees of cross-reaction between related antigens and of specificity for different antisera, as has been done in the past indirectly using linear single diffusion.

[6] For example, development of multiple rings of precipitate in a reversed test is more likely the result of the antiserum precipitating different antigens than of one antigen precipitating different varieties of antibodies (Stiehm, 1967).

[7] Added to this complication is the nonantibody macromolecular heterogeneity of an antiserum. Antisera with comparable titers of precipitins by conventional test might, for instance, become quite dissimilar in a reversed test as proportions of precipitate-enhancing or precipitate-inhibiting ingredients (cf. Chapter 1) to precipitins of different efficiencies became altered by diffusing radially at different rates. In a conventional test all would be present in uniform concentration.

of antibodies, of antibodies with widely differing capacities to bind with or precipitate antigen, and of antibodies having differing avidities for different determinants on the one kind of antigen being used as the internal reactant. Furthermore, there is a greater heterogeneity of antigen–antibody complex composition across the disc of precipitate in the reversed test than in the conventional test (Stiehm, 1967).

Despite these several potential hazards, the reversed test can be put to practical use for simple, relative quantitation of precipitins (Döhner, 1970; Becker, 1969). There is usually a straight-line relationship between precipitin titer in antisera of similar source and precipitate disc size (Stiehm, 1967; Nariuchi *et al.*, 1970). Indeed, the "hazards" of reversed tests can provide qualitative information not readily obtained from other kinds of immunodiffusion test, such as subtle specificity differences between presumably equivalent commercial antisera employed for quantitating one kind of antigen (Reimer *et al.*, 1970). In this manner they can reveal characteristics of an antiserum which affect its capacity to precipitate antigen but which are not precipitins.

Selected Single Diffusion Techniques

Each type of immunodiffusion technique has many varieties. Attempting to describe all these would be both impractical and wasteful. Instead, representative varieties will be explained both to illustrate a general type of method and to provide the reader with a working, useful model of it. A rationale for operations that are not self-explanatory and brief descriptions of important alternative techniques or styles will supplement each account. The reader should refer to Chapter 2 for explanation of minor operations common to several kinds of immunodiffusion test and therefore simply mentioned here.

Single Diffusion Tube Tests

Now seldom used, the classic Oudin test is set up in a small tube by layering antigen solution over a long column of gel, usually agar although agarose would be better now that it is so readily available, charged with just sufficient antiserum to perceptibly precipitate antigen at its front as it diffuses through the antiserum gel column. The general procedure is explained in the following paragraphs.

GENERAL PROCEDURE

Dip previously cleaned glass tubes into hot 0.2% agar, shake out excess and drain them well, and then air-dry them (alternatively, siliconize them;

see Chapter 2). This precoating suppresses capillary movement of external reactant solution around the antiserum column between the contacting surfaces of glass and gel.

Dissolve agar in a buffer of suitable pH and ionic strength to double its final required concentration. This solution will be mixed after subsequent cooling with an equal volume of diluted antiserum; therefore, for a final concentration of 0.6%, as is usually used, make the original solution 1.2%. Physiologic phosphate buffer of pH 7.4 is an appropriate solvent; the antiserum to be mixed with the agar is diluted in the same buffer. Ionic strength and pH can be varied according to the precipitating characteristics of the antiserum being tested or the solubility characteristics of its antigen (see Chapter 2), but external and internal reactant solvents should be the same. Transfer enough of this warm liquid mixture into an agar-coated tube to half fill it.

The transfer technique will depend on the internal diameter of the test tube. Capillary tubes can be used for micro tests, transfer being effected by capillary attraction of the gel–antiserum mixture up into the tube (Huntley, 1963). But because precipitin bands are difficult to either observe or resolve in capillary tube single diffusion tests, larger tubes with an internal diameter of 2 to 4 mm are more frequently used. The gel–antiserum column should have no air bubbles, and none of it should contaminate the upper portion of the tube which later will receive the antigen solution.[8] Transfer therefore is effected by injecting gel–antiserum mixture into the test tube with a pipet drawn to a long, fine tip (e.g., Pasteur pipet), or with a hypodermic needle and syringe. The procedure is facilitated by warming both the test tube and the transferring instrument to approximately 56°C for this manipulation. Alternatively, if the internal diameter of the tube is too small for a pipet or needle but is open-ended, the column of gel–antiserum can be sucked gently up into the tube and held there until it gels, or injected up into the tube from its lower tip.

After the agar–antiserum layer has gelled, antigen solution is layered upon it without trapping air at the interface. The concentration of antigen should be high enough to serologically overbalance the antiserum in the gel below it throughout the duration of the test, yet not so high that the wave of precipitation will pass through the antiserum column too fast and will be too ill defined for careful observation. The antigen–antibody ratio must be high enough to prevent significant back-diffusion of antibody while movement of the antigen diffusion front is being meas-

---

[8] "Contamination" from a moderately curved meniscus is insignificant (Van Oss, 1963).

ured, since, if it is not, the linear relationship between antigen concentration and $\sqrt{t}$ will fail, and Liesegang precipitation may develop.

The Oudin test should be kept at constant temperature during reaction development and observation, because its results are highly temperature-dependent, and it is very susceptible to temperature artifacts. An ideal container for one of these tests is a constant-temperature water bath built to permit observation of the tube *in situ* (Glenn, 1962a). Incubators, water baths, cold boxes, or refrigerators with temperature stabilization sufficient for all but the most critical Oudin tests are found in most laboratories, but means for observing the tube without removing it from its incubator are not. To circumvent this problem, immerse the tube in a suitable container of water. The thermal inertia of this water will smooth out fluctuations in temperature due both to the cooling–warming cycling of the incubator or refrigerator and to removing the tube in its container of water to room temperature for a few minutes of observation (Lueker and Crowle, 1963). Oudin tests can be developed at any constant temperature from 4°C to body temperature. Refrigerator temperatures permit leisurely observations, enhance antigen–antibody precipitation, and minimize reactant deterioration; temperatures of 20°C or more accelerate development of results, which is desirable for the higher-molecular-weight antigens like γ-globulins, but antiseptic chemicals may have to be added to the gel.

OBSERVATIONS OF RESULTS

Usually, one of three kinds of observation is made. One is to determine how many precipitin bands develop; the other two are concerned with the rate of movement of the antigen into the antiserum column. The first observation is for qualitative analyses: the number of "moving" bands usually corresponds to the presence of at least that many different antigens in the mixture being analyzed. But if the precipitin bands are counted when they have become or are about to become immobile, then there is a high risk that some may be secondary precipitates (Lueker and Crowle, 1963; Crowle, 1963).

The other two types of observation are more useful, yielding information not only on the number of antigens present but also on their concentrations, their interrelationships if any, and some of their physical properties. These observations are meant to determine the diffusion rate of an antigen. For one, measurements of the advance of the precipitating front from the meniscus are made and plotted against time. For the other, just one measurement of this distance is made at a time set by previous standardization; by comparing this with measurements made at the same time under identical conditions for the same antigen in different known concentrations, one can estimate the concentration of this antigen in the tested sample.

Other kinds of observations can be useful. For instance, because the density of a precipitin band depends largely on how many antibodies are precipitating antigen, and these antibodies increase in proportion as the antiserum is stronger and as a greater number of antibodies in a given antiserum recognize and precipitate the antigen, the precipitate formed by a homologous reaction (e.g., antiserum to human serum albumin– human serum albumin) is denser for a given amount of antigen than that formed by a heterologous reaction (e.g., antiserum to human serum albumin–chimpanzee serum albumin). This observation, which can be made objectively in various types of immunodiffusion test with densitometers, is useful for studying interrelationships between various antigens and their sources (i.e., taxonomy: Leone, 1964).

The antiserum–gel column can be extruded from an open-ended Oudin tube for washing, fixing, and staining, either to constitute a permanent, original record of the results or for more convenient photographic and/or densitometric registration. This procedure is facilitated by using agarose instead of agar (stronger gel) and silicone-coated rather than agar-coated tubes.

Interactions between reactants analogous to those in double diffusion plate tests can be observed in comparative single diffusion tube tests when these are set up to feed separated antigens to be compared into a common area of gel charged with antiserum containing antibodies to both (Oudin, 1971). But this technique has been too cumbersome to compete with double diffusion plate tests and so is very rarely used. Reversed single diffusion tube tests using antiserum as the external reactant are not often used because of the interpretative problems discussed above for reversed radial single diffusion plate tests, which appear to be compounded in linear tests if migration of the precipitate front is measured, as is usual in these tests. But for this very reason they may be especially useful in the future for studying these problems and their general significance in the use and interpretation of immunodiffusion tests just as the conventional Oudin test has been in the past.

Radial Single Diffusion Plate Tests

Although first performed some 40 years ago (Chapter 8), this kind of immunodiffusion test did not become popular until it was miniaturized and adapted to ready quantitation of serum antigens (Fahey and McKelvey, 1965; Mancini et al., 1965). Macro single diffusion plate tests (e.g., 5-mm-diameter wells cast or cut in agar gels several millimeters thick in petri dishes) are obsolete because they waste reactants, are difficult to convert to permanent records of the original test, develop slowly, and offer no advantage over micro methods (i.e., tests performed in gels ≤ 1 mm thick from wells approximately 1 to 2 mm in diameter). Therefore, only a micro procedure will be described here. The steps are the same as for a single diffusion tube test but adapted to a flat surface. Various precautions which were mentioned for the single diffusion tube test regarding buffers, gels, and antisera apply equally to a radial diffusion test.

GENERAL PROCEDURE

Use an agarose-coated microscope slide to support the reaction gel, and cast an absolutely flat and uniformly thick (Masseyeff and Zisswiller, 1969; Hill, 1968) layer of agarose–antiserum mixture on it to a thickness of about 0.5 mm using the sandwich technique described in Chapter 2 (cf. also Mancini *et al.*, 1965). Prepare 2% agarose in suitable buffer, and cool it to 60°C. Warm antiserum, diluted appropriately in the same buffer, to 55°C. Mix the two thoroughly but without creating bubbles, and then cast the mixture on the support slide. After the gel has set and been cooled, remove the casting slide, cut 2-mm wells, and add antigen at various dilutions in the same buffer to different wells but in identical volumes. Allow antigen solution to soak into the gel in a moist chamber, and then store the plate under mineral oil for development of the discs of precipitate.

Precipitate development can be in the refrigerator (Fahey and McKelvey, 1965) or, if preservatives are being used (e.g., sodium azide in the agarose, thymol in the oil), at 37°C (Mancini *et al.*, 1965). The reactions are usually read as diameters of fully developed discs of precipitate measured directly or, more easily and accurately, indirectly by measuring the projected images of the discs. If the discs are not round, project and trace their images on paper, cut out the tracings, and weigh these for accurate objective measurement of disc "area" (Mancini *et al.*, 1965). Discs that are too faint for adequate observation can be intensified by specific (antiserum to antiserum) or nonspecific (lowered pH) means as described in Chapter 2.

VARIATIONS AND SUPPLEMENTARY INFORMATION

Whenever agar or agarose solutions are warm enough to be fluid and are mixed with antiserum at this temperature, some antiserum constituents become insoluble and fixed within the gel (Masseyeff and Zisswiller, 1969). These add to background turbidity of the gel and interfere somewhat with readings, and with subsequent staining and differentiation of the immunodiffusion patterns if they are to be kept as permanent original records. Moreover, an antiserum–agar solution must be used at a temperature no higher than 56°C to prevent denaturation of the antibodies, and, since agar solutions gel at about 44°C, casting becomes complicated by possible premature congealing of the gel, especially in thicknesses used for micro tests. An alternative technique for avoiding these problems while charging gel with antiserum—a technique made practicable by the thinness of these gels in micro tests—is to soak antiserum into the surface of the already cast gel as described for electroimmunodiffusion in Chapter 6 (cf. also the alternative micro technique described below).

The concentration of antiserum which must be used in the gel is determined empirically, and also according to the purpose of the test (Fahey and McKelvey, 1965; Sandor et al., 1967). For quantitative tests it should be the least that will form a sufficiently evident disc of precipitate to be measured accurately (typically 5%: Fahey and McKelvey, 1965; McCracken et al., 1969); for qualitative analyses it should be as strong as is compatible with expansion of rings of precipitate sufficient for these to be resolved from each other. In antigen comparisons, a low concentration of antiserum will be best to permit maximum interaction of potentially cross-reactive antigens with each other and the antiserum (Mancini et al., 1970). Homologous antiserum should be used, but if it is not available heterologous antiserum (i.e., one against a cross-reacting antigen) can be substituted for certain single diffusion plate tests, providing the homologous and heterologous antigens are of similar diffusion coefficient (e.g., in quantitation of rodent α_{2M}-globulin using antiserum to human α_{2M}-globulin: Nash et al., 1970).

However antiserum is incorporated into the gel for a single diffusion plate test, its concentration must be uniform throughout and consistent from one test slide to another. Thus, for quantitative reproducibility the external reactant must always face the same environment of internal reactant within a series of compared tests. Each test also should employ the same batch of internal reactant; if a new batch is to be used, it must be standardized against the old one or against known amounts of the external reactant. For quantitative tests, the volume of the internal reactant should be "infinite" relative to expansion of the external reactant to minimize aberrations in total expansion of the latter. This qualification is associated with placement of the external reactant wells as discussed below. Exceptions to this rule are in comparative single diffusion plate tests in which discs of precipitate purposely are meant to overlap, and in certain kinds of quantitative tests in which readings are made before reactions have reached equilibrium, or in which antiserum strength or quality is being assessed.

Antiserum-charged agar gel for single diffusion plate tests can be stored as long as it suffers no microbial contamination, significant drying, or deterioration of antibodies. Such gels are sold ready for use, these requirements being met by various devices for preventing water evaporation, by inclusion of antiseptics like sodium azide, and by instructions to the buyer to store the gels at 4°C.

Commercial plates already have wells which are to receive external reactant cut or cast in them. The user making his own plates will have to cut wells himself. Various techniques for doing this have been described in Chapter 2. If the test is to be used on a large scale, it should be performed on double-width microscope slides or on photographic plates, and mechanically assisted hole-cutting (e.g., a Plexiglas template with holes in it to guide the gel punch: Fahey and McKelvey, 1965; or one of the commercial multiple-punch cutters) will be desirable. Alternatively, one can lay a multiple-hole Plexiglas template upon the surface of the gel containing the antiserum and simply charge the holes in the template with the external reactant (Crowle, 1960b).[9] Such templates also can be used on cellulose acetate membranes instead of agar gels (Agostoni *et al.*, 1970).

The well pattern on a radial single diffusion plate should not place two wells near enough to influence each other's reactions (unless intended, for comparative analyses) nor should the wells be close enough to the corners of the edges of the plate for the atmosphere of antibody locally to become uneven during diffusion of antigen and its reaction with the antibody, or for the diffusion rate of the antigen to be altered by evaporation of water from the edges of the plate. For an unknown antigen–antibody system being studied on a microscope slide, it is best to use only three wells spaced across the midline of the slide about 1.5 cm apart (Fahey and McKelvey, 1965).

For freshly cast and cut antiserum gels, the external reactant should be added to the wells as soon as possible because liquid from the surrounding gel may accumulate in the wells and thus interfere with charging each well with the same volume of reactant. Fluid that has accumulated in these wells in gels that have not been used immediately should be removed. Gels that have been stored for longer periods may not have this accumulation because they have dried somewhat. To a certain extent this drying can influence initial movement of the external reactant into the surrounding gel and can cause different results in otherwise identical

[9] The gel used in this fashion with a template can be charged with antiserum by surface application as described in Chapter 6 for electroimmunodiffusion (see also Chapter 2) with considerably increased convenience and, possibly, sensitivity (Lueker, personal communication).

plates which have been stored for different intervals. This is a major reason for using known standards for each plate if utmost reliability is desired (Patnode *et al.*, 1966).[10] Although fairly uniform volumes of external reactant can be added to wells cut in uniformly thick gel with a fine capillary tube by just filling each well, a calibrated micropipet is preferable for uniform results although not for convenience.

Conventionally, the external reactant diffuses into the internal reactant-charged medium. Similar tests with somewhat different meaning and interpretation can be performed by not charging the gel with the internal reactant until diffusion of the external reactant is complete. Since this variant of single diffusion plate tests has been used primarily as a quantitative immunoelectrophoretic method (Afonso, 1964b; Afonso, 1966a,b) it is discussed more extensively in Chapter 5 (see also Chapter 7). The most obvious difference between this and a conventional technique is that the external reactant will diffuse away from its source indefinitely, since there is no internal reactant to complex with and eventually arrest it. When the internal reactant is finally added to such a test, it has the primary role of specifically detecting the extent of external reactant diffusion which has already occurred, although it may interfere with further diffusion in a more conventional manner. The utility of this type of single radial diffusion test has not yet been much explored.

As is indicated above, radial single diffusion plates usually are set up with antigen as the external reactant. However, reversing this and using antigen as the internal reactant is especially convenient for comparing different antisera to a given antigen, both in overall capacity to precipitate the antigen and in relative contents of antibodies for different determinants (e.g., light versus heavy chain determinants of IgG) and varieties of these (e.g., *k* versus λ light chains: Reimer *et al.*, 1970; Vaerman *et al.*, 1969; Stiehm, 1967). Antibody titers can be expressed in micrograms of antigen with which antibodies in 1 ml of antiserum are equivalent (Becker, 1969).

Radial single diffusion tests can employ any medium that can hold internal reactant and into which external reactant can diffuse. For example, both quantitative and qualitative tests have been performed on cellulose acetate membranes (Vergani *et al.*, 1967; Agostoni *et al.*, 1970).

---

[10] Preparing and storing an adequate standard often may be a considerable problem in itself (McCracken *et al.*, 1969). For instance, standard solutions of IgG vary in determinant quality, if not in absolute quantity of protein, and they are stable for only short periods at 4°C. Once a standard has been prepared, it is most likely to be kept intact by freezing and storing it at −70°C in small one-use portions. Antigens that can be harmed by freezing (Chapter 2) must not, of course, be stored in this manner but rather by whatever method is empirically found to preserve them.

The membrane is sprayed or wiped uniformly with internal reactant. Small droplets of external reactant are applied and allowed to soak into the surface of the membrane, and then the membrane is incubated under oil. Later this is rinsed off, the membrane is washed, and the reactions are stained for measurement of disc size. In a similar test with a different kind of end point, the dry membrane is marked off with a ball-point pen into squares, soaked in a dilution (e.g., 10%) of antiserum, blotted lightly, and then charged at the middle of each square with a microdrop of antigen from various samples, or in various concentrations (Feinberg, 1962). After a short incubation (e.g., 1 hour) in a humid atmosphere or under oil followed by washing and staining for protein, the membrane is examined for the presence or absence of spots of antigen fixed to the membrane by antibody. The reverse of this "microspot" technique can be used to detect and titer antibodies (Feinberg, 1963). The microspot test can be performed also on very thin layers of agar supported on microscope cover slips instead of cellulose acetate (Feinberg, 1961).

ULTRAMICRO TESTS

One can use minute single radial diffusion tests to identify antigens produced by single cells (Daufi and Rondell, 1969). For one of these "cytoimmunodiffusion" tests, suspend the cells (e.g., erythrocytes, white blood cells) in physiologic buffer in 1% agarose, cast this between a microscope slide and a tape-supported cover slip (sandwich technique) in a very thin layer (25 to 30 microns), allow the gel to stand enough time for reactant (e.g., antigen)[11] to be produced or released into the gel surrounding individual cells, and remove the cover slip. Cut 3-mm discs of gel, transfer them to the opposite reactant (e.g., antiserum) on a spot plate, and let them stand for about 30 minutes at room temperature. Then let them develop precipitates around the "producing" cells for 12 hours at 4°C. The resulting precipitate can be observed by light or electron microscopy, before or after staining, and with or without enhancing indicators like those labeled with fluorescence or radioactivity (Daufi and Rondell, 1969).

This kind of technique also has been used to show that precipitins in trichinosis are directed against antigens originating orally rather than anally from *Trichinella spiralis* larvae (Castro and Fairbairn, 1969). On a much larger scale, transverse sections of potato tubers laid on antiserum-containing gel produced radial spots of precipitate corresponding anatomically to areas of highest antigen concentration in the tubers (Lester,

---

[11] In a reversed procedure using a low-temperature gelling agent, the technique could detect production of antibodies (cf. Coffino *et al.*, 1970).

1965). The scale of this type of technique therefore can be made to fit the problem.

In a different kind of ultramicro test, a *tour de force* more than a practical technique, a 2-mm disc of cellulose acetate is cut with a glass tube and is pushed about 1 cm into this same glass tube where it is held vertically by contact with the sides of the tube. A small piece of wet filter paper is placed in the tube to maintain humidity, and each end of the tube is closed with a droplet of paraffin oil. With a micromanipulator, enough antiserum is pipetted through the oil in one end onto the micro disc to just saturate it, and then a small quantity of antigen is deposited in the center of the disc. The unit is allowed to react overnight (Ringle and Herndon, 1965). Subsequent procedures are routine but scaled down accordingly.

APPLICATIONS

Certain particular applications of single diffusion tests further illustrate interesting technical variations. For instance, antibodies with biological effects can be assayed by diffusing them into gel charged with substrate and applying indicator reagent to measure the antibody concentration by the diameter of its diffusion. Hemolysins diffused into erythrocyte-charged agar or agarose were detected by guinea pig complement as indicator for their presence (i.e., lysis of the erythrocytes: Weiler *et al.*, 1965; Nariuchi *et al.*, 1970; McGhie *et al.*, 1971).

In an antiserum, the proportion of one immunoglobulin class with antibody activity to a selected antigen can be determined by incubating the antigen with the antiserum overnight at 4°C and then testing the antiserum for loss of the immunoglobulin by the following procedure. Precipitating antiserum to the same antigen but from an unrelated species of animal is added to the mixture of antigen and test antiserum to ensure precipitation of all antibody that has complexed with the antigen. The mixture is centrifuged, and the supernatant fluid is assayed with radial single diffusion plates specific for each different class of immunoglobulin. Measuring the reduction of total immunoglobulin of each class in the test antiserum resulting from these procedures will indicate the percentage of each class of immunoglobulin having antigen-binding capacity, whether or not it happens to be a precipitin (Nash and Heremans, 1969; Nash *et al.*, 1969).

Radioimmunodiffusion can accomplish a similar purpose. Test antiserum is diffused into gel containing antibodies to one or another of its classes of immunoglobulin. After the disc of precipitate has formed and nonprecipitated substances have been washed from the gel, radioactive antigen for which the original antiserum had antibodies is infused into the gel. There, it complexes with discs of a precipitated immunoglobulin in proportion to the amount and quantity of antibody in that class of immunoglobulin. Thus, both the identity and the combining capacity of each class of antibody in an antiserum can be measured for a radioactive antigen by this technique (Heiner *et al.*, 1970). Fluorescein-labeled reagents can be used similarly and without the special precautions needed for working with radioactivity (Centifanto and Kaufman, 1971).

Conclusion

The single diffusion test can be very sensitive.[12] Because of this and the simplicity of micro radial diffusion techniques, single diffusion tests will remain useful despite evidence that for most purposes they are obsolescent. They have been used principally for determining diffusion coefficients of selected antigens, and for quantitating antigens. The first can be accomplished more easily now by double diffusion tests, and the second can be effected nearly as easily but with greater accuracy and versatility by electroimmunodiffusion. Single diffusion tests can be used for qualitative analyses, but other types of immunodiffusion test are much superior for this purpose (Naylor and Adair, 1962). There are two tasks to which they seem better suited than other kinds of immunodiffusion test: detailed studies of the mechanics of antigen–antibody precipitation (single diffusion tube tests), and very simple, very sensitive field tests for the presence of antigen or antibody (micro spot tests).

[12] A conventional quantitative radial diffusion test in agar gel can detect 1.25 to 3.0 µg of antigen per milliliter (i.e., 2.5 to 6 ng; Fahey and McKelvey, 1965; Mancini *et al.*, 1965). The micro spot test in cellulose acetate is said to detect as little as 0.02 ng of antigen (Feinberg, 1962).

Chapter 4

Double Diffusion Tests

Immunodiffusion tests in which both antigen and antiserum diffuse toward each other significantly are known as double diffusion tests. Like single diffusion tests, these double diffusion tests can be radial or linear. In addition, because both reactants diffuse, they can also be angular.

Characteristics and Mechanisms

Although in double diffusion tests both antigen and antibody must migrate toward a common reaction area before they begin to precipitate each other, if they are employed greatly out of proportion serologically, any double diffusion test becomes a form of single diffusion test governed by conditions affecting the latter (Crowle, 1960c). In fact, the two reactants initially are rarely in balance, but the moderate differences usually encountered are compensated for soon after antigen and antibody fronts meet (Meffroy-Biget, 1967a, 1968; Aladjem *et al.*, 1968). Since a steep gradient of each reactant tends to form on either side of the precipitin zone, the initially stronger reactant, by forcing its way across the developing precipitate, both dilutes itself and encounters rapidly increasing quantities of the opposite reactant. Consequently, the zone of precipitation shifts slightly toward the weaker reactant and becomes stabilized as the respective reactants feed into it at equivalent rates (Meffroy-Biget, 1967a). If an antigen, because of large initial concentration or low molecular weight, diffuses much more rapidly than its antibody, in all but exceptional instances it loses its "advantage" by spreading itself across so much gel that at its front, which meets the antibody, it has become quite dilute, while the antibody, having diffused scarcely

247

at all, meets it at no particular serologic disadvantage. Hence, by its nature the double diffusion test tends to adjust itself to balanced conditions (Kaminski and Meffroy-Biget, 1961). This balancing effect can be overrun as mentioned above; or it can be defeated if, for example, one of the reactants is exhausted long before the other, or one is replenished out of proportion to the other (Wachendörfer, 1965; Barber and Taga, 1964; Parlett, 1961; Casman et al., 1969; Van Oss and Heck, 1963).

Types of Double Diffusion Test

Double diffusion tests can be performed in tubes or on flat surfaces, in the three varieties illustrated in Figure 1.5. In one, antigen and antibody diffuse face-to-face into a common reacting arena, as in the double diffusion tube technique. In a second, antigen and antibody diffuse across each other, usually at 90 degrees. An example of this method, sometimes called a double diffusion gradient test (Elek, 1949a), is that in which two strips of filter paper impregnated with the two respective reactants are laid upon agar at right angles to form an L or a T, and antigen–antibody precipitate forms at an angle extending away from the hypothetical intersection of the two reactant sources (see Fig. 1.8). In the third variety, the radial test, some advantages of both linear and angular tests are blended. Antigen and antibody approach each other at various angles, ranging from 180 degrees in the centers of forming precipitin bands to less than 90 degrees at band tips in some extreme instances. Convergence of reactants at angles considerably less than 180 degrees favors identification of secondary precipitates (Liesegang bands) when they occur, for reasons explained below.

General Considerations

The number of precipitin bands developing in a double diffusion test usually can be interpreted as representing the minimum number of precipitating systems present (Maurer et al., 1963b); however, they do not necessarily represent the maximum number (Fujio et al., 1959; Kaminski, 1954b; Richter et al., 1958; Ouchterlony, 1958). If several systems are present, the double diffusion test generally is capable of detecting more of them than the single diffusion test because its resolution is inherently greater (Wilson, 1958; Pierce, 1959; see below). Occasionally, the number of bands appearing may exceed the number of individual precipitating systems taking part in a double diffusion test (Van Oss and Heck, 1963). These secondary precipitates are readily identified in most variations of this test, particularly in the double diffusion gradient test, but not in the tube test (Crowle, 1960c; Lueker and Crowle, 1963; Crowle, 1963).

Most factors governing the development of single diffusion tests play similar roles in the double diffusion test (Ouchterlony, 1958; for mathematical descriptions of the events of double diffusion precipitation, see Meffroy-Biget, 1966, 1967b,c,d; Kaminski and Meffroy-Biget, 1961; Meffroy-Biget, 1968; Aladjem *et al.*, 1968; Aladjem and Palmiter, 1965; Aladjem, 1964). However, in the latter there is no distinction between internal and external reactant; both diffuse and neither remains at a constant concentration during the test (Fig. 4.1). Both edges of a precipitin zone formed in the average double diffusion test, regardless of the type of antibody or antigen employed, tend to be sharp. When H-type antibody is being used, marked unilateral diffuseness of the border of a precipitin band suggests that the reactant on the side of the diffuseness is excessive in respect to the other reactant (Ouchterlony, 1948a, 1958). However, when antibody is excessive this may be untrue, particularly with R-type antibody (Korngold and Van Leeuwen, 1959b). Thus, at antigen excess against either R- or H-type antibody, both edges of the precipitin line will tend to move in a situation analogous to a normal single diffusion test, but if antibody is in excess and is of R type, the band edge nearer this reactant will remain stationary and only that facing the antigen will move, causing the existing band to broaden (Oudin, 1952). Unilateral band diffuseness also may indicate either that precipitation in the presence of the proximal reactant is somewhat unstable or that it can vary considerably in the proportions at which antigen and antibody combine. Bilateral band diffuseness hints that the particular precipitin system being studied might consist of rather wide ranges of antigen and antibody types—that is, that the antigen is not entirely homogeneous in combining ability with available antibody, and that several kinds of antibody with varying specificity and avidity are present (Lapresle, 1959). It also could suggest reaction between antiserum and a heterologous but cross-reacting antigen, instead of a homologous antigen against which the antiserum originally was made (Jennings, 1959d). If the system being observed were studied in an aqueous precipitin test, it probably would have a rather broad range of optimal proportions (Becker, 1953). Finally, bilateral diffuseness can occur also if the reactants are diffusing into the reaction zone faster than they can form nondiffusible aggregates, so that even as aggregates they will continue to diffuse a small distance to either side of the middle of the precipitin zone before accumulating sufficient mass to become immobilized and visible (Barber and Taga, 1964; Wachendörfer, 1965).

Comparatively little attention is paid to band movement in double

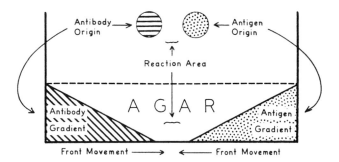

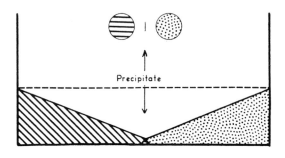

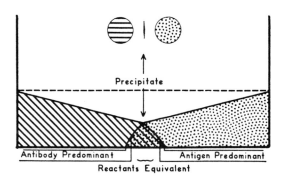

Fig. 4.1. A diagrammatic representation of how precipitin bands develop in agar and of their composition. In the first drawing at the top of the figure, antigen and antibody diffusing from their respective origins toward the reaction area in agar have set up concentration gradients, the tips of which have not yet met but continue with time to move toward each other. Both reactants are assumed to be present in proportions which are optimal for this hypothetical double diffusion test. In the second, these tips have just met and have formed a thin band of precipitate which is slightly thicker at its center than at its extremities. In the third drawing

diffusion tests (cf. Meffroy-Biget, 1967a; Van Oss and Heck, 1963). Consequently, many of the factors affecting band movement in the single diffusion test have attracted only secondary interest in using and interpreting it. For example, results from the gradient double diffusion technique employed to ascertain an antigen's diffusion coefficient are not of the rate of band movement but rather of the angle at which its precipitin band forms with respect to either the antigen or the antibody source, since the tangent of this angle is determined by the ratio of the antigen diffusion coefficient to the antibody diffusion coefficient (Allison and Humphrey, 1959, 1960; Ouchterlony, 1949c). Thus, if the ratio is unity (diffusion coefficients equal) and the original concentrations of antigen and antibody reasonably approach equivalence, and if the reactant sources are troughs laid out at right angles to each other, the angle of the precipitin band formed by the two will be 45 degrees. However since the angle of this band depends ultimately on relative rates of reactant diffusion, factors affecting these rates unequally for antigen and for antiserum can interfere with the reliability of this test just as they can by affecting the rate of only one reactant in the single diffusion test (see Fig. 4.2).

Factors Directly Affecting Sensitivity

The double diffusion test inherently is more efficient than the single diffusion test, because it does not depend on whether sufficient antibody is present in the reaction zone initially to yield a visible precipitate, but rather on how much can be fed into this zone against an equivalent quantity of antigen arriving from the opposite direction (Aladjem *et al.*, 1959; Elek, 1949a; Ouchterlony, 1958; Oudin, 1952; Wilson and Pringle, 1954; Aladjem, 1964). As antigen–antibody complexes form, each of these reactants will go out of solution locally, and more from the adjoining agar will diffuse into this area to replace the deficit, only to be precipitated in turn (Aladjem, 1964; see Fig. 1.7). If complexes forming in this zone (where, visibly, nothing is happening at first) are not diffusible, theoretically there is almost no lower limit to the sensitivity of the

---

the precipitin band is well developed but still has its spindle cross-sectional shape, and the precipitate represented graphically in the reaction area is shown to consist of antigen–antibody complexes mostly formed in or near equivalent reactant ratios but also partly, at the precipitin zone's respective edges, formed under conditions of either antibody or antigen excess. The type of reaction illustrated here would occur between human serum γ-globulin and its rabbit antibody, but it would be different in some details if horse antiserum were used, or if the antigen were human serum albumin.

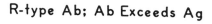

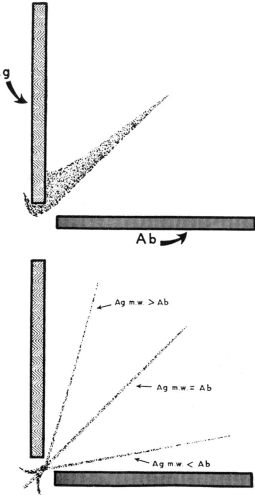

Varying Ag Mol. Weight;
Ag Equivalent to Ab

Fig. 4.2. Various forms of precipitin patterns as they develop in double diffusion
gradient tests. The top two patterns contrast the thin, slightly curved precipitin band
formed by H-type antiserum with the broad-based, lance-shaped band formed by
R-type antiserum, when both are used in excess against antigen. The lower left
diagram shows how this type of test can be used to estimate antigen molecular
weight when antibody of known molecular weight is used. Thus, antigen with a lower
molecular weight and hence greater diffusion coefficient than antibody will form a

H-type Ab: Ab Exceeds Ag

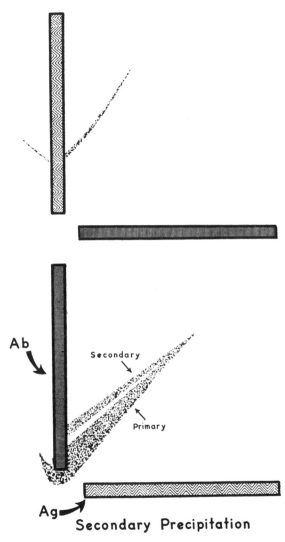

Secondary Precipitation

precipitin band with a small angle between it and the antibody source, while a
large-molecular-weight antigen forms a precipitin band with a large angle. For this
type of experiment, the reactants should be used at equivalence so that band positions
will be influenced solely by the relative diffusion coefficients of each reactant, and
so that the tangent of the angle formed by one of these can be measured accurately
for use in subsequent calculations. The lower right diagram shows how a secondary
precipitate can form with R-type antiserum in the gradient double diffusion test,
and how it is distinguished from the primary precipitate (see text).

double diffusion test.[1] Practically, its sensitivity as defined by visible precipitation is governed by the quantity of reactants placed and maintained in their depots, assuming that conditions reasonably close to those of equivalent proportions are maintained (Aladjem et al., 1959; Ouchterlony, 1958).

The time lapse preceding visible precipitation in the double diffusion test is controlled by three main factors (Aladjem et al., 1959; Aladjem, 1964; Jameson, 1969a; Kaminski and Meffroy-Biget, 1961). The first and second govern the diffusion rates of the two reactants and therefore the rapidity with which they meet. These are their respective diffusion coefficients and their absolute concentrations. The third factor is how soon antigen and antibody form visible complexes after their fronts have met. Assuming that antigen and antibody in a hypothetical system are employed in equivalent proportions, the time passing before a visible precipitate appears is proportional, in a mathematically predictable way, to their concentrations, to the distance between their sources, and to factors mentioned in connection with single diffusion tests which govern the diffusion rates of antigen and antibody molecules, such as temperature, agar concentration, and additives to the agar gel (Aladjem et al., 1959; Wilson and Pringle, 1954). If the reactant sources are too far apart, antigen and antibody fronts may meet, but the concentration of antibody at this front may never accumulate sufficiently to form a visible precipitate (Aladjem et al., 1959; Augustin, 1957; Wilson and Pringle, 1954). Both this fact and the predictability of the time required for a given precipitate to appear under standardized conditions have been applied to double diffusion quantitative analyses, and also to determining a reactant's diffusion coefficient, since this is intimately concerned with its quantitation (Aladjem et al., 1959; Kaminski and Meffroy-Biget, 1961; Meffroy-Biget, 1966; Jameson, 1969a). From these considerations it is obvious that, if other factors are held constant, the visible precipitation sensitivity (but not the resolution when complex antigen mixtures are being analyzed) of a double diffusion test for a given system is directly proportional to the closeness of antigen and antibody depots (Fig. 4.3; Aladjem et al., 1959; Wilson and Pringle, 1954).

Cross-reacting antigens in a mixture can interfere with each others' precipitation in double diffusion tests much as they do in the single diffusion test. However, the adaptability of double diffusion tests to comparison of antigen preparations, varied either qualitatively or quantitatively, makes these tests somewhat more versatile in contending with

---

[1] If one does not depend solely on visible precipitation as an indicator for complex formation but instead uses auxiliary means (e.g., radioautography, enzymatic labeling), theoretical and practical lower limits coincide.

this potential problem. This is doubly true if the technique is combined with electrophoresis in immunoelectrophoresis. Comparing reactants has been the foremost function of double diffusion tests and hence will be discussed in detail below.

Antigen–Antibody Equivalence

Equivalent proportions of antigen to antibody determined by the double diffusion test agree better with those in aqueous medium than the aqueous medium values agree with proportions obtained with the single diffusion test. Probably, this is because double diffusion reactions have a tendency to adjust themselves to equivalence and to compensate for differences in reactant diffusion coefficient (i.e., molecular weight). In double diffusion tests the lower-molecular-weight reactants lose their serologic advantage which they obtain from being able to diffuse more rapidly than those of higher molecular weight in single diffusion tests and which makes their equivalence values in the latter spuriously low, because by diffusing farther during a given time in the double diffusion test they become proportionally more diluted. With steep reactant concentration gradients facing each other across the reacting zone, any initial tendency, except for a very marked one, for one reactant to predominate over the other, either by diffusion coefficient or by concentration, is readily neutralized as this reactant simultaneously dilutes itself by diffusion and encounters succeeding planes of the opposite reactant's gradient. However, this very tendency for self-adjustment makes band movement itself so insignificant in double diffusion tests that usually other means must be employed to determine accurately when the reactants truly are being used at equivalence (cf. Meffroy-Biget, 1967a). When H-type antiserum is employed this is simple, since, in a series of tubes with a constant quantity of one of the reactants used against varying concentrations of the other, equivalence produces a sharply defined precipitin band, while an excess of either reactant causes the band to be fuzzy on the side of the excess reactant (Boerma, 1956). For R-type antibody, however, this criterion is faulty for reasons already explained, but other criteria have been employed which yield quantitative or diffusion coefficient data of quality matching or exceeding the best obtainable by other serologic methods (Augustin and Hayward, 1955; Hayward and Augustin, 1957; Ouchterlony, 1958; Polson, 1958; Van Regenmortel, 1959). For example, one may make very accurate measurements of the distance between the precipitin band and the antigen meniscus and correlate these either with the varying antigen concentration or with the antigen diffusion coefficient, assuming that the diffusion coefficient of

256

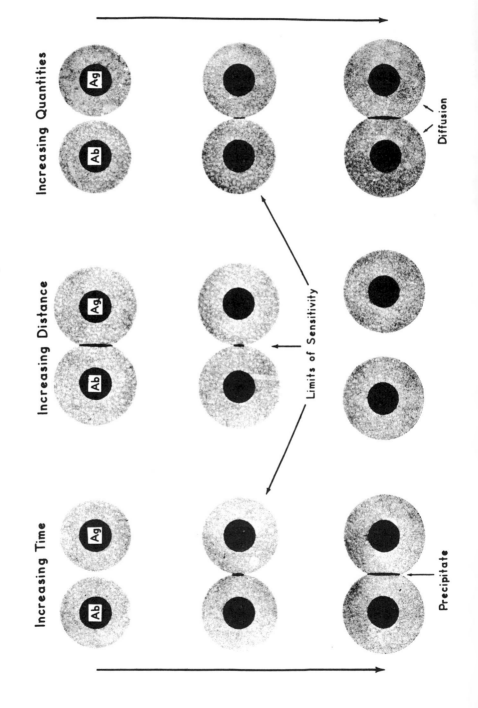

the antibody is known (Polson, 1958; Van Regenmortel, 1959). Alternatively, one can adjust the quantity of antigen so that in a series of tubes used against a given antibody concentration or antibody concentration gradient, previously established in the gel separating antigen from antibody, the unmoving precipitin band forms just barely below and in contact with the antigen meniscus (Augustin and Hayward, 1955; Hayward and Augustin, 1957; see Fig. 4.4).

The ratio of antigen to antiserum that is equivalent for one kind of double diffusion test will tend to be equivalent also for other varieties. But in some varieties reactant placement can void this tendency (Casman *et al.*, 1969). For instance, a large volume of one reactant in a large central well surrounded by smaller satellite wells is prone to "wash" the central reactant into the surrounding gel faster than it would move by diffusion alone, and tip the balance in favor of this reactant (Kirst, 1966; Löfkvist and Sjöquist, 1963).

Patterns of Precipitation in Comparative Radial Double Diffusion Tests

The patterns of interacting antigen–antibody precipitation classically seen in and described for radial double diffusion tests are prototypical of similar patterns seen in all varieties of immunodiffusion test. Some of the rationale for their development was discussed in Chapter 3 in the section on interacting antigen–antibody systems. Here this discussion is extended to explaining various associations between approaching and connecting bands of antigen–antibody precipitate (Finger, 1964). Note that it can be applied to any comparative immunodiffusion test, whether compared reactants are placed in adjacent wells or are brought close to each other electrophoretically or by other means (Deckers, 1967).

The Classic Comparative Test

In this test (cf. Wilson and Pringle, 1955), two antigens are compared using one antiserum. Suppose that one solution of antigen B is being compared with another against As/B (i.e., antiserum to B) in a double diffusion plate with three reactant depots. If in each antigen well

---

Fig. 4.3. Three factors that affect the sensitivity and resolution of double diffusion tests and govern precipitin band formation all have in common the distance across which the reactants must diffuse before reacting. They are shown here in hypothetical double diffusion plate tests. The discs of reactant diffusion represent areas over which these have spread in quantities sufficient to form visible precipitates; if the discs of opposing reactants do not overlap, no precipitate will form. Overlapping may fail for lack of incubation time, if the distance between two reactant sources initially is too great, or if the quantities of reactants originally used is too small.

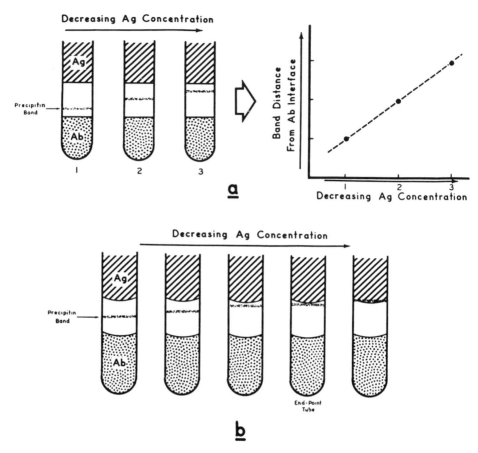

Fig. 4.4. Two forms of quantitative double diffusion tube test which have been used with considerable accuracy. In the first (*a*), the tubes are set up with special techniques to have flat menisci, so that the distance between a precipitin band and a meniscus can be measured accurately. When decreasing antigen concentrations are used in a series of tubes containing constant quantities of antibody, the distance from the antibody meniscus to precipitin bands forming in these tubes increases in proportion to the decrease in antigen concentration as depicted in the graph. The second form of double diffusion quantitative test takes as its end point tube in a series that in which the precipitin band forms just below and touching the upper of two menisci, the antigen meniscus in the example given (*b*). This test can be used, for example, to compare very accurately the quantities of an antigen in various test solutions; it also has been used to quantitate antibody.

the antigen concentration is equal, the molecular weights of antigen and antibody are the same, and equivalent concentrations of antigen and antibody are used to charge their respective wells, two straight precipitin bands arching into a chevron, as shown in Fig. 4.5*a*, will be formed be-

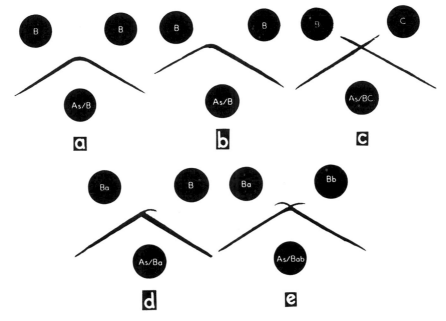

Fig. 4.5. Precipitin patterns commonly observed in double diffusion plate tests and related tests in which two antigen solutions are compared using antiserum as the analytic agent. Pattern *a* (of identity or fusion) develops when the compared antigens (B) are identical serologically and are used in equal concentrations against their specific antiserum (As/B). A skewed pattern results when the same antigens are compared, but one of them is less concentrated than the other (*b*). When two serologically different antigens are compared using an antiserum that contains antibodies to both of them, each antigen–antibody system precipitates independently of the other, so that the resulting precipitin bands cross in the pattern of nonidentity or intersection (*c*). An antigen that is similar enough to another to be capable of precipitating some antibodies in the antiserum against the latter (the homologous antigen) will form a precipitin band which is arrested at its juncture with the band formed by the homologous antigen. The latter band, however, continues to grow, forming a "spur" (pattern of partial identity or partial intersection) whose length is inversely proportional to how closely related the cross-reacting antigen is to the homologous antigen and whose curvature and faintness are directly related to this relationship (*d*). A double spur forms if two antigens are compared which are different but are related to a third antigen, and antiserum to this third antigen is employed (*e*).

tween the antigen wells and the antibody well (Ouchterlony, 1958). The coalescence of the proximal band tips constitutes a *reaction of identity*, since it implies, as is so in this instance, that the two antigens being compared are identical serologically. However, since two nonidentical antigens sometimes will give a spurious reaction of identity because of indirect relationships they may possess (Wilson and Pringle,

1955; cf. also Butler and Leone, 1968), this precipitin band pattern might more cautiously be termed *pattern of fusion* (Wilson and Pringle, 1956).[2]

In this example, if the antigen concentration in one depot is less than that in the other, but other conditions remain unchanged, the same type of pattern will develop (Fig. 4.5b). The precipitin bands will be straight, but the band formed by antigen in the lower concentration will not be midway between antigen and antibody wells but rather will be shifted toward the antigen depot, so that an asymmetrical chevron forms (Kaminski, 1954b; Ouchterlony, 1948a; Wilson and Pringle, 1954, 1955).

A different pattern develops when two nonidentical antigens are compared using an antiserum with antibodies against both (Fig. 4.5c). Antigen B compared with antigen C against As/BC produces a precipitin band *pattern of intersection* (i.e., nonidentity) in which bands B and C cross with complete indifference to each other (Wilson and Pringle, 1956; Finger, 1964). Rarely, a pattern of intersection can be produced by identical antigens (Feinberg, 1957; Korngold, 1956a), but this happens only when the concentrations of the two antigen solutions are highly disproportionate (Jameson, 1969b).

In addition to patterns of fusion and of intersection, there is the intermediate pattern of *partial intersection,* or partial identity, which is produced most commonly when cross-reacting antigens are compared with respect to antiserum to one of them (Fig. 4.5d; Finger, 1964). For example, if different antigens Ba and B are compared using As/Ba, then heterologous antigen B will form a precipitin band somewhat more diffuse and weaker than that produced by homologous antigen Ba. This band results from interaction between antigenic determinants the same as those constituting the B component of Ba and just those antibodies in the antiserum with affinity for these determinants. Where the B and Ba bands meet, the B band terminates, but the Ba band extends further, though weakly, as a *spur* (Wilson and Pringle, 1956). The main Ba band is formed by Ba antigen and precipitins reactive with determinants of both B and *a* components of the antigen, but the Ba spur is the product of reaction between only the *a* component and the corresponding anti-

---

[2] Two antigens may be immunologically identical but physicochemically quite different (e.g., 75 S and 140 S derivatives of foot-and-mouth disease virus: Cowan and Graves, 1968). A pattern of fusion is as much a product of the analytic antiserum as of the compared antigens: if the antiserum lacks antibodies to the different determinants on the two antigens and has only antibodies to the shared determinants, it will indicate wrongly that the two antigens are identical (Finger *et al.,* 1963). As a corollary, if two antigens are shown to be different with any single antiserum used for their comparison, they can be considered different even though numerous other antisera may have shown them to be "identical" (Finger, 1964).

bodies with *a* specificity. This is because only these antibodies will have escaped reaction with cross-reacting B antigen, diffused through the B precipitin band, and be available on the other side of it to precipitate Ba antigen by means of its *a* component alone. Hence, the appearance of two precipitin bands, one interrupted at their junction and the other continuing as a weakened spur of precipitate, suggests that an antigen similar to but not identical with the homologous antigen is being studied (Fig. 4.6).

In a serologically balanced system, the length and the intensity of a spur are inversely proportional to the degree of antigenic determinant

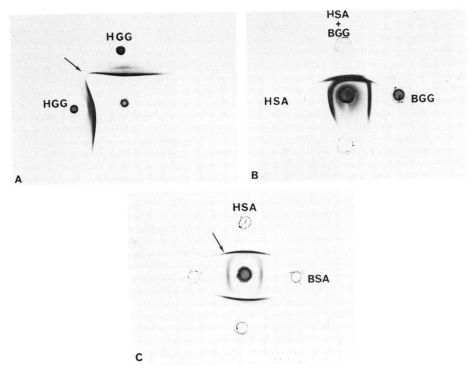

Fig. 4.6. Double diffusion plate tests using human and bovine serum albumins (HSA, BSA) and human and bovine γ-globulins (HGG, BGG) and corresponding antisera to illustrate reactions of identity (A), nonidentity (B), and partial identity or spurring (C). Thus, in A, precipitin bands produced by the compared antigens fuse (arrow); in B, identical antigens from different sources form fusing bands and are undisturbed by precipitation by nonidentical antigens in the same area; in C, the homologous antigen HSA forms a strong spur (arrow) beyond the cross-reacting antigen BSA, indicating that the antiserum to HSA contained only a modest titer of precipitins reactive with BSA.

similarity between two antigens being studied (Jennings, 1959c; Weigle, 1960; Kaminski, 1962; Finger, 1964). Two intersecting spurs sometimes form and resemble true patterns of intersection, but usually they can be identified by their characteristic weakening in extending beyond the point of junction (Fig. 4.5e). Bands that will form double spurs share with bands forming uncomplicated fusion patterns a tendency to bend toward each other as they come into juxtaposition (Korngold, 1956a), and the spurs themselves also tend to bend in the same direction (Wilson and Pringle, 1955, 1956). A pattern with double spurs indicates, as Fig. 4.5e suggests, that the two antigens being compared share some determinant groups (B) in common with each other and with the third against which the antiserum being used was made, but that each also cross-reacts with the third antigen by some other different determinant groups (a and b) which they do not share with each other.

Interpretations of spur patterns must be made carefully because spurs can form under different conditions, and, moreover, the length and intensity of a spur and even the likelihood of its appearance are governed by the type and quantity of antibodies present in an antiserum (Fig. 4.7). Antiserum containing antibodies too nonspecific to differentiate two similar but not identical antigens forms no spur (e.g., hyperimmune horse antiserum to human serum reacting with serum albumins from numerous other species); when two antigens are compared that cross-react equally with the third, against which the antibody is directed, but which themselves are different, no spur forms (Crowle, 1960c). Cross-reactions between related antigens are best observed with near-optimal

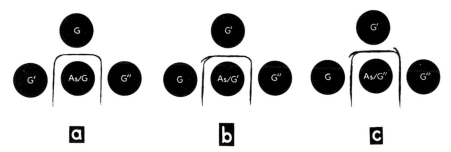

Fig. 4.7. The importance in any critical study of closely related antigens of using an antiserum capable of differentiating them is illustrated here. Three hypothetical antigens G, G′, and G″ are compared using antiserum against each, respectively. Only antiserum to G″ (c) shows that G″ has reactive sites lacking on G′ and G. Although antiserum to G′ cannot show this and it falsely indicates that antigens G′ and G″ are identical, it does show that both of these have greater antigenic complexity than G (b). To antiserum against G, all three antigens appear to be identical (a).

reactant proportions (Burtin, 1954; Kaminski and Ouchterlony, 1951), since artifacts resembling spurs can be produced by use of grossly disproportionate reactant quantities (Van Oss and Heck, 1963; Finger, 1964).

Double diffusion plate patterns of intersection, partial intersection, or fusion are the most readily interpreted when factors affecting their formation are understood (Finger, 1964; Weigle, 1961). When an antigen and its antibody react in the double diffusion plate under ideal conditions, particularly when they are used in equivalent proportions, the precipitin band which they form often is said to be a "barrier" to passage of either reactant through it. However, more accurately, this band (Wilson and Pringle, 1955; Aladjem, 1964; Van Oss and Heck, 1963) merely indicates the site at which antigen and antibody bar each other's passage.[3] On one side of the zone of precipitation is an excess of antigen, and on the other an excess of antibody (Fig. 4.1). Any antigen diffusing through this precipitin zone toward the antibody excess becomes increasingly likely to be precipitated by antibody molecules until at the edge of the antibody excess zone its chances for continuing diffusion freely are nil (Feinberg, 1957). The species of antibodies in an antiserum are not uniform, some, for example, having less avidity and less specificity than others (see Chapter 1). But, by contrast, antigens are fairly homogeneous, so that this antibody variation has little practical effect on formation of the precipitin band and on its barrier effect, although the band's physical appearance (i.e., sharpness or fuzziness) may be affected. It is the barrier effect in a zone of precipitation which gives the reaction of identity (fusion) its meaning. Antibody variation will be evident, however, when a heterologous but cross-reacting antigen is employed against an antiserum. Thus, if this heterologous antigen is homogeneous, its molecules will not be able to diffuse through the zone of reaction with antibody, but on the other hand those antibodies in the antiserum that are too specific to react with this heterologous antigen are not barred from penetrating the zone, and they diffuse freely beyond it where they are precipitated only if they encounter homologous antigen and form a spur (see Fig. 4.5d). The efficiency of a heterologous antigen in barring diffusion of a range of antibodies is proportional to how closely related it is to the homologous antigen. The most closely related but still heterologous antigen will sieve out the most antibodies, permitting formation of only the smallest spur across its precipitin band by the homologous antigen.

---

[3] Rarely, precipitin bands can be dense enough to present a physical barrier to reactant diffusion (Chen and Ely, 1968).

The selectivity of the zone of precipitation as a serologic barrier is further exemplified by the fact that if two heterologous antigens are tested with antiserum to the homologous antigen, and one of these cross-reacts more with the homologous antigen than the other (i.e., is serologically more similar), the antigen more closely resembling the homologous antigen will be the one to form a spur. This spurring by one of two heterologous cross-reacting antigens can suggest wrongly that this antigen is the homologous antigen, a mistake not readily caught when natural antigen mixtures are being studied.

Purely mechanical forces can cause precipitin bands to align themselves in positions falsely indicating some relationship between them (Burtin, 1954; Wilson and Pringle, 1955; Finger, 1964; Crowle, 1963). As has been mentioned above, identical antigens from adjacent depots can form a pattern of intersection (nonidentity). This can happen if in one depot antigen is used at low enough concentration so that in the area approaching the point of line juncture it cannot precipitate all antibodies diffusing against it, and these penetrate to precipitate antigen diffusing from the more concentrated source behind the line formed by the weaker antigen and thereby produce a spur of precipitate (Korngold, 1956a; Van Oss and Heck, 1963). False spurring also can occur with H-type antibody if one antigen solution is much more concentrated than the other (Ouchterlony, 1958). In this instance, the band formed by the more concentrated antigen solution will "migrate" toward the antibody depot more rapidly than that produced by the weaker antigen solution and so break the original loop of fusion unevenly, forming a spur. Similar effects can be seen when the diffusion coefficient of one of the compared antigens is very low. Its precipitin band may not grow long enough to cross that of the other antigen, and so partial fusion and spurring appear to develop (Dudman, 1965a).

Another mechanical cause of false spurring is precipitation by two different antigen-antibody systems in one plane so that what appears to be a single line extending into a spur really is a double line, one of its components being the same as the compared antigen solution and fusing with it but the other not fusing and therefore extending beyond the point of fusion (Ouchterlony, 1953; Löfkvist and Sjöquist, 1963; Finger, 1964). Some particularly lucid experiments on spur formation have been performed by Wilson and Pringle (1956) and by Korngold (1956a).

False reactions of nonidentity (intersection) produced by identical antigens appear to be rare, but they can occur. In one particular instance (Feinberg, 1957), crystallized ovalbumin was used to charge small wells in serial dilution surrounding a much larger central wall, charged with antibody, in a petri dish. A pattern of intersection appeared between the wells with the strongest and weakest antigen concentrations. The particular type of test being used was not designed to allow antigen to diffuse very far from its source, and so in its lower concentrations it tended to become exhausted rapidly. On the other hand, antibody in the large central well purposely was used in large excess and furthermore was allowed to diffuse into the surrounding agar toward the potential reaction areas for some time before antigen wells were charged, to give additional physical advantage to the antibodies. Intersection resulted from the inability of exhausted antigen from one well to block antibody diffusion through its precipitate to an area behind the precipitate where it could react with antigen still diffusing from the adjacent antigen well which was originally heavily charged. Penetration of reactants through precipitin bands under such conditions as these has been well established (Korngold and Van Leeuwen, 1958, 1959b; Van Oss and Heck, 1963). False spurring can occur similarly if one of two compared antigens is too concentrated relative to the other (Jameson, 1969).

A pattern of this kind also could be interpreted as one of double spurring, because in the photographs presented of it (Feinberg, 1957) the short bands extending beyond the point of intersection curve rather sharply toward the antibody source, a characteristic of spur formation.

Identical antigens being compared can form "false" spurs if the antiserum contains complement-dependent precipitins in addition to the more usual complement-independent precipitins (Paul and Benacerraf, 1966). The former do not become immobilized by antigen except in the presence of complement and therefore act as a semi-independent precipitating system.

False reactions of identity can occur between two antigens reacting with an antiserum, usually clearly able to distinguish them, if physical conditions are such that insufficient antibody is available to foster precipitin band formation with either antigen beyond their point of intersection. The bands, growing no further than this point, then appear to coalesce. False identity reactions also may develop in comparison of entirely different antigens reacting with different populations of antibodies if the two different precipitating systems have a third factor in common for precipitation to occur, such as a requirement of complement (Paul and Benacerraf, 1966). Band fusion then only indicates this shared property. This seems to be a rather uncommon situation.

Such spurious patterns of fusion wrongly indicating identity of antigens also are common, and in fact are difficult to avoid even consciously, when antiserum specifically directed against the antigens being analyzed is not available (Crowle, 1960c; Korngold and Lipari, 1956b; Korngold and Van Leeuwen, 1957). In practice, this is exemplified by experiments in which "abnormal" human serum γ-globulins are analyzed using some antiserum produced against pooled normal human serum or normal γ-globulins. Such an antiserum might show two abnormal globulins to be alike which actually differ in minor but significant aspects antigenically, or they might seem to be identical with a normal, comparable γ-globulin. On the other hand, an antiserum prepared against these abnormal globulins would demonstrate these antigenic differences, since animals injected with them probably would produce antibodies capable of making these distinctions. This can be shown schematically if normal γ-globulin is designated Ga and two abnormal ones are designated Ga′ and Ga″, the prime marks indicating minor antigenic differences (Fig. 4.7). Antibody to Ga would recognize Ga′ and Ga″ as identical; reactions of false identity would be rendered in double diffusion plate tests in which any two of these antigens were compared with one of the others using this antiserum (Fig. 4.7a). On the other hand, if antibody produced specifically against Ga′ were available, then such tests would show Ga′ and Ga to be related but not identical, the Ga′ having an antigenic determinant not present on Ga. But still Ga′ and Ga″ would appear to be identical to this antibody (Fig. 4.7b). Only if antibody specific for Ga″ were utilized would the slight differences between Ga″, Ga′, and Ga be elucidated (Fig 4.7c). The practical importance of these sometimes very elusive differences may be small in many instances; on others, it may be weighty but completely overlooked. Such interpretive subtleties counsel cautious interpretation, reference to the type of antiserum employed, and, on most occasions, formation of only tentative conclusions. One is not justified in stating, for example, that a given antigen in bacterium X is identical with a comparable antigen in closely related bacterium Y if the conclusion is based solely on experiments employing antiserum prepared only against bacterium X; a mixture of antisera against both should be utilized.

COMPARISON OF ANTISERA

In the discussion above, only antigen comparison was considered. When, in the opposite situation, two antisera are compared with respect to a given antigen, interpretations are similar but they may be more complicated (Crowle, 1960c, 1963; Jennings, 1956; Robbins and Summaria, 1966; Darbyshire and Pereira, 1964). Largely, this is because no two animals injected with antigen in the same manner are likely to produce exactly the same species of antibody against a given antigen in the same quantity or ratio, and because the specificity of antibodies produced by one animal may differ from that of another (Crowle, 1960c; Wilson and Pringle, 1956). If two compared antisera, seemingly identical because they produce a pattern of fusion against an antigen, are used inter-changeably with an understanding that they truly are identical sero-logically, the results may be confusing (Milgrom and Loza, 1967). Thus, the range of antibodies in one of the antisera might show two antigens analyzed with it to be similar but not the same, while the other anti-serum with a range of antibodies of narrower specificity could indicate that these two antigens were identical (see Fig. 4.7). Two different anti-sera can produce a reaction of identity when compared with respect to one antigen but have antibodies of entirely different specificity. One antiserum might react with determinants x and y and the other with determinants a and b, but since all four determinants are on one species of antigen, to this antigen the two antisera would "look" identical (Grogan *et al.*, 1964; Fig. 4.8).

The ephemeral value of comparing antisera as contrasted to comparing antigens in double diffusion tests is illustrated by matching the kind of results expected in each case. For example, if chicken ovalbumin and duck ovalbumin are compared, using several different good antisera against the former antigen, precipitin patterns probably will differ in minor details, such as line intensity and spur length produced by the chicken ovalbumin. But generally from test to test they will be very similar, invariably showing the pattern of partial intersection and a spur produced by the homologous antigen. By contrast, suppose that two of these antisera are compared with each other using chicken ovalbumin,

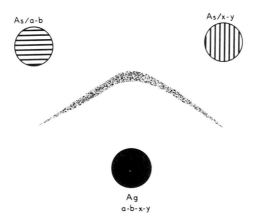

Fig. 4.8. Diagram illustrating formation of reaction of identity which might in-correctly be interpreted as indicating that the two antisera (As) compared are serologically identical. Actually, they have precipitins to entirely different antigenic determinant sites, but since the determinants with which they both can react are all found on one population of antigen molecules, the precipitin bands that they form coalesce.

duck ovalbumin, turkey ovalbumin, pheasant ovalbumin, and other similar but not identical fowl ovalbumins. The antisera would be "identical" with reference to the chicken ovalbumin, but while one might produce a spur over the other with turkey ovalbumin, the second could form a spur over the first with duck ovalbumin. There is a definite but, at first, not too obvious difference between such comparisons of antisera using antigens, and antigens using different reference antisera. In the latter instance, the antigens are being tested against reactants (antisera) formed in response to one of them. Hence, the reference reactants have induced common features. However, when two antisera are tested against several different antigens, there is no common denominator except the chance content of antibodies formed in response to immunization with the original antigen which happen to cross-react with the heterologous antigens. Mention hardly need be made that two antisera compared with respect to a crude antigen mixture and shown thereby to react with the same antigens similarly should not, on this basis, be used interchangeably for analyzing other similar mixtures of antigens. Compared with respect to one of these, one antiserum is likely to show content of antibodies not indicated in the first test comparison and absent from the other antiserum; or regarding an antigen not present in the first antigen mixture used for antiserum comparison, antibodies in one may differ significantly from those in the other in specificity or avidity.

These problems do not, of course, prevent comparison of two different antisera for potential to precipitate the same antigen (Robbins and Summaria, 1966). Such a comparison is valid in showing by reaction of fusion that two antisera have precipitins to the same antigen. Nevertheless it does not show that the respective precipitins are the same kind of immunoglobulin.

Precipitin Band Curvature

This characteristic often reveals important qualitative and quantitative properties of the reactants in immunodiffusion tests. It depends importantly, and more-or-less self-evidently, on the shape and arrangement of reactant sources (Wilson, 1964). The following discussion reveals its basic principles.

In a two-well double diffusion plate test using antigen and antibodies at equivalent concentrations, if both have approximately the same diffusion coefficient, their precipitin band will form midway between antigen and antibody depots, and it will be straight (Wilson, 1964; Van Oss and Heck, 1963; Fig. 4.9a). Lowering the concentration of one or the other reactant will cause the band to shift its position toward the weaker re-

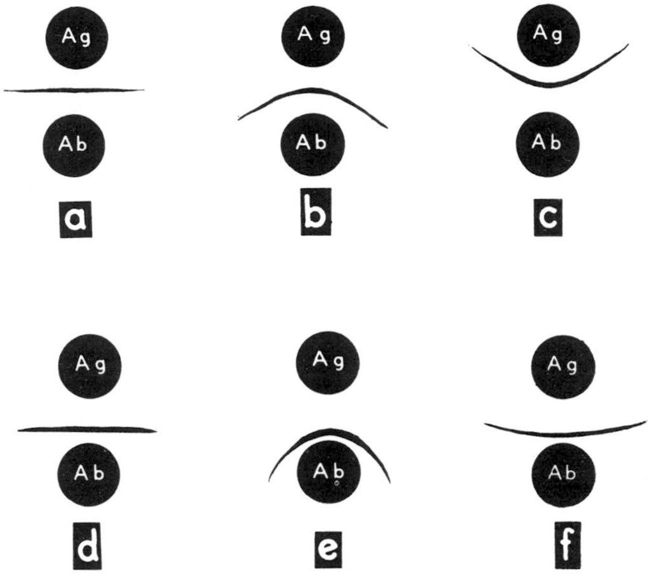

Fig. 4.9. The curvature of a precipitin band between reactant sources in double diffusion plate tests depends on the relative diffusion coefficients of antigen and antibody, even when these two are not used in exactly equivalent proportions. In diagrams *a* and *d,* antigen and antibody have equal diffusion coefficients (i.e., probably equal molecular weights), and they form straight precipitin bands. When they are used at equivalence, their band forms midway between them (*a*); when antigen concentration initially exceeds that of antibody the band is formed closer to the antibody source (*d*). The precipitin band formed by an antigen with a higher diffusion coefficient (lower molecular weight) than antibody curves toward the latter at serologic equivalence (*b*). This curvature is accented if antigen excess is employed (*e*). The opposite effects prevail when antigen has a lower diffusion coefficient than antibody (*c, f*).

actant, but except for extreme concentration differences the band will remain straight (Korngold and Van Leeuwen, 1957c). The straightness or curvature of a precipitin band reflects the relative diffusion coefficients of the two reactants.[4] Thus, if the diffusion coefficient of antigen is greater than that of its antibodies, the precipitin line will curve toward the antiserum source in proportion to the difference between the reactant diffusion coefficients (Fig. 4.9*b*). This effect is most obvious in plates utilizing cylindrical reactant depots, since then the reactants diffuse radially, and any tendency toward curvature is magnified for the following reasons.

[4] Characteristics of the test itself, like salt concentration, can significantly affect results (Wachendörfer, 1965; cf. Chapter 1).

When the two reactants diffuse through agar gel at equal rates, they will reach a serologically equivalent reaction plane in equal time to form a precipitate. Since each will be diffusing radially from its cylindrical source at the same rate, the precipitin band must grow laterally between the two depots in a straight line. If one of these reactants with equal diffusion coefficient is used at higher concentration than the other, its diffusion rate (not diffusion coefficient) will be greater, so that it will have moved farther from its source than the weaker reactant before the two meet and precipitate, and the precipitin band will begin to form closer to the weaker reactant (Fig. 4.9d). However, since serologic equilibrium is established at this plane, this equilibrium exists equally at succeeding points along a straight plane where the circles of diffusion for each reactant make first contact. This equilibrium thus exists not only for antigen and antibodies at the plane of precipitation but also for their relative ratio of dilution by radial diffusion, and a straight precipitin band again will be formed (Korngold and Van Leeuwen, 1957c). From this reasoning, it is easy to see that if one reactant has a greater diffusion coefficient (lower molecular weight) than the other, although the two will meet in the precipitin zone at serologically equivalent rates, the reactant of higher diffusion coefficient will increase its circle of diffusion more rapidly for a given concentration than the other. Then the serologic equivalence plane shifts slowly away from the faster diffusing reactant, curving the forming precipitin band toward the reactant of lower diffusion coefficient. As a general rule, then, a precipitin band in the double diffusion plate is concave toward the reactant of higher molecular weight; if the molecular weight of one reactant is known, then, that of the other can be estimated (Korngold and Van Leeuwen, 1957c). But as Figs. 4.9e and 4.9f suggest, serologic imbalance between antigen and antiserum can affect the meaning of this type of test.

Patterns of Precipitation in Angle Double Diffusion Tests

In angle double diffusion tests (i.e., double diffusion gradient tests), reactants diffuse across each other at less than 180 degrees (Elek, 1949a; Ouchterlony, 1949c). Consider the reaction between equivalent quantities of antigen and antibody of approximately equal molecular weight placed in troughs in agar as an L, the antigen in the vertical trough and the antibody in the horizontal one. The diffusion front from either trough into the reaction area will be straight, and hence the reactant concentration gradients will extend outward from each trough parallel to it (cf. Fig. 1.6). Since the two troughs are not made to join where they converge but only to approach each other closely, the reactants will make first contact between these two proximal trough ends to begin forming visible precipitate there very soon (sometimes minutes) after the troughs have been charged. As time passes and each diffusion front advances farther into the reaction arena, the tip of the zone of contact will move away from the trough convergence area in a straight line exactly bisecting the 90-degree angle of the troughs (see Figs. 1.6 and 4.2). The plane of agar traversed by this continual succession of points of contact will contain the precipitin band formed by the intermingling reactants, and under the hypothetical conditions considered here this band will be narrow and sharply defined. If large enough quantities of antigen and antibody are employed, the base of this band will be substantially broader than its very fine tip, because by their large quantities not diluted by diffusion over a considerable distance, each respective reactant will tend to diffuse through already formed and serologically inert precipitate to form additional precipitate on either side of the band's central plane. On the other hand, at the outermost actively growing end of the precipitin band, the reactants will be first encountering each other in minimal concentrations and will form the visible tip of the precipitin zone only by sufficient accumulation (Elek, 1949a). Thus, just ahead of the tip of the visibly growing precipitin line there will be a zone of antigen–antibody complexes in the process of aggregating into visible quantities but not yet visible unless brought out or observed by some auxiliary means.

When R-type antibodies are employed, the state of equivalence between two reactants can be ascertained by the shape of the precipitin band base formed in the double diffusion gradient test. Since the band always is formed by growth at its tip where antigen and antibody continually meet in optimal proportions for precipitation, this tip will be sharp. However, if antibody is used in excess, it will tend to diffuse through specific precipitate to form more precipitate on the antigen side of the initially sharp zone. The result is that at its base the precipitin band will broaden toward the antigen source while remaining fairly sharply defined on the side facing antibody diffusion (Fig. 4.2). A relative excess of antibody has progressively less time to accumulate at increasing distance along the precipitin band from its base, so that the maximum broadness of the base gradually diminishes toward the sharp point of the precipitin zone (Elek, 1949a). The effect of using excess antigen is similar (Jochim and Chow, 1969). If H-type antiserum is employed, the broadening of the precipitin band base is small, because excess reactants with this type of antiserum readily dissolve specific precipitate. Rather, there is a wholesale shift of the precipitin band up the plane of the weaker reactant, so that if only one observation is made this appears to originate not from the angle of the trough convergence but rather from some point up that trough itself (Fig. 4.2; Elek, 1949a). This point of insertion represents a definite ratio between the concentrations of reactants originally used, since in a given time this point will rise along the axis of the weaker reactant a distance proportional to the ratio of stronger to weaker reactant.

When equivalent antigen and antibody are utilized in a gradient double diffusion test, the slope of the precipitin band formed by them is proportional to the ratio of their diffusion coefficients (Stollar and Levine, 1963; Tokumaru, 1965b). Hence, if this value is known for an antibody,[5] then it can be estimated very closely for an antigen, and vice versa. When the slope is small—for example, when the band forms closer to the antibody source than to the antigen trough—the diffusion coefficient of one reactant (e.g., antigen) is greater than that of the other (e.g., antibody), and its molecular weight is less (Fig. 4.2). If the slope is steep, then the antigen has a lower diffusion coefficient than the antibody, and its molecules are larger. These data can be treated mathematically (Allison and Humphrey, 1959, 1960).

Double Diffusion Tube Tests

The double diffusion tube test was at one time highly regarded because of its excellent sensitivity. But with the development of other kinds of immunodiffusion tests of increased sensitivity and convenience, and especially of less susceptibility to secondary precipitation (Lueker and Crowle, 1963; Crowle, 1963), this type of test has become obsolete (Casman et al., 1969). Therefore, it will be discussed only briefly (cf. Augustin, 1957; Boerma, 1956; Polson, 1958; Augustin and Hayward, 1955; Hayward and Augustin, 1957).

The linear (tube) double diffusion test resembles single diffusion tube tests (cf. Fig. 1.6). Usually it is set up in a glass tube by casting three succeeding layers of agar gel, the lowest containing antigen, and the topmost antiserum; the middle layer provides a reaction arena. Antigens and antibodies diffuse from their respective sources into the middle layer, meet, intermingle, and precipitate at or close to the plane of their original meeting. Precipitation accumulates in this narrow area because both reactants migrate into the reaction layer at rates determined by their respective diffusion coefficients and original concentrations, and they continue to do so after adjusting themselves to each other somewhat, if they were not balanced to begin with. Hence, unless large dis-

---

[5] For rabbit antibodies it is 3.8×10^{-7} cm^2/sec (Stollar and Levine, 1963).

proportions exist, serologically, forming bands of precipitate will not migrate as they do in a single diffusion tube test.

If antigen and antiserum are not used at approximate immunologic equivalence, as their precipitin band forms it will shift away from the excessive reactant. This shift will continue until it compensates for the excess of the overbalancing reactant by making it diffuse both further and through an increasing gradient of the weaker reactant. The characteristics of precipitin band formation and movement during this equilibration are the same as those for the formation and movement of such a band in a single diffusion test, resembling them especially in a single diffusion tube test which has developed for a long time and hence retains only a small excessive amount of external reactant over internal reactant. The more disproportionate one reactant is to the other serologically, the longer will be required for their equilibration and stabilization of their precipitin band, the farther the forming band will move away from the excess reactant and their initial plane of precipitation, and the more the characteristics of this double diffusion tube test will resemble those of a single diffusion tube test. This is true also for double diffusion angular and radial tests, but because precipitin bands in these two tests grow laterally between the two sources of reactants, their results are somewhat easier to interpret (see below).

The tendency for a precipitin band to move away from its original position in an unbalanced double diffusion test is readily evident for R-type antibodies because their precipitates with antigen dissociate poorly in reactant excess. Hence, a trail of incompletely dissociated precipitate will remain nearer the excessive reactant, while the freshly forming edge of precipitation nearer the weaker reactant will be sharp. This is just as is observed in the single diffusion tube, and the reasons are the same. Of course, a sharp precipitin band formed by R-type antibodies in a double diffusion tube test indicates that antigen and antibody have been used at or near equilibrium. H-type antibodies will tend to form a sharp precipitin band even when the reactants are out of serologic proportion because of the ready solubility of antigen–antibody precipitates produced by H-type antibodies; hence, disproportionate conditions are more difficult to detect in tests using these antibodies.

Occasionally, the excess of one reactant may be large enough and its diffusion rate high enough so that, after some initial precipitation where it first meets the opposing reactant, it escapes continued precipitation for a short distance until, by the dilution of its further diffusion and by the gradient of opposing reactant that it encounters during this additional diffusion, it once again arrives at precipitating proportions with the other reactant. The result will be development of a second precipitin band very much like the first; that is, two precipitin bands will have been formed by this single antigen–antibody system (Lueker and Crowle, 1963; Crowle, 1963). This secondary precipitation is an important problem in all immunodiffusion tests. But it is especially troublesome in double diffusion tube tests because it occurs frequently, and yet it cannot be identified directly. The following discussion may be helpful to the reader in understanding, identifying, and avoiding this phenomenon.

Secondary Precipitation

The formation of more than one precipitin band by one kind of antigen and its antibodies because of a serologic imbalance of the reactants in the area where precipitation is taking place can occur in any immunodiffusion test (Wilson, 1958; Lueker and Crowle, 1963; Crowle, 1963). Basically there are two types of secondary precipitation. One is a reactant concentration artifact. It is caused by sudden changes in relative rates at which the reactants are arriving in the area of precipitation due to sudden changes in reactant concentrations at their origins of diffusion (e.g., recharging a well) or to changes in ambient temperature of the test and therefore of reactant diffusion rates. The other kind of secondary precipitation is the Liesegang phenomenon.

Since both types of secondary precipitation occur only when the two opposing reactants are serologically unbalanced (see Chapter 3), linear immunodiffusion tests will be more susceptible to them than radial or angle tests. In linear tests the imbalance prevails longer and across more of the reactant arena because neither reactant is diluted as rapidly or within as small a length of agar as in angle and radial tests. In the latter, serologic imbalance usually cannot be maintained for long directly between the reactant origins, and it recedes even more rapidly lateral to this area. Hence in angular and radial tests secondary precipitation fades out (concentration artifact) laterally, or melds into only primary precipitation (Liesegang precipitation).[6] These effects, illustrated in Figs. 1.8 and 4.10, cannot occur in linear immunodiffusion tests, and they account for the inability of the experimenter to detect secondary precipitation directly in these tests (Lueker and Crowle, 1963; Crowle, 1963).

[6] Merging of the lateral tips of Liesegang bands in radial double diffusion plate tests is the primary means of identifying them. However, two truly different antigen–antibody precipitating systems occasionally will give the appearance of merging lateral tips in such a test merely by coincidence (Jennings, 1959b,d). This situation can be revealed by changing the respective concentrations of the two different antigens (Grabar, 1957c; Salvinien and Kaminski, 1955b), or by immunoelectrophoresing or electroimmunodiffusing the antigen mixture, since the two antigens are not likely to have identical electrophoretic mobilities.

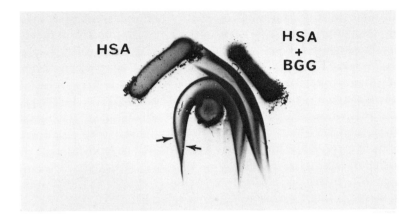

HSA

HSA + BGG

Fig. 4.10. Illustration of Liesegang precipitation in a double diffusion plate test in which human serum albumin (HSA) and a mixture of this antigen and bovine γ-globulin (BGG) were reacted with antiserum to both. The arc forming acutely around the central antiserum reservoir was developed by the HSA. Because of HSA excess, this arc is double (arrows) around most of its extent, but at its tips, which are too far away from the antigen sources for such excess to be maintained, its double bands merge into a single band characteristic of the Liesegang phenomenon as seen in double diffusion plate tests or immunodiffusion tests similar to these.

A sudden surge of one reactant over the other in the area of precipitation favors concentration-change secondary precipitation. A relative surge can occur if one reactant well is recharged and the other is not, or if both are recharged but not in the same proportions as they were originally (Kaminski, 1954a). It can develop with a temperature change of from 1 to 5 degrees, apparently by changing the local concentration of free predominating reactant (i.e., increasing it with a rise in temperature resulting in less efficient precipitation, and decreasing it with a drop in temperature resulting in its more effective insolubilization) and therefore shifting the serologic balance between the two reactants to temporarily either interfere with precipitation or enhance it, depending on whether the temperature is raised or lowered. The effect develops most readily with easily dissociable antigen–antibody precipitates, such as those formed by H-type antisera; this factor associated with antibody characteristics appears to be more important than a disparity in diffusion coefficients of the two reactants in secondary precipitation. But secondary precipitation does tend to occur more readily with fast- than with slow-diffusing reactants, because local changes in concentration of the latter are slow enough and in so small an area physically that secondary precipitation may not be distinguishable from primary precipitation.

Liesegang precipitation tends to occur when one reactant is diffusing into the precipitation area faster than the other can meet it in precipitating conditions, but not so fast that diffusion of the weaker reactant is negligible (see Fig. 1.7). Therefore, it appears only when there is a moderate excess of reactant (Lueker and Crowle, 1963). It is favored also by a difference in diffusion coefficients between the two reactants, most often being noticed with low-molecular-weight antigens like human serum albumin. It occurs as readily with R-type as with H-type antisera. But it is more readily identified when developing with the former because the stability of the precipitate formed by R-type antibodies gives clues to conditions of reactant excess and changes in precipitin band position upon simple visual inspection which are missing without more exacting observations and measurements with H-type precipitins.

Selected Double Diffusion Techniques

There are many varieties of double diffusion test, especially of the radial type. Many have virtues justifying their special use; others are simply novel designs of reactant arrangements or well shapes; still others, once useful, now are obsolete. Just as for the single diffusion tests discussed in Chapter 3, it is practical here to describe only a few representative and most useful of the double diffusion techniques. Supplementary methods with special uses are mentioned briefly at the end of this section. Obsolete techniques are omitted; the reader with a historical curiosity about these is referred to the first edition of this book for their description.

Double Diffusion Tube Tests

There are both macro and micro varieties. A macro test is easier to perform but uses more reactants; it is easier to observe and interpret. The macro test is more satisfactory unless the investigator is forced by circumstances to use very small amounts of reactants.

One may use a tube of any internal diameter to perform the macro test; one of 3 to 5 mm is convenient. The tube may be open at both ends or closed at one. The smaller its internal diameter, the more important are its precoating with agar solution (if agar or agarose is to be used for the gel, as is usual) as described already for the single diffusion tube test (Chapter 3), its charging with reactants that do not touch the sides of the tube which they are not meant to cover, the uniformity of its gel layers with flatness of menisci, and its development at constant temperature.

In a typical double diffusion tube test a column of antigen-charged gel is overlaid with a column of gel without reactant, and this in turn is overlaid with antiserum solution or antiserum in more gel. The length of antigen- and antiserum-charged columns is less important than the concentration of reactant which each contains; the middle column of gel without reactant, which will serve as the reaction arena, typically will be 1 cm long and 3 mm in cross section. The classic way of preparing a. double diffusion tube is to stand it in modeling clay if the bottom of the tube is left open, or in some other convenient holder if that end has been sealed shut, mix a double-strength solution of antigen warmed to 56°C with 2% agar dissolved in appropriate buffer and cooled to this temperature, and deposit a 1-cm column of this solution in the bottom of a 4-cm-long tube with a long-tipped Pasteur pipet. After this column of antigen-charged agar has gelled, a 1-cm length of 1% agar, cooled to 56°C to prevent denaturing antigen at its interface of contact in the tube, is layered upon the antigen-charged gel, and after this reaction layer has congealed it is in turn covered with an appropriate volume of either liquid antiserum or antiserum that has been incorporated in agar as was done for antigen. The double diffusion tube then is set in a water bath at 4°C for development over several days.

Double diffusion tube length varies according to the whims of the user. Long tubes and gel columns develop precipitates slowly but usually offer better band resolution than short tubes; but they are also less sensitive. If more than 1 cm of reaction column length is needed to resolve the different precipitating systems, then an immunodiffusion technique of higher resolution should be employed. The 3-mm width indicated here is a compromise between reactant economy and the ease with which reactants can be deposited in the tube. One of the two reactants usually is gelled to provide a support for the reaction column of gel, and this reactant usually is antigen because it tends to be more heat-stable than antiserum. If both reactants are heat-labile, gelatin can substitute for agar; alternatively, polyacrylamide or low-gelling-point agarose can be used, or one can dispense with incorporating the reactants in a gel altogether.[7] One must avoid touching the upper reaches of the double diffusion tube with the antigen–gel mixture when placing the mixture in the bottom of the tube, and avoid injecting any bubbles into the tube with this mixture.

Although a reaction may become visible within 24 hours in one of these double diffusion tube tests developed at 4°C, precipitin bands

---

[7] Both reactants can be used liquid in a U- or J-shaped tube in which the bottom of the U contains the reaction area and its two arms are charged with the opposing reactants (Ouchterlony, 1968; Naylor and Adair, 1962).

generally continue to appear and intensify for 1 to 3 weeks (Morton and Dodge, 1963). Higher temperatures promote faster development but also decrease sensitivity, risk microbial contamination, and thus require addition of preservatives to prevent such contamination. The tubes should be observed several times during development, because the number of visible bands can change from one time to another (Morton and Dodge, 1963). For maximal sensitivity and least possibility of artifactual precipitation, reactants should be used at or near serologic equilibrium (Parlett, 1961), and the distance between the reactant layers should be the least that is enough to resolve the several separate bands of precipitation expected to develop.

Results usually consist of sharply defined discs of precipitate within the reaction column (Fig. 4.11). However, immunologic excess of antigen or antibody, usually antigen, will cause fuzzy bands to develop. Indeed, the sharpness of a disc of precipitate is an indicator for immunologic balance and can be used in quantitative analyses (see below). Precipitin bands can form within either the antigen or the antiserum column, if these are cast as gels, when one of the reactants is in great excess to the other or diffuses much more rapidly. However, this is unusual. Some antiserum components, especially those associated with lipids, tend to precipitate at the antiserum–reaction column interface and should not be confused with specific antigen–antibody precipitates. Misinterpretation can be avoided by setting up control tests in which antigen is replaced with buffer alone or with an unrelated antigen, and in which antiserum is replaced by a similar normal serum. Gaps induced by temperature change and striae developing with R-type antiserum usually can be recognized by their occurrence in a wide disc of precipitate which looks as though it has broken into sections, and by their developing in association with conditions of immunologic excess of one reactant or the other. Unfortunately, there is no direct way of identifying Liesegang precipitation in a double diffusion tube test, and no sure way of avoiding it except by carefully regulating the proportions of already reasonably well-characterized antigen–antibody systems.

Results from double diffusion tubes usually are recorded as number of precipitin bands developing, their intrareactant locations, and their individual characteristics (fuzzy, sharp, trailing, etc.). Appropriate drawings may suffice, but dark-field photography is more convenient and reliable.

Micro Double Diffusion Tube Tests

One enters the "micro" range of these tests by using tubes with internal diameter of 2 mm or less. In tubes with these diameters, incorporat-

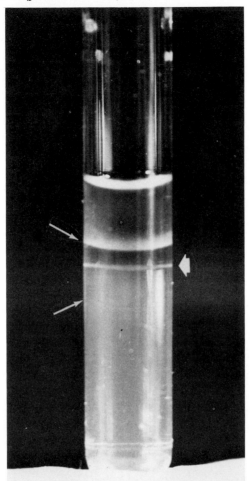

Fig. 4.11. Double diffusion tube test in which 0.1% human serum albumin antigen (lower turbid column) was reacted with undiluted rabbit antiserum (clear upper column) to form a disc of precipitate seen from the side as a turbid band (heavy arrow) in a slightly turbid middle column. Interfaces between the three different columns are indicated by the smaller arrows. The precipitate at the bottom of the antiserum, which was not incorporated in agar, presumably in serum lipoprotein precipitating as it diffuses into and reacts nonspecifically with the agar gel of the middle layer.

ing the reactants in a gel can be dispensed with because capillarity will keep the reactants in place within the tube (El-Marsafy and Abdel-Gawad, 1962). For instance, inject enough hot 1% agar into the middle of a 50-mm-long tube to fill its center. After this has solidified, inject

0.02-ml quantities of antigen and antiserum into contact with opposite ends of this column of gel without entrapping air bubbles. Seal each end with melted wax, and then allow the reactions to develop in the usual manner.

Ultramicro adaptions of double diffusion tube tests using either agar gel or minute cellulose acetate strips within 3-mm lengths of glass capillary tubes, micromanipulation equipment, and volumes of reactant solution as small as 0.03 μl can be employed when the available volume of reactant is very small (Ringle and Herndon, 1965). The contents of these tubes are kept from dehydrating by closing each end of the capillary tube with a microdrop of paraffin oil. Reactants are delivered into a tube from either end with microsyringes through the oil seals. Ultramicro techniques probably have more esthetic than practical value because they are difficult and exacting to perform and have no demonstrably greater sensitivity than is readily within the reach of more conventional micro methods.

Preparatory Linear Double Diffusion

In immunodiffusion tests, antigen is concentrated by specific precipitation with its antibodies in a narrow plane of gel. The precipitate that forms is stable enough to be washed repeatedly with physiologic saline to rid it of nonspecific adsorbates. The precipitin band therefore is a source of modest amounts of very highly purified antigen. The quantity of antigen in a precipitin band of conventional micro or macro immunodiffusion tests is small. But immunodiffusion can be scaled up for preparatory purposes to obtain yields of antigens in milligram rather than microgram quantities (Smith et al., 1962b). For example, the reaction area in a preparatory cell can be 1 cm wide and 2.5 × 2.5 cm in cross section. This is filled with 1.5% gelatin because this forms a gel at 0° to 5°C but will liquefy at room temperature. Antigen and antiserum are placed on opposite sides of this reaction area in volumes of 1.5 ml, and the cell is held for 1.5 to 3 weeks at 4°C for deep ribbons of antigen–antibody precipitate to form. Then, the cell is disassembled, the gelatin block containing the precipitin bands is frozen, and sections of this block 120 microns thick are cut from it with a freezing microtome. These sections are transferred to separate tubes by brush and brought to room temperature, whereupon the gelatin melts and the precipitate in each section may be collected by centrifugation. Conventional immunochemical methods next can be employed to wash the precipitate and to dissociate antigen from its antibodies. Antigen obtained in this manner is reported to be 25% of that originally applied to this type of preparatory cell (Smith *et al.*, 1962b).

The principle of this technique is to obtain large, flat planes of antigen–antibody precipitate in a medium from which they later can be harvested.

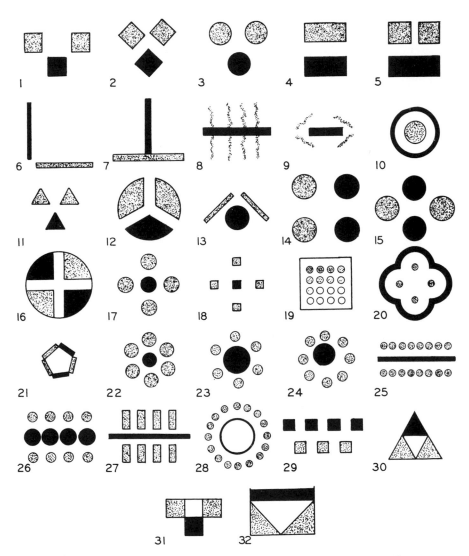

Fig. 4.12. Schematic representation of various forms of double diffusion tests (except form 19). Solid black shading represents antibody, and stippled areas represent antigen.

The method described above requires specially made cells, a long development time, and the use of gelatin which, as was indicated in Chapter 2, has distinct disadvantages as a gelling medium for immunodiffusion tests. The preparatory technique could be improved by casting a vertical stack of antigen–gel–antiserum layers in wide tubes, in disposable petri dishes, between glass plates with temporary walls, or in other similar conventional apparatus. Additional improvements might include employing a low-melting-point agarose or carrageenin instead of gelatin, or forcing all of each reactant to participate rapidly in precipitation by electroimmunodiffusion (Chapter 6). A primitive form of this type of preparatory electroimmunodiffusion in agar columns within glass tubes has been described previously (Crowle, 1956).

Radial Double Diffusion Tests

There are many varieties of this type of test, perhaps more than of any other kind of immunodiffusion technique (Fig. 4.12). Classic conformations, originally in petri dishes but more recently also in "micro" variations, are referred to as Ouchterlony plates in honor of the immunologist who did the most to earn due recognition for this excellent analytic technique (Ouchterlony, 1946a). Others have special names, usually referring to their particular uses or their physical characteristics. There are macro and micro and even ultramicro varieties. The principle, and therefore basic, procedure for all is the same: diffuse antigen radially from one source and antibodies similarly from another source nearby, and then observe their precipitation between these two sources as their respective areas of diffusion merge.

CLASSIC MACRO OUCHTERLONY TEST

This technique is obsolescent because it wastes reactants, its bands of precipitate develop slowly, its resolution generally is inferior to that of micro tests, and the original test is inconvenient to process for staining and preservation. Nevertheless, because it has been so important in the development of immunodiffusion and because it is so easy to set up, it will be described (Fig. 4.13).

Enough hot 1% agar in saline is poured into a 9-cm petri dish to cover the bottom and form a flat surface. After this has gelled, molds (e.g., short glass cylinders of 5-cm outside diameter, short plastic rods of similar size) are placed on the surface of this gel, usually three to a group in the shape of an equilateral triangle. Several groups can be placed on a single petri dish. A second layer of 1% agar 3 to 5 mm thick is poured, allowed to gel at room temperature, and then to set harder at

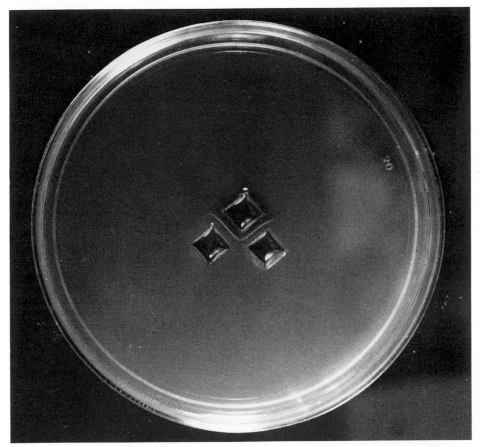

Fig. 4.13. Classic macro double diffusion (Ouchterlony) test performed in a petri dish. Bovine antiserum to human IgG (top well) has formed two precipitin bands with the compared antigens (lateral wells) which have fused in a reaction of identity. One antigen was a 0.1% solution of Cohn Fraction II from human serum, and the other was a 1:20 dilution of normal human serum. (Antiserum courtesy ICL Scientific, Fountain Valley, California.)

4°C. The molds are removed from the gel, and the resulting wells are filled with reactants. Usually one of the wells is charged with undiluted antiserum and the other two of the typical pattern of three are charged with antigen solutions (e.g., of different concentrations, or containing antigens to be compared qualitatively). The petri dish is placed in a refrigerator for the immunodiffusion patterns to develop, which, typically, is complete in 3 to 5 days. Precipitin bands are observed or photographed by dark-field lighting. Although the agar gel can be removed from the petri dish, washed and stained, and later dried as an original record of the reactions that developed, for a macro test this is tedious and seldom done.

Results are recorded in numbers of precipitin bands developing, their relative intensities, their positions between reactant wells, whether they are sharp and well-defined or are fuzzy, whether they are fuzzy on one side and not the other, and how they interact with each other. The potential interpretations of these results were discussed earlier in this chapter.

Although agar is the usual medium for these macro Ouchterlony tests, other media can be employed, notably polyacrylamide and gelatin. The purposes of the first layer to be poured in a macro test are to level the second layer (cf. Darcy, 1961) and to provide agar gel at the bottom of each well instead of bare glass: on bare glass reactants occasionally will be drawn from the bottom of a well between the agar and the glass with development of abnormal patterns of precipitate. However, only a single layer of gel need be poured if the petri dish has been leveled, and if the bottoms of wells cast or cut in the agar are sealed with a drop of hot agar before reactants are added.

The shape of the reactant source which is cut (Feinberg, 1956; Schubert et al., 1961), cast, or applied as a reactant-saturated piece of filter paper (Schaebel, 1962; Duquesnoy, 1966; Lueker and Crowle, 1963) may be important to accomplishing the purpose intended of a double diffusion test. Circular wells are better for qualitative analyses, and because they are adequate and also easier to prepare they are the most often used for quantitative analyses. Various sizes and patterns of round hole cutters for immunodiffusion tests are readily available. However, square, rectangular, or triangular wells are superior for comparing antigen for immunologic cross-reactivity or identity. Reactant wells of different sizes can be used in a single test. For example, using a large central well surrounded by a circle of regularly placed smaller satellite wells guards against overwhelming the reactant in the larger well by opposing reactant collectively diffusing against it from all the surrounding satellite wells (Hitzig, 1961). This large central well also can make enough volume of a weak reactant available for positive reactions to develop, whereas with a smaller central well there would be no evidence of precipitation (Shulman et al., 1966b). Distances between opposing reactant wells usually affect resolution and sensitivity oppositely. Thus, placing the wells farther apart usually increases resolution and decreases sensitivity, but if one of the reactants is very weak relative to the other, then moving the wells closer together may decrease instead of increase sensitivity (Anderson et al., 1962a).

The arrangement and number of wells also are determined partly by the purposes of a test. The triangular placement of three wells is intended mostly for comparing two antigens and an antiserum. A variant of this which sometimes yields more definitive data is to arrange four wells at the points of a square, two charged with antiserum and two with antigens to be compared. But for qualitative analyses to enumerate multiple antigen–antibody systems or to detect a given antigen–antibody system, any arrangement placing the reactant origins close enough together for good sensitivity without undue loss of resolution will suffice (5 mm·between the near edges of reactant wells in common). To study several different solutions of antigen or antiserum at once, four to eight wells are placed around a central well containing the common reactant (e.g., four antigen wells around one charged with antiserum); six is the most frequently used number. There are arrangements for comparing still more solutions at once. For instance, a large number of antigen wells can be set equidistant along a path parallel to a trough charged with antiserum (e.g., arrangement 25, Fig. 4.12).

The reactants usually are applied to their respective wells simultaneously. But when diffusion of one is considerably faster than that of the other (by its nature, quantity, or volume), then the slower reactant

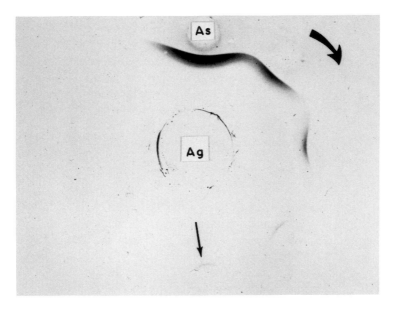

Fig. 4.14. Micro quantitative double diffusion plate test set up with a template such as that shown in Fig. 4.17. The titer of the antiserum tested was 16 because the 1:16 dilution of antiserum was the last of the succeeding doubling dilutions tested (clockwise from the top) which could form a visible band of precipitate (small arrow).

can be added minutes to hours ahead of the faster (Kunter, 1963; Distler and Roseman, 1964; Long and Silverman, 1965; Feinberg, 1956). If the time delay is in hours, then the empty wells eventually to receive the faster reactant should be filled with the same buffer as was used to prepare the gel while the slower reactant is diffusing into the gel.

Double diffusion plate tests can quantitate either antigen or antibody. The commonest well arrangement for such quantitations is eight small wells around a large central well (Fig. 4.14). Multiple well cutters or templates should be used for these tests to achieve the necessary reproducibility of technique.

The gel in macro Ouchterlony plates usually contains an antimicrobial preservative because of the several days required for full reaction development. The bulk of gel in these tests usually suffices to protect them against undue dehydration without auxiliary humidification such as is necessary for micro tests.

In classic Ouchterlony tests most reactant from each source is wasted by diffusion radially away into the gel where it will not encounter anything with which to react. Special immunodiffusion tests have been designed to prevent this by enclosing reactant sources on their "outsides" so that their reactants can diffuse only into the mutual reaction arena (see Fig. 4.15 for an example). They have been used especially to compare antigens with each other (Jennings and Kaplan, 1962). But because the advantages they offer seldom outweigh their need for special equipment and procedures, and because it is now possible to involve entire quantities of reactants in ordinary apparatus by electroimmunodiffusion, they will not be described further here. The interested reader may consult the following references for additional details: Crowle (1961), Ouchterlony (1968); Smith (1967), Lieberman et al. (1970), and Iványi and Valentová (1966).

MICRO DOUBLE DIFFUSION PLATE TESTS

The greater economy, rapidity, simplicity, and sensitivity of micro double diffusion plate tests make comparable macro techniques obsolescent (Mansi, 1958; Fox et al., 1963; Widra et al., 1968; Milgrom and Witebsky, 1962). There are approximately as many varieties of micro as of macro tests, and for similar reasons. The information given above on well shapes and arrangements for macro tests applies in general also to micro tests. In addition to varieties of the macro test which have been miniaturized, there are some micro techniques which are unique because they cannot be applied practically on a macro scale. The biggest difference among varieties of micro immunodiffusion tests is whether or not they employ a template to position and deliver the reactants.

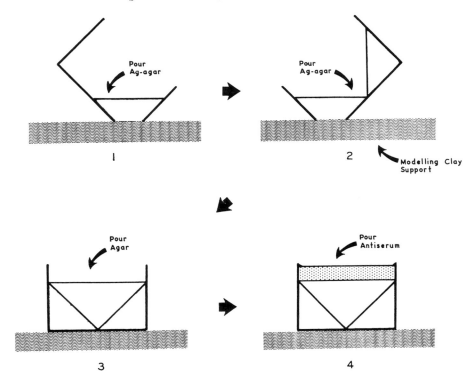

Fig. 4.15. Steps taken in setting up double diffusion gradient test in cell 32 of Fig. 4.12. The angles of the clear reaction arena can be varied, while still using the same type of cell, by varying the angle at which this is held in its modeling clay support during pouring of antigen-agar mixtures.

Micro tests using no template are simply small-scale macro tests: small wells are punched in a thin layer of gel usually cast on a microscope slide but sometimes also in other containers like small, disposable petri dishes (Centeno *et al.*, 1965). The following is a typical procedure for setting up such a test (cf. Mansi, 1958).

Prepare a 1% solution of agar in suitable buffer and pipet enough onto a level agar-precoated glass slide to make an even layer 1 to 2 mm thick. The slide should be resting on appropriate supports (e.g., applicator sticks, match sticks, thin glass rod) on a water-saturated piece of filter paper in an open petri dish during this procedure. The supports protect against capillary loss of the melted agar between slide and bench top as it is being cast; the moist filter paper and petri dish protect against dehydration and dust during the time that the agar is gelling. After the gel has set at room temperature, it is hardened for several minutes at 4°C. Slides with agar gel cast on them in this manner can be kept for several days at 4°C before use but must not become dehydrated or contaminated with bacteria or fungi. Next, wells are cut in the hardened gel according to whatever pattern is required.[8] These wells need be only 1 or 2 mm in diameter and usually are spaced 2 to 4 mm apart. They are charged with capillary tubing of external diameter slightly less than the well diameter: reactant solution is drawn up into one of these tubes, held at a low angle, by capillary attraction, and then fed into a well from the tube held at a higher angle with its tip touching the inner surface of the well. All wells should be filled with the same volume— for example, by filling each well just level with the surface of the gel.

Once the wells have been charged, the glass slide is returned in the humidified petri dish to a refrigerator for development at 4°C. Precipitin bands begin to appear within a few hours, and frequently the pattern will be adequately developed within 24 hours. Results can be observed and photographed with dark-field lighting, as is done with macro tests. In addition, the glass slide can be soaked in reaction-enhancing agents to intensify antigen–antibody precipitation, often bringing out precipitates that were not originally visible. Subsequently, the micro test is easily washed free of nonreacting serum and antigen components, stained, and dried to provide a permanent record of the original test itself. Precipitin band patterns in micro tests are interpreted in the same way as are those in macro tests.

Precipitation develops rapidly in micro tests because the reactants need diffuse only a short distance (Omland, 1963a). The gel in these tests is too shallow for the precipitin bands to form ribbons with much of an angle; in macro tests, such ribbons of precipitate may overlap and prevent good precipitin band resolution. Because micro test reactions develop rapidly, they can be held at 4°C with the advantages of more sensitivity, diminished chances of artifact formation, and minimal chance of microbial contamination. This, in turn, eliminates a need for adding preservative to the gel. Employing capillary tubes to deliver reactants to the wells is inexpensive, convenient, and clean.

Some precautions peculiar to micro tests must be observed. The gel is thin enough to require special protection against dehydration, and especially against uneven dehydration which can cause uneven reactant migration by hydrodynamic transport (cf. Chapter 7). This problem is solved by developing these tests at 4°C in a highly humidified chamber,

---

[8] With appropriate apparatus, uniform patterns of wells can be cast in the gel instead of cut (Omland, 1963a). With very thin layers of gel, reactant alternatively can be applied directly as a droplet to the surface of the gel (Wilson, 1964; Crowle and Hu, 1967), or in paper or absorbent membrane discs, squares, or strips (Liu, 1961c).

especially if the slide is supported upside down. Alternatively, the slide can be submerged in light mineral oil, a technique that is especially useful if reactions are to be observed frequently (e.g., for time-lapse photography) or must be developed at higher temperatures (Kohn, 1961). The mineral oil can be rinsed off later with petroleum ether, or some other such volatile hydrocarbon, and the slide processed for staining as it would be ordinarily. The slide also can be set in a layer of the same buffer as was used in the gel, deep enough to just make contact with the edges of the gel (Omland, 1963a).

Since micro test wells are much smaller than those of a macro test, they are more difficult to charge with equal volumes of reactant solution. However, with reasonable care this is not a significant problem except in quantitative tests, and for these tests one of the template micro techniques described below could be used to eliminate most of this risk of error. Equivalent filling of the wells can be effected by observing the level of added reactant by reflected light and bringing it just even with the surface of the surrounding gel.

Micro tests hitherto usually have employed agar gels; but today, agarose is beginning to predominate. Other semisolid media have been used, including gelatin (Crowle and Hu, 1967), polyacrylamide, and cellulose acetate (Kohn, 1961; Hayashida and Grunbaum, 1962; Rhodes, 1960). Of these, only polyacrylamide is likely to enjoy increasing popularity (cf. Chapter 2).

TEMPLATE MICRO DOUBLE DIFFUSION PLATE TEST

This term is applied to any of several techniques in which reactants are located upon and fed into a thin layer of gel by templates resting upon the surface of the gel. Templates provide the greater sensitivity obtained by second recharging of wells with reactants as is sometimes done in conventional micro tests (Murty and Hanson, 1961; Croisille, 1962; Remington and Finland, 1961; Wadsworth, 1962), without the disadvantages of procedural inconvenience and possible secondary precipitation resulting from a change in concentration. The templates are made from inert plastics like Plexiglas. Template techniques improve on nontemplate methods in uniformity of reactant source patterns built into the rigidity of the template itself and not requiring cutting of the gel, in greater uniformity of gel thickness and application of predetermined volumes of reactants, in greater resolution and sensitivity, and in easier washing and staining of the precipitin patterns (Crowle and Lueker, 1962; Wadsworth, 1957, 1962; Crowle, 1958; Zwartouw *et al.*, 1965; Styk and Schmidt, 1968; Schmidt and Styk, 1968; Casman *et al.*, 1969; Marquardt *et al.*, 1964; Peterson and Good, 1963; Auernheimer and

Atchley, 1962). These last two advantages stem from the facts that very thin (200 to 400 microns) gel is used, and yet reactant reservoirs can contain ten times as much reactant volume as will fit into a well of the nontemplate test.

There are several ways of applying a template. It can be rested on spacers on a microscope slide. Then hot agar solution is run between it and the slide (Krause and Raunio, 1967). Or, hot agar is spread between spacers on such a slide and the template is laid upon the agar and the spacers before the agar gels (Mäntyjärvi, 1965). Alternatively, a predetermined volume of hot agar is placed upon a glass slide and a template with spacers built onto it (Markowitz, 1964) or attached to it (Wadsworth, 1962) as legs is laid down upon the still liquid agar. But the most reliable and reproducible technique in our experience is to cast a thin layer of absolutely flat gel as described in Chapter 2 and then, after this has solidified and the top (casting) slide has been removed, replace it with the template. Briefly, the technique is as follows (cf. Figs. 2.4 and 2.5).

Small polyethylene spacers as thick as the agar is intended to be are placed on opposite ends of an agar-precoated glass slide. A noncoated glass slide is laid upon these, slightly offset to provide a pouring "lip" for the hot gel to be cast. This is pipetted upon the lip and allowed to flow evenly between the two slides. A slight excess is used to offset any tendency for shrinkage, and before this gels the top slide is nudged back into position directly over the lower slide. The gel is allowed to solidify and then is held at 4°C to harden, and the top slide is removed. Onto the resulting moist and absolutely flat surface of gel one or two templates are slid (Fig. 4.16A). Some workers find it more convenient to place them upon the gel, laying them down from one end to the other (Fig. 4.16B). Air bubbles between the lower surface of the template and the agar gel on which they are resting must be avoided.

After the templates are in place, reactants are added to their various wells. Reactant solution should be delivered from the bottom of each well upward, so that no air bubbles will be trapped in the bottom of the well. Such a bubble will prevent contact between the reactant solution and the gel and prevent reactant diffusion. Because template wells usually have considerably larger capacities than wells punched in gels of the nontemplate micro tests, either a syringe and needle (bent and with tip cut off, for convenience) or a micropipet rather than capillary tubing is used to charge template wells.

After the wells have been charged, the microscope slide–template sandwich is placed in a petri dish along with water-moistened filter paper

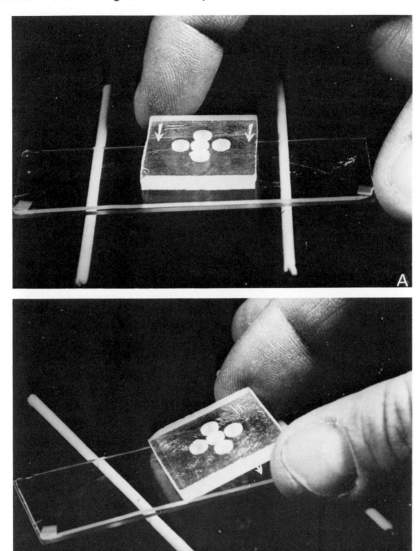

Fig. 4.16. Alternative ways of laying Plexiglas templates on agar gel for micro immunodiffusion tests. In one (A) the template is slid over the surface of the gel into position; in the other (B) it is lowered gently onto the gel. The gel has been precast by the sandwich method (see text) before the templates are applied and serves as their sole support. Two templates can be placed on one microscope slide, as is shown in Fig. 4.17.

and allowed to develop its reactions in this humid atmosphere for 24 to 48 hours at 4°C. These reactions can be seen through the bottom of the glass slide, which can be inverted with a rapid motion without dislodging its templates. After development of the reaction is complete, the slide is tilted to a vertical position, and the template(s) allowed to slide off by their own weight. Observations and subsequent processing of the slide are similar to those for the nontemplate micro tests, although they are somewhat easier because the gel for the template tests is thinner and more uniform.

Templates usually are custom-made, but some are also available commercially. For use on microscope slides they are generally made from Plexiglas $\frac{1}{8}$ inch (3.2 mm) or $\frac{1}{16}$ inch (1.6 mm) thick and 2.5 cm square. However, templates as thick as $\frac{1}{4}$ inch also have been used (Casman et al., 1969). The thicker templates are better for qualitative analyses, the thinner for quantitative analyses (Cline, 1967). Two of the most useful well patterns for qualitative and quantitative analyses are shown in Fig. 4.17. But many others analogous to those described above for macro tests also can be employed (Flandre and Damon, 1961; Holm, 1965). Large templates with multiple sets of patterns have been used on areas of agar the size of a petri dish (Taymor et al., 1965). Wells for templates used for qualitative analyses are funnel-shaped to permit feeding of a large volume of reactant into the agar gel from a small-diameter source; this contributes to the excellent resolution of micro template tests. The wells in templates used for quantitative analyses have uniform diameter through the template (Fig. 4.17). Sliding or laying a template onto an already cast flat surface of agar ensures that the capacity of individual wells is identical because there is no gel to rise into the well, as there is when the template is placed in contact with the agar before it has gelled.

The thickness of the gel under a template can be varied considerably. At one extreme it can be as little as 50 to 100 microns (Casman et al., 1969; Auernheimer and Atchley, 1962); at the other, large templates have been used in macro tests on agar gels several mm thick. A thickness between 200 and 500 microns probably is best for both convenience and utility. The gel must support the template and so should be reasonably rigid. This rigidity is obtained with 1% or more agar and 0.7 to 0.8% or more agarose. Polyacrylamide should be used at 3%; at higher concentrations it is more rigid, but sieving of reactants begins to occur. It is too sticky to slide a template onto, but with appropriate care a template can be laid upon it without trapping air bubbles. It can also be cast and gelled under a template (see Chapter 5). Cellulose acetate has been used with templates (Johnson et al., 1964). A wet strip is

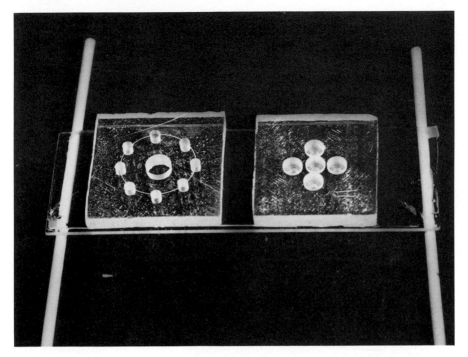

Fig. 4.17. Two types of templates commonly used for immunodiffusion tests on microscope slides. The left template is for quantitative analysis, and the right for qualitative analysis. Note the funnel-shaped wells in the latter, and compare with the diagram in Fig. 2.5.

placed on a microscope slide and a template is slid into position on it, as is done on agar gel. Excess water is blotted from the end of the acetate strip with filter paper, and reactants are added to the template wells. Further procedures are similar to those of micro template techniques for agar gel.

Immediately after removal from a test, a Plexiglas template should be soaked in water containing a moderately strong detergent, rinsed with tap and then with distilled water, and finally rinsed with 95% ethanol (Casman *et al.*, 1969). It should not be boiled or exposed to plastic solvents; and it should be dry when used for another test.

Template micro double diffusion plate tests are used less often than comparable nontemplate tests because they are somewhat more difficult to set up and because templates have not been as vigorously commercialized as have various cutters or precast immunodiffusion plates. Nevertheless, when highest sensitivity, resolution, and quality are required of a double diffusion plate test, the template should be employed.

ULTRAMICRO DOUBLE DIFFUSION PLATE TESTS

Minute tests executed with the aid of micromanipulation equipment can be performed in either cellulose acetate or gels (Ringle and Herndon, 1965). But, as was indicated previously, such extreme miniaturization is more of academic than practical interest. One particular disadvantage is that, because reactions are confined to so small an area, they must be observed with considerable magnification. The result is similar to observing a greatly magnified printed photograph: the overall meaning of the photograph is lost as the eye becomes preoccupied with the black and white dots of the printing itself. That is, in observing such ultramicro tests one sees antigen–antibody aggregates instead of bands of precipitate.

ANGLE DOUBLE DIFFUSION PLATE TESTS

Like linear and radial double diffusion tests, angle tests have both macro and micro varieties; and they can be performed with or without templates. The object of one of these tests is to have antigen and antiserum produce a sharp, well-defined precipitin band which is long enough for its angle between the reactant sources to be accurately measured. In length and breadth the test is of macro scale to permit most accurate measurement of the precipitin band; but the gel is cast as in a micro test by the sandwich technique for thinness and uniformity, and for ease of washing and staining. A template is used to feed a large volume of reactant into the gel so that the precipitin band will continue to grow over a longer distance than it would if troughs were used. The test is set up on a double-width microscope slide (75 × 50 mm) using a 200- to 400-micron layer of 1% agar (or equivalent) and a 4 × 4-cm Plexiglas template 3.2 mm thick. This has two slots 2.5 cm long and approximately 2 mm wide cut at right angles. The template is positioned on the gel as described for the micro template technique. The two slots are charged with antigen and antibody solutions, respectively, and the test is developed in a humidified petri dish at 4°C. Development to completion will take longer for this test than for micro template tests because the reactants have considerably farther to diffuse; 4 or 5 days may be required, although the precipitin line will begin to appear within a few hours, and therefore humidification is especially important. After the necessary time for reaction development, the template is removed and the reaction is observed.

Often, adequate information can be obtained by a simpler technique. Prepare a flat-surfaced gel on a double-width slide as already indicated. But, instead of using a template, cut two strips of filter paper about 1 mm thick, 2 mm wide, and 2.5 cm long. Lay these on another double-width microscope slide which has been silicoated to make it water-repellent, and arrange them in the same configuration as the slots of the template described above. This is facilitated by resting the support slide on a pattern diagram. Just saturate each strip with appropriate reactant, invert the glass slide which has the agar gel on it, and then carefully and gently press it down upon the filter paper strips. These will adhere to its agar when it is lifted back up. It should be pressed onto the strips only hard enough to make them adhere. Transfer this slide, still upside down, to supports for each of its two 50-mm edges in a petri dish over a water-saturated disc of filter paper. The precipitin band in this type of test will not be quite so sharp, intense, or long as that developing in a template test, but its angle of development can be readily determined.

Quantitative Tests

Double diffusion tests can quantitate antigen and antibodies in several ways, depending on such effects as position of a precipitin band between the antigen and antiserum sources, time required for band development, shifting of the band from one position to another with changes in reactant concentration, alteration in band appearance from fuzzy through sharp to fuzzy, or simply its appearance or nonappearance. All these effects depend on antigen–antiserum balance. They are most clearly evident in double diffusion tube tests, which are therefore worth considering although now seldom used.

Quantitative Double Diffusion Tube Tests

Quantitative experiments with this method generally depend upon (1) whether a precipitin band tends to move from the plane in which it originally formed and what balance of antigen and antibody make it immobile (Fig. 4.4*a*; Augustin, 1957; Boerma, 1956; Polson, 1958; Glenn, 1961a, and (2) what quantity of a given reactant will form a precipitin band diffusing into a previously prepared increasing gradient of the other reactant at some clearly defined plane, such as at the meniscus between the uppermost reactant in a tube and the agar upon which it lies (Fig. 4.4*b*; Augustin, 1957; Augustin and Hayward, 1955; Hayward and Augustin, 1957). For the first method, slight movement of the band is most readily detected if R-type antiserum is employed, since, for reasons already discussed, the band will be somewhat ragged on the side facing the stronger reactant (Augustin and Hayward, 1955; Hayward and Augustin, 1957). However, H-type antibody can be used if its peculiarities are recognized in advance (Boerma, 1956). When the two reactants are utilized at equivalence, each side of the zone is sharp. Since in the second method the precipitin band should remain practically immobile, R-type and H-type antisera can be equally well used without particular precautions.

OTHER QUANTITATIVE DOUBLE DIFFUSION TESTS

Although not so frequently used as radial single diffusion tests or electroimmunodiffusion for reactant quantitation, some techniques of quantitative double diffusion deserve description because they are reliable and simple, and they may be the best for certain applications.

In the simplest and most popular quantitative double diffusion test, a central well charged with one reactant is surrounded by a circle of equally spaced satellite wells charged with regularly diminishing concentrations of the reactant to be quantitated (cf. Fig. 4.17). The central well usually is considerably larger than the satellite wells (Jameson, 1969).[9] Most frequently, the end point in this test is that concentration of reactant used in one of the satellite wells which first fails to form a distinct precipitate, or at which the precipitate forming just touches the edge of or just surrounds the satellite well (Heiner *et al.*, 1962; Dameshek, 1963; Feinberg, 1956; cf. Fig. 4.14). Data so obtained are related to previously established standards of antigen or antiserum concentration. For instance, different antisera can be compared with each other for precipitin content against one or more antigens placed in the central well, and in comparison with some standard reference antiserum (Heiner *et al.*, 1962; Cline, 1967; Alexander and Moncrief, 1966). Or, the relative concentrations of one or more antigens in unknown solutions can be determined similarly by using them at various dilutions in peripheral wells against a standard antiserum in the central well (Hitzig, 1961; Terr and Bentz, 1965; Collins-Williams *et al.*, 1967).

This type of test has been performed on both macro (Dameshek, 1963) and micro scales with or without templates (Crowle, 1960b), and in gels or on cellulose acetate (Kohn, 1960). Its results are reliable and reproducible, and it can be made quite sensitive to detecting even small changes in reactant concentration (Dameshek, 1963; Darcy, 1961; but see also Glenn and Becker, 1969, reporting that 75% changes in antigen concentration are the lowest reliably detectable in routinely used micro double diffusion plate tests). It is capable of quantitating several antigen–antibody systems at one time. However, because in common with several other kinds of quantitative immunodiffusion tests it detects the overall precipitating capacity of antisera, its results must be inter-

[9] A test for conveniently and quickly determining the optimal precipitating ratio for a given antigen–antiserum system uses two parallel lines of wells cut in agar on a glass slide, well sizes in one string progressing from large to small, and opposing wells in the other string progressing conversely from small to large (Piazzi, 1969).

preted with the precaution that what appear to be quantitative differences in precipitins may sometimes be as much qualitative differences (see Chapter 1). On the other hand, if this seeming disadvantage is appropriately recognized, it can be used to reveal important information about changes in quality of antisera to a given antigen which will not be so readily evident in classic quantitative precipitin tests performed in liquid medium (Cline, 1967).

Quantitative tests similar to those just described but with different end points have been used. For instance, one may measure the distance between the source of one reactant and a precipitin band (Darcy, 1963; Darcy, 1960; King *et al.*, 1964; Collins-Williams *et al.*, 1967); note which in a series of changing concentrations of one reactant against a constant concentration of the other produces the sharpest and most stationary (i.e., serologically best balanced) precipitate (Cline, 1967; Sewell, 1964); record changes in precipitin band position between two reactants with time; or match shape and/or appearance of precipitin band patterns for unknown and standard solutions of antigen or antiserum (Micheli and Aebi, 1965; Crockson, 1963). But these techniques generally are more tedious and require more care and experience to perform than those using extinction end points as mentioned above, and they do not provide any better results practically.

A distinctly different variety of double diffusion plate quantitation, also adaptable to other kinds of immunodiffusion technique, is an inhibition test which relies on changes in precipitin band intensity or position under standardized conditions when various quantities of one reactant are added to the other. For example, precipitins can be quantitated by mixing twofold dilutions of an antiserum with a standard small quantity of antigen to determine at what antiserum dilution this antigen prevails in neutralizing the antiserum and preventing its precipitating the same antigen in a double diffusion test (Ray and Kadull, 1964; Gold and Freedman, 1965b). In a refinement of this technique, reference antigen and reference antiserum are placed in opposite wells, a third well is placed between them but offset somewhat, and then this third well is charged with unknown antiserum or unknown antigen mixed with known quantities of opposing reactant (see Fig. 4.18). The precipitin band formed between reference reactants will bend in one direction if precipitins predominate in the offset well, and in the other if free antigen predominates (Deckers, 1967).

Applications of Special Technical Interest

As was mentioned before, there are many varieties of double diffusion test. Space limitations curtail the number that can be described or even

Antigen Predominates

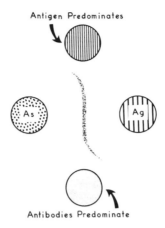

Antibodies Predominate

Fig. 4.18. Diagram depicting detection of antigen and antibody by precipitin band bending. If antigen predominates in a mixture of antigen and antiserum, for instance, then the tip of the precipitin band formed by reference antigen (Ag) and antiserum (As) will bend to enter the area between the antiserum reservoir and the test well (upper); but if antibodies predominate (lower), the band will bend in the opposite direction.

mentioned here. The following tests therefore are touched upon because they have some special application.

Precipitin reactions for the same antigen–antibody systems can be compared in different media by casting the media adjacent to each other and then cutting reactant wells astride their interface so that precipitation develops across them. Comparing gelatin and agar in this way revealed that gelatin strongly interferes with diffusion of some antigens and also suppresses antigen–antibody precipitation (Dudman, 1965b).

Reactants usually are applied to a gel mechanically; that is, a well is charged, or a reactant is deposited on the surface of the gel. But they also can be applied electrophoretically for such purposes as separating the reactant from substances in solution with it which may interfere with its precipitation, or placing it in the gel at a particular position or without marring the gel structure (Deckers, 1967). In this manner, serum antigens in hemolyzed serum were moved away from the hemoglobin. which tends to precipitate nonspecifically and confusingly in agar (Berg, 1964). Though obviously similar to immunoelectrophoresis, this technique nevertheless does not attempt to achieve significant separation of antigens from each other as is done in immunoelectrophoresis.

Double diffusion tests usually employ solutions of reactants prepared before the test. But the solution can be "prepared" during the test. For example, the antigen well can be charged with a thick suspension of bacteria from which soluble antigen will leach and then diffuse (Otto, 1960; Slaterus, 1961). Meningococci are readily typed this way (Slaterus, 1961). As in Elek's early tests of 1948 (see Fig. 4.19), toxigenic bacteria can be grown in immunodiffusion gel enriched with appropriate nutrients, used aseptically, and to which of course no antibacterial preservatives have been added. The species-specific exotoxin of pathogenic species of *Pseudomonas* can be identified by placing an antiserum-soaked strip of filter paper on nutrient agar on which the bacteria are being grown (Liu,

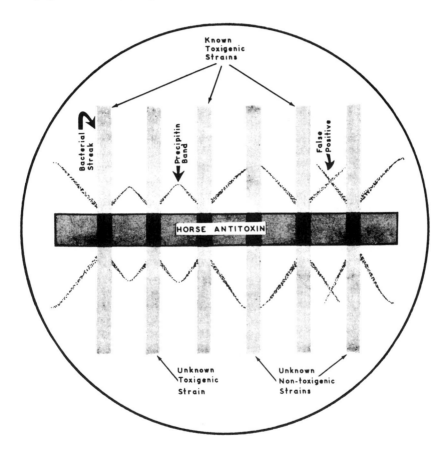

Petri Dish of Nutrient Agar

Fig. 4.19. Diagram showing how the diphtheria bacillus toxigenicity test is set up. Unknown toxigenic strain produces toxin which forms precipitin band with horse antitoxin fusing with similar band produced by known toxigenic reference strain. Nontoxigenic strain may produce precipitin band by exuding some other antigen, but this band crosses true toxin band produced by known reference strain.

1961b). Success in this kind of test depends partly on bacteriologic skills; peptone concentration in the medium, for instance, affects bacterial production of exotoxin (Maximescu and Saragea, 1964).

The Elek test, like most other immunodiffusion tests, also has been miniaturized (Liu, 1961c). An antiserum-impregnated strip of sterile filter paper is laid aseptically along the center of a sterile microscope slide, and this is overlaid with a thin layer of appropriate culture medium agar. After this has solidified, it is inoculated with spots of bacterial suspension at appropriate intervals and parallel to but offset from the embedded strip of paper. On incubation at appropriate temperature, the bacteria grow and produce antigens which diffuse into the gel and precipitate with antiserum diffusing meantime from the paper strip. After precipitation has developed satisfactorily, the microscope slide can be washed, stained, and dried as is done with other microimmunidiffusion tests to produce a permanent record of the test.

Intact mammalian cells and viruses have also been used in immunodiffusion tests. Lymph node cells taken from immunized mice were cultivated in a double diffusion tube test to detect their *in vitro* production of precipitins (Egdahl *et al.*, 1962). The presence and multiplication of viruses were observed directly in double diffusion tests by inoculating a well with mammalian cells and culture medium and allowing it to stand for 2 days, adding virus and waiting 4 to 9 days more for the virus to multiply in the mammalian cells and release its antigen, and then charging nearby wells with antiserum to the virus (Mata and Weller, 1962).

In most varieties of double diffusion test, reactants are detected directly by precipitation. But interference with precipitation of a reference antigen–antibody system (i.e., precipitation inhibition) by either kind of reactant is an alternative and generally underestimated technique for the same purpose but with advantages of improved sensitivity and a capacity to detect nonprecipitating reactants (see Chapter 7). In its simplest form, the presence of antigen or antibodies is signaled by inhibition of precipitation in a known reference antigen–antiserum system made by adding unknown to the opposing known reactant (e.g., adding unknown antigen to reference antiserum). The sensitivity of this test is maximized by employing only enough of each reference reactant to barely precipitate. Tumor-specific antigen was revealed in various specimens of tissue, for example, by placing tumor antigen in a central well, charging satellite wells with precipitins to this antigen, and then mixing extracts of the various tissues with these different deposits of antiserum (Gold and Freedman, 1965b). An extract found to contain this antigen could be further tested in serial dilutions by the same technique to determine its relative concentration of tumor antigen. Precipitation requires both reactants to be at least divalent (Chapter 1). But univalent reactants can be detected in an inhibition test by adding a solution of these to the appropriate one or another of a reference precipitating system (Malley *et al.*, 1964).

The effect of inhibition can be measured with some increase in sensitivity by observing its influence on the shape or location of a forming precipitin band (cf. Fig. 4.18). Thus, a well charged with unknown antigen solution is set next to an area in gel where the growing tip of a precipitate between a precipitating concentration of the same antigen and appropriate antiserum will approach it (Heiner and Rose, 1970b). The presence of a small amount of this antigen causes a specific, distinct bending in the tip of this band; if no antigen is present in this well, precipitin band growth will continue laterally along its normal course. This type of test has been useful for detecting bacterial endotoxin (Casman *et al.*, 1969). Sometimes the physical presence of a well to which the unknown specimen is added interferes mechanically with this type of test, giving false results (i.e., bending not due to the presence of specific reactant). This can be avoided by using a template instead of making wells in the gel, by electrophoresing the unknown into the vicinity of the partially formed reference precipitin band (Deckers and Abelev, 1963), or by adding a droplet of the unknown onto the surface of the gel after the reference precipitate has begun to form.

This precipitation–inhibition technique can increase the sensitivity of the double diffusion test as much as 200-fold (Deckers and Abelev, 1963). But it can also be deleterious in serial quantitations if wells containing dilutions of the reactant being measured are too near each other: a falsely high end point will be reached because of aid (i.e., inhibition) that reactant sufficing in one well to produce a precipitate may give to that present in an adjacent well in sub-precipitating quantity (Klontz *et al.*, 1962; Anderson *et al.*, 1962a). Occasionally, the opposite effect is seen; that is adjacency of a strong antiserum may obscure the precipitating capabilities of a weak antiserum (Anderson *et al.*, 1962).

Conventionally, determinant groups on a species of antigen are analyzed and enumerated in double diffusion tests by progressively degrading the antigen chemically and comparing the resulting products with the original antigen against an appropriate antiserum. But, determinant composition of related antigens can be compared and much can be learned about these determinants without degrading the antigens by measuring their relative reactivities at equal concentrations with several different antisera, such as by band position between antigen and antiserum in a double diffusion tube test. Since the position of the band in such a test depends on the total concentration of antibodies able to react with the antigen, differences in profile obtained for a given antigen analyzed with several antisera reflect differences in the number of antigenic determinants on different antigens able to react with corresponding antibodies (Finger and Heller, 1963). Presumably, similar differences also might be seen between two identical antigens in different states of polymerization, since, although identical in number and variety of determinants (providing none depended on tertiary or quaternary structure), the more polymerized antigen might have less determinants "exposed" for reaction with antibodies than the monomeric antigen.

In a classic comparative Ouchterlony test two antigens are compared with respect to an antiserum by placing the three reactants at the points of an imaginary triangle (cf. Fig. 4.5). Each antigen forms its own precipitin band with the common antiserum, and their interrelationships, if any, can be observed by noting how their respective precipitin bands affect each other as they grow across each other. But in this kind of test the antigens must diffuse rather far before, by their reacting with the antibodies, these interrelationships can be seen. Usually this is no problem because the antigens most often analyzed are small enough molecules to diffuse reasonably rapidly. However, viruses or portions of them, while diffusible, are too large to be compared readily by this technique. This problem was solved in comparing foot-and-mouth disease viruses by placing a mixture of the viruses to be compared in a single well and then charging another well with antiserum to one virus and a third well with antiserum to the other (Van Oss et al., 1964). The viruses had only a short distance to diffuse; each antiserum reacted only with antigen which it could recognize. The resulting precipitin bands therefore had the same meaning as they would have had in a classic Ouchterlony test. Although differences between the compared antigens noted in this type of test are most likely to be genuine, antibody response invariably also is being compared. Hence, some "differences" may reside more in the antisera because of differences in individual animal response to the same antigen, than in the compared antigens themselves. Hence, in using this technique one should use antisera produced under as nearly identical conditions as possible, and also use several antisera rather than just two.

Sensitivity of Double Diffusion Tests

The sensitivity of a given test depends on many factors including its own physical nature, the nature of the antigen, and the efficiency of the antiserum being used (Soothill, 1962; Graf and Rapport, 1965). Therefore, the following data are only suggestive.

Immunoelectrophoresis is frequently thought to be more sensitive than double diffusion tests because it usually reveals more precipitin arcs. However, its superiority is in resolution and not in sensitivity (Holland *et al.*, 1962; Dodin, 1963; Crowle and Lueker, 1962).

Macro tests appear to be the least and micro template tests the most sensitive of double diffusion tests, but this observation is true only on the basis of absolute quantities of reactants employed and relative capacities to detect larger numbers of antigen–antibody systems. These in turn are characteristics of antigen–antibody apposition: micro tests develop reactions with much smaller volumes of reactants than macro tests, but not with smaller concentrations of reactants; template tests reveal many more precipitating systems than macro or micro nontemplate tests only because they feed large quantities of reactants into very thin layers of gel where precipitates can build to the threshold of visibility, not because they are inherently more sensitive. Thus, if neither auxiliary means of revealing antigen–antibody reactions nor special concentrating techniques are used, the sensitivity of all varieties of double diffusion test appears to have a lower limit of about 1 μg of antigen per milliliter (Darcy, 1961; Krause and Raunio, 1967); but usually only one-tenth of this degree of sensitivity is achieved (Krause and Raunio, 1967; Heiner and Rose, 1970b; Soothill, 1962; Dudman, 1965a). Sensitivity for detecting antibody is about the same, 1 μg/ml (Silverstein *et al.*, 1963b).[10]

Before immunoelectrophoresis became widely used, double diffusion tests were primary tools for general qualitative analysis (see review by Wodehouse, 1956a). Because of the greater resolution and informativeness of immunoelectrophoresis for such analyses, double diffusion tests in more recent years have been reserved for more specialized tasks like critically comparing individual antigen–antibody systems, detecting very weak precipitating systems, or simple routine quantitations. Their use probably will become still less common as new developments in electro-immunodiffusion are more widely known and applied.

---

[10] By way of comparison, diphtheria antitoxin assay can detect 0.003 μg of antibody per milliliter; and passive hemagglutination, phage neutralization, and bacterial agglutination can detect 0.005 μg, 0.001 μg, and 0.01 μg/ml, respectively (Silverstein *et al.*, 1963).

Chapter 5

Immunoelectrophoresis

Single and double diffusion tests are unable to resolve more than a few coexisting antigen–antibody systems; although different antigen–antibody systems should precipitate in different planes of the reaction gel, there is not enough space in these tests for the planes to be physically separate. Immunoelectrophoresis partially circumvents this problem by separating many of the reactants (usually antigens) from each other laterally before they are exposed to immunoprecipitation. The essential happenings of immunoelectrophoresis are illustrated in Fig. 5.1.

Theory and Interpretation of Immunoelectrophoresis

Immunoelectrophoresis tests are interpreted in the same way as double and single diffusion tests, except for some novel effects connected with the preliminary electrophoresis. Most of the following discussion of these peculiarities of immunoelectrophoresis is based on information and ideas in several papers and reviews (Whipple, 1964; Schwick and Störiko, 1964; Ferri, 1961; Cawley, 1969; Ouchterlony, 1968; Girard, 1963; Ventruto *et al.*, 1963; Burtin and Grabar, 1967; Longsworth, 1967; Neuzil and Masseyeff, 1959; Wieme, 1959a).

General Characteristics

In a typical form of immunoelectrophoresis, a microscope slide is flooded with an even layer of agar gel in an appropriate buffer, and the ends of the gelled agar on the slide are connected with buffer vessels. A hole is punched in the agar and charged with antigen and, after electrophoresis, slots are cut parallel to the path of electrophoretic migration

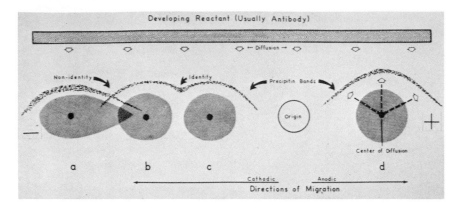

Fig. 5.1. Precipitin band patterns in immunoelectrophoresis have essentially the same meaning that they have in other double diffusion tests, except that the position and curvature of each depends largely on the electrophoretic characteristics of its electrophoresed reactant. Thus, the shape of a precipitin band reflects the shape of the spot formed by such a reactant under electrophoresis (*a* vs. *d*). The apex of a band indicates the hypothetical center of a fraction's diffusion (*d*). Two antigens which without electrophoresis might never form more than one precipitin band may be sufficiently different electrophoretically to separate and to form distinct precipitin bands, which show the relationship of the two fractions by fusing into a "gull-wing" (*b* and *c*).

on either side of it far enough away to permit development of precipitin arcs in the intervening agar. An antigen fraction usually has one of three shapes (Fig. 5.1): it is round or symmetrically ellipsoid, it is drawn out on either side of its center equally or unequally, or it assumes the shape of a comet with a trail either before or behind it (Hirschfeld, 1960a). Its shape controls the shape of the precipitin arc it will form with antibody diffusing against it. After antibody is placed in its trough (antigen sometimes also is used as the developing or indicator agent when antiserum is being studied by immunoelectrophoresis), it diffuses toward the path of electrophoresis as a straight front. Meanwhile, each fraction which has been electrophoresed expands radially by diffusion from its source, part of it moving toward the antibody as a curved front corresponding to the original curvature of the spot of electrophoresed antigen. Thus, if the final shape of the antigen spot is round, it presents a semicircular front; if it has the form of a symmetrical ellipse, its front will be symmetrically ellipsoid. An antigen spot that is asymmetrical will present a corresponding asymmetrical curved front. The acuteness of curvature also depends largely on the relative diffusion rates of antigen and antibody (in turn depending on their respective concentrations and molecular weights), for if the antigen does not diffuse very rapidly from its origin by comparison with the rate of antibody diffusion, the precipitin arc it forms will curve around it more acutely than if opposite conditions prevail. A long arc of only moderate curvature suggests that it has been formed by an antigen which electrophoretically is heterogeneous and consists of a population of molecules with smoothly graduated differences in electrophoretic mobility. This happening is typified by serum γ-globulin, which forms an elongated curve stretching evenly and thinly as far as the α-globulin area at its anodic end but curving suddenly inward at its cathodic end (Grabar, 1955c). Most γ-globulin molecules, then, have mobilities familiarly observed for γ-globulin on paper electrophoresis; but others, although serologically similar, have mobilities sometimes as great as those of the α-globulins.

There are antigens which by double diffusion tests produce only a single precipitin band but which on immunoelectrophoresis divide into two distinctly different fractions. If these have remained close enough during electrophoresis, each forms its own arc, but the tips of these arcs fuse to form the so-called "gull-wing" pattern (Crowle, 1960b; Fig. 5.1).

Electrophoresis in Immunoelectrophoresis

The form and location of precipitin arcs in immunoelectropherograms are determined by two predominating factors—electrophoretic migration of the reactants, and their later diffusion and immunologic interaction. The general nature of electrophoresis and its use in various kinds of immunodiffusion test were explained in Chapter 1. The following paragraphs expand on this information with a discussion of some aspects of electrophoresis more specifically related to the development of immunoelectropherograms and to their interpretation (cf. Fine, 1968).

THE ELECTROLYTE

The pH of the buffer determines the direction of reactant movement: reactants with isoelectric point above the pH of the buffer tend to move toward the cathode, those with lower isoelectric point are repelled by the cathode, and those with the same isoelectric point as the pH of the buffer remain electrophoretically immobile. This knowledge can be employed, along with empirical learning, to formulate buffers for optimal resolution of given antigen mixtures.

Barbital buffers of pH 8.2 to 8.6 are the most often employed for immunoelectrophoresis of serum antigens because long experience has proved them generally to be superior to buffers of other composition or pH. However, appropriate alterations in buffer composition may improve on their performance. Immunoelectrophoretic resolution of human serum antigens is aided by adding calcium lactate to the formula. Human serum α_2-globulins are especially well resolved with a discontinuous buffer system, in which the composition of buffer in one electrode vessel differs from that in the other (Hirschfeld, 1960b). Rat serum α_1-globulins were resolved increasingly well from albumin by increasing pH and ionic strength of the buffer, optimal composition being pH 9.0 and molarity 0.05 (Escribano, 1962). Faster and better separations of human hemoglobins are obtained at pH 8.8 with a discontinuous buffer (Heller et al., 1962).

Resolution of antigen mixtures different from human serum is best effected with buffers matched to their tasks. Acid buffers are not uncommon. For the pineapple enzyme bromelin, a pH of 5.5 was used (Cawley et al., 1966). To resolve streptococcal antigens which could not be distinguished at more neutral pH, electrophoresis was performed at pH 5.3 in acetate buffer. The problems associated with subsequently performing immunodiffusion reactions at a pH this low were avoided by soaking the electropherogram for 30 minutes in a physiologic buffer before adding antiserum (Wahl et al., 1965). Hemoglobin was separated from other erythrocyte lysate antigens by immunoelectrophoresing it at pH 6.4 in citrate buffer (Rachmilewitz et al., 1963). An eye lens enzyme which decomposes at alkaline pH was stabilized and detected at a mildly acid pH (Rathbun et al., 1967). Antisera to *Pasteurella pestis* were studied at pH 6 (McNeill and Meyer, 1965), microbial extracts at pH 7 or 7.4 (Wright and Lockhart, 1965; Wehmeyer, 1965), and human precipitins to DNA at pH 7.6 (Atchley, 1961). The marked electroosmosis which occurs in agar gel at pH 7.2 was employed for improved resolution of milkweed bug hemolymph (Terando and Feir, 1967).

Buffers more alkaline than pH 8.6 also are employed. For instance, glycolic acid mixtures of pH 9.5 and 10.5 were used to immunoelectrophorese streptococcal antigens by the stepwise electrophoresis–electropherogram soaking–precipitation sequence mentioned above (Wahl et al., 1965).

Buffer pH alters during immunoelectrophoresis in proportion to the intensity and length of electrophoresis (Jouannet, 1968). This ordinarily undesirable effect is minimized mechanically by using continually renewed buffer, large volumes of buffer, and baffles in the electrode vessels, and by reversing electrode polarity for each electrophoretic run. It is suppressed in addition by composing the buffer with constituents providing maximum pH stabilization, and using these at the highest concentrations compatible with an acceptable speed of electrophoretic migration and heating of the electrophoresis medium (Jouannet, 1968). Using a poorly ionizing buffer like tris favors achieving maximum electrophoretic migration with minimum practical conductivity (Fredrick, 1964). On the other hand, a physically "ideal" buffer such as this may not resolve antigens as well as another. For instance, the relative mobilities of albumin and α_1-globulins in rat serum were changed, and they could be separated from each other by using a buffer of increased ionic strength and pH (Escribano, 1962). Interestingly, this study showed the α_1-globulins all to retain the same relative mobilities among themselves during these changes in buffer. By contrast, using a low ionic strength improved corneal antigen resolution by decreasing the solubilities, and therefore mobilities, of some antigens (Kawerau and Ott, 1961). Incidentally, the electrical conductivity of a buffer is affected by temperature as much as electrolyte concentration; it is an exponential function of temperature (Wunderly, 1960). Consequently, for greatest reproducibility electrophoresis should be done at a single standard temperature.

What may seem to be improved antigen resolution resulting from a change in pH may instead sometimes be an effect of changing electrolyte solutes. Such changes could act by providing either better electrophoretic resolution or better immunoprecipitation. Since both of these reasons for improvement are only partially understood, they are best explained by example.

Using lactate in barbital buffer for sharper electrophoretic resolution of human serum globulins has been mentioned (Hirschfeld, 1960d; Nerstrøm, 1963a; Hirschfeld, 1962; Cleve and Bearn, 1961). Both barbital and phosphate buffers excelled over tris at pH 7.4 for resolving salmon serum antigens (Krauel and Ridgway, 1963). At equivalent pH values and molarities, barbital and carbonate buffers both distinguished between albumin and α_1-globulins of rat serum better than borate buffer (Escribano, 1962). On the other hand, eye lens antigen resolution was so much better with a combination of tris, EDTA, and borate that this combination was referred to as a "high-resolution buffer" (Zwaan, 1963). Differences like these among buffers in achieving good electrophoretic separations are conditioned partly by the type of medium in which they are being used. For example, because borate ions complex with polysaccharides, a borate buffer may suffer as much as a fivefold loss of conductivity when used in agar, which is, of course, a complex polysaccharide (Escribano, 1962).

The potential effects of immunoelectrophoresis buffers on the immunoprecipitation portion of immunoelectrophoresis are most evident in extremes of pH which may cause spontaneous antigen precipitation on the acid side, or prevent specific antigen–antibody precipitation in the alkaline range (see Chapter 1). Hence, the pH of an electropherogram may have to be adjusted up or down before it is exposed to antiserum

(Wahl *et al.*, 1965). But there are also more subtle effects. For instance, better precipitation usually develops with barbital-containing buffers in immunodiffusion analyses of serum antigens than in phosphate buffers (Krauel and Ridgway, 1963). On the other hand, this usual superiority of barbital over phosphate buffers may fail for some serum antigens. Thus, human precipitins to human serum low-density lipoprotein were demonstrable with phosphate but not with barbital buffer (Berg, 1965b).

The superiority of certain buffers may derive from effects that the additives to them may have on the antigens being analyzed. One such effect is chelation. For instance, copper-containing ceruloplasmin produces only one precipitin arc in immunoelectrophoresis with nonchelating buffers, but in a borate–tris–EDTA buffer it develops two (Kasper and Deutsch, 1963; cf. also Poulik, 1963a). This is a direct effect of chelators on antigen. By a less direct effect of chelating Ca^{++} ions, EDTA-containing buffer drastically alters the mobilities of human serum complement components (Peetoom *et al.*, 1964; Mardiney and Müller-Eberhard, 1965). This may explain why calcium lactate–barbital buffer permits so fine a distinction among complement components as detection of the nonfunctional esterase inhibitor diagnostic of hereditary angioneurotic edema (Rosen *et al.*, 1965). Direct and indirect effects may function jointly to improve immunoelectrophoretic resolution of casein fractions in mammalian milks when a supplement of 10 mM EDTA is added to barbital buffer (Lyster *et al.*, 1966).

Immunoelectrophoresis buffers may include additives for other specific functions like protecting labile antigens or achieving and maintaining solution of antigens. Mercaptoethanol was added at 0.01 M to 0.05 M tris phosphate buffer, pH 7.5, to study the effects of univalent cations on structurally labile pyruvic kinase (Sorger *et al.*, 1965). IgA myeloma protein was electrophoresed in starch gel with a buffer containing 8 M urea (Osterland and Chaplin, 1966). The electropherogram had to be washed for 90 minutes in tap water before being embedded in agar gel for the immunodiffusion step of two-step immunoelectrophoresis. Detergents like deoxycholate, used at 0.3%, help to solubilize cell mitochondrial antigens and increase their immunoelectrophoretic mobility and separation (D'Amelio *et al.*, 1963a). Reducing agents like cysteine minimize spontaneous interaction between antigens (Zwaan, 1963).

THE MEDIUM

Some general effects that changes in the medium used for immunoelectrophoresis can have on the results of this technique have been discussed in Chapters 1 and 2. They are discussed more explicitly in the following paragraphs.

Electroosmosis is an effect most evident in various agars. It is greatest in those that are the least pure (see Table 5.1) and is due principally to the agaropectin constituent of agar. Electroosmosis usually is a nuisance, but sometimes it helps by increasing immunoelectrophoretic resolution. Indeed, it is essential for certain electroimmunodiffusion tests (see Chapter 6). Interestingly, resolution of antigens moving in the direction of electroosmosis (i.e., toward the cathode) is less than that of antigens moving against it (Hase, 1964). By comparison with agar, agarose gels exhibit only modest electroosmosis. Hence, although immunoelectrophoretic patterns of serum in agarose resemble those in agar, all antigens are shifted farther toward the anode relative to the origin (Masseyeff and Josselin, 1965). Other media that are used for immunoelectrophoresis, like polyacrylamide, cellulose acetate, starch, and gelatin, do not develop electroosmosis (Crowle, 1961). On the other hand, some of these, including polyacrylamide, starch, and gelatin, do achieve molecular sieving (see Chapter 1), the degree of which depends on their characteristics and concentrations.[1] This property is useful in immunoelectrophoresis for selecting and identifying antigens and antibodies.

Agar and gelatin interact with certain kinds of antigens, sometimes thereby improving immunoelectrophoretic resolution, and sometimes interfering with it by preventing antigen migration or altering the migra-

TABLE 5.1

POSITION OF ORIGINS IN RESPECT TO HUMAN SERUM COMPONENTS AFTER THEIR
ELECTROPHORESIS IN DIFFERENT AGAR PREPARATIONS[a]

Experimenter	Agar	Origin	pH
Wieme	Difco special agar-Noble	Between α_2 and β_1	8.4
Wieme	Behring Rein-agar	At β_1	8.4
Wieme	Difco Bacto-agar	At α_2	8.4
Crowle	Difco Bacto-agar	At α_2	8.2
Crowle	Deionized Difco Bacto-agar	Between β_2 and γ	8.2
Williams and Grabar	Washed Difco Bacto-agar	At β_1	8.2

[a] These data obtained from the following sources: Wieme (1959a); Crowle (1956); Crowle and Lueker (unpublished); Williams and Grabar (1955a).

[1] Although not sieving in a conventional sense, agar gels used at ordinary concentrations may seem to impede free migration of some macromolecules. For example, taking the migration rate of serum albumin in 1% Nobel agar as equivalent to a value of 100, this rate was 180 in 0.75% agar but only 60 in 2% agar under otherwise similar conditions (Jordan and White, 1965). This effect probably is due to increased electroosmostic flow with increased agar concentration rather than to true sieving (Bennett and Boursnell, 1962).

tion into abnormal configurations. Agar, for instance, interacts with basic proteins, lipoproteins, and IgM globulin (Süllmann, 1964). Gelatin reacts with polysaccharide antigens (see Chapter 2). The effects of such interactions on the appearance of an immunoelectropherogram will be elongated, often asymmetrical antigen–antibody precipitation (see Fig. 5.2; Süllmann, 1964).

THE SAMPLE

The nature of the sample and the way in which it is applied to the medium at the beginning of electrophoresis both affect development of immunoelectropherograms (Jouannet, 1968). Ideally, sample antigens should be completely dissolved and dissociated from each other; they should migrate out of their origin into the electrophoresis medium uniformly across the width of the origin and with no change in rate; and two identical samples should migrate the same in two different immunoelectropherograms (Schumacher et al., 1965). The first objective is best achieved by working with dissolved, nonassociating antigens, or by adding to the antigen solution detergents or other agents that preserve association-prone antigens in their dissociated state (see Chapters 1 and 2; Zwaan, 1963). The second is attained by avoiding any physical differences between the origin and the surrounding medium (Wieme, 1959a). Thus, ideally the antigen solution should have been dialyzed against the buffer to be used in the medium, and physical distinction between the origin and the medium should be avoided either by diffusing the sample of antigen into the medium, or by mixing sample and medium itself and casting this mixture in the origin well. The origin of the sample on each of several electropherograms which are to be compared should be in the same position between cathode and anode. Often, ideal application of the sample is impractical; the possible consequences of such deviation will be discussed briefly so that they can be recognized.

The result of not dialyzing the sample solution against electrophoresis

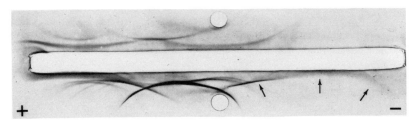

Fig. 5.2. Immunoelectropherogram of human saliva (upper) and tears (lower) developed with rabbit antiserum to tears and showing in particular the elongated cathodic arc of precipitate formed by lysozyme (courtesy G. J. Revis).

buffer is illustrated in Fig. 5.3, which also illustrates the importance of sample origin shape. The "bat-wing" pattern in the upper electropherogram in this figure developed because the ionic strength of the sample was higher at the beginning of electrophoresis than the ionic strength of the electrophoresis buffer. As this began to equilibrate with the surrounding medium, sample ionic strength dropped faster at the edges of the origin than in the middle. This caused antigens to migrate away more rapidly peripherally than centrally. This effect was suppressed somewhat by using a round hole instead of a slot, as well as by using less sample. Note that antigens have migrated farther in the same time from the hole than from the slot because sample ionic strength in the hole equilibrated sooner with the electrophoresis buffer. The effects shown directly in Fig. 5.3 would also be evident, but more confusingly, in aberrant arc formation in immunoelectropherograms.

If the sample is not to be dialyzed against the electrophoresis buffer (e.g., because only a minute volume is available), bat-wing development can be minimized by using a small sample and letting this equilibrate with the surrounding gel for a few minutes before beginning electrophoresis. However, protracting equilibration for more than 30 minutes may dilute some weaker antigens in a mixture by diffusion so much that later they are not detectable (Jordan and White, 1965).

The faster migration of serum antigens away from a more cathodic

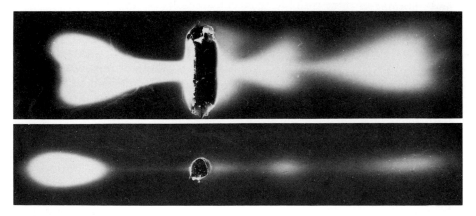

Fig. 5.3. Photographs comparing effects of origin shape on electrophoresis of undiluted, undialyzed human serum in agar. Irregular ("bat-wing") shape of fractions in slide with slot origin (top) apparently is due to the influence of serum electrolytes on current carried in unequal quantities through the origin at the beginning of electrophoresis. Circular origin is less affected because quantities of salts at its lateral edges are relatively small; excess electrolyte in center merely causes elongation of fractions into "tear-drop" shape. Electrophoresis above was carried out in BBL laboratory agar.

than anodic origin, and their progressive slowing as they move farther away from the cathode, are both familiar to most users of zone electrophoresis and immunoelectrophoresis. Presumably, they are due to a drop of voltage along the length of the electropherogram, although electroosmosis also may be involved (Hermans *et al.*, 1960). These effects are accentuated in long electropherograms, or in shorter ones connected in series (Reinskou, 1966b). To avoid them, short electropherograms arranged in parallel should be used (Ornstein, 1964). However, long electropherograms may have to be used to separate antigens migrating very close together (Reinskou, 1963, 1964; Grumbach and Kaplan, 1962).

OTHER FACTORS INFLUENCING ELECTROPHORESIS IN IMMUNOELECTROPHORESIS

Antigens affect each others' migrations; mixed with others, a given antigen may migrate differently than it would electrophoresed alone. For example, the presence of albumin in serum affects the position of other antigens, especially of α_1-globulins in the albumin area, by altering pH, conductivity, field strength, and ionic composition locally (Raymond and Nakamichi, 1962b). Albumin can affect its own migration rate, for it tends to migrate faster when it is dilute than when it is concentrated (Depieds *et al.*, 1963; Russell, 1966). Serum β_1 lipoprotein, IgM globulin, and fibrinogen also exhibit concentration-dependent electrophoretic mobility but probably for the different reason of concentration-dependent changes in interaction with agar (Dencker and Swahn, 1961; Süllmann, 1964; Berglund, 1962a; Russell, 1966; Zwaan, 1963; Seligmann and Marder, 1965). The immunoelectrophoretic mobilities of prealbumin and γ-globulins in normal mouse serum are concentration-dependent (Sassen *et al.*, 1963). Serum α and β lipoproteins change mobility by reacting with each other in different degrees determined by their relative concentrations (Beaumont *et al.*, 1965; Levy and Fredrickson, 1965).

Electrophoretically different antigens in mixtures frequently exist as complexes (Zwaan, 1963; Aurand *et al.*, 1963; Roche *et al.*, 1965); or an antigen may be attached to some nonantigen with a different electrophoretic mobility (Grieble *et al.*, 1965; Hannouz, 1965). The results observed from the presence of complexes depend on the relative mobilities of the complexed molecules (Korngold, 1963a), their stability, and the voltage of electrophoresis (high voltage tends to dissociate weak complexes: Lawrence and Melnick, 1961; Roche *et al.*, 1965; the effect being proportional to the square of the voltage gradient: Ornstein, 1964). Effects may range from subtle differences in electrophoretic mobility at different voltages, through larger differences—the development of gull-wing precipitates, precipitates with multiple apexes, skewed precipitates, long uncurved lines of precipitate (Seligmann, 1959), or arcs of precipitate at opposite ends of the immunoelectropherogram joined in between by a long band (Nielsen *et al.*, 1963; Clausen *et al.*, 1963; Parker and Bearn, 1962; Lawrence and Melnick, 1961; Hadden and Prout, 1964; Patterson, *et al.*, 1964; Beaumont *et al.*, 1965).[2] Two or more isomers of one antigen may exist in a mixture of antigens (Beckman *et al.*, 1961; Atchley *et al.*, 1962; Boffa *et al.*, 1967; Brummerstedt-Hansen, 1962).[3] The proportions of one to the other, which may vary according to their chemical or biological states (Fine *et al.*, 1962b; Poulik, 1963a; Peetoom *et al.*, 1964; Anzai *et al.*, 1965; Yagi *et al.*, 1962), the age of the antigen mixture (Crowle, 1961), or the characteristics of their source (Dencker, 1963; Aurand *et al.*, 1963; MacPherson and Saffran, 1965),[4] will determine which predominates, even to the occasional extent of suggesting that an antigen has changed its electrophoretic mobility (Zimmer, 1960; Dencker and Swahn, 1961).

The length and strength of electrophoresis must be selected for unknown mixtures from preliminary trials lest fast-migrating antigens be lost off the electropherogram. Some antigens move very rapidly: a toxin from *Naja nigricollis* venom, for instance, has six times the mobility of human serum albumin (Jouannet, 1968).

Because so many factors affect the characteristics of electrophoresis in immunoelectrophoresis, greatest consistency from run to run will be obtained by using one or more internal controls on the extent of electrophoretic migration for each run (see Techniques section).

Immunodiffusion

Electrophoretically separated constituents are detected after electrophoresis in immunoelectrophoresis by single and double diffusion reac-

---

[2] As a rather extraordinary example, IgA-globulin has been observed to associate with albumin, haptoglobin, β lipoprotein, α_1 glycoprotein, and even itself (Glueck and Hong, 1965; Creyssel and Richard, 1966; Beaumont *et al.*, 1965). Serum IgG-globulin, by contrast, does not associate with other serum proteins (Glueck and Hong, 1965).

[3] Many serum polymorphisms are known, including those of pre-albumin, a "variable" α-globulin, amylase, α_{2M}-globulin, ceruloplasmin, haptoglobin, and transferrin (Brummerstedt-Hansen, 1967).

[4] Serum albumin and IgM-globulin may develop long, asymmetrical precipitin arcs in carelessly prepared serum samples because they complex with platelets and platelet constituents (Seligmann, 1961).

tions interpreted like those described in Chapters 3 and 4. However, there are some novel aspects to these reactions due to lateral electrophoretic spreading of reactants before immunoprecipitation develops. These will be explained in the following paragraphs.

PRECIPITIN ARC FORMATION AND CHARACTERISTICS

Most varieties of immunoelectrophoresis are double diffusion tests: after the antigens in a mixture are electrophoresed laterally, they are precipitated by a long front of antiserum diffusing from a trough parallel to but offset a few millimeters from the path of antigen electrophoretic migration (cf. Fig. 5.1). These events have been described mathematically (Aladjem et al., 1962). The precipitin arc for any single antigen in the mixture develops like the precipitin arc of any single antigen in a mixture tested in a double diffusion plate. The same factors govern such characteristics of precipitation as band sharpness or fuzziness and movement or stability. Liesegang and temperature artifacts can develop in immunoelectropherograms just as in single and double diffusion tests (Crowle, 1963; Lueker and Crowle, 1963; Griffiths et al., 1965; Seligmann, 1961; Betsuyaku et al., 1964). As in double diffusion tests, precipitin arcs are sharpest and best defined with H-type antiserum, but such arcs also are less stable in reactant excess than arcs formed by R-type antiserum (Ursing, 1965; D'Amelio et al., 1963a, see Fig. 5.4).

However, because the source of antiserum is a long trough instead of a well, all precipitin arcs curve toward the antigen. Estimating antigen molecular weight therefore is difficult in immunoelectrophoresis. In general, arcs formed by high-molecular-weight antigens tend to develop nearer the path of electrophoresis than arcs formed by low-molecular-weight antigens, but antigen concentration, antigen interaction with the medium, and medium concentration are equally important in determining arc position (Ursing, 1965; Seligmann, 1959). Arc shape in immunoelectropherograms is more informatively an indicator of the electrophoretic characteristics of an antigen, as illustrated in Fig. 5.5.

In development of a double diffusion test, all antigens in a mixture are diffusing into the reaction area where they can affect each others' precipitation by antibodies specifically or nonspecifically (see Chapter 1); but in development of an immunoelectropherogram they are separated from each other and therefore cannot interact. Thus, two antigens which share determinants but are electrophoretically different might form only one precipitin band in a double diffusion test but could form two in immunoelectrophoresis. The protein concentration in a mixture of antigens nonspecifically may aid precipitation of a particular antigen in a double diffusion test, but it could not in immunoelectrophoresis. This

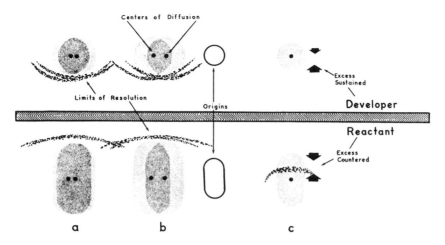

Fig. 5.4. Sensitivity and resolution in an immunoelectrophoresis test depend partially upon origin shape. More reactant to be electrophoresed can be used in an oblong origin than in a circular one of the same diameter, so that while indicator reactant excess may preclude precipitin band formation by a weak fraction originating from a circular origin, it might not if an oblong origin were employed (*c*). On the other hand, resolution obtained with a circular origin probably is superior to that obtained with the oblong origin, because the former offers more acute curvature of precipitin bands (*a* and *b*). Immunoelectrophoresis provides fraction resolution far better than that obtainable with other forms of electrophoresis, because the centers of closely overlapping fractions can be distinguished with the aid of their individual precipitin arcs. By its curvature, each arc clearly points to a small hypothetical center of diffusion for its electrophoresed reactant.

latter distinction is common in reversed immunoelectrophoresis, in which antiserum is electrophoresed instead of antigen (see below).

RESOLUTION

Distinction among different antigens in immunoelectrophoresis depends both on their electrophoretic resolution and on certain aspects of their precipitation by antiserum. Reasons for the better resolution of immunoelectrophoresis than zone electrophoresis, and for the superiority of small antigen mixture origins, are illustrated in Fig. 5.4. Best resolution in the immunodiffusion step of immunoelectrophoresis usually is obtained by reacting antiserum with the antigens as soon as possible— that is, by electrophoresing at maximum speed and applying antiserum soon after electrophoresis (Ornstein, 1964; Jordan and White, 1965; Zwaan, 1963). But there are exceptions. Some weaker antigens are resolved better if antiserum is not applied until 15 to 30 minutes after ceasing electrophoresis (Jordan and White, 1965). The paradox com-

1 Prealbumin

2 Albumin

3 Acid α_1 Glycoprotein

4 α_{-1} Lipoprotein

5 α_{-1} Antitrypsin

6 α_{-1x} Glycoprotein

7 Gc Globulin (1-1)

8 Ceruloplasmin

9 Haptoglobin (1-1)

10 α_2 - Macroglobulin

11 α_2 - Lipoprotein

12 Hemopexin

13 Transferrin

14 β_{1c} - Globulin

15 IgA

16 IgM

17 IgG

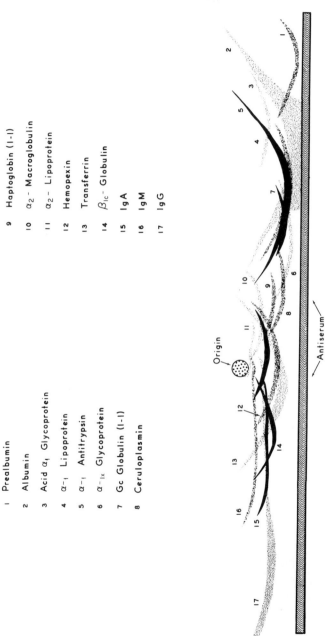

Fig. 5.5. Diagram showing locations of the more prominent antigens of normal human serum in agar gel immunoelectrophoresis. The cathode is to the left. (Adapted from a diagram published by Schwick and Störiko, 1964.)

plicating this principle is that, if electrophoresis is short enough to prevent undue diffusion of adjacent antigens, they may not have separated sufficiently from each other electrophoretically, but if electrophoresis is prolonged, they will not be distinguishable because of intermixing by diffusion (Jouannet, 1968). Solutions to this paradox include using buffers of different formulations (see above, and Gräsbeck *et al.*, 1963), using diffusion-restricting media or medium additives (Korngold, 1963b; Poulik, 1964), using a series of wells for antiserum instead of a trough (Kaminski and Gajos, 1962), employing different concentrations of antigens (Goetinck and Pierce, 1966; Seligmann, 1961; Betsuyaku *et al.*, 1964), or employing electroimmunodiffusion (see Chapter 6).

Despite electrophoresis, several antigens in a mixture such as serum α_2-globulins still may be together in one area at the beginning of immunodiffusion. Clearest resolution of these is achieved as in double diffusion plates, by using a strong antiserum or lots of it (as from a template, Fig. 5.6: Crowle and Lueker, 1962), by prolonging development, and by using an H-type antiserum. Some auxiliary means for increasing resolution were described in Chapter 2.

SINGLE DIFFUSION IMMUNOELECTROPHORESIS

This undeservedly overlooked technique, also called "direct immunoelectrophoresis," is related to conventional immunoelectrophoresis as single radial diffusion plate tests are related to double diffusion plate tests (Wilson, 1964). Antigens are electrophoresed and then reacted with antiserum infused uniformly into the medium around them. Typical results are illustrated diagrammatically in Figs. 5.7 and 5.8. Developed especially to make immunoelectrophoresis quantitative (Afonso, 1964b, 1966a,b), this technique is also capable of providing qualitative information on diffusion coefficients, electrophoretic characteristics, and the effects of antigen interactions on each other (Córdoba *et al.*, 1966; see Yokoyama and Carr, 1962, for a two-dimensional technique). It avoids the notoriously poor resolution of single diffusion tests for mixtures of antigens. With polyvalent antiserum it can quantitate different antigens simultaneously in one test.

Little research has been done on theoretical aspects of this interesting and esthetically pleasing technique. Its use and interpretation probably can be predicted on combined background knowledge from single diffusion tests and double diffusion immunoelectrophoresis. However, this combined information might not predict effects that nonantibody antiserum components might have in possibly complexing with electrophoretically purified antigens during or before immunoprecipitation and thus altering their physical and immunological properties.

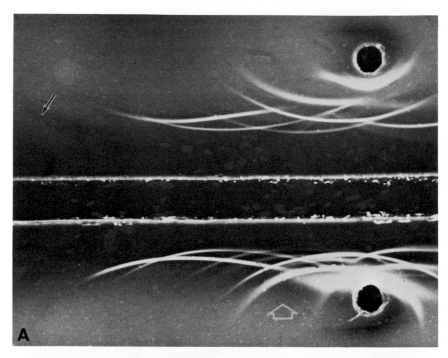

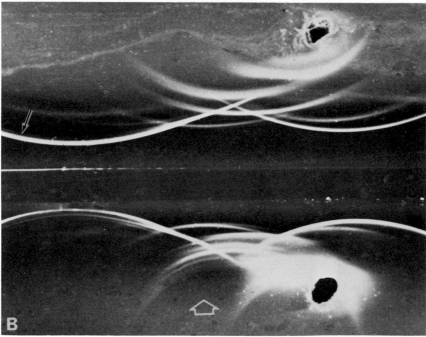

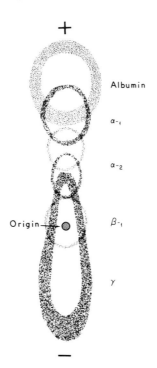

+

Albumin

$\alpha\text{-}_1$

$\alpha\text{-}_2$

Origin

$\beta\text{-}_1$

γ

—

Fig. 5.7. Diagram of results from single diffusion immunoelectrophoresis of normal human serum. (Redrawn from Yokoyama and Carr, 1962).

Reversed Immunoelectrophoresis

Usually in immunoelectrophoresis antigens are electrophoresed and then detected with antiserum. But in reversed immunoelectrophoresis the antibodies of an antiserum are electrophoresed and then are detected with antigen. The goal generally is to identify electrophoretically the precipitating types of immunoglobulin (Kuwert and Niedieck, 1965; Paluska, 1963; Da Silva and Ferri, 1965b; Krywienczyk, 1962; Burstein, 1969; Cline, 1967).

Reversed immunoelectrophoresis is more difficult than conventional immunoelectrophoresis for several reasons. Its resolution is poorer because most precipitins are closely related γ_1- and γ_2-globulins, and be-

---

Fig. 5.6. Contrast in capabilities of nontemplate (*A*) and template (*B*) immunoelectrophoresis techniques for detecting minor antigens in a mixture. The latter revealed nine antigen arcs in the α_2-globulin region (large arrow), where the former detected only five. Excess albumin in the nontemplate slide prevented formation of a visible precipitate (see small arrow; horse antiserum was being used), but the volume of antiserum delivered by the template was sufficient to avoid this problem.

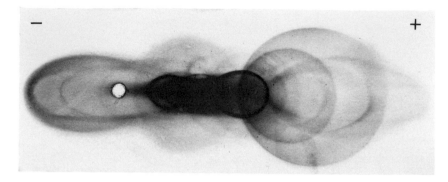

Fig. 5.8. An example of single diffusion immunoelectrophoresis in which human serum was electrophoresed on a microscope slide of 0.75% agarose in pH 8.2 barbital buffer of ionic strength 0.025 and then was precipitated with rabbit antiserum applied undiluted for 10 minutes by the method shown in Fig. 2.6. Prominent components from cathode to anode are IgG, transferrin, α_1-antitrypsin, albumin, and at the extreme anodic end of the pattern an elongated loop of α_1-lipoprotein.

cause individual types of precipitins tend to be electrophoretically heterogeneous. Occasionally precipitins are found in anodic areas of an immunoelectropherogram, but because some immunoglobulins complex readily with various other serum constituents and may owe their anodic mobility to these (see above), proving that a precipitin has nongamma mobility is complicated. Since detecting two different species of antibodies against the same antigen depends on availability of antigen to both for precipitation, if one diffuses faster than the other, the slower one may go undetected. This is a lesser problem in single diffusion-type reversed immunoelectrophoresis, since antigen is applied to the top of the electropherogram; it is insignificant for the same reason in reversed radioimmunoelectrophoresis (Samloff and Barnett, 1967; cf. Chapter 7).

Antigen–antibody precipitation does not develop as well in reversed as in conventional immunoelectrophoresis. One reason is that precipitation is poor or absent in antigen excess, which is frequently present in this technique (Raynaud *et al.*, 1965). This is because the developing reactant, antigen, usually is applied in a trough as a large volume, whereas only a small volume of antiserum can be used. Solutions to this adversity include using concentrated antiserum (da Silva and Ferri, 1965b), a slot origin instead of a hole, dilute antigen, or antigen applied in a series of wells parallel to the path of electrophoresis rather than in a trough (Cline, 1967).

Another prominent problem of reversed immunoelectrophoresis is that antibodies are electrophoresed away from other antiserum constituents which directly or indirectly can aid the antibodies to precipitate antigen (Cline, 1967). These accessory constituents may be cofactors like complement or low-avidity antibodies which stabilize and enlarge a forming antigen–antibody lattice, or substances like serum albumin which protect against the solubilizing effects that some antigens have on these lattices even as they are forming them. This problem is overcome by restoring the missing constituents by mixing normal serum with the antigen in its trough, by infusing normal serum into the reaction area at the same time that antigen is diffusing into it, or by using substitutes for whole serum similarly (Cline, 1967).

Immunoelectrophoresis Techniques

In immunoelectrophoresis a mixture of antigens is electrophoresed in suitable semisolid medium, usually agar or agarose, and then detected by precipitation with antiserum diffusing from a trough laid parallel to the path of electrophoresis (Lawrence, 1964). Originally, immunoelectrophoresis was performed on large glass plates. But such macro techniques are wasteful, their sensitivity and resolution are not better than and usually are inferior to those of microvariations, and processing for staining and preservation of macro immunoelectropherograms is slow and cumbersome. Consequently, the macro method (see Grabar, 1960) will not be described here.

Microimmunoelectrophoresis

The method originally described by Scheidegger (1955) was so good as to have undergone little change. The following current variation is nearly as easy to use as a micro double diffusion plate test.

Pipet an even layer of 1% agarose in pH 8.2 to 8.6 buffer of ionic strength 0.025 to 0.05 onto a microscope slide, previously coated with 0.2% agarose in distilled water as described in Chapter 2.[5] After this has gelled and the gel has hardened for a few minutes at 4°C, punch a well out of the gel about one fourth of the distance across the length of the slide and in its middle plane.[6] Charge this with antigen solution in the same way as in a non-template micro double diffusion plate test. Invert

[5] Better resolution is obtained in agar electrophoresis and immunoelectrophoresis if the support slide is silicone-treated (e.g., with Siliclad, or by polishing with a silicone-base stopcock grease) instead of agar-coated (Crowle and Lueker, unpublished work). But the gel on such a slide will tend to float off it during later washing and staining procedures.

[6] In inert media like agarose, polyacrylamide, and cellulose acetate, cationic antigens migrate as freely as those that are anionic. Detecting both is more certain if two origins are used at both cathodic and anodic ends of the slide, placed so that their respective paths of electrophoresis will be equidistant on opposite sides of the antiserum trough subsequently to be cut between them (Stephen, 1961).

the slide and place it on the electrophoresis apparatus with its origin nearest the cathode (see Fig. 5.9). Electrophorese it at 8 to 10 volts/cm of gel in a humidified atmosphere at 4°C for about 1 hour (e.g., to allow serum albumin to migrate 2.5 to 3.0 cm). Remove the slide from the electrophoresis apparatus, and cut 1- to 2-mm-wide troughs on either side of the plane of the electrophoretic separation, preferably at different distances such as 3 and 5 mm to detect a wider range of antigens, and charge these with antiserum. Keep the slide in a humid atmosphere for 24 to 48 hours at 4°C for the immunodiffusion pattern to develop. Observe and/or photograph the pattern; wash and stain the slide for permanent preservation.

Electrophoresis apparatus designed expressly for immunoelectrophoresis tests can be purchased; it can be adapted from paper or zone electrophoresis equipment; or it can be assembled from readily available apparatus by the investigator. There are many designs (cf. Zydeck *et al.,* 1965b; Barrett *et al.,* 1963; Uriel, 1966), but basically the apparatus need be no more than two electrode vessels each with sponge contacts as shown in Figs. 5.9, 5.10, and 1.12.

TECHNICAL VARIATIONS

Using 1.5% or 2.0% agarose makes a stiffer, easier-to-cut gel which develops sharper precipitin arcs, but some sieving develops,[7] and precipitation takes longer. Agarose can be employed at concentrations as low

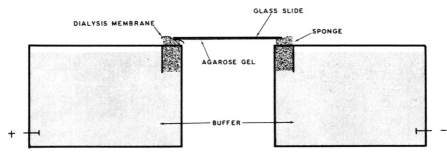

Fig. 5.9. The basic elements of electrophoresis apparatus required for gel electrophoresis, immunoelectrophoresis, and electroimmunodiffusion. Sponges serve as both contacts and baffles against pH change. The dialysis membrane is used to prevent serum macromolecules from migrating into buffer as they would, for example, without the membrane in place during single electroimmunodiffusion. The glass slide is inverted both to provide good contact with sponges and to minimize evaporation. The entire apparatus usually is enclosed in a humidified chamber and is used at 4°C.

[7] Macroglobulins were eliminated selectively from immunoelectropherograms by placing a disc of 4% agar in the path of serum antigens being electrophoresed in 1% agar (Kořínek, 1964).

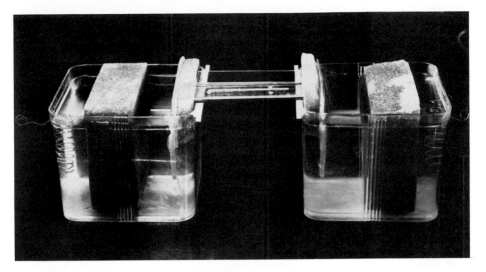

Fig. 5.10. Simple micro immunoelectrophoresis setup consisting of (from left to right) buffer vessel, electrode in first compartment, sponge to prevent electrolysis products from changing pH of second compartment of buffer vessel, second compartment, sponge connector, microscope slides on which electrophoresis takes place. The uppermost slide is covered simply with a layer of gel, while the lower slide is covered with Plexiglas template.

as 0.5%, but its gels then become inconveniently weak. Agar still is frequently used instead of agarose and at equivalent concentrations. Increasing or decreasing the concentration of agar alters electroosmosis and interaction with certain antigens more than analogous changes in agarose concentrations.

Sandwich casting the electrophoresis gel to a uniform thickness of 200 to 500 microns as described in Chapter 2 is worth the slightly greater time and effort required. It increases immunoelectrophoresis sensitivity, versatility, resolution, and uniformity; it saves reagents and time; and it facilitates observation, photography, washing, staining, and storing of immunoelectropherograms.

Barbital buffer at pH 8.2 is most frequently used as something of a comparative standard, especially for serum antigen analyses, but buffer pH and composition should be chosen to effect optimal antigen separation. An ionic strength of between 0.025 and 0.05 is most common[8] because this strength offers the best compromise for most buffering agents

---

[8] Because calculated ionic strength may differ from effective ionic strength as measured by conductivity, an alternative way of describing useful ranges of buffer composition is by conductivity itself. Uriel finds the optimal range for immunoelectrophoresis as described in this manner to be between 1/700 and 1/900 Ω^{-1} cm^{-1} (Uriel, 1966).

of stable pH, rapid electrophoretic migration without undue heating of the electrophoresis medium, protection against exceptional gel distortion (Bennett and Boursnell, 1962), and reasonable stabilization of antigens against either spontaneous aggregation or interaction with the electrophoresis medium. Double-strength buffer sometimes is used in the electrode vessels, but the minor increases that this practice offers in stabilized pH and better conductivity may be offset by the irregularities of what thereby becomes a discontinuous buffer system, by exaggeration of electroosmosis, and by such changes in the medium as local dehydration (Bennett and Boursnell, 1962; Jouannet, 1968).

In our apparatus used at 4°C, 8 to 10 volts/cm of the electropherogram (i.e., 75 volts for a 75-cm microscope slide) is the largest voltage that can be used with buffer at ionic strength 0.025 without overheating the electropherogram (cf. also Zwaan, 1963). Lower voltages can be used, but they require longer electrophoretic runs and permit more diffusion of antigens. Nevertheless, a lower voltage is required for electrophoresis at room temperature. With special cooling devices, higher voltage can be used (Aurand et al., 1963; Bon, 1966; Van Furth et al., 1966b).[9] In one such technique a thin electropherogram on a 2½ × ⅞-inch cover slip is floated on mercury for cooling, and electrophoresis is completed in 5 minutes (Traill, 1968).

For serum analyses this voltage arbitrarily is applied long enough to move serum albumin about 3 cm from its origin in agarose, so that serum antigens will be reasonably well separated from each other but neither the prealbumins nor the γ-globulins will be too near the edges of the slide to make undeformed arcs. If agar is being used instead of agarose, the origin should be placed closer to the anode than the cathode to offset electroosmosis, and allowable albumin migration will be approximately 1.0 to 1.5 cm instead of 3 cm.

By common practice, electropherograms generally are placed in the electrophoresis apparatus gel upward (see Fig. 5.10). But applying them gel downward, instead (Bennett and Boursnell, 1962; see Fig. 5.9), is better because it decreases drying during electrophoresis, it makes labeled indicators easier to see, it minimizes dust contamination, and

[9] The voltage across the electropherogram and that indicated on the power supply meter may not be the same. Differences in contact between electropherogram and electrode vessels or distances between electrodes (due to larger buffer vessel size or the use of numerous baffles therein) make different designs of electrophoresis apparatus perform differently (Jouannet, 1968). The best empirical indicator of proper electrophoretic voltage is a labeled marker for electrophoretic migration (Reinskou, 1966b). Whether the power supply is built to maintain constant voltage or to maintain constant current is immaterial if such an indicator is used (Jordan and White, 1965).

in an apparatus with contacts like that in Fig. 5.9 for the buffer vessels, it is easier and more effective.

There are many potentially useful antiserum trough and antigen well arrangements; some of the more important are described later. That mentioned above with two troughs set at different distances from the antiserum well will detect the most antigens. Another has the trough cut down the center of the slide between two antigen wells. This usually is employed to compare two mixtures of antigens using a single reference antiserum.

The mixture to be electrophoresed usually is placed in a small well cut in the gel, but better results sometimes are obtained by letting it soak into the gel for a few minutes either from a droplet placed on the surface of the gel (Goullet, 1964) or from a disc of filter paper or cellulose acetate saturated with it. If a disc is used, it must be removed before beginning electrophoresis. When the mixture is dilute (e.g., cerebrospinal fluid), an origin well can be refilled three or four times before electrophoresis to increase the mixture's concentration in the gel (Brill and Brönnestam, 1960; Ursing, 1965). Antiserum usually is applied by charging troughs cut in the gel, but an excellent, easy alternative is to apply it with narrow but thick strips of antiserum-saturated filter paper.[10]

Indicators for Electrophoretic Migration

Internal indicators for electrophoresis not only facilitate comparisons of different immunoelectropherograms (Reinskou, 1966b) but also indicate the electrophoretic mobilities of constituents being analyzed.

Three kinds of colored indicator are used in immunoelectrophoresis: colored components of the electrophoresed mixture, charged dyes or dyed materials used to observe and regulate the progress of electrophoresis,

---

[10] Waterproof a microscope slide with a polish of silicone grease. Lay a strip or strips of filter paper in the approximate positions required for the immunoelectropherogram. Saturate each with antiserum until it glistens. With a dissecting needle, adjust each to exactly the correct position required (e.g., over markings drawn on a paper under this slide). Lower the gel slide on which electrophoresis has been completed gently and evenly down upon these strips of filter paper; then lift it. The antiserum-saturated strips will adhere to the gel and come away with the electropherogram. This technique is simple and versatile and avoids trough-associated problems like antiserum spillage and irregular washing, staining, and drying of the immunoelectropherogram. Different antigen–antiserum arrangements fitting different analytic problems are easier to employ in this way than by cutting troughs and wells. Furthermore, an occasional antigen present in excess will precipitate under a filter paper antiserum source, whereas when a trough has been used it will precipitate in the liquid within the trough and may not be observed.

and electroneutral substances used to measure electroosmosis. In addition, there are noncolored indicators which are employed both as landmarks for identifying less well-known constituents of a mixture after immuno-electrophoresis and for accurately measuring electrophoretic mobilities.

COLORED INDICATORS FOR ASSESSING ELECTROPHORESIS

The most common is dye-labeled serum albumin, because serum is so frequently a subject of immunoelectrophoretic analysis, because albumin has a natural affinity for acid dyes, and because this antigen is so prominent and electrophoretically reliable a constituent of serum. It is labeled with Evans blue, for instance, by adding approximately 1 mg of the dye per milliliter of serum. After the dye has been mixed with the whole serum, or with purified albumin if this is being used separately, excess unbound dye is removed either by dialysis against the electro-phoresis buffer or by Sephadex G-25 column chromatography (Hanson et al., 1966a). When this cannot be done (e.g., in electrophoresing very small volumes), then two spots of color may be seen migrating toward the anode during electrophoresis; the more cathodic is the labeled albumin. One must not use more than 1 mg of Evans blue dye per milli-liter of antiserum, because concentrations larger than this begin to change the apparent mobility of the albumin (Crowle and Jarrett, unpublished work).

Other dyes are used like Evans blue, including amido black B (Hanson et al., 1966a; Reinskou, 1963; Nerstrøm, 1963a), bromphenol blue (Williams, 1962a), 2(4'-hydroxybenzazo)benzoic acid (Burtin and Grabar, 1967), and orange G (Schur and Sandson, 1963). Amido black-stained human serum albumin in whole serum has been reported not to pre-cipitate with its antibodies in immunoelectrophoresis (Reinskou, 1963). We have not had this trouble using Evans blue as a label for it; indeed, the precipitin arc that forms is itself blue. Nevertheless, this observation should warn that dye labeling may affect the antigens being studied directly or indirectly.

Sometimes one antigen of a mixture may be an obvious enough pig-ment to provide a native marker for electrophoresis. Transferrin, hemo-globin, and ferritin are examples, although in thin electropherograms they may be too faint to see easily. Serum albumins from different species of animals migrate at somewhat different rates (Reinskou, 1963; Fig. 5.11); hence, they cannot be used as indicators interchangeably. Intra-specific variations of the electrophoretic characteristics of albumin also have been observed (Burtin and Grabar, 1967).

Charged dyes alone are inexpensive and reliable markers to use for observing and regulating electrophoresis. They are run alongside the antigens being electrophoresed. We use thiazine red because it is easy

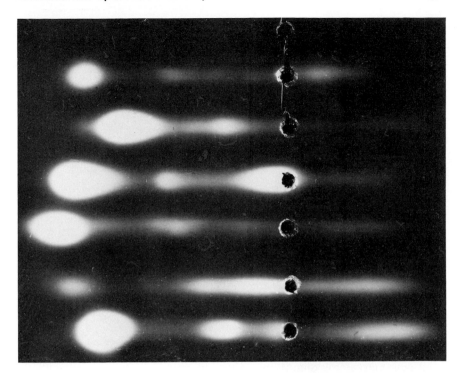

Fig. 5.11. Photographic print showing differences in electrophoretic mobilities of proteins in chicken, guinea pig, horse, rabbit, mouse, and human sera (top to bottom). All sera were electrophoresed simultaneously on one glass plate in agar and barbital buffer at pH 8.2, ionicity 0.1, and their fractions then stained with thiazine red R.

to see and migrates slowly (Crowle, 1961). Other acid dyes also can be used in agar, and either acid or basic dyes can be employed in agarose or polyacrylamide. Pyronine is said to have a γ-globulin-like mobility (Khramkova and Abelev, 1963).

Measuring electroosmosis is sometimes necessary during electrophoresis in agar gels. Indicators with ready visibility and electroneutrality are needed. Orthonitroaniline (Ragetli and Weintraub, 1964, 1966) and colored dextran (e.g., Macrodex: Zwaan, 1963) have been used. Dextran, glucose, other polysaccharides, and polyvinylpyrrolidone can be employed uncolored if after electrophoresis they are detected by precipitation or by staining (Wunderly, 1960). Polyvinylpyrrolidone, for instance, can be stained with bromphenol blue.

MARKERS AND IMMUNOELECTROPHORETIC MOBILITY

In a completed immunoelectropherogram, the center from which an antigen has diffused to form its arc of precipitate can be determined

330 IMMUNOELECTROPHORESIS

accurately by noting where a line drawn from the apex of its arc perpendicular to the path of electrophoresis crosses this path (cf. Fig. 5.1). The position of one antigen therefore is easily compared with that of another as a standard, both to identify the former and to determine its immunoelectrophoretic mobility. For example, to determine the mobility of unknown antigen x, one relates it within an immunoelectropherogram to those of two others, a and b, whose mobilities are known:

$$m^x = m^b + (m^a - m^b)\frac{x - b}{a - b}$$

in which m^a and m^b are the mobilities of the reference antigens in 10^{-5} cm^2 $volt^{-1}$ sec^{-1}, $x - b$ is the distance measured on the immunoelectropherogram between the unknown antigen and reference antigen b, and $a - b$ is the distance measured between the two reference antigens themselves (Weiner et al., 1963). Alternatively, relative mobility can be recorded as the position of the unknown antigen relative to that of albumin taken arbitrarily as 100, either from the origin, or from the position of an indicator for electroosmosis if this is a significant effect in the medium being used (Zwaan, 1963).

Although albumin is the more prominent, transferrin is more often used as a marker for identifying other antigens in serum immunoelectropherograms (see Fig. 5.5) because it also is easily evident, because it can be identified more certainly by iron content (Keutel, 1960), and because it has a consistent electrophoretic mobility. γ-Globulin (IgG) is another landmark frequently employed because of its prominence in the cathodic region; ceruloplasmin is a useful marker within the complex α_2-globulin region. Albumin and IgG usually are identified by location, intensity, and shape; ceruloplasmin and transferrin can be more definitely identified by differential stains for copper and iron, respectively (Schen and Rabinovitz, 1966b).

All such markers must be used cautiously for abnormal or unfamiliar mixtures of antigens. For example, the most prominent precipitin arc in the IgG region of a human saliva immunoelectropherogram is not IgG but amylase, and, also in saliva, albumin is the lesser of two arcs in the albumin region (Revis, 1968; cf. also Nash and Schwab, 1968). Transferrin is a familiar β_1-globulin in human serum and has the same location in horse and mouse serum, but in guinea pig and sheep sera it is an α_2-globulin, and in rat sera it is a γ_1-globulin (Havez et al., 1965; Ślopek et al., 1966; Watkins et al., 1966; Ślopek et al., 1965b). Transferrin exists in two forms in human cerebrospinal fluid and therefore develops an unfamiliar gull-wing precipitin arc (Parker and Bearn, 1962; Dencker and Swahn, 1961). As indicated in the section of this chapter on different media, it is polymorphous in the sera of certain lower mammals.

Template Microimmunoelectrophoresis

Template microimmunoelectrophoresis refers to techniques in which a template is laid on the electrophoresis gel before or after electrophoresis to position reactants and, especially, to feed them in large volumes into the thin layer of gel. Sensitivity and resolution are increased in this manner, as was explained for template double diffusion tests in Chapter 4. Although the template technique has not often been used because it is harder to set up and less easily changed for different antigen–antibody configurations, it is unexcelled for maximum resolution and sensitivity (Crowle and Lueker, 1962).

On an agarose precoated slide, cast a flat 500-micron-thick layer of 1.5% agarose using the sandwich method. Remove the casting spacers before electrophoresis. Punch one or two origins, as required by the ultimate reactant arrangement, charge them with antigen mixture to be analyzed (or make no wells and simply use the surface application technique, Chapter 2), and electrophorese the inverted slide as described above. After electrophoresis, carefully lay or slide the template onto the gel as related in Chapter 4, positioning the antiserum troughs alongside the path(s) of antigen migration exactly as required. Charge these troughs with antiserum, and allow precipitin arcs to develop in a normal manner.

Agarose at 1.5% is used to minimize distortion of the gel during electrophoresis and thereby ensure good contact between the gel surface and a subsequently applied template. The casting spacers are removed so that a template rests only on the gel surface and will not draw away from it if it shrinks some from drying during precipitin arc formation. The templates are made from 3-mm (⅛-inch) Plexiglas or similar water-repellent transparent plastic in the same dimensions as the microscope slide (see Fig. 5.12). Antiserum slots cut or cast in them should be as wide as the template is thick; they are placed to feed antiserum into the surface of the electropherogram at an appropriate distance from the origin(s) cut in it.

The overriding advantage of using a template, as mentioned above, is that it can deliver unusually large volumes of antiserum into a developing immunoelectropherogram. The same principle can be achieved less neatly with flexible plastic film (e.g., Mylar) templates with slots cut in them. A bead of antiserum is used to cover the slot in one of these and with time gradually sinks down into the gel as the level of fluid does

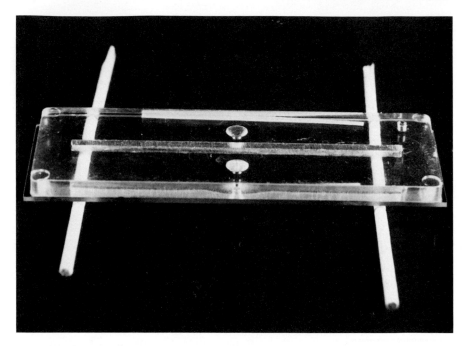

Fig. 5.12. Template immunoelectrophoresis, showing one form of template in place on a 0.3-mm-thick layer of agar on a microscope slide. Samples to be analyzed are placed in wells in the agar through the two funnel-shaped access holes in the template; electrophoresis tracking dye is placed in the agar similarly through the hole in the upper right corner. After electrophoresis the central trough is filled with antiserum.

from the slot of a Plexiglas template. A polyvinyl chloride sheet with slots and holes cut in it can be used as a template to cut the holes and, after electrophoresis, also for feeding antiserum into the thin layer of gel under it (Feinberg *et al.*, 1964). The sheet is laid on the molten agar during casting and is left in place until antigen–antibody precipitation has been completed.

Immunoelectrophoresis in Media Other Than Agar or Agarose

Agar or agarose gels are usually used in immunoelectrophoresis because they yield excellent results and are easy to obtain and work with. The techniques described above are meant primarily to be used with these two gelling agents, but with some modification they can be employed also with other media which differ from the traditional gels in sometimes advantageous ways. The characteristics and preparation of these other media (e.g., polyacrylamide, cellulose acetate, gelatin, starch) have been described in Chapter 2. The following paragraphs discuss some examples of their use in immunoelectrophoresis.

POLYACRYLAMIDE

The use of this medium for immunoelectrophoresis was described over a decade ago (Crowle, 1961). Five percent Cyanogum (a commercial mixture of acrylamide and bisacrylamide; see Chapter 2) is polymerized with heat under heptane within a petri dish containing a microscope slide. Ammonium persulfate and β-dimethylaminopropionitrile are used as catalysts (see Chapter 2 for details). The slide in the petri dish is cut free of the surrounding gel, antigen mixture is applied from a square of filter paper laid on the surface of the gel for a few minutes, electrophoresis is performed as in agar gel electrophoresis, antiserum is fed into the gel from antiserum-soaked filter paper strips, and immunodiffusion arcs are allowed to develop for several days at 4°C (see Fig. 5.13).

This technique still remains the simplest to use with polyacrylamide. It might be improved somewhat by using the more efficient catalysts currently available, although those originally used did not seem to affect immunoelectropherograms adversely and, if deemed so for some critical analyses, can be replaced by dialyzing the gel against immunoelectrophoresis buffer overnight.

However, this method is not well suited to producing the very thin gel layers now routinely used with agarose. Furthermore, gel not actually resting on the microscope slide in the petri dish used for casting is wasted. These problems have been solved, at the expense of some addi-

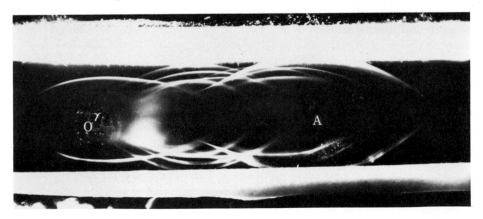

Fig. 5.13. Micro immunoelectrophoresis of human serum in 5% Cyanogum 41 gel under conditions similar to those employed with gelatin (Fig. 5.14). Immune precipitation required 72 hours. Note both the lack of electroosmosis and the unusual clarity of the gel.

tional complication, by using a Plexiglas template and photographic plate in a modified method for sandwich casting (Keutel, 1964; Keutel *et al.*, 1964; cf. also Antoine, 1962). The template is made in a pattern of alternating pegs and slightly shorter bars. When it is laid on a photographic glass plate of 3¼ × 4-inch dimensions it rests on the pegs 1 mm above the plate, and when polyacrylamide gel is formed between it and the slide, the pegs cast antigen holes and the bars cast antiserum troughs (Keutel *et al.*, 1964). A 2.8% concentration of photopolymerized polyacrylamide is employed rather than a higher concentration because the templates can be removed without lubrication, electrophoresis time is shortened and migration of macromolecular antigens is not inhibited (Keutel *et al.*, 1964), diffusion and reaction of antigens and antibodies are faster, and there is less shrinkage from drying (Keutel, 1964). Electrophoresis of human serum can be completed in 20 minutes under conditions requiring 45 to 50 minutes in agar; but precipitin reactions require 72 hours to develop fully, whereas in agar only 14 hours are required. In 2.8% polyacrylamide the relative positions of human serum antigens appear to be the same as in conventional agar immunoelectropherograms (Keutel *et al.*, 1964). An interesting new variety of polyacrylamide immunoelectrophoresis, applicable also to other kinds of gel, has been described recently and named "immunodisc electrophoresis" (Makonkawkeyoon and Haque, 1970). Acrylamide is polymerized in tubes as for routine disc electrophoresis except that a Plexiglas rod is left in the center of the polyacrylamide column which therefore is actually a long cylinder. After electrophoresis, the Plexiglas rod is removed and replaced with a warm mixture of antiserum and molten agar. Each separated disc of antigen in the exterior cylinder of polyacrylamide then is revealed by reaction with corresponding precipitins in the enclosed columns of antiserum–agar gel mixture.

POLYACRYLAMIDE–AGAROSE

The difficulty of working with soft and sticky polyacrylamide gels has discouraged their use, especially at concentrations used to avoid sieving. Casting them with agarose avoids these difficulties and somewhat improves agarose gels as well, because the combination is more flexible and less fragile than agarose alone (Uriel, 1966). Polyacrylamide–agarose gels are nearly as easy to use as agarose, but they have the valuable sieving versatility of polyacrylamide.

As described in Chapter 2, the combination gels are cast with the sandwich technique, the acrylamide being polymerized chemically at 50°C and the agarose set later at 4°C. The resulting gel then is soaked in electrophoresis buffer to leach out catalysts and secondary products of polymerization which might harm certain antigens like enzymes. This gel can be kept after preparation for up to 2 weeks in the buffer at 4°C.

Two-Step Polyacrylamide Immunoelectrophoresis

Although judging from results described in the literature two-step immunoelectrophoresis with polyacrylamide has not been very successful, it is useful when the electrophoresis buffer is incompatible with the immunodiffusion step of immunoelectrophoresis. The antigens are electrophoresed in a column of polyacrylamide (i.e., submitted to "disc" electrophoresis), and then the column is extruded and embedded in agarose gel, and troughs are cut alongside and charged with antiserum (Bednařík, 1967). Antigens diffusing out of the polyacrylamide column then react in the agarose with their antibodies diffusing from the troughs. If the electrophoresis buffer will allow normal antigen–antibody precipitation, the polyacrylamide column is embedded without intermediate treatment; if the buffer is incompatible, then the column must be washed with a compatible buffer or tap water before embedding (see starch immunoelectrophoresis, below). The column can be sliced into halves, one being stained and the other analyzed with antiserum to correlate immunoprecipitation arcs with zones of protein or other substance detected by the stain (Bloemendal, 1967). The disc electrophoresis column also can be embedded in antiserum-charged agar in a tube (El-Sharkawy and Huisingh, 1971) in what could be considered an inverse immunodisc electrophoresis (Makonkawkeyoon and Haque, 1970). In just a few minutes, rings of precipitate form around corresponding discs of antigen. These can be quantitated by densitometry. Examples of this two-step method include detecting C-reactive protein isomers (Riley *et al.*, 1965), identifying growth hormone and prolactin (Kwa *et al.*, 1965), and resolving seven antigens in an extract of squid axioplasm different from antigens in squid blood (Huneeus-Cox, 1964).

Because antigens diffuse more slowly in polyacrylamide gels than in those of agarose, better results usually are obtained by incubating the embedded column in agarose overnight at room temperature before cutting and charging antiserum troughs (Pettersson and Höglund, 1969). Still better resolution and sensitivity would result from submitting the polyacrylamide column to electroimmunodiffusion (see Chapter 6).

Cellulose Acetate Immunoelectrophoresis

Contrasted with older macro methods for agar gel immunoelectrophoresis, cellulose acetate immunoelectrophoresis offered remarkable speed, sensitivity, and economy (Hayashida and Grunbaum, 1962). But today this speed, sensitivity, and economy can be matched and surpassed by techniques using agar or agarose; such techniques are easier to perform more reproducibly, and precipitin arcs can be observed in these gels as they form. The advantage of cellulose acetate of being inert to cationic antigens such as lysozyme (Allerhand *et al.*, 1963) also is a property of agarose. For these reasons, cellulose acetate immunoelectrophoresis now is only infrequently used.

The essence of this technique is to moisten a strip of cellulose acetate evenly, soak a small spot of antigen solution into an appropriate point of origin, electrophorese this for a few minutes in a very humid atmosphere, make a uniform strip of antiserum parallel to and appropriately spaced from the path of electrophoresis, incubate the strip overnight under oil for immunoprecipitation to develop, wash off the oil, and stain the strip for proteins to observe the reactions that have developed (Allerhand *et al.*, 1963; Kohn, 1961; Atchley, 1960, 1961; Nelson *et al.*, 1964; Grunbaum *et al.*, 1963; Lomanto and Vergani, 1967).

A film of the acetate can be moistened by floating it on the electrophoresis buffer, then submerging it, and then removing and blotting it very lightly. It should be stretched tightly or supported on water-resistant points, like the bristles of a nylon brush, during electrophoresis; and drying must rigorously be prevented (Allerhand *et al.*, 1963; Nelson *et al.*, 1964). Strips of antiserum can be added after electrophoresis by gently dragging a capillary tube charged with antiserum and guided by a ruler along the area of the membane to be charged (Kohn, 1961), doing the same along the edge of a narrow strip of filter paper previously placed on the membrane (Grunbaum *et al.*, 1963), applying antiserum-impregnated filter paper strips (Kohn, 1961; Allerhand *et al.*, 1963), or touching the antiserum onto the membrane with an applicator made with two parallel wires (Grunbaum *et al.*, 1963). Additional manipulations of developing the immunodiffusion reactions, washing off oil, and washing, staining, and drying the membranes are the same as those described for double diffusion tests with cellulose acetate in Chapter 4.

If a wide strip of the membrane is employed with an elongated origin, a length of the membrane can be cut off at the end of electrophoresis for staining of the separated antigens to compare their electrophoretic and immunoelectrophoretic locations (Atchley, 1960, 1961). Cellulose acetate can be used in two-step immunoelectrophoresis in essentially the same manner as that described for polyacrylamide (Kohn, 1967). Because of the ease with which cellulose acetate electropherograms can be handled relative to those made with various gels, they may be especially useful for the first electrophoresis in two-dimensional electroimmunodiffusion (see Chapter 6).

IMMUNOELECTROPHORESIS IN GELATIN

Immunoelectrophoresis using gelatin, originally described in the first edition of this book (Crowle, 1961), apparently has not been used since. Although a gelatin immunoelectropherogram of human serum closely resembles that in agar (Fig. 5.14), recent findings that gelatin strongly inhibits diffusion and precipitation of polysaccharide antigens suggests that critical comparisons would reveal differences between these two different types of immunoelectropherogram. Gelatin is not likely to see much use for immunoelectrophoresis in the future, because for nearly all purposes there will be an alternative medium which is better, but it may possibly be uniquely useful for experiments with polysaccharide or polysaccharide-associated antigens as is suggested in more detail in Chapter 2.

IMMUNOELECTROPHORESIS WITH STARCH GEL

Before polyacrylamide gel was used for electrophoresis, starch was unsurpassed as a sieving medium for sharply resolving populations of molecules from each other, and even from their own isomers. Therefore, it was potentially interesting to users of immunoelectrophoresis (Korngold, 1963b; Brummerstedt-Hansen, 1962). But its turbidity and resistance to ready diffusion of antigen and antiserum prevented its ever

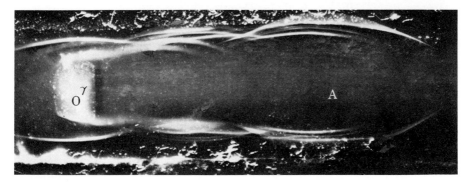

Fig. 5.14. Micro immunoelectrophoresis of human serum in 2% gelatin gel made up in barbital buffer at pH 8.2, ionicity 0.05. Serum was allowed to soak into a 1-mm-thick layer of gelatin on a microscope slide for 20 minutes from a piece of filter paper at origin (O). Then the filter paper was removed, and 50 volts of direct current was applied for 1 hour and 45 minutes. Finally, strips of filter paper soaked with Pasteur Institute horse antihuman serum were placed parallel and to either side of the expected path of electrophoretic separation, and immunoprecipitation was allowed to develop for 48 hours. Albumin (A) and γ-globulin areas are indicated; note lack of electroosmosis. All procedures were carried out at 4°C.

being practically useful in one-step immunoelectrophoresis. Nevertheless, its utility in two-step immunoelectrophoresis is well established.

The two-step technique is the same as that used for polyacrylamide: antigen mixture is electrophoresed in the starch gel, and then this is applied to or embedded in agar or agarose gel for immunoprecipitation (Poulik, 1966). The extra effort of using starch in this two-step technique frequently will be amply rewarded. For example, it resolved serum haptoglobins, which produced only one symmetrical precipitin arc in agar gel immunoelectrophoresis but are known to vary in molecular weight from 85,000 to 400,000, into four or five different but coalescing precipitin arcs (Korngold, 1963b). It can separate transferrin from serum immunoglobulins completely, for in starch gel electrophoresis transferrin is more anodic than in agar (Korngold, 1963b). It can detect five varieties of transferrin simultaneously in cattle serum (Brummerstedt-Hansen, 1967). Immunoglobulins are more distinctly resolved in starch immunoelectrophoresis than in agar or agarose (Pierce and Feinstein, 1965); human serum β lipoproteins are clearly distinguished from each other in starch but not in agar (Lawrence and Shean, 1962); two anterior pituitary hormones of 5000 and 10,000 molecular weight have been separated and detected (Friesen et al., 1962); and subunits of complex proteins like the immunoglobulins can be distinguished by using additives like urea in the starch during the electrophoresis (Gräsbeck et al., 1963; Poulik, 1963b; Putnam et al., 1962; Thorpe and Deutsch, 1966). Human serum albumin in Cohn Fraction V appearing by agar immunoelectrophoresis to be monomeric was shown by starch gel immunoelectrophoresis to consist of four polymers; and polymers of IgG-globulin in human myeloma sera were evident with starch but not with agar immunoelectrophoresis (Poulik, 1964). A chromatographically purified o-diphenyl oxidase from sweet potato roots was shown to consist of two electrophoretically different but antigenically similar constituents in starch gel immunoelectrophoresis (Hyodo and Uritani, 1965).

For a detailed review of starch immunoelectrophoresis technology, see Poulik (1966). The following micro technique gives excellent results (Korngold, 1963b; Bloemendal, 1967; Poulik, 1966). Prepare a 15% suspension of hydrolyzed starch (e.g., Starch, Hydrolyzed, Fisher Scientific Co.) in a tris–citrate buffer of pH 8.5 (composition of Appendix III) by heating it with constant swirling. Just before it boils, de-gas it for a few seconds with a slight vacuum. Cast the hot viscous liquid on a preheated, leveled 3¼ × 4-inch photographic glass plate by decanting 15 to 20 ml from the dissolving flask into a preheated beaker, pouring from this onto the plate, and smoothing out any unevenness with a glass rod. Cool the gel to room temperature, and let it stand overnight in a humidified container. Cut four or five well-separated holes in a row across the plate about 1 inch from what will be the cathodic edge, charge these with antigen solution to be analyzed, and electrophorese across the length of the plate as described previously for agar gel electrophoresis. Best results are obtained by using a borate buffer for the electrode vessels (formula in Appendix III). If serum is being analyzed, the albumin should be electrophoresed to within about 1 inch of the anodic edge of the plate.

After electrophoresis, the starch gel can be used entire or in sections containing individual electrophoretic components for either staining or immunodiffusion (i.e., two-step immunoelectrophoresis). Loosen the gel by running a razor blade between it and the glass plate around the edges, and transfer it or whatever strip portions of it are being used to 1% agarose gel already sandwich-cast on another slide of appropriate dimensions, being careful in laying the starch gel on the agarose not to trap air bubbles, and to place the portion of the starch gel originally in contact with its glass plate in contact with the agarose. After 1 hour, use a two-razor blade cutter to cut troughs through both starch and agarose alongside the path of electrophoretic separation, charge these with antiserum, and allow immunoprecipitation to develop for 24 hours at room temperature. Finally, remove the starch gel from the agarose gel, and observe and record the immunoelectrophoretic results as with an agarose immunoelectropherogram.

When a buffer that will interfere with antigen–antibody precipitation is employed, like 8 M urea in formate, the starch electropherogram should be dialyzed against tap water and/or immunodiffusion buffer before it is applied to or embedded in agarose for immunodiffusion (Poulik, 1963b, 1966). If running tap water is used and the gel is 1 to 2 mm thick, washing for 2 to 3 hours should suffice; a urea-containing gel will turn from relatively clear to opaque as the urea is washed out. Prolonged washing will begin to wash out electrophoresed antigens and so should be avoided.

IMMUNOELECTROPHORESIS WITH PAPER

Although resolution of antigen–antibody precipitates in immunodiffusion tests performed on filter paper is poor because of the texture of the paper, paper, like starch, can be used for preliminary electrophoresis followed by application to or embedding in agarose gel for immunodiffusion (McCully *et al.*, 1962; cf. also Sarcione and Aungst, 1962). However, since there are no obvious advantages to using it and there are some disadvantages, such as adsorption of proteins to the paper, it will not be described further here.

Qualitative Immunoelectrophoresis

Immunoelectrophoresis is primarily a qualitative technique—that is, one that detects, characterizes, and identifies antigens and antibodies. It has rather limited quantitative capabilities, as will be described below. Immunoelectrophoresis detects antigens (or antibodies) by specific immunologic precipitation or fixation; it characterizes them electrophoretically, histochemically, by biological features, and by immunologic comparisons; and it identifies them by these various characteristics. The following paragraphs will discuss only the ways in which immunoelectrophoresis is used to characterize substances by immunologic comparisons, since other methods of characterization such as specific staining and enzymatic activity already have been discussed in Chapter 2.

COMPARATIVE IMMUNOELECTROPHORESIS

In simplest form, this consists of comparing precipitin arc shape, intensity, general appearance, and electrophoretic location on two different immunoelectropherograms developed similarly. For well-known mixtures of antigens, like human serum, this technique readily identifies more prominent constituents such as IgG- and IgM-globulins, transferrin, and albumin,[11] but increasingly more exacting techniques must be used to identify succeedingly less familiar antigens, or to relate them to each other or similar antigens in other mixtures. The following examples are illustrated in Fig. 5.15 in order of discussion.

Two antisera can be compared with the arrangement in diagram *A*, Fig. 5.15, for scope and approximate strength of reactivity with a mixture of antigens, the two antisera being used in troughs equidistant on either side of the electrophoresed antigens (Zlotnick and Landau, 1966). If the two antisera have been obtained from different species of animals (e.g., rabbit and horse) which were immunized with serum proteins (e.g., human serum), they may cross-precipitate each other's serum antigens. This complication is avoided by cutting away a narrow strip of gel through the center of the electropherogram; then each antiserum will develop a full pattern of precipitin arcs, but it cannot diffuse into the other's domain.

By a slight modification of this technique (diagram *B*), two mixtures of antigen can be compared against a single antiserum or two different antisera (from the same species of animal) to determine, for example, whether they have similar numbers and concentrations of antigens, or

---

[11] Individual antigens need not be identified for some applications. This technique can be used with a superimposed grid to identify a person, such as for forensic purposes, by his serum's immunoelectrophoretic "fingerprint" (Laudel *et al.*, 1962).

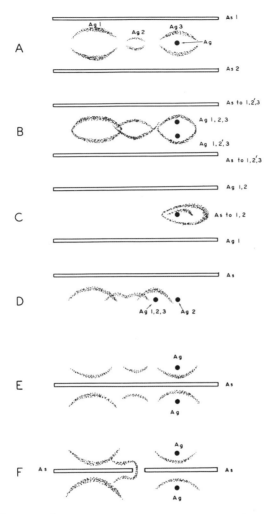

Fig. 5.15. Varieties of reactant arrangement in immunoelectrophoresis drawn usually to indicate analyses of three hypothetical antigens of increasing electrophoretic mobility. These are electrophoresed from right to left (cathode to anode), and then are revealed in any of various different ways by appropriate antisera (As). In example *Q*, however, antiserum itself is electrophoresed in immunoelectrophoretic analysis of its enzyme-neutralizing antibody. Each variety of immunoelectrophoresis is discussed more fully in the text.

what the antigenic relationships for individual antigens in the mixture might be. Reactions of identity, nonidentity, or partial identity develop as they do in comparative double diffusion plate tests, and they have the same meaning (see Chapter 4). Diagram *C* indicates that antigens

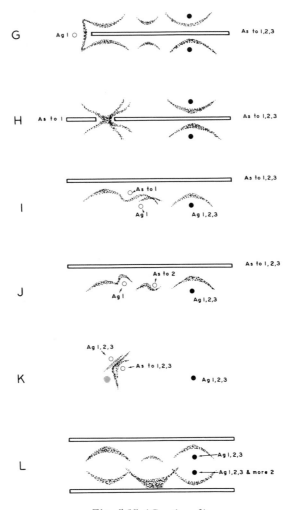

Fig. 5.15 (Continued).

also can be compared by reversed immunoelectrophoresis (Cuadrado and Casals, 1967).

Another technique for comparing antigens, which is especially useful for identifying one among many in a mixture if the one already has been purified, is illustrated in diagram *D*. Reference antigen is deposited to one side or the other of the unknown mixture in the direction of electrophoresis. After electrophoresis, the reference antigen will develop an arc of precipitate which selectively coalesces with the arc of its analog in the mixture. Reference and test solutions should be applied without leaving holes in the gel (i.e., as droplets, by diffusion from sample-saturated paper discs, or in holes but mixed with gel) so that there will

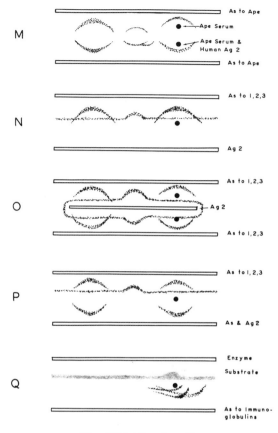

Fig. 5.15 (Continued).

be no gel discontinuity to distort the electrophoresis of the more cathodic mixture as it migrates through the area where the more anodic mixture was deposited. Two relatively simple mixtures also can be compared with each other by this technique to learn how many of their antigens are identical and what relationships their nonidentical antigens bear to each other. This technique is illustrated more fully in Chapter 6 for electroimmunodiffusion in which it is considerably more effective.

Several varieties of immunoelectrophoretic comparison are based on the reactant arrangement shown in diagram *E* in which two mixtures of antigen to be compared are electrophoresed on either side of a central trough later charged with antiserum. This arrangement enumerates the antigens in both mixtures, compares their electrophoretic mobilities, and, if the precipitin arcs in one mixture are known, also tentatively identifies corresponding arcs with each other. For more definitive immunologic identification, the antiserum trough can be divided into two sections as shown in diagram *F* ("interrupted trough technique": Clausen and Heremans, 1960); or it can be cut short and reference antigen placed in a well at one end of it (diagram *G*, "short trough technique": Lévy and Polonovski, 1958). Diagram *H* shows a combination of the previous two: the trough is interrupted, the longer section is filled with polyvalent antiserum, and the shorter with monovalent antiserum (Hanson, 1962).

In the form of analysis depicted in diagram *I*, routine immunoelectrophoresis is complemented by two-way identification using both purified reference antigen and monospecific antiserum to the same antigen placed in wells cut in the immunoelectrophoretic pattern slightly lateral to the expected distal region of the developing precipitin arc (Burtin and Grabar, 1967). For a similar but slightly simpler technique illustrated in diagram *J*, a droplet of antiserum or a droplet of antigen is deposited on the immunoelectropherogram early during its development, so that if the growing precipitin arc picked out for study is related to either it will develop an acute turn near the appropriate deposits (Nelson *et al.*, 1964). With somewhat greater risk of not accurately placing reference reactants, reactant troughs can be dispensed with as shown in diagram *K* (Norman and Kagan, 1966) by arranging a comparative double diffusion plate test on an electropherogram, with wells of reference reactants placed near the area where the electrophoresed antigen is expected to be.

There are several additive and subtractive variations of comparative immunoelectrophoresis. In one (diagram *L*), purified antigen is added to a mixture, and this is analyzed in comparison with the same mixture without this addition. The supplemented mixture should develop the same number of precipitin arcs as the unsupplemented, but that formed by the added antigen should be stronger because of the additional antigen (Schultze *et al.*, 1963). This technique is useful for identifying antigens by homology. Thus, the many antigens of human serum which are known and have been purified can be used in this way for identifying homologous antigens in lower animal sera (diagram *M*: Seligmann, 1961; Grumbach and Kaplan, 1962; Beckman *et al.*, 1961). These comparisons also usually indicate the relative immunoelectrophoretic mobilities of the homologous lower animal antigens and their rough taxonomic relationships to the human antigens.[12]

Diagrams *N* and *O* depict varieties of antigen absorption techniques

[12] One should be cautious about accepting a measure of electrophoretic mobility for an antigen added to a mixture of other antigens without knowing whether the added antigen will react spontaneously with one of the others. Elastase, for instance, mixed wih serum complexes with a β_1-globulin carrier and so shows β_1 mobility in mixture unless added to the serum in excess of what will be taken up by the carrier (Baumstark, 1967).

which are useful for immunoelectrophoretically identifying some selected arcs of precipitate among many (Osserman, 1959). In diagram *N*, reference antigen diffusing from the lower trough forms a straight band of precipitate with antibodies against it diffusing from the upper antiserum trough except where the same antigen is located in the immunoelectropherogram. Here the added antigen will bulge this band. Elsewhere in the immunoelectropherogram immunologically unrelated precipitin arcs will form undisturbed. The variant of this technique shown in diagram *O* may be easier to observe (Berglund, 1962a). Diagram *P* represents a dual test in which antiserum is mixed with known antigen for charging the lower trough so that two complementary effects will be evident: this added antigen absorbs antibodies to itself specifically among the antibodies present against all the antigens in the unknown mixture and thus prevents development of the corresponding arc of precipitate by antiserum from this trough. And by the phenomenon illustrated in diagram *N*, it also forms a straight line of precipitate which coalesces with and thus identifies the arc of precipitate produced by the same antigen in the mixture of all the antigens. Diagram *Q* illustrates a way in which neutralization can be employed in qualitative immunoelectrophoresis to identify antibodies rather than antigens, and also the general principle of using biochemical and biological methods for immunoelectrophoretic quantitation (Mansa and Kjems, 1965). For this technique different populations of antibodies are moderately separated from each other by electrophoresis, and then they are identified on the one hand by precipitation in which they serve as antigens (i.e., immunoglobulins) and on the other by the capacity that some have to neutralize an enzyme. In illustration *Q*, β-staphylolysin was locally prevented by lysin-neutralizing antibodies from disrupting rabbit erythrocytes. The immunoelectrophoretic mobility and other characteristics of fibrinolysin have been studied similarly by substituting a mixture of fibrin and agarose for the erythrocyte–agarose mixture (Herman, 1970).

AGGLUTININS

Various characteristics of antibodies besides that of precipitation can be identified by qualitative immunoelectrophoresis. The technique of Hanson *et al.* (1960) illustrates this, showing that appropriately modified immunodiffusion tests readily can detect agglutinins (cf. Fig. 7.1). This technique is described in Chapter 7 as a specific test.

NONPRECIPITATING REAGENTS

Agglutinins and precipitins make themselves visible by their effects on their antigens. But, as was pointed out in Chapters 1 and 2, immunodiffusion tests can detect both antigens and antibodies which are unable to generate the directly visible manifestations of antigen–antibody precipitation. For example, the immunoelectrophoretic mobility of guinea pig antibody to insulin was determined by precipitating the antibody, as an immunoglobulin, in the presence of radioactive insulin (Yagi *et al.*, 1962). An antigen available in only very small quantity but radiolabeled (e.g., manufactured by a few living cells *in vitro* from radiolabeled amino acids) can be detected by a "carrier" technique: when this labeled antigen is added to a mixture of antigens including its own kind used in sufficient quantity to form precipitin arcs with specific antiserum, the radioactive antigen will coprecipitate in the arc formed by the more plentiful nonlabeled antigen in the mixture and thus radiolabel this arc (Asofsky and Thorbecke, 1961). As little as 0.2 ng of IgG-globulin manufactured *in vitro* by splenocytes could be detected (Van Furth, 1966). Substances that do not even qualify as antigens can be revealed. The affinity of uric acid for β lipoprotein, β_2-macroglobulin, and an α-globulin in addition to albumin was demonstrated by adding it in small amounts, after radiolabeling, to human serum and then immunoelectrophoresing the serum (Alvsaker, 1966).

Quantitative Immunoelectrophoresis

Single and double diffusion tests are sensitive, accurate, and reliable for quantitating antigens and antibodies providing they are employed with adequate standards and controls. Since immunoelectrophoresis tests are themselves either single or double diffusion tests, depending on technique, they too should be useful quantitatively. Early workers hoped, for instance, that a routine clinical immunoelectrophoretic test would be able to determine simultaneously the relative and perhaps absolute quantities of each of twenty or thirty different constitutents of any sample of human serum. But difficulties in devising the appropriate multiple standards and sufficiently rigid controls, as well as adequate techniques for making measurements, have been much greater than anticipated. Hence, progress toward practical achievement of this goal has been very slow. The trend of current research in immunodiffusion techniques suggests that it may be reached more easily by electroimmunodiffusion than by immunoelectrophoretic tests.

QUANTITATION BY SERIAL DILUTION

Serial dilutions of the unknown mixture of antigens are electrophoresed. The dilution at which a given precipitin arc just fails to develop visibly, becomes sharpest, or otherwise acquires some exactly recognizable change can be used as an end point for the antigen forming that arc (Griffiths *et al.*, 1965; Medgyesi and Koch, 1964).

Serial dilution tests can compare unknown mixtures with a standard mixture in which the antigens being quantitated may or may not have been identified. They can provide absolute instead of relative quantitations for individual antigens which are available pure and have been employed separately to set up comparative standards (Bentz, personal communication). However, because each of the many antigens in an immunoelectropherogram is likely to be related to its antibodies differently from every other, serial dilution immunoelectrophoresis will not be very accurate for more than a few antigens in a mixture without being rendered unwieldly by the large number of dilutions and corresponding analyses that have to be made. Of course, if the mixture of antigens consists of only four or five, then serial dilution immunoelectrophoresis can be practical.

This type of test is simplified somewhat by diluting reference antigens to match the unknown, instead of diluting the unknown mixture to match the reference antigens (Robyn *et al.*, 1963). For example, a battery of immunoelectropherograms using serial dilutions of a standard mixture of antigens[13] can be prepared, and the immunoelectropherograms washed, dried, and stained. Then, these can be used to make visual comparisons with immunoelectropherograms of unknown mixtures similarly prepared but at only one concentration.

QUANTITATION BY PRECIPITIN ARC POSITION

As was described in Chapter 4, the measured position of a precipitin band between sources of antigen and antiserum can be used to quantitate antigen in double diffusion tests (cf. Fig. 4.4). This technique also can be used for quantitative immunoelectrophoresis (Russell, 1965; Betsuyaku *et al.*, 1964). But its shortcomings just in double diffusion plate tests are so magnified for immunoelectrophoresis tests as to make it impractical for all but the simplest systems.

[13] Defining a "standard mixture" has been one of the largest obstacles to quantitative immunodiffusion tests of all kinds. Because the concentrations of several antigens in the sera of normal people vary over wide ranges, to refer to a "normal serum" is impractical (Krøll *et al.*, 1970). An arbitrary solution to this problem is to use a pool of normal sera to prepare a standard in which individual differences average out. But a more definitive solution might be to synthesize a "normal" serum by mixing purified samples of each of the component antigens together in absolute concentrations and relative proportions which have been determined to be normal median values for each, individually—no mean undertaking.

QUANTITATION BY RADIOIMMUNOELECTROPHORESIS

The technique of microdensitometrically scanning precipitin bands has been adapted to reliably determining the amount of radiolabeled antigen in a precipitin arc by scanning the darkened area corresponding to the precipitate on the radioautograph negative (Von der Decken, 1967). This sophisticated technique requires reagents and equipment not readily accessible to most laboratories, and it adds to the several immunologic variables, which must be recognized and controlled, several more relating to producing and scanning the radioautograph. For example, acceptable results are obtained when only a moderate amount of carrier (i.e., nonlabeled) antigen is used and the density of the radioautograph image is measured during linear increase of reduction of the silver grains in the photographic emulsion. This method therefore is mainly suited to careful quantitation of a few antigens separable and identifiable by electrophoretic fractionation.

QUANTITATION BY ABSORPTION

The principle of adding increasing quantities of antigen to succeeding samples of antiserum and testing these samples for residual capacity to precipitate the same antigen in an immunodiffusion test can be applied also to immunoelectrophoresis (West et al., 1961; Mackiewicz and Fenrych, 1965). Thus, if a known quantity of antigen is required to neutralize corresponding antibodies in an antiserum, then determining the concentration of an unknown mixture of antigens containing this one which will just neutralize the same antiserum indirectly indicates how much of this antigen is present in the mixture. For this technique, the capacity of immunoelectrophoresis to clearly resolve many different antigens in a complex mixture is a large advantage, because even if these are not known by name they can all be quantitated relatively by adding the entire mixture in increasing quantities to a standard antiserum and comparing the immunoelectrophoretic pattern developed by this mixture with that developed by the unabsorbed antiserum. This method therefore offers simultaneous multiple quantitative analyses which can be either absolute or relative. However, it is handicapped by the same major problem affecting quantitations by serial dilution—namely, that several tests must be performed to quantitate several antigens in just one mixture.

A self-adjusting exception to this handicap is to use this technique for qualitative analyses in which two similar mixtures of antigens are compared with each other for relative contents of individual antigens. For example, different strains of sea herring which were too similar to be distinguished by qualitative differences of individual antigens in their sera could be differentiated by variations in relative quantities of their serum antigens (Di Capua, 1966). These differentiations were achieved by noting that sera from different kinds of herring were more effective in absorbing antibodies from homologous than from heterologous antisera as detected by immunoelectrophoresis. Absorption immunoelectrophoresis tests used in this manner thus are both quantitative and qualitative. Potentially they are very powerful, because they can detect and identify quantitative differences among individual antigens in a complex mixture and can be used for such purposes as studying taxonomic relationships, identifying antigenic markers diagnostic of certain diseases, and detecting tumor-specific antigens in a complex mixture of nontumor antigens.

RADIAL SINGLE DIFFUSION QUANTITATIVE IMMUNOELECTROPHORESIS

The single radial diffusion plate test has become a routine clinical laboratory technique for quantitating several human serum antigens because it is easy and its results are clear. Since the diameter of the disc of precipitate developing in this test is proportional to the amount of antigen forming the disc (see Chapter 3), any of many antigen concentrations can be measured directly and from just one test. After appropriate preliminary standardization, it does not require multiple dilutions or absorptions and a corresponding number of separate tests to adjust the concentration of an unknown antigen to a certain level before it can be measured accurately. Probably first suggested for such use by Backhausz in 1961 (Seligmann, 1961), quantitative immunoelectrophoresis tests based on the principles and practice of the radial single diffusion plate test indeed have been developed (Afonso, 1964b, 1966a,b). Unfortunately, their potential has yet to be exploited.[14]

The principles of this technique, illustrated in Figs. 5.7 and 5.8, were discussed earlier in this chapter. The procedure itself is simple. Antigen mixture is electrophoresed conventionally in agar gel. For instance, residual fluid from the origin hole is withdrawn and replaced with molten agar of the same concentration as the electrophoresis gel. Edges of the gel which will not be involved in the subsequent immunoprecipitation are trimmed away and discarded to conserve antiserum and to avoid the irregular thickness characteristic of edges. An appropriate

---

[14] This technique also is used for qualitative analysis (Wilson, 1964; Cordoba *et al.*, 1966). The electropherogram is covered with a thin layer of agar, this is flooded with antiserum, and electrophoretically separated antigens are detected by specific immunoprecipitation. A two-dimensional variation of this technique (Yokoyama and Carr, 1962) is described in Chapter 7.

volume of antiserum trace-labeled with bromphenol blue is dropped on the surface of the remaining gel; between 0.3 and 0.45 ml will be required for a 6×5-cm area. This is spread evenly on the surface with a bent glass rod which is rubbed lightly on the gel in all directions until the antiserum has worked in. Even distribution is indicated by even coloring of the gel with bromphenol blue. The plate then is held for 16 hours at room temperature for immunoprecipitation to develop. Finally, to facilitate readings, the immunoelectropherogram is washed for 2 hours or more in 0.9% saline and then soaked in 1% acetic acid for 10 minutes to intensify antigen–antibody precipitates.

Better results sometimes can be obtained by allowing electropherograms to stand for 4.5 hours at 30°C before applying antiserum at 4 to 5 μl/cm^2 to the trimmed agar surface, reapplying antiserum 1 hour later at the same concentration, and then letting immunoprecipitation continue to develop at 30°C for 10 to 12 hours more (Afonso, 1966a). The diameter of a halo of precipitate is measured in millimeters on a 2.5$\times$ photograph of the plate, and it can be transformed into quantity data with a nomogram (Afonso, 1966a).

If all the precautions that experience has shown necessary for quantitative radial single diffusion plate tests also are taken with this similar quantitative immunoelectrophoretic technique, it will give reliable data (cf. Afonso, 1966a). A criticism that two substances diffusing in the same region may influence each other's diffusion rates and therefore mutually distort their respective quantitations (Benaš, 1967) is more theoretical than practical when a mixture of antigens is used for standardization (see footnote 13). Perhaps the step in this technique most vulnerable to error is that of infusing antiserum into the gel after electrophoresis, but if a positive standard control always is run with the unknown, as is recommended for radial single diffusion plates too, then measurements of the discs of precipitate for antigens in the unknown mixture can be compared with those of analogous discs in the reference mixture, and this problem will be minimized.

From some experience with this technique we have devised the following minor alterations and improvements. Double-width microscope slides are used rather than the larger plates originally suggested. These are used with 1% agarose instead of agar and are precoated with agarose. Their gel is cast by the sandwich technique for flat uniformity. The sample to be analyzed is soaked into the surface of the gel from a saturated disc of paper for a defined period of time at 4°C, and the disc is removed before electrophoresis. After electrophoresis, antiserum is applied evenly to the surface of the gel by the technique described in detail in Chapter 6 for two-dimensional single electroimmunodiffusion. Essentially, this is to spread and hold it evenly over the surface of the gel layer for several minutes at room temperature (time and temperature vary with antiserum strength) by resting an uncoated glass plate on spacers a fraction of a millimeter above the surface of the gel. Alternatively, the antiserum is spread evenly by laying a film of Mylar slightly smaller than the electrophoresis slide on the antiserum (about 0.3 ml) placed on the gel: as the Mylar is laid down from center out, it will spread the antiserum evenly over the surface of the gel. Film of this kind can be cut and used to spread a smaller volume of antiserum only over the areas of electrophoresis so that none is wasted on the edges of the electropherogram. After the Mylar film or glass slide is removed, any excess fluid remaining on the surface of the gel is rinsed off with a jet of distilled water, the slide is drained briefly, and immunoprecipitation is allowed to develop overnight at 4°C instead of room temperature. Following this, the slide is washed, stained for proteins, and dried; then the results are read.

Radial single diffusion immunoelectrophoresis can, of course, be used for just qualitative analyses (Yokoyama and Carr, 1962). Because the effect of antibodies on antigens is similar to the effect of protein-precipitating fixatives but is different in being immunologically specific, this technique recently was termed "immunofixation electrophoresis" (Alper and Johnson, 1969). As such it has been used with starch, as well as agar gel, with the attendant advantages of starch for molecular sieving.

IMMUNOELECTROFOCUSING

The principle of isoelectric focusing, as explained in Chapter 1, is to separate populations of charged antigens from each other by rapidly creating a stable pH gradient in the electropherogram so that each population will migrate to an area corresponding to its isoelectric point (Longsworth, 1967). This technique is especially useful as a preparatory tool because of the relatively large quantities of macromolecules which it can handle without strain (cf. also Svendsen and Rose, 1970). Isoelectric focusing also has been used on a reduced scale in place of conventional zone electrophoresis to separate antigens before they are precipitated by their antibodies—that is, in what is called "immunoelectrofocusing" (Catsimpoolas, 1969). In a two-step procedure, antigens are electrofocused in a column of polyacrylamide, and then this is embedded in agar for immunoprecipitation with antiserum (Catsimpoolas, 1969). A one-step procedure was performed in the following manner (Riley and Coleman, 1968).

A microscope slide was covered with 1.5% agarose gel prepared in 2% Ampholine (trademark name for mixtures of small peptides which create the required pH gradient during electrophoresis), at pH 3 to 10, charged with human serum as in routine immunoelectrophoresis, and electrophoresed for 5 hours at 15 volts between a 2% ethylenediamine cathode buffer and 1% phosphoric acid anode buffer. After electrophoresis the slide was submerged in neutral 1.0 M phosphate buffer for 4 minutes, to adjust it throughout to the same pH, and drained briefly. Then antiserum wells were filled, and precipitin arcs were allowed to develop as in conventional immunoelectropherograms.

An agarose immunoelectrofocusogram of serum antigens looks like a conventional agarose immunoelectropherogram, except that arcs of precipitate are found on both sides of the origin because they are formed by antigens segregating by isoelectric point in the pH gradient spreading across the entire length of the electropherogram (Riley and Coleman, 1968). Resolution does not seem to be any better than in immunoelectrophoresis, and, since antigens separate in agarose immunoelectrophoresis mostly by difference in electric charge (i.e., isoelectric point) too, isoelectric focusing does not at present seem to offer any special advantages for antigen separation in nonsieving gels over ordinary zone electrophoresis in immunoelectrophoretic analyses. It does cost more and is slightly more complicated to perform.

From the time of its invention in 1953 until just recently, immunoelectrophoresis has been the most versatile and effective technique available for analyzing complex antigens and their mixtures. Although currently it is being challenged strongly for this position by its close relative electroimmunodiffusion, it is sure to continue being used for many years as the reliable and powerful immunochemical tool it has so often proved itself to be.

Chapter 6

Electroimmunodiffusion

In the immunodiffusion technique described in previous chapters, antigen and antiserum are mixed solely by diffusion. This chapter discusses electroimmunodiffusion techniques in which either antigen or antibodies or both are intermingled electrophoretically.

The basic idea for this potent variety of immunodiffusion test has been known for nearly two decades, but until recently it has received scant attention. This is because earlier, generally simpler immunodiffusion techniques were themselves so effective that the outstanding potentialities of electroimmunodiffusion were not yet needed and were overlooked. Now, its reintroduction with improved technology, and a growing acquaintance of its capabilities as demonstrated by the still relatively few but striking published examples of its use, are sure to attract intense interest, and electroimmunodiffusion will become the foremost technique for immunochemical analyses.

History

The following is a passage from the first edition of "Immunodiffusion" (Crowle, 1961), pp. 239–240:

> Several years ago Macheboeuf and co-workers (1953) showed that if antigen solution were streaked across the width of a strip of filter paper at one place and antiserum at another, so that upon subsequent electrophoresis antigen and antibody would cross each other, they would complex and become fixed to the paper. Other antigens and antiserum constituents not entering into this reaction remained soluble and could be washed from the paper strip leaving only the fixed aggregate demonstrable by later staining. A procedure resembling this but capable of locating electrophoresed agglutinins or anti-

353

bodies which react only with insoluble antigens, which cannot be used in routine immunoelectrophoresis, consists of electrophoresing an antiserum on a slip of paper and then spraying antigen suspension onto the strip (Bustamante, 1957; Buttery, 1959). As in Macheboeuf's technique, antigen and antibody form fixed, insoluble, stainable complexes. Macheboeuf's technique of causing antibody to cross antigen during electrophoresis and precipitate it also has been used in agar gel. Tuberculoprotein, with an affinity for the anode, was placed in a column of agar in a glass tube behind its antiserum. During electrophoresis, the protein migrated toward the anode and the antibody toward the cathode, both invisibly, and upon meeting they formed a heavy, immobile precipitin band between their respective origins and nearest the antiserum origin (Crowle, 1956). This reaction was complete within about 20 minutes. The practical uses of this technique have not yet been explored, although Bussard and Huet (1959) point out, on the basis of similar experiments which they carried out, that its forceful acceleration of immunodiffusion reactions may be useful when heavy molecular weight antigens and antibodies are used, cutting the time required for them to diffuse and precipitate from days to minutes. The technique's greatest shortcoming is that several antigens in a crude mixture might migrate in the same direction as antibody and therefore not ever encounter it. Libich (1959) independently has developed this kind of technique into a method for demonstrating graphically, and in one experiment, precipitation under optimal reactant ratios as well as the breadth of the optimal reaction range. He believes that his method can be used advantageously to study the nature of antigen–antibody reactions. Conceivably, the basic technique of causing antigen to migrate electrophoretically across antibody might be used in other media, particularly in starch gels in which immunodiffusion reactions so far have not been demonstrated, perhaps because reactant diffusibility is so low in this medium.

Slight modifications of these early one-dimensional double electroimmunodiffusion tests, in which both antigen and antibodies migrate electrophoretically, now are used routinely for such purposes as rapidly screening transfusion bloods for hepatitis-associated virus (see below). Two-dimensional double electroimmunodiffusion apparently was first described independently by Bon and Swanborn (1965) and by Crowle and Hu in 1965. It does not appear to have been used since that time.

In 1960 Newton Ressler described the forerunner of present single electroimmunodiffusion tests, analogous to single diffusion with only one reactant migrating electrophoretically, and also demonstrated its application to two-dimensional analyses (Ressler, 1960a,b). In 1962 (Ressler et al., 1962) he used this technique to detect cancer-specific antigens in human serum.

Ressler's reports excited little of the attention that they deserved because his techniques were more difficult than those of conventional immunoelectrophoresis which at that time was undergoing its widest and most rapid development, and because no practical techniques for producing a nonelectroosmotic gelling agent which would be suitable for immunodiffusion reactions, like agarose, were yet known. This second problem probably is the principal reason that development of double electroimmunodiffusion antedated development of single electroimmuno- diffusion, since the electroosmosis of agar gels aided performance of the former but detracted from application of the latter. Fortunately, at about the same time that Ressler was performing his experiments, Hjertén was working out a suitable means for preparing agarose from laboratory agar. When in 1961 he described his technique, and the properties of agarose as well, this problem was surmounted and Ressler's technique became practical.[1]

While double electroimmunodiffusion unobtrusively was becoming es- tablished as a very rapid and more sensitive alternative to double diffusion plate tests which also could detect antigens too large to diffuse readily through agar gels (e.g., Jameson, 1968; Merétey, 1969; Nasz et al., 1967; Howe et al., 1967; Regetli and Weintraub, 1964; White et al., 1971; Bon and Swanborn, 1965; Rawstron and Farthing, 1962; Gocke and Howe, 1970; Watson and Whinfrey, 1958), interest in single electroimmunodiffu- sion lay dormant until 1966, when Laurell showed how this technique could be used for quantitating antigens in place of and with several advan- tages over single diffusion plate tests (Laurell, 1966). Hartley et al. (1966) made the same development almost simultaneously and also in- vented the term "electroimmunodiffusion" and its abbreviation EID (Hartley et al., 1966; Merrill et al., 1967). One year earlier Laurell had been able to resurrect Ressler's two-dimensional technique in a form made practical by the availability of agarose (Laurell, 1965a,b).

One- and two-dimensional double electroimmunodiffusion tests origi- nally were developed as miniaturized techniques, because they were adapted directly from corresponding micro double diffusion or immuno- electrophoresis. This was also true of one-dimensional single electro- immunodiffusion tests. But two-dimensional single electroimmunodiffu- sion tests evolved more along traditions of two-dimensional starch block electrophoresis and until recently therefore have been performed on large glass plates often requiring expensive quantities of reagents. Lately two laboratories (Crowle, 1972; Firestone and Aronson, 1969) have used variations of the Yokoyama-Carr (1962) and Afonso (1964b) methods for applying antiserum to gel medium to reduce the scale of two-dimensional single electroimmunodiffusion to that of conventional microimmunoelectrophoresis.

The technology of electroimmunodiffusion thus has developed enough

---

[1] Techniques are now available for chemically altering agar to either decrease or increase its electronegativity or even to change it to a positively charged gel (Ragetli and Weintraub, 1966; see Chapter 2).

to make of it a practical, valuable, and versatile addition to the family of immunodiffusion tests. That basic understanding of its unique characteristic of antigen–antibody interaction within an electric field still is only fragmentary (cf. Merétey, 1969; Jameson, 1969b) will not deter its empirical and effective application.

Theory and Mechanisms

As has already been indicated, there are four varieties of electroimmunodiffusion, these being analogous to similar varieties of immunodiffusion. One-dimensional single and double electroimmunodiffusion correspond, respectively, to single and double diffusion tests; used in two-dimensional form, these become analogs of the single diffusion and double diffusion immunoelectrophoresis tests described in Chapter 5 (see Figs. 6.1 through 6.5). Understanding these comparisons facilitates both theoretical comprehension and practical application of an otherwise rather bewildering array of electroimmunodiffusion tests. They are recognized, then, as having only one really new and rather unexplored characteristic—antigen–antibody reactions occurring during electrophoresis. Most other aspects of electroimmunodiffusion can be understood from general information which can be interpolated directly from simpler varieties of immunodiffusion.

Antigen–Antibody Precipitation in Electroimmunodiffusion

The basic principles of antigen–antibody precipitation affecting various other types of imunodiffusion test also affect electroimmunodiffusion, but there are some additional peculiarities to the latter. The two most distinct are, first, that antigen and antibodies are forced together very rapidly, and, second, that antiserum antibodies are separated from other antiserum components more than in other kinds of immunodiffusion tests.

As has already been explained in Chapter 1, the primary stage of antigen–antibody precipitation occurs quite rapidly. Presumably,[2] then, this reaction develops as well in electroimmunodiffusion tests as in other immunodiffusion tests. In the latter, other than during the earliest stages of a single diffusion test, the second stage of antigen–antibody complex aggregation into stable, visible precipitates has considerable time to mature, and conditions for this maturation are ideal in double diffusion tests. But in electroimmunodiffusion, conditions for growth of secondary

---

[2] Some speculation is necessary for this chapter because little theoretical information is yet available on the mechanisms of antigen–antibody precipitation in electroimmunodiffusion.

complexes can range from almost nil, when a cloud of antigen molecules passes rapidly through a cloud of antibody molecules migrating equally fast in the opposite direction and complexes have no time to grow large enough to precipitate (e.g., in one-dimensional double electroimmunodiffusion effected at high voltage), to excellent, when the front of one reactant migrates into a field of the other, becomes progressively weaker, and finally reaches equilibrium with the other (e.g., in one-dimensional single electroimmunodiffusion.)

ONE-DIMENSIONAL SINGLE ELECTROIMMUNODIFFUSION

Antigen solution is deposited in a well in agarose gel charged with an appropriate concentration of antiserum (Laurell, 1966; Fig. 6.1). Electrophoretic current is applied, and the antigen (e.g., human serum albumin) migrates out of its origin toward the anode and into the antiserum-charged gel. At a pH of 8.2 to 8.6, usually used, the antibodies meanwhile either remain stationary or migrate slightly toward the cathode (Krøll *et al.*, 1970). As the concentrated spearhead of antigen migrates into the diffuse and uniform surrounding field of antibodies, its advancing front complexes with antibodies that it encounters. But even at the relatively low voltages typical of electroimmunodiffusion, this spearhead moves quite rapidly in comparison with migration of antigen in immunodiffusion, which is solely by diffusion. Consequently, in the center of the direction of electrophoresis, complexing of antigen with antibody occurs in conditions of extreme antigen excess during most of the test. Indeed, there is frequently no visible precipitation at the anodic tip of antigen migration (Salvaggio *et al.*, 1970). Individual antibody molecules are complexing with pairs of antigen molecules, and these triads remain soluble and moderately diffusible, and probably acquire

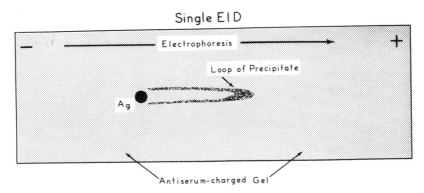

Single EID

Electrophoresis

Loop of Precipitate

Ag

Antiserum-charged Gel

Fig. 6.1. Diagram showing one-dimensional single electroimmunodiffusion as it can be performed on a microscope slide.

electrophoretic characteristics intermediate between those of the antigen and antibodies individually.

While this is occurring, antigen molecules lateral to the central path of electrophoretic migration also are combining with antibodies, and the farther lateral they are, the less they are reenforced by succeeding influx of fresh antigen, since the main stream of antigen movement is along the central path of electrophoretic migration. Consequently, antibody molecules along the edge of this path have more chance to complex antigen in precipitating ratios, the complexes formed therefore are larger and have lower mobility, and antigen–antibody complexes have more time to equilibrate into a stable precipitate. Moreover, the formation of this nondiffusible precipitate steepens the gradient of relative antigen decrease toward the edges of the path of electrophoresis by the sink effect (see Chapter 1) and thus further encourages balancing of antigen with antibody laterally. Hence, although there is frequently no visible precipitation of antigen in the immediate path of antigen electrophoresis, during single electroimmunodiffusion two lateral lines of precipitate do appear and grow upward and inward toward each other as the test develops.

Precipitation of the antigen along the periphery of electrophoretic migration and, especially, its complexing with antibody more centrally dilute the population of free antigen as it migrates farther and farther into the antibody-charged gel. Consequently, there is progressively less to diffuse laterally, which is why the two lateral lines of precipitate converge. When antigen is used at a concentration that is only moderately excessive relative to its antibody, and optimal for antigen quantitation by electroimmunodiffusion (Laurell, 1966; Merrill *et al.*, 1967), the population of antigen molecules will be depleted and will narrow fairly rapidly and steadily by attrition of complexing with antibodies; and it will form a loop of precipitate, resembling the trail of a comet or rocket, as it is electrophoresed (hence the name "rocket electrophoresis").

If the original quantity of antigen is very large, or if the antibody concentration is very small, or if antigen and antibody develop H-type precipitation, convergence of the lateral lines of precipitate will be negligible for the duration of electrophoresis, and they will end diffusely without joining (cf. Fig. 6.7). If electrophoresis is sufficiently prolonged to dilute the excessive reactant to a range of beginning moderate excess, they may converge toward each other anodally in various patterns ranging from a diffuse blunt-ended front of precipitate to one that begins to resemble the rocket of precipitation in the better balanced tests. When antibody is excessive, no precipitate will form outside the origin at all. Figure 6.2 illustrates the appearance of loops of precipitate formed by

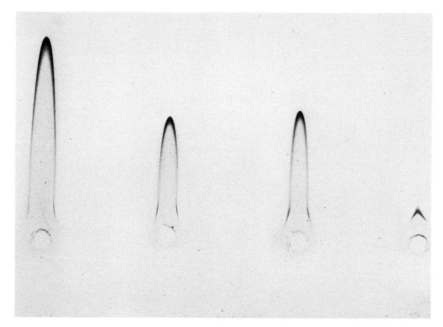

Fig. 6.2. Example of quantitative one-dimensional single electroimmunodiffusion as performed with human serum on a microscope slide in agarose charged with antiserum to α_1-antitrypsin. The left loop was produced by serum with a normal level of this antigen. The one on the right indicates a 90% deficiency of this antigen. The two central loops indicate moderate deficiencies. The badly deficient serum **was** obtained from a patient with severe emphysema, and the moderately deficient sera from his two daughters. Results from this type of test can be returned to a physician in less than 3 hours after blood was drawn. (Antiserum courtesy ICL Scientific, Fountain Valley, California.)

different concentrations of antigen over a range balanced well enough with antiserum to provide useful quantitative data.

The preceding description of events fits antigens like human serum albumin which move rapidly toward the anode during electrophoresis. But other antigens, like serum β-globulins, migrate less rapidly in that direction because they have lower net negative electric charges. Under given conditions of electrophoresis,[3] these antigens will have proportionally longer to react with their antibodies; therefore, they will tend to form heavier, stronger, more slowly elongating loops of precipitate, and

---

[3] Changes in buffer pH or ionic strength, or in voltage applied to the electropherogram, can profoundly affect the outcome of an electroimmunodiffusion test by promoting or impairing the secondary aspects of precipitation, either directly by changing reactant mobilities or indirectly by affecting growth of antigen–antibody lattices.

the lateral borders of these precipitates will tend to converge more sharply. Practically, this is important because on the one hand quantitative conditions for these antigens to form chevrons of precipitate which are closed-ended and sharp-tipped and therefore appropriate for quantitating them will be broader; but on the other hand, these chevrons will be shorter and quantitative differences therefore will physically be less easily measurable (Salvaggio et al., 1970).

The data above apply primarily to antigen–antibody systems with R-type precipitating characteristics. Systems with H-type characteristics tend to form parallel-sided, open-ended "loops" of precipitate because forming antigen–antibody complexes are so labile that very little antigen is lost from the migrating front. On the other hand, using an H-type antiserum will not necessarily result in H-type precipitation. Thus, whether a horse antiserum will precipitate in this manner appears to depend vitally on the nature of the antigen being precipitated (cf. Fig. 6.9). Antigen quantitation by electroimmunodiffusion will be more difficult with H-type than with R-type precipitation.

At pH 8.2, usually used for serum antigen analyses, some antigens like serum γ_1-globulins remain stationary in agarose. If they are electrophoretically homogeneous they do not form practically measurable rockets of precipitate. However, if they consist of a moderately heterogeneous electrophoretic population, again like serum γ_1-globulins, they will develop modest loops of precipitate on both anodic and cathodic sides of the origin. Human serum IgG can be quantitated at its mean isoelectric point by measuring the final distance between anodic and cathodic tips of the loops of its precipitate in single electroimmunodiffusion (Krøll, 1970; Grubb, 1970). Raising or lowering buffer pH (Rebeyrotte et al., 1969), or using agar instead of agarose (Merrill et al., 1967), will make such an antigen migrate. Since these alterations in technique also will affect the precipitins being used similarly, these antibodies must be applied either all around the source of antigen (Merrill et al., 1967) or as nearly so as is practical (Rebeyrotte et al., 1969). There are alternative frequently better ways of studying antigens with the same electrophoretic mobilities as precipitins in electroimmunodiffusion. One is to select precipitins with different electrophoretic mobility from an alternative species of animal (see Chapter 2 and Fig. 6.17). Another is to change the isoelectric point of either antigen or of precipitins artificially, such as by carbamylation (Weeke, 1968a,b).[4]

Basic antigens like lysozyme will migrate toward the cathode at pH

---

[4] One volume of antigen solution is mixed with 2 volumes of $2\,M$ potassium cyanate, allowed to stand for 18 hours at room temperature, and then dialyzed against electrophoresis buffer to remove most of the potassium cyanate (Weeke, 1968a).

8.2 or less and can be detected, studied, and quantitated by single electroimmunodiffusion in agarose like the more often studied acidic antigens which migrate toward the cathode (Grubb, 1970).

Two-Dimensional Single Electroimmunodiffusion

The phenomena and conditions affecting antigen–antibody precipitation in one-dimensional single electroimmunodiffusion tests are similar to those in two-dimensional single electroimmunodiffusion. In this technique, also called "antigen–antibody crossed electrophoresis" (Laurell, 1965a), a mixture of antigens is separated electrophoretically and then, by a second electrophoresis at right angles to the first, the separated antigens are moved into gel charged with analytic polyvalent antiserum (Krøll, 1970; Fig. 6.3). The chevron of precipitate formed by each separate antigen is similar to that which would have formed had this antigen been used alone in a one-dimensional single electroimmunodiffusion test. One significant interpretational difference between the one- and two-dimensional tests, the same as that between analogous single diffusion and immunoelectrophoresis tests, is that cross-reacting antigens which affect each others' precipitation in the one-dimensional test may not do so in the two-dimensional test because they have been separated from each other electrophoretically before being analyzed immunologically. Hence, the two-dimensional test can detect and quantitate two or more electrophoretically distinct isomers of a given antigen which to the one-dimensional test appear to be a single antigenic population (Laurell, 1965b).

One-Dimensional Double Electroimmunodiffusion

This type of test is known also as "countercurrent immunoelectrophoresis" and "counterimmunoelectrophoresis" (Crowle, 1961; Howe *et al.*, 1967), "electroprecipitation" (Rawstron and Farthing, 1962; Watson, 1960; Zydeck *et al.*, 1966), "electrosyneresis" (Merétey, 1969), and "immunoosmophoresis" (Bon and Swanborn, 1963, 1965).[5] In it, the properties of buffers, semisolid media, and reactants are employed to electrophorese antigen and antibody in opposite directions simultaneously so that, analogous to a double diffusion test, they will meet, react,

[5] In a medium like cellulose acetate (Zydeck *et al.*, 1966), polyacrylamide (Fitschen, 1963), or filter paper (Lang, 1955), antibodies either are stationary or move slightly toward the anode at pH 8.2 to 8.6. A negatively charged antigen placed cathodic to the antibodies therefore overtakes them during electrophoresis and is precipitated during this transmigration. This variety of double electroimmunodiffusion therefore has been called "transmigration electrophoresis" (Lang, 1955) or "immunotransmigration" (Zydeck *et al.*, 1966).

2-D Single EID

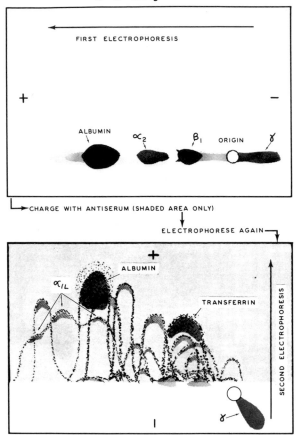

Fig. 6.3. Diagrammatic explanation of two-dimensional single electroimmuno-diffusion as described in the text. The pattern of separated human serum antigens shown in the upper rectangle was drawn directly from a photographic projection of the antigens after they had been stained; the pattern of loops of precipitate in the lower rectangle was drawn similarly after second electrophoresis into horse antiserum. Tests from which these patterns were drawn were performed on double-width microscope slides in 0.75% agarose in pH 8.2 barbital buffer of ionic strength 0.025.

and precipitate somewhere between their respective origins (Fig. 6.4). A classic example is to react serum albumin with its antiserum in agar gel at pH 8.2. The albumin moves electrophoretically toward the anode while the γ-globulin precipitins of the antiserum migrate by electro-osmosis toward the cathode. Under suitable conditions antigen–antibody precipitation develops within a few minutes (cf. Fig. 6.20).

Double electroimmunodiffusion is more susceptible to such adverse

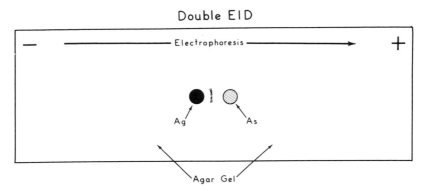

Fig. 6.4. Diagram showing one-dimensional double electroimmunodiffusion such as can be performed on a microscope slide as explained in the text.

conditions as antigen excess than single electroimmunodiffusion because both reactants are migrating at once as finite zones. Little time is available for visible second-stage antigen–antibody complexes to accumulate; and since the two reactants confront each other as two zones nearly the same size as their origins, if these are short (e.g., coming from round wells), precipitating proportions of reactants may not be achieved in the consequently modest range of antigen–antibody ratios that will develop as the zones intermingle (contrast Figs. 6.14 and 6.22). The reactants must be used at nearer to precipitating ratios in their origins than in other kinds of immunodiffusion test, since they originally meet in nearly the same concentrations as they were at their origins. Only during the brief course of their encounter do they have a chance to adjust themselves to precipitating ratios as some of each becomes immobilized or altered electrophoretically by reaction with the other. Obviously, for these tests origins elongated in the direction of electrophoresis are better than round holes for optimal capacity to detect the largest number of several different antigen–antibody systems, or for detecting a single system in a single test when its optimal proportions ratio is unknown (Jameson, 1968). Moreover, if reactants used in hole origins are not electrophoretically in line with each other, oppositely migrating zones of antigen and antibodies may miss each other and not react, or they may graze each other and form a slanted trace of precipitation in the gel which can be misinterpreted as some kind of artifact (Nasz *et al.*, 1967).

If precipitation does not occur, or if it reverses before it is noticed, the test becomes irretrievably negative because each zone continues its migration independently on toward the electrode attracting it (Merétey, 1969).

Double electroimmunodiffusion therefore exhibits considerable disadvantages. Why, then, should it ever be used instead of other immunodiffusion tests? The reason is that it also has large advantages. It is faster and more economical (Culliford, 1964; Ragetli and Weintraub, 1964; Bon and Swanborn, 1965); it is more sensitive (Culliford, 1964; Ragetli and Weintraub, 1964; Jameson, 1968); it can be used with antigen molecules too large to simply diffuse appreciably through agar gels (Nasz et al., 1967; Ragetli and Weintraub, 1965); and it can detect inefficient antibodies which in routine immunodiffusion tests form too diffuse and ephemeral a precipitate to be seen (Crowle and Hu, 1965).

Most of its disadvantages can be minimized mechanically (Jameson, 1968). Thus, the rate of electrophoretic migration can be kept low by using lower voltage and higher ionic strength than is employed in immunoelectrophoresis. One or both reactant origins can be rectangular instead of round, and one or both can be elongated along the path of electrophoresis or even wedge-shaped (see Fig. 6.21). None of these artifacts circumvents the still largely unexplored problem of reacting antigen with antiserum antibodies that have been separated from other antiserum constituents which may in some instances have a significant capacity to enhance precipitation of the antigen–antibody complexes (see Chapter 1). As was mentioned earlier in a discussion of reversed immunoelectrophoresis (Chapter 5), this may be a more important problem than is generally recognized. Therefore, it is discussed independently below.

Two-Dimensional Double Electroimmunodiffusion

Also called "two-dimensional immunoosmophoresis" (Bon and Swanborn, 1965), this technique resembles classic immunoelectrophoresis. A mixture of antigens[6] is separated electrophoretically, and then the separated antigens are detected by moving them electrophoretically against oppositely migrating precipitins (Crowle and Hu, 1965; Bon and Swanborn, 1965; Fig. 6.5). The pattern of arcs of precipitate which develops is like that in immunoelectrophoresis except that it develops in staggered array because of the progressively faster mobilities of the more anodic antigens, and the arcs and their interrelationships are revealed better (cf. Fig. 6.22).

The problems of one-dimensional double electroimmunodiffusion are somewhat muted in the two-dimensional technique because the antiserum is used in relatively large volume in a trough and chances for

[6] The reversed test in which antibodies are electrophoresed and detected by antigen, analogous to reversed immunoelectrophoresis, apparently has not yet been performed.

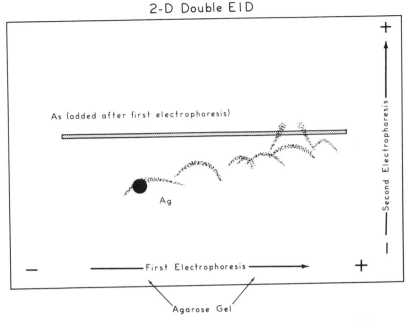

Fig. 6.5. Diagram showing two-dimensional double electroimmunodiffusion such as can be performed, for example, on a double-width microscope slide.

overwhelming antigen excess conditions to develop therefore are minimized. The resolution of this test for complex mixtures of antigens appears to be superior to that of classic immunoelectrophoresis. In other respects it seems to have the same advantages over immunoelectrophoresis as one-dimensional double electroimmunodiffusion has over conventional double diffusion tests, particularly that of speed, a double electroimmunodiffusion test being finished within as little as 30 minutes.

Isolation of Antibody during Electroimmunodiffusion

During single electroimmunodiffusion, antibodies are stationary while most other antiserum constituents migrate anodally leaving the antibodies alone to react with the influx of antigen(s). As was discussed in Chapter 1, reaction between antigen and antiserum in immunodiffusion tests often depends importantly on constituents of the antiserum other than the antibodies primarily involved in the specific reaction with antigen, formation of a precipitating complex is the net effect (both negative and positive) of all the antibodies present in an antiserum that are reactive with the antigen, and among these antibodies there will be electrophoretic heterogeneity. Indeed, normal serum is added to antigen being quantitated in radial single diffusion plates employing very dilute antiserum in order to achieve maximum sensitivity (Mancini, 1965). In electroimmunodiffusion, ammonium sulfate-purified rabbit antibodies are generally less effective for precipitating antigens than whole antiserum from which they have been derived; their effectiveness is restored by mixing them with normal rabbit serum (Crowle and Jarrett, unpublished observations). Consequently, significant differences probably will be seen between results obtained with electroimmunodiffusion tests and those obtained with comparable single diffusion tests. However, these probably will not be consistent because they themselves will depend on the nature of the antigen. Thus, antigen–antibody interaction may occur in a single electroimmunodiffusion test in the presence of most other antiserum constituents if the antigen is fast-migrating, in the presence of several if it is only moderately anodic, or in the presence of only γ_2-globulin antibodies if it tends to be cathodic. Hence, even if an antiserum has the same kind and quantity of antibodies for two different antigens, these may react somewhat differently in single electroimmunodiffusion because they develop in somewhat different milieu.

Apart from these considerations, there is also the probably significant difference of sequential reaction for antigen in an electroimmunodiffusion test. In classic single and double diffusion tests, antigen encounters most varieties of antibodies in an antiserum simultaneously, since these have the same diffusion coefficient.[7] But in single electroimmunodiffusion an antigen will encounter antibodies in cathodic–anodic sequence. Two antisera adjusted to equivalent precipitin titers by a single diffusion test for a given antigen could react differently in an electroimmunodiffusion comparison because in one the precipitins might be predominantly γ_1-globulins and in the other predominantly γ_2-globulins, and each might also contain substantial amounts of nonprecipitating antibodies of opposite globulin class.

This kind of sequential reaction may make electroimmunodiffusion tests more susceptible to secondary precipitation (see Chapter 1) than comparable immunodiffusion tests (note large number of "double" loops in Figs. 6.9 and 6.10). In addition to Liesegang precipitate-like phenomena and electrophoresis-induced gap–stria precipitation, one antigen–antibody system could generate more than one band of precipitate by sequential encounters with electrophoretically different classes of antibodies, and sequential exposure to other serum factors which can either interfere with or enhance precipitation.

[7] Exceptions in which 19 S antibodies constitute a significant proportion of the precipitins in an antiserum sometimes produce unexpected results; see Secondary Precipitation, Chapter 1.

These various effects probably will be bigger in double electroimmuno-diffusion tests; they probably also will be harder to recognize. For example, it is easy to conceive of the development of two precipitin bands by a single kind of antigen reacting with two electrophoretically different classes of antibodies in one antiserum. The more cathodic class would encounter and precipitate some of a fast-migrating anodic antigen but not be able to precipitate it all, whereupon this antigen might precipitate in a second band with a less cathodic class of precipitins. If the test were set up with hole origins, as is most commonly done, there would be little change in antigen–antibody ratio laterally and therefore no direct means for identifying two precipitin bands formed in this manner as being due to just one kind of antigen, as there is in the precipitin arc tip coalescence of Liesegang precipitation in double diffusion plate tests (cf. Chapter 4). It is also easy to imagine, on the basis of similar observations for double diffusion tests (Chapter 1), the formation of antigen–antibody complexes with a γ_2-globulin class of antibodies which become fixed in agar but do not precipitate, the precipitation of complexes of the same antigen and γ_1-globulin precipitins further toward the anode, and then the precipitation of the fixed γ_2-globulin–antigen complexes as antiserum complement (or complement from the antigen mixture itself if it is whole serum) migrates into the area of reaction.

The preceding inferred speculations on the effects of sequential reaction in electroimmunodiffusion tests remain yet to be rigorously proved, but until this has been done and our understanding of the mechanics of electroimmunodiffusion has been increased proportionally, users of this technique should interpret their data conservatively.

TECHNICAL FACTORS AFFECTING ELECTROIMMUNODIFFUSION

Conventional immunodiffusion and immunoelectrophoresis tests are affected by such factors as antigen concentration, reactant volumes, gel viscosity, the presence of various solutes like colloids, proteins, and detergents, and interactions of reactants with themselves. This is because the development of their reactions depends on intermingling of antigen and antibodies by diffusion alone, and all these factors affect reactant diffusion. In electroimmunodiffusion these factors are less important because reactant migration has a different, stronger motivation which overrides the generally weaker effects of these factors. However, they are significant when a sieving medium like polyacrylamide or starch gel is being used, and when electroimmunodiffusion is followed by a period of conventional immunodiffusion to allow precipitates to develop or to become more intense. Within practical limits compatible with electrophoresis, variations in temperature are of only minor importance in comparison with their weighty effects in other kinds of immunodiffusion test.

By contrast, using constant voltage probably is as significant to preventing gap–stria secondary precipitation during an electroimmunodiffusion test as maintaining constant incubation temperature is to the same end in single diffusion tests (see Fig. 1.11). Susceptibility to voltage change secondary precipitation appears to vary among different antigens even when they are reacting with the same antiserum in the same test. Thus, only one of three principal loops of precipitate shown in Fig. 6.6 has developed them (cf. also Fig. 6.7). True Liesegang precipitates also can develop in electroimmunodiffusion tests when antigen and its antibodies are approaching equilibrium from antigen excess, just as they do in conventional single and double diffusion tests (Fig. 6.6; cf. also Libich, 1959).

Because reaction between antigens and precipitins occurs so rapidly in electroimmunodiffusion tests, the location and distribution of re-

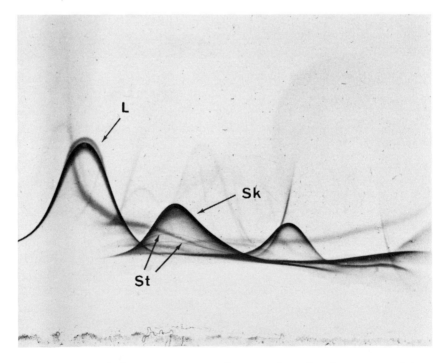

Fig. 6.6. Detail from a micro two-dimensional single electroimmunodiffusion analysis of human serum showing in particular Liesegang (L) precipitation, the formation of a skewed (Sk) loop of precipitate, and development by the antigen producing the skewed loop of two gap–stria artifacts (St).

actants is more important in electroimmunodiffusion than in conventional immunodiffusion. For instance, if antiserum is not evenly distributed for secondary electrophoresis in a two-dimensional single electroimmuno-diffusion analysis, waves may form in a loop of precipitate mimicking the presence of antigen isomers with different electrophoretic mobility (cf. Fig. 6.7).

INTERPRETING PATTERNS OF PRECIPITATION IN ELECTROIMMUNODIFFUSION

Classic patterns of precipitin band coalescence, partial coalescence, or crossing are evident in electroimmunodiffusion tests and have the same meaning as in other kinds of immunodiffusion test. However, the appearance of these patterns will be somewhat unfamiliar to the user of more conventional techniques, and some precipitin band shapes are unique to electroimmunodiffusion. A number of illustrations therefore accompany

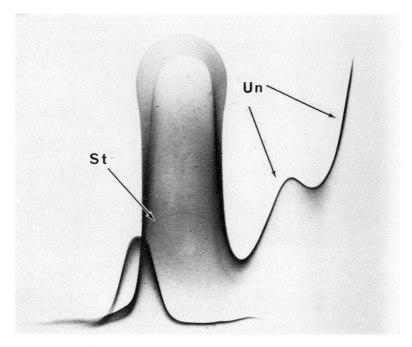

Fig. 6.7. Micro two-dimensional single electroimmunodiffusion of human serum using antiserum with antibodies to human serum albumin and to α_1-antitrypsin. This figure indicates a serologically balanced reaction (the antitrypsin loop) and one of large antigen excess (the high albumin loop and halo), a voltage-change stria (St), and abnormally rising loops of precipitate due to uneven distribution of antiserum in the gel during secondary electrophoresis (Un). (Antitrypsin antiserum courtesy ICL Scientific, Fountain Valley, California.)

the following discussion. They have been prepared from two-dimensional single electroimmunodiffusion tests in which most of these are best seen.

The greater the antibody–antigen ratio with antibody as the stationary phase in single electroimmunodiffusion, and/or the lesser the electrophoretic mobility for antigen, the more acutely and abruptly will a loop of precipitate peak (Laurell, 1966; Fig. 6.7; cf. also Fig. 6.2). Extremes of antibody–antigen ratio may range from so large as entirely to prevent antigen migration (Fig. 6.8) to so small as not significantly to impede it (cf. albumin, α_1-antitrypsin, transferrin, Fig. 6.9). For optimal quantitation of antigen by its interaction with a standardized quantity of antibody in single electroimmunodiffusion, the ratio should be intermediate between these two extremes (Figs. 6.2 and 6.7), so that the advance of the antigen front (i.e., peak of the loop of precipitate) in a given period of electrophoresis will be predictably proportional to the concentration of the antigen (Merrill *et al.*, 1967; Laurell, 1966). For qualitative analyses, such as in two-dimensional single electroimmuno-

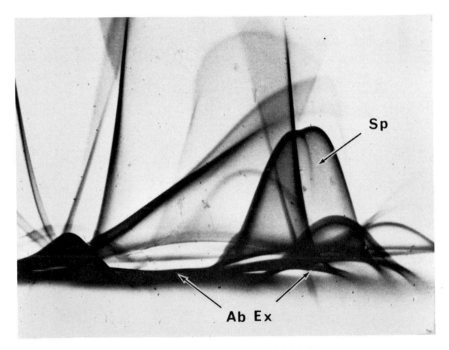

Fig. 6.8. Detail in the β_1 region of a micro two-dimensional single electroimmunodiffusion analysis of human serum showing in particular loops of precipitate kept flat during secondary electrophoresis by excess antibody, and the formation of a spur (Sp) in a reaction of partial identity between two electrophoretically and antigenically closely related β_1-globulins.

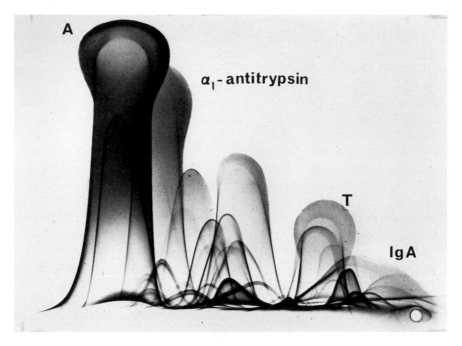

Fig. 6.9. Micro two-dimensional single electroimmunodiffusion pattern of human serum as analyzed with horse antiserum in agarose using pH 8.2 barbital buffer of ionic strength 0.025. The antiserum was applied by the technique shown in Fig. 2.6. A and T indicate albumin and transferrin, respectively. (Antiserum courtesy ICL Scientific, Fountain Valley, California.)

diffusion, variations in concentrations of antibodies in an antiserum to different antigens in either direction are advantageous because they increase resolution of different antigens from each other. Notice the excellent resolution thus attained with horse antiserum as shown in Fig. 6.9.

When the ratio of antigen to antibody is high, antigen will migrate at what is essentially its normal electrophoretic rate, not being significantly impeded by antibodies. Two lines of precipitate will form to either side of its migration as explained above, and at the end of electrophoresis there may be no visible evidence of its most advanced position. However, if the electroimmunodiffusogram is allowed to stand for several hours, a radial single diffusion reaction will develop around this position and a halo of precipitate will appear (Laurell, 1966; Figs. 6.7 and 6.9). The halo may form asymmetrically on a relatively symmetrical loop indicating, like the skewed loop (below), electrophoretic heterogeneity of the antigen (IgA, Figs. 6.9 and 6.14).

Skewed loops, in a background of symmetrical loops formed by unrelated antigens, indicate the presence of electrophoretically gradually varying heterogeneous antigen molecules (Fig. 6.6). The symmetrical loops indicate that this skewing is not an artifact of uneven contact between the electropherogram and electrode vessels during electrophoresis or uneven distribution of antiserum in the gel (cf. Fig. 6.7). A symmetrical loop itself (Fig. 6.7) indicates, of course, the presence of an electrophoretically homogeneous population of antigen molecules. Loops that coalesce with each other (Fig. 6.10; cf. also α_1 lipoprotein in Figs. 6.3 and 6.14) indicate the presence of two electrophoretically different but antigenically related populations of molecules (e.g., isomers, degradation products, electrophoretically different molecules complexed with a common antigen; Laurell, 1965b). Reactions of nonidentity (loops of precipitate crossing each other) are illustrated in many of the accompanying figures. Reactions of partial identity also may be observed; one is pointed out in Fig. 6.8.

Dropping a line from the apex of a loop of precipitate in two-dimensional single electroimmunodiffusion perpendicular to the path of first electrophoresis indicates the electrophoretic mobility of a given antigen somewhat more precisely than does the comparable technique in im-

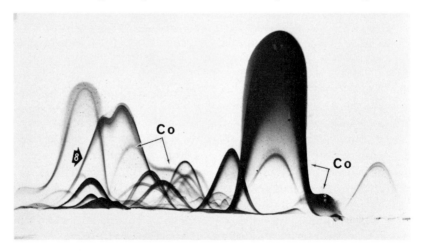

Fig. 6.10. Micro two-dimensional single electroimmunodiffusion pattern of human serum electrophoresed from left to right (the large, dark loop of precipitate is albumin) through 1% agarose containing 6% starch in pH 8.2 barbital buffer of ionic strength 0.025. Using the added starch during the first electrophoresis (second electrophoresis was through antiserum-charged agarose alone) revealed isomers of several antigens better than using agarose alone. Several pairs are readily evident as coalescing (Co) loops. One, as indicated by the large arrow, developed a loop of precipitate with a series of eight coalescing peaks.

munoelectrophoresis. Independent values for diffusion coefficient or quantity of a given antigen can be obtained by measuring the distance between the "legs" of a loop just above the path of first electrophoresis, and the diameter of the halo of precipitate which forms on standing of an electroimmunodiffusogram in conditions of antigen excess. The first measurement is of a purely physical value, since it results from diffusion of the antigen during the time of primary electrophoresis; the second measurement is of both immunological and physical effects and is analogous to measuring precipitate disc diameter in a quantitative radial single diffusion plate test (Chapter 3). In appropriate ranges of anti-body–antigen ratio when the loop of precipitate peaks sharply and is high enough to be measured accurately, the quantity of a given antigen can be determined by the height or, preferably, the area of its loop of precipitate (Firestone and Aronson, 1969; Laurell, 1966; Merrill *et al.*, 1967); and in two electroimmunodiffusograms prepared under similar conditions with the same antiserum, relative quantities of all antigens forming sharply peaking loops of precipitate can be determined simultaneously (Krøll, 1968a).

Since the characteristics of precipitin loops in electroimmunodiffusion tests depend as much on the characteristics and concentration of the antibodies in an antiserum specifically reacting with a given antigen, some of the interpretations mentioned above for characteristics of antigens also provide information on their antibodies. For instance, using two different antisera for preparing comparable electroimmunodiffuso-grams of the same mixture of antigens compares them for varieties and specificities of precipitin content, and for the quality and quantity of these precipitins. As in other immunodiffusion tests, the nature of the loops of precipitate (e.g., fine versus broad) indicates whether the pre-dominating precipitin to a given antigen in an antiserum is H-type, R-type, or some intermediate type. Contrast Figs. 6.9 and 6.14.

Techniques

One-Dimensional Single Electroimmunodiffusion

This technique most frequently has been used to quantitate antigens, but it can also be used for identifying antigens in a mixture and for quantitating and comparing antibodies against individual antigens in different antisera. Differences in origin arrangements are made according to the purpose of the individual test, but the essential idea is to electro-phorese antigen(s) into antibody-charged gel.

ANTIGEN QUANTITATION

Onto a double-width (75 × 50-mm) microscope slide precoated with 0.2% agarose in distilled water and dried, cast a thin layer of 1% agarose in suitable buffer, and containing antiserum, using the sandwich method described in Chapter 2. Across the length of this slide about 1 cm from its cathodic edge punch a row of five wells 1 cm apart, and fill each with antigen solution level with the surrounding gel surface. Invert the slide on its electrode contacts (cf. Fig. 5.9), and submit it to electrophoresis until the tips of the loops of precipitate formed by the migrating samples of antigen become sharp (Laurell, 1966; see Fig. 6.2). Remove the slide and measure the lanceolate precipitates which have developed; or wash it for 24 hours in saline and for 1 hour in distilled water, and then dry and stain it for more critical observations and to obtain a permanent record of the test (Merrill *et al.*, 1967).

Agarose usually is better than agar for this technique because it develops less electroosmosis. Consequently, there is no chance of a change in antibody concentration in the path of antigen migration during a run, since the antibodies remain static. The loops of precipitate for anodic antigens also will be higher and easier to measure in agarose. On the other hand, although antigens used at isoelectric pH sometimes can be quantitated by this technique in agarose gels (Grubb, 1970), better results can be obtained using agar instead of agarose. This is because relative to such antigens the atmosphere of precipitins undergoes no movement, since both reactants migrate equally rapidly toward the cathode electroosmotically, and a long, readily measurable spearhead of precipitate will form from the antigen–antibody complexes being immobilized in the wake of the cathodally moving antigen. Lateral edges of the spearhead converge because the concentration of antigen is being decreased by precipitation with antibodies, whereas practically the surrounding concentration of antibodies remains constant. Immunoglobulins, for example, are readily quantitated in agar gel by electroimmunodiffusion (Merrill *et al.*, 1967).

Cellulose acetate also has been used for single electroimmunodiffusion (Krøll, 1968c), but the disadvantages of using it for other kinds of immunodiffusion tests apply to its use in this technique also.

The quantity of antiserum to be used in the gel depends on the strength of its precipitins for the antigen to be measured and is determined most easily by trial and error using concentrations of antigen in the range likely to be encountered in subsequent samples. It should be just enough to form a sharp loop of precipitate long enough for a given period of electrophoresis to readily reveal 50% differences in antigen concentration (Laurell, 1966). With this precaution, quantitations can be made with a standard error of approximately 2% (Laurell, 1966; Grubb, 1970; Krøll *et al.*, 1970). Under given analytic conditions antigens that migrate more slowly produce proportionally lower peaks of precipitate with corresponding decreases in accuracy with which they can be measured and the antigen quantitated (Salvaggio *et al.*, 1970). Typically, the antiserum is used at between 1% and 10% if it is mixed with warm agar or agarose solution before the solution is cast (Laurell, 1966; Merrill *et al.*, 1967); if it is infused into the gel already cast (see two-dimensional single electroimmunodiffusion, below), it may have to be used at higher concentration or even undiluted. Buffer composition for the gel usually has been the same as that employed for classic immunoelectrophoresis tests, such as ionic strength 0.025 to 0.05 and pH 8.2 to 8.6. The purposes of this buffer are to maintain a constant pH, to allow an easily measurable length of antigen migration in suitable time without causing the gel to overheat, to hold the antibodies immobile, and to promote precipitation of the antigen by its antibodies. More latitude in selecting the ionic strength of this buffer is allowable in quantitations of just one or two antigens than in immunoelectrophoresis because electrophoresis can be milder. Selecting an appropriate pH to maintain zero mobility for the analytic precipitins is an empirical task because antibody mobilities in different antisera can differ, and because electroosmosis varies somewhat from batch to batch of agarose (Krøll *et al.*, 1970).

The length of electrophoresis depends on such factors as the mobility of antigen and the conditions of electrophoresis like voltage, buffer ionic strength, and ambient temperature. It can vary from 30 minutes (Merrill *et al.*, 1967), through 2 hours (Laurell, 1966), to overnight (Krøll *et al.*, 1970). It is selected to obtain linearity over a wide range of antigen concentrations between the height of the loop of precipitate and the concentration of the antigen (Krøll *et al.*, 1970). This proportion will not be linear if electrophoresis extends beyond the time required for the smallest concentration tested to reach equilibrium with its antibodies (i.e., the loop ceases to grow) unless it is continued long enough for all other concentrations tested also to reach equilibrium (Laurell, 1966). Therefore, it should either be short enough for none of the concentrations to reach equilibrium or long enough for all of them to. If only relative values are being sought, this restriction is less important.

An antigen is quantitated by this technique by comparing the penetration of its loop of precipitate into the antiserum-charged agarose with that of a standard concentration of the same antigen run in the same test or under identical conditions (Krøll *et al.*, 1970; Merrill *et al.*, 1967; Miller and Anderson, 1971; Laurell, 1966). The comparison must be made with known concentrations of antigen rather than with supposedly equivalent antisera because of the greater heterogeneity of antibodies among antisera than of antigen among samples of the same kind of antigen (Krøll *et al.*, 1970). With a symmetrical sharp loop of precipitate, produced by an antigen migrating toward either the anode or the cathode, measuring the distance from origin to tip of the loop and plotting this on semilog paper against known antigen concentrations will provide a straight line over a wide range of antigen concentrations. From such a graph can be derived knowledge of the quantity of the same antigen in an unknown sample (Merrill *et al.*, 1967, 1971). If portions of the antigen population being analyzed migrate simultaneously in opposite directions toward both electrodes (e.g., IgG in agarose), then similar quantitation can be achieved by measuring the distance between opposite tips of the bilateral loop of precipitate (Krøll *et al.*, 1970). Planimetric measurement of the area within a loop, or the mechanical equivalent projection of the loop on paper in standardized enlargement and subsequent weighing of the area of paper encompassed by this loop and cut away from the rest of the paper, is an alternative way of using this technique quantitatively.

The basic understanding and technology of quantitating antigens by one-dimensional single electroimmunodiffusion tests are still sparse. These tests appear to be more sensitive and versatile than comparable single diffusion plate tests (Salvaggio *et al.*, 1970). But being quite similar to single diffusion tests, they share similar problems. For example, two antigens can be quantitated at once if they are not cross-reacting, for then they precipitate independently. But if, like isomers of complement, they cross-react, then the foremost peak of precipitate indicates the total of both antigens, and the inner loop of precipitate indicates only the presence but not the quantity of the cross-reacting antigen (Krøll and Thambiah, 1970). In mixtures of antigens like serum there are several antigens that cross-react with each other, and therefore this is a serious disadvantage. Fortunately, it is readily overcome by the two-dimensional electroimmunodiffusion tests described below.

The presence of two precipitin loops in a single electroimmunodiffusion test usually indicates detection of two different antigens. But these also can be formed by reaction of antibodies with a single population of antigen by Liesegang precipitation, because the origin was recharged during electrophoresis (Krøll and Thambiah, 1970), or because electrophoresis was interrupted or its voltage changed in mid-course.

One-dimensional single electroimmunodiffusion also can be used for qualitative analysis, as is illustrated in Fig. 6.11. However, its two-dimensional derivative (see below) is superior for this purpose.

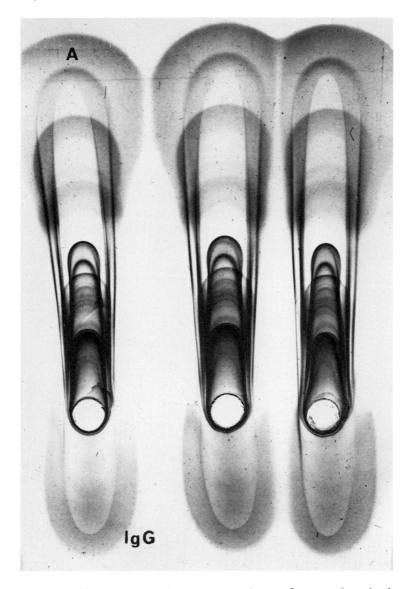

Fig. 6.11. Qualitative analysis of human serum by one-dimensional single electro-immunodiffusion performed in agarose and pH 8.2 barbital buffer of ionic strength 0.025 on a double-width microscope slide. Before the samples of serum were applied for electrophoresis the agarose was charged with a 50% concentration of rabbit antiserum by a 30-minute exposure (cf. Fig. 2.6) and then rinsed briefly with distilled water. IgG and albumin are indicated for purposes of orientation.

SOME USEFUL VARIATIONS OF ONE-DIMENSIONAL
SINGLE ELECTROIMMUNODIFFUSION

This test can be used to quantitate several antigens simultaneously, to compare several antigens with each other at one time, to compare precipitins in mono- or polyvalent antisera, and to perform various kinds of qualitative analysis. The best results in these various applications have been achieved by a modification of the technique facilitating resolution and identification of multiple precipitating systems in a single test (see Krøll, 1968b).

Cast a flat, thin layer of agarose in electrophoresis buffer on an agarose-precoated double-width microscope slide by the sandwich method. After the gel has set and hardened and the upper, uncoated casting slide has been removed, apply antigens and antiserum in the following manner. Across the width of the slide approximately 1 cm from

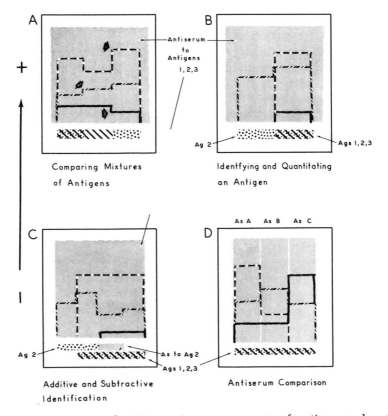

Fig. 6.12. Diagrams depicting various arrangements of antigens and antisera described in the text for one-dimensional single electroimmunodiffusion analyses.

the cathode end apply three samples of antigen solution in 10 × 4-mm areas, and extending 3 mm from anodic edges of these samples to within approximately 1 cm of the anodic edge of the slide, and across its width apply an even layer of dialyzed antiserum (see Figs. 6.12A and 6.12B). Electrophorese the slide to obtain a "ladder" of bands of precipitate across the length of the slide for each of the samples of antigen mixture. Identical antigens in the different mixtures will interconnect in reactions of identity (Fig. 6.13), and by their relative distances of migration reveal their comparative concentrations.

Although the antigens can be cast in agarose and the antiserum mixed with the agarose before the antiserum layer is cast with excellent results (Krøll, 1968b), a less time-consuming technique is to let the reactants

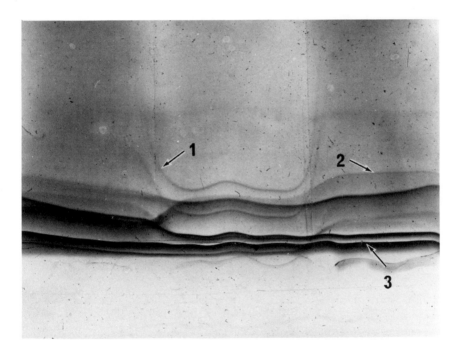

Fig. 6.13. Comparative one-dimensional single electroimmunodiffusion test set up on a microscope slide as indicated in diagram D, Fig. 6.12. Three different guinea pig antisera to rabbit serum are being compared. Precipitins to antigen 1 are present in the middle antiserum but absent from the lateral two. The titer of precipitins to antigen 2 is highest in the left antiserum and lowest in the right antiserum. The titer of precipitins to antigen 3 is the same in all three antisera. The three vertical areas of antiserum and a horizontal area of antigen were charged by a 10-minute overlay exposure to reactant-saturated strips of filter paper, as described in the text. Agarose at 0.75% concentration in pH 8.2 barbital buffer of ionic strength 0.025 was used, and the slide was electrophoresed for 2 hours at 10 volts/cm.

diffuse into a thin layer of already cast gel. The reactants can be placed by using reactant-saturated filter paper as described in Chapter 2. A less wasteful alternative, since no reactant is lost within the applicator material, is to use strips of waterproof plastic (e.g., Mylar[8]) as guides for spreading each reactant over a sharply defined area. Thus, to apply the samples of antigen arrange three 10×4-mm rectangles of Mylar in line, separated from each other by 1-mm distances on a corresponding guide diagram drawn on an index card. At the same time also lay a square of Mylar film 4.5×4.5 cm on the guide index card parallel to and 3 mm away from the three antigen strips. Place 0.15 ml of dialyzed antiserum on the middle of this square of film and 1.0 μl of antigen solution on each of the three smaller rectangles of film. Then, invert the slide with the agarose cast on it, and gently and evenly lower it into contact with the pieces of Mylar and their respective reactants. Lift it away, and the Mylar will adhere to the gel and will have spread the antigen samples and antiserum evenly about their respective appropriate areas. If a strip inadvertently has been moved slightly out of position in this procedure, it can be pushed back to proper position with a dissecting needle. Best results are obtained in applying the samples of antigen and antiserum if there is no free water on the surface of the gel, as there is immediately after removing the casting slide (see Chapter 2).

Following this, the slide should be held in a humidified petri dish at room temperature for 1 hour for reactants to soak into the gel. Then it can be electrophoresed upside down with the Mylar films left on it; or these can be removed, the surface of the agarose rinsed briefly with distilled water any excess of which should be thoroughly shaken off, and the slide electrophoresed. After electrophoresis, usually requiring 2 to 3 hours at 10 volts/cm but determined empirically, reactions can be observed and recorded, or the slide can be set aside overnight at 4°C in a humid atmosphere for precipitin bands to intensify and then be observed.

The technique described above is a miniaturization and simplification of that originally described by Krøll (1968b). It is easier to use with the various antigen and antiserum configurations described below. Factors affecting the "rocket" variety of one-dimensional single electroimmunodiffusion as discussed above also apply to this technique, whichever way it is employed.

Krøll invented several variations of comparative one-dimensional

---

[8] Mylar film can be purchased from drafting supplies stores in large sheets and cut to required size. Appropriate pieces of thin microscope cover slips, either glass or plastic, also can be used. The reactant guide should be composed of material that is light and will not curl when moistened.

single electroimmunodiffusion for purposes not only of quantitating antigen but also of identifying individual antigens and comparing antisera (Krøll, 1968b, 1969a,b). These are illustrated in Fig. 6.12. Diagram *A*, for instance, shows how the relative concentrations of the same antigens in different mixtures can be determined (Krøll, 1968b, 1969b). Three hypothetical antigens are distinguishable across the electropherogram by reactions of identify, and their relative quantities are indicated by the respective distances into the antiserum-charged gel that their fronts of precipitate have penetrated. Antigen 3 is shown to have the same concentration in mixtures 1 and 2 but a lower concentration in mixture 3; by contrast, the concentration of antigen 1 is demonstrated to be higher in mixtures 1 and 3 than in mixture 2.

Diagram *B* illustrates identification of one among several bands of precipitate by comparison with purified antigen (Krøll, 1969b). Discounting interpretational problems, like the effect of a cross-reacting antigen or nonspecific accelerated migration of antigens, this diagram also indicates that the concentration of identified antigen in the mixture is higher than that in the reference solution.

Diagram *C* extends the comparison suggested by diagram *B* by using comparison, addition, and subtraction all in one test, to identify a selected antigen (Krøll, 1969b). Placing some purified antigen in the path of migration of the unknown mixture increases the migration distance for the same antigen in the mixture without affecting the other two. Interposing antiserum specific for this antigen has the opposite effect. Identification, addition, and subtraction all are associated with the antigen being studied as it occurs in "natural state" by including the whole mixture itself in the electroimmunodiffusogram. Conversely, this type of test also assesses the purity of the isolated antigen, investigates its immunologic relationship to the native antigen, analyzes the specificity of the absorbing antiserum, and measures the relative quantities and strengths of absorbing and developing antisera.

Relative antibody quantitation and comparison of polyvalent antisera are the primary objectives of the test shown in diagram *D* (Krøll, 1969a). In this, antiserum A is observed to contain less precipitins to antigen 1 than antiserum B, more to antigen 2, and the same to antigen 3. The test shows antiserum C to contain precipitins to antigens 2 and 3 but not to antigen 1. These comparisons assume that precipitins being compared have the same isoelectric point. But this may not be true for antisera of different animal species, or even strains, or for antisera obtained at different intervals from the same animal (see Chapter 1), and must be recognized as a possible complication of comparative tests like this.

Two-Dimensional Single Electroimmunodiffusion

Originally developed as a large-scale derivative of two-dimensional starch block electrophoresis (cf. Clarke and Freeman, 1966, 1968; Laurell, 1965a), this technique now can be employed on a scale comparable to microimmunoelectrophoresis (Crowle, 1972; Firestone and Aronson, 1969). Only micro tests will be described, since they offer several advantages in convenience and economy over macro tests without sacrificing any analytic capabilities.

SINGLE ANALYSIS ON A DOUBLE-WIDTH MICROSCOPE SLIDE

Two varieties of this technique will be described. The first is a two-step method similar to macro techniques currently used; the second is a one-step method in which, after primary electrophoresis, antiserum is diffused into the portion of the gel to be used for secondary electrophoresis.

For both methods, a 0.5-mm-thick layer of 1% agarose in suitable electrophoresis buffer is cast on an agarose-precoated 75×50-mm microscope slide by the sandwich method, and the casting slide is removed (see Chapter 2). Antigen mixture to be analyzed is placed in a well 2 mm in diameter cut 1 cm in from one of the corners of the slide. The slide is inverted and submitted to primary electrophoresis upside down at 4°C (Fig. 5.9), typically for 1 hour at 10 volts/cm with barbital buffer at pH 8.2 and ionic strength 0.025. This electrophoresis should be across the length rather than width of the slide (cf. Fig. 6.3).

For the two-step method, the slide next is removed from the electrophoresis apparatus, a straight cut is made parallel to and near but not touching the path of first electrophoresis, and the large portion of unused agarose is scraped off the slide and discarded. A casting slide is laid upon supports on the workbench (see Chapter 2), 0.5-mm spacers such as used for casting the original gel by the sandwich technique are positioned along its two shorter edges, and the slide on which the first electrophoresis has been effected is inverted and rested on these supports in essentially the same manner as is depicted for antiserum application in Fig. 2.6. The agarose slide must be offset from the casting slide to exactly align the inner edge of its strip of agarose with the edge of the casting slide, again in a manner similar to that shown in Fig. 2.6. Then agarose mixed with antiserum and at 56°C is run rapidly from a pipet onto the uncovered lip of the lower casting slide and between it and the inverted upper slide. By this arrangement the agarose will flow evenly between the two slides to constitute a flat layer which fuses with the edge of the agarose already on the agarose slide without overrunning it.

The flow of agarose will be facilitated if the casting can be performed over a warm surface (e.g., a slide warmer), and if the spacers are short to permit free escape of air from between the slides. After the gel has hardened, the casting slide is removed as in the sandwich casting technique, and the original slide with its newly cast expanse of antiserum-charged agarose is returned to the electrophoresis apparatus for secondary electrophoresis which, typically, will be for 3 hours at 5 volts/cm in the same buffer.

Good results are obtained with this technique using only a little antiserum (e.g., 0.2 ml, if antiserum is used at 10% and some wastage of unused antiserum–agarose mixture is allowed for). Advantages of this technique over that below in which antiserum is diffused into the surface of the agarose instead of being mixed with it before casting are that it is somewhat faster, uniformity of antiserum distribution throughout the gel may be more certain, and there is less chance for premature antigen–antibody precipitation which might develop during the antiserum diffusion period in the alternative technique if the concentration of one of the antigens being analyzed is very high or if the antiserum is placed too close to the path of first electrophoresis. This two-step technique also is usually the more convenient when conditions for primary and secondary electrophoresis purposely are meant to differ. When only one portion of an electropherogram need be analyzed, this can be cut away from the rest after primary electrophoresis and analyzed by transfer to antiserum-containing agarose and subsequent one-dimensional single electroimmunodiffusion (Briscoe *et al.*, 1966).

The two-step technique also has some disadvantages which prompted development of a one-step alternative (Crowle, 1972). For instance, antiserum mixed with melted agarose is harder to wash out later when an electroimmunodiffusogram is to be stained. A significant loss of precipitin titer frequently occurs in sera mixed with warm agarose; this can be especially confusing in the quantitative analyses which can so conveniently be performed simultaneously for several antigens by electroimmunodiffusion. The procedure of cutting away unused agarose and replacing it with a good casting of antiserum–agarose mixture (a bad casting cannot be corrected and must be discarded) is more complicated and requires more expertise than the procedure of diffusing antiserum into the surface of the unused agarose gel. Variation in the placement of reactants, such as for detecting cathodic as well as anodic antigens as illustrated in Figs. 6.17 and 6.18, usually is not so easy.

As was already mentioned, initial casting of the agarose, applying the sample of antigen to be analyzed, and primary electrophoresis all are the same for both one-step and two-step procedures. But for the one-step technique, at the end of primary electrophoresis the agarose-carrying slide is inverted and placed upon two lengths of 0.3-mm spacers which in turn are resting on another glass slide as shown in Fig. 2.6. The agarose slide should be offset both to provide a lip for applying antiserum to the lower slide and to allow this antiserum to be spread parallel to but not over the path of primary electrophoresis (also shown in Fig. 2.6). Antiserum immediately is run between the two slides, and they are allowed to stand within a humidified petri dish for 45 minutes at room temperature for precipitins to diffuse into the portion of agarose to be used for the second electrophoresis. Alternatively, an appropriate volume (e.g., 0.25 ml) of antiserum can be placed on the lower slide before the inverted agarose slide is laid on it, and then the latter is laid upon the spacers from one end to the other, flattening and spreading the antiserum as it comes to rest on the spacers. After the 45-minute incubation period, the slides are gently pulled apart, the surface of the antiserum-exposed agarose is rinsed briefly with a jet of distilled water which immediately is drained off, and the slide is returned upside down to the electrophoresis apparatus for second electrophoresis as was described above for the two-step technique.

Mylar or similar film also can be employed to direct the spread of antiserum as in one-dimensional single electroimmunodiffusion, but care must be taken that the film does not curl enough to spread the antiserum unevenly. Antiserum can be applied quite simply by overlaying the area of second electrophoresis with antiserum-soaked filter paper (Yokoyama and Carr, 1962), but this wastes antiserum, since much is absorbed by the paper.

Agarose also can be charged with antiserum by rubbing the antiserum into the surface of the gel with a bent glass rod (Afonso, 1964b). For instance, at the end of primary electrophoresis, cover the zone of agarose through which this was effected with a strip of Saran Wrap (cf. Firestone and Aronson, 1969), place 0.3 ml of antiserum in the center of the area of agarose to be charged, and then gently massage this into the surface of the agarose with a bent glass rod, using only the weight of the rod for pressure on the gel surface. In this manner the antiserum is worked into the gel within only a minute or two. Allow the slide to stand for 30 to 45 minutes at room temperature in a humid container for the antiserum to diffuse evenly into the gel. Remove the Saran Wrap and perform secondary electrophoresis.

Whether a one-step or two-step technique is used, at the end of the second electrophoresis a number of precipitin loops will have developed, but several that are faint and others not even seen at this time can be developed by allowing the plate to stand at 4°C overnight.

Following overnight incubation, the slide can be observed by dark-field lighting and/or photographed. If it is to be kept for permanent record, it can be washed for 1 hour in physiologic phosphate buffer, for 4 to 5 hours in running tap water, and for 1 hour in distilled water, and then can be stained for proteins and dried in routine manner (Fig. 6.14).

Undiluted antiserum is necessary to analyze the stronger antigens in a heterogeneous mixture like human serum, but it prevents several weaker antigens from forming loops of precipitate high enough to be evident. For these, diluted antiserum should be used. The time required to infuse antiserum into the surface of the gel, and the temperature, can be varied empirically to optimize results. Secondary electrophoresis over a period of approximately 3 hours is appropriate for the conditions of

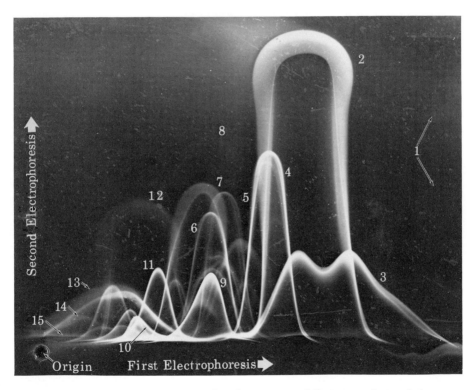

Fig. 6.14. Two-dimensional single electroimmunodiffusion analysis of human serum using rabbit antiserum and conditions as described for this technique for Fig. 6.9. Some of the more readily identifiable antigens are indicated by number as follows: prealbumin (1), albumin (2), α_1 lipoprotein (3), α_1-antitrypsin (4), Gc-globulin (5), ceruloplasmin (6), α_2 HS glycoprotein (7), hemopexin (8), α_2-macro-globulin (9), β lipoprotein (10), β_{1C}-globulin (11), transferrin (12), IgA (13), IgD (14), IgM (15).

voltage, temperature, and ionic strength described here; but for other situations, and for other systems or purposes, its conditions should be devised by trial and error. Overnight incubation of electroimmunodiffusograms at 4°C reveals more loops of precipitate than are evident immediately after a 3-hour secondary electrophoresis, and it intensifies those already evident. Although secondary electrophoresis sometimes is much longer (e.g., overnight) with full development of precipitin loops for optimal antibody–antigen ratios, shorter electrophoresis as recommended here followed by overnight standing will more clearly detect loops developed in antigen excess (cf. albumin and transferrin loops in Fig. 6.14).

MULTIPLE SIMULTANEOUS ANALYSES

In 1969 Firestone and Aronson developed a micro technique permitting completion of eight analyses on a single glass plate of approximately 10×20 cm. With this technique one technician was reported to be able to produce sixty-four patterns in an 8-hour period. A thin layer of 1.2% agarose is cast with a modification of the sandwich technique on a 10×20-cm glass plate previously covered with a sheet of Mylar 0.0075 inch thick. Eight sample wells are cut in two rows of four across the length of the slide, and samples are electrophoresed across its width for 1 hour at approximately 1.4 volts/cm with 0.05 M barbital buffer at pH 8.8.

The areas of primary electrophoresis are tightly covered with Saran Wrap, 1 ml of antiserum diluted with distilled water to 1.3 ml is applied to the gel, and then this is worked into the gel surface uniformly by rolling a glass tube gently over the surface until all the antiserum has been absorbed. Following this, the Saran Wrap strips are removed, the electropherogram is cut into two equal 10×10-cm squares, these are rotated 90 degrees with the support of the underlying Mylar film and replaced on the supporting glass plate, and secondary electrophoresis is effected for 2 hours, also at approximately 1.4 volts/cm.

This method reduces two-dimensional single electroimmunodiffusion to the practical simplicity, economy, and rapidity required in the clinical laboratory. Although 1 ml of antiserum is used, since there are eight patterns run at once only 0.125 ml is actually expended per pattern.

Precipitin loop "area" in these electroimmunodiffusograms, or projections of them to a standard degree of enlargement, can be measured quickly and conveniently by means of a sliding wedge scale which simultaneously indicates the height of a loop and points of intersection on its legs at half its height. The height of a loop is multiplied by its width at these points of intersection, and an area in square millimeters is obtained and used for quantitation (Firestone and Aronson, 1969; see Fig. 6.15). These area values can be used simply as relative, or by comparing

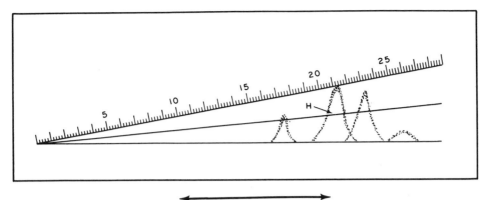

Fig. 6.15. Sliding wedge as devised by Firestone and Aronson (1965) for obtaining comparative area measurements of loops of precipitate in two-dimensional single electroimmunodiffusion quantitative analyses. The wedge, etched on Plexiglas or similar transparent material, is fitted to a loop of precipitate as shown, the height of the loop is read from the scale, and the "width" of the loop at half its height (H) is measured. The product of height and width is the value used for quantitative comparisons. The electroimmunodiffusion pattern usually is enlarged by projection for suitably accurate use of the wedge.

them with values derived from standards using known quantities of a given antigen they can also provide absolute values of quantity.

These measures should be applied, for most reliability, to symmetrical loops which have become stabilized (i.e., to loops with sharp peaks equilibrated with their antibodies and therefore no longer lengthening during electrophoresis). Since the range of antigen concentrations in a mixture like human serum is wide, empirically determined variations in antiserum concentration and antigen dilution will have to be used if all the antigens in such a mixture are to be quantitated. Sensitivity in this type of test increases with progressive dilution of antibodies, because this permits progressively greater penetration of antigen into the antibody-charged gel, with development of higher, more accurately measurable loops of precipitate. This characteristic is especially important for quantitating weaker, more cathodic antigens. Its principal limitation is the progressive weakening of the precipitate which also occurs with dilution of antibody. As was mentioned in Chapter 2, it is possible partly to counteract this weakening to invisibility by enhancing the antigen–antibody precipitation, such as by overlaying the electroimmunodiffusogram with more antiserum after secondary electrophoresis (Firestone and Aronson, 1969).

Some comments on this technique of Firestone and Aronson for multiple analyses may be useful. If two plates 10 cm square are used instead of a rectangular one of 10×20 cm, then neither the gel-supporting film of Mylar nor cutting the gel in half to rotate it after primary electrophoresis is necessary. Furthermore, the plates then can be electrophoresed upside down to minimize dehydration. As was mentioned in Chapter 2, if electropherograms are run in series, antigens will migrate more slowly in anodic than in cathodic areas. Although Firestone and Aronson do not indicate that they encountered any problems from this effect, such problems could be present.

COMPARATIVE TWO-DIMENSIONAL SINGLE ELECTROIMMUNODIFFUSION

The already most gratifying potentialities of two-dimensional single electroimmunodiffusion can be extended still further for qualitative and quantitative immunochemical analyses by such variations as those diagrammed in Fig. 6.16.

Comparative electroimmunodiffusion (diagram A) is performed by using two origins, one for the unknown and the other for the reference system (Krøll et al., 1970; Krøll, 1968a, 1969b). The origins for this and similar tests (e.g., diagrams B and C) should not be physical interruptions in the structure of the gel, lest the migration of the more cathodic component thus be disturbed.[9] Diagram A shows an antigen being identified in a mixture of three by classic reaction of identity using a known sample of the antigen for comparison.

All variations of comparative double diffusion plates described in Chapter 4 and their interpretations apply also to this type of comparative electroimmunodiffusion, and data are also provided in these tests on electrophoretic mobility and relative or absolute quantity. Thus, in diagram A, the quantity of antigen 2 in the mixture is revealed to be approximately the same as that in the known reference solution. If the native antigen in the mixture were different from the purified antigen (e.g., because of its attachment to a molecule of different electrophoretic mobility, or because during purification the reference antigen has polymerized), this would be evident from a corresponding aberration in the electrophoretic location of one of the loops, from multiple loop development, or from development of skewed shapes as was discussed earlier in this chapter. This technique can be used to compare two different complex mixtures of antigen, such as urine and serum, to reveal quanti-

---

[9] If wells are used, samples should be mixed with agarose before being added to the wells. Preferably, the samples should be applied without wells, such as in small droplets, in paper or cellulose acetate discs, under discs of Mylar, or through holes in Mylar templates. Primary electrophoresis is begun after antigens from such sources have been allowed to diffuse into the surface of the gel for a few minutes. See Chapter 2 for more technical details.

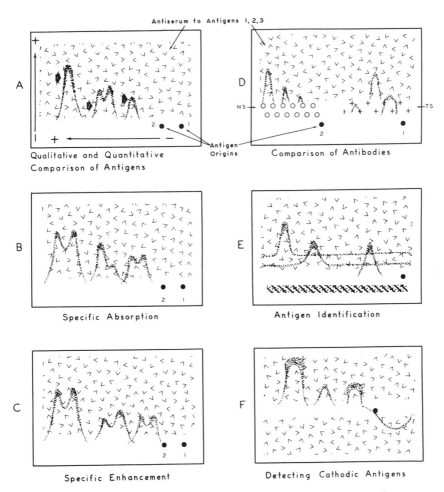

Antiserum to Antigens 1, 2, 3

A — Qualitative and Quantitative Comparison of Antigens

Antigen Origins

D — Comparison of Antibodies

B — Specific Absorption

E — Antigen Identification

C — Specific Enhancement

F — Detecting Cathodic Antigens

Fig. 6.16. Diagrams depicting variations in location of antigens and antiserum which can be made in two-dimensional single electroimmunodiffusion as described in the text.

tative and qualitative differences in one or more of their many constituents (Krøll, 1971).

Diagram *B* shows the principle of reversed absorption used in a test set up similarly (Krøll, 1969b). Thus, when the anodic origin is charged with antigens 1, 2, and 3 and the cathodic origin is charged with the same mixture but mixed with antiserum containing antibodies to antigen 2, the antibodies to this antigen become evident by depression of the loop of precipitate formed by this antigen in the mixture containing antibody. The reason for this is that either the antibodies have precipitated some of antigen 2, or they have complexed with it to impede its migration during primary electrophoresis so that there is less or none to form a loop of precipitate during secondary electrophoresis. This technique also can be used to quantitate both antigen and antibodies. It can detect antibodies that are not precipitins; that is, it can be used as a primary binding test for all kinds of antibodies. In forming primary complexes with antigen, nonprecipitating antibodies will significantly decrease the mobility of that proportion of antigen with which they bind, and if antibodies to these antibodies either are included in the original antigen–antiserum mixture or are incorporated themselves in the path of electrophoresis between the two origins shown in diagram B, primary antigen–antibody complexes will be precipitated and prevented from electrophoretic migration altogether. This technique can be refined by using as antibodies to the antibodies those selected to react with defined classes of immunoglobulin, so as to determine not only whether antibodies are present but also to what immunoglobulin class they belong.

Whereas diagram B depicts specific absorption for identifying antigen, diagram C shows how this is accomplished by the opposite effect of enhancement (Krøll, 1969b). For example, if the pattern formed by antigen mixture 1, 2, and 3 is compared with that formed by the same mixture to which extra antigen 2 has been added, the loop of precipitate formed by antigen 2 in the second mixture will be higher than that formed by the unsupplemented quantity in the first mixture.

Diagrams D and E depict somewhat different approaches to comparative electroimmunodiffusion in which after primary electrophoresis analytic reactants are placed in the paths of the separated antigens during secondary electrophoresis (Svendsen and Axelsen, 1972). The technique shown in diagram D probably can achieve better simultaneous qualitative and quantitative analysis of different antibodies in an antiserum to multiple antigens than any other comparative electroimmunodiffusion test. The principle of this technique is that, whereas electrophoretic migration of the several antigens in a mixture will not be impeded during secondary electrophoresis by a long, narrow area of gel containing either no antibodies or antibodies unrelated to any of the antigens migrating through this area, if the area is charged with antiserum containing antibodies that will react with one or more of these antigens, they will be precipitated and their migration retarded proportionally. For example, in diagram D two tests are being performed on one plate. The left test shows antigens 1, 2, and 3 migrating freely through an area of gel without antibody and then precipitating with antiserum to all three infused into the gel beyond this area, as would occur in a routine two-dimensional single electroimmunodiffusion test. But in the test at the right a strip of gel between the primary electrophoretic pattern and that charged with analytic antiserum to all three has been charged with a test antiserum containing antibodies only to antigens 1 and 3.[10] The result is that, although antigen 2 migrates through this area unimpeded, as it did also in the left test, antigen 1 is precipitated in a loop too short to extend into the upper analytic region, and antigen 3 reaches this region in only a small fraction of its original concentration. These results indicate, then, that the test antiserum contains a high titer of antibodies to antigen 1, a good titer to antigen 3, and no antibodies to antigen 2.

This technique can be used to compare two antisera both quantitatively and qualitatively for all the antigens detectable by either. For instance, it was used to identify nineteen precipitins to different antigens of *Candida albicans* in antisera from candidiasis patients which corresponded to precipitins to the same antigens in hyperimmune rabbit antiserum (Svendsen and Axelsen, 1972). The titers of seven were equal to and those of twelve were lower than analogous titers in the rabbit antiserum. Had free *Candida* antigen been present in the antisera of any of the patients, it also could have been detected by this test. This technique should be excellent for comparing polyvalent antisera to a given mixture of antigens with each other for such purposes as blending mixtures suitable for comprehensive balanced analyses, or for observing simultaneously the rise and fall of responses to individual antigens in a mixture with changes in immunization protocol or time, or with aging of the animal. It can compare antisera to related mixtures of antigens (e.g., extracts of normal and cancerous tissues; sera from closely related animals) to identify one or more unique characterizing antigens from among many. Its potentialities for utilization thus are excellent.

Closely related to this test and with similar utility is one in which a strip of antigen solution instead of antiserum is laid across the path of secondary electrophoresis. However, as is shown in diagram *E*, better results are obtained by placing this cathodic rather than anodic to the path of primary electrophoresis (Krøll, 1969b). Some possible effects of this arrangement are illustrated in the diagram. For example, the test mixture consists of antigens 1, 2a, 3, and 2c; antigens 2a and 2c are the same immunologically, but electrophoretically the first is more anodic than the second. The reference mixture consisting of antigens 1 and 2 migrating during secondary electrophoresis with the test antigens separated during primary electrophoresis identifies antigen 1 as electro-

---

[10] For this technique, antiserum can be infused from beneath a strip of Mylar film at the same time as analytic antiserum is being infused from beneath a rectangle of the film. This is more convenient than casting succeeding mixtures of plain agarose and antiserum-containing agarose.

phoretically homogeneous but shows antigen 2 to be electrophoretically heterogeneous. By ordinary electroimmunodiffusion the two loops formed by antigen populations 2a and 2c would have been interpreted as being due to two separate antigens because they would not have been close enough to coalesce in a reaction of identity. Antigen 3 forms a loop of precipitate undisturbed by the presence of the reference antigen mixture and therefore is not present in this mixture.

In these various examples of comparative electroimmunodiffusion as well as in the description of the basic techniques themselves, attention has been focused on anode-migrating antigens because these are the most frequently analyzed. But cathode-migrating antigens also can be analyzed, as is depicted in diagram F. One way is to perform both primary and secondary electrophoresis at pH 7.8 (Rebeyrotte *et al.*, 1969). Another is to use horse antiserum with γ_1-globulin precipitins at the usual pH of 8.2 instead of the γ_2-globulin precipitins, because γ_1 precipitins remain stationary at this pH (cf. Figs. 6.17 and 6.18). Primary electrophoresis was directed across a more central area of the slide to permit

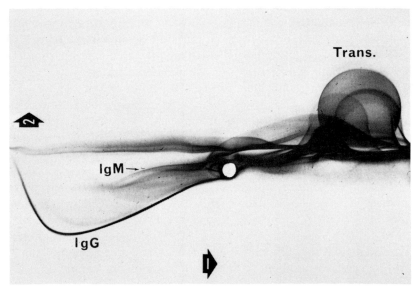

Fig. 6.17. Detection of human serum immunoglobulins, especially IgG and IgM, with a horse antiserum to human serum in a micro two-dimensional single electroimmunodiffusion test set up as in Fig. 6.16F, using the antiserum both above and below the path of primary electrophoresis. Transferrin also is indicated as an aid to orientation. Electrophoresis was performed as described in the legend of Fig. 6.9 with primary separation for 1.5 hours at 10 volts/cm and secondary electrophoresis for 1.5 hours at 5 volts/cm, antiserum being applied for 45 minutes between the first and second runs. (Antiserum courtesy ICL Scientific, Fountain Valley, California.)

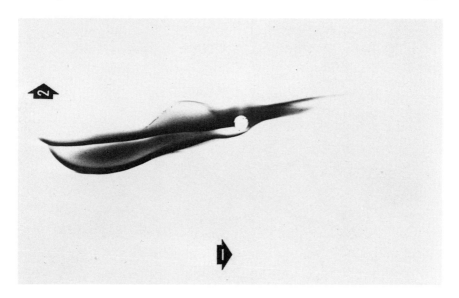

Fig. 6.18. Detection of IgG in micro two-dimensional single electroimmunodiffusion using goat antiserum to IgG in the agarose above and below the path of primary electrophoresis; experimental conditions otherwise were as described for Fig. 6.17. (Antiserum courtesy ICL Scientific, Fountain Valley, California.)

charging both anodic and cathodic regions with antiserum for secondary electrophoresis. Little has been done in analyzing basic antigens by immunodiffusion in the past for lack of adequate techniques (cf. Crowle and Hu, 1967); but obviously this should no longer be a deterrent.

An example of comparative two-dimensional single electroimmunodiffusion performed to compare migration in agarose and in agarose–starch mixture of human serum antigens is illustrated in Fig. 6.19. As is explained in the figure legend, the technique employed necessarily was somewhat different from those shown in Fig. 6.16.

One-Dimensional Double Electroimmunodiffusion

This simple technique is very popular for screening sera from potential blood donors for hepatitis-associated antigen (White *et al.*, 1971; Gocke and Howe, 1970; Nordenfelt *et al.*, 1970) because it gives results rapidly and economically. Anode-migrating antigen is placed in the electro-osmotic path of cathode-migrating antibodies in agar gel; during subsequent electrophoresis the two precipitate each other within a few minutes (Crowle, 1956; Bussard and Huet, 1959; Ragetli and Weintraub, 1964; John, 1965; Howe *et al.*, 1967; Jameson, 1968, 1969b; Nasz *et al.*, 1967; Culliford, 1964; cf. Fig. 6.3).

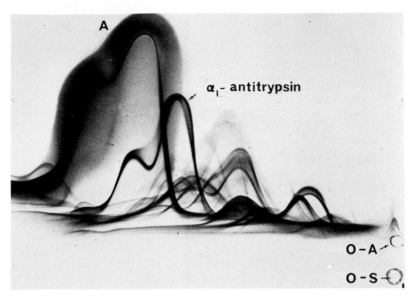

Fig. 6.19. Micro two-dimensional single electroimmunodiffusion test comparing mobilities of human serum antigens in a mixture of 6% starch and 1% agarose with those in 1% agarose alone (conditions as in Fig. 6.10). The agarose origin (O-A) was charged 30 minutes after the beginning of electrophoresis of serum from the origin in starch (O-S); total time for primary electrophoresis was 1.8 hours. Albumin (A) and α_1-antitrypsin are indicated for orientation. The pattern indicates loss of some antigens within the starch, and differences in relative mobilities in the two media for several antigens. It also shows excellent examples of reactions of identity in electroimmunodiffusion tests.

BASIC TECHNIQUE

Using the sandwich technique, cast a thin layer of 1% agar in appropriate buffer on an agar-precoated microscope slide, and punch two 2-mm wells about 3 mm apart in the center of the slide and directly in line with each other electrophoretically (Nasz *et al.*, 1967; Culliford, 1964). For multiple tests on one slide, from six to eight pairs of wells can be used simultaneously (John, 1965; Culliford, 1964). Charge the cathodic one with antigen solution and the anodic one with antiserum, and submit the slide to electrophoresis in the same manner as for classic immunoelectrophoresis. In a few minutes a band of antigen–antibody precipitate will develop, and the test is complete (cf. Culliford, 1964; Fig. 6.20).

Agar is frequently used for one-dimensional double electroimmunodiffusion because in it precipitins migrate vigorously toward the cathode in commonly used buffers like barbital at pH 8.2 to 8.6 and ionic strength

0.05 (cf. Fig. 6.20). Under these same conditions, many of the most frequently studied antigens migrate toward the anode. Consequently, conditions are appropriate for antigen and precipitins to meet, mix, and precipitate between their respective origins. However, there are many antigens which, like precipitins, also migrate toward the cathode in agar gels. Even though they may do so less rapidly and thus be overtaken and precipitated by precipitins (i.e., immunotransmigration: Zydeck *et al.*, 1966), in agar the precipitins may have to migrate through the antigen well before overtaking the antigen. Agarose then is a better medium, and, by varying pH conditions, nearly any antigen can be precipitated somewhere between reactant origins by its antibodies. The only exception will be that in which both antigen and antibody migrate identically, or nearly so, electrophoretically. For this situation, one can resort to such solutions as using a sieving medium like polyacrylamide to retard the migration of one of the reactants more than the other, or changing one

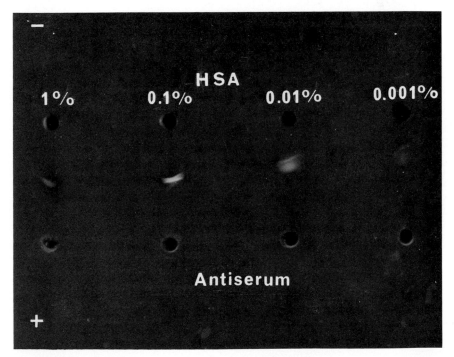

Fig. 6.20. Example of one-dimensional double electroimmunodiffusion performed on a microscope slide using various concentrations of human serum albumin antigen, as indicated, against undiluted rabbit antiserum. Electrophoresis was for 50 minutes at 10 volts/cm in 1% agar in pH 8.2 barbital buffer of ionic strength 0.025, and the reactions seen were photographed with dark-field lighting immediately thereafter.

or the other chemically to different characteristics of electrophoretic migration, such as by carbamylation, sulfonation, or carboxymethylation (Weeke, 1968a; Ragetli and Weintraub, 1965).

As in other kinds of immunodiffusion test, one kind of gel may be found empirically to be better than another for a given antigen–antibody system. For instance, alfalfa mosaic virus produced two bands of precipitate in agarose but only one in agar (Ragetli and Weintraub, 1964). Apparatus used for this test can be exceedingly simple. It is sufficient, for example, to rest opposite ends of the microscope slide electropherogram on two petri dishes filled with buffer, use filter paper wicks to connect each end of the slide with this buffer, and use a platinum wire stretched across the bottom of each dish and clamped to its edge as an electrode (John, 1965).

VARIATIONS OF ONE-DIMENSIONAL DOUBLE ELECTROIMMUNODIFFUSION TESTS

The most important variations are in shape and orientation of reactant origins. Some of these are diagrammed in Fig. 6.21. The two-origin basic microscope slide test (diagram A; Culliford, 1964) can be varied slightly to use three origins.[11] The added origin can be charged with sulfonated antibodies which will migrate toward the anode (Ragetli and Weintraub, 1965). Thus, both anodic and cathodic antigens will be detected. In diagram A, the first test detected anodic-migrating antigen 1, and the second test detected both anodic-migrating antigen 1 and cathodic-migrating antigen 3.

Another variation of this test is to use a glass tube in a technique resembling disc electrophoresis (Crowle, 1956; Fig. 6.21B). In addition to ensuring reactant alignment and complete interaction, this method can be scaled up for preparatory electroimmunodiffusion (cf. similar double diffusion technique, Chapter 4).

Utilizing rectangular origins, as in diagram C, makes electrophoretic alignment of reactants less critical and evanescent reactions less likely to go undetected (Bussard and Huet, 1969). A similar arrangement (diagram D) employing three elongated antiserum origins minimizes

[11] Origins most frequently have been wells cut in the gel. However, better results frequently are obtained when the origins do not physically interrupt the gel. Wells should be avoided for additional reasons. Precipitation in some tests will occur within the origin of a reactant. Origin arrangements and shapes can be selected and used with more versatility if origins are not cut. All the varieties of one-dimensional double electroimmunodiffusion shown in Fig. 6.21 can be used with reactants applied to the surface of a thin gel as described previously in this chapter; simply placing a droplet of reactant on the surface often suffices (John, 1965; Bon and Swanborn, 1965).

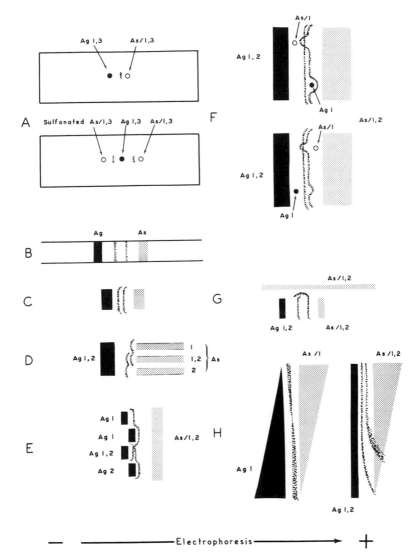

Fig. 6.21. Diagrammatic illustrations of the varieties of one-dimensional double electroimmunodiffusion discussed in the text.

chances of falsely negative results due to antigen excess, and also increases the sensitivity of the test by feeding a train of antibody molecules into the precipitate developing at the front of opposite-migrating antigen (Jameson, 1968). This test can compare several antisera at once for antibodies to the same antigens.

Diagram *E* shows a similar test used for comparing antigens by one-dimensional double electroimmunodiffusion (Bon and Swanborn, 1965; Denis, 1964). Staggering the origins of antigens makes interactions of their precipitin bands more distinct. Immunologic addition and subtraction can be employed in double electroimmunodiffusion as in other kinds of immunodiffusion. Exemplary arrangements are shown in diagram *F* in which antigen 1 is identified by subtraction of reactants in the first arrangement and by addition of reactants in the second.

Many more arrangements are theoretically possible in which double electroimmunodiffusion is used in conjunction with other kinds of immunodiffusion test. Diagram *G* illustrates one that has actually been used (Merétey, 1969). Thus, after electroimmunodiffusion was completed, antigens were also detected by double diffusion, using a trough of antiserum placed parallel to the path of original electrophoresis. As is shown in the diagram, electroimmunodiffusion detected antigen 2, but double diffusion did not; and antigen 1 detected by electroimmunodiffusion developed a reaction of identity with the same antigen as was detected by double diffusion.

Early in the history of one-dimensional double electroimmunodiffusion, Libich (1959) described a gradient test which ensures use of a wide range of antigen–antibody ratios and thereby detection of a given precipitating system (diagram *H*). In addition, this test provides quantitative data from a single test on conditions of electroimmunodiffusion which guide the selection of optimal conditions for screening tests with the system to be set up by the simpler technique of diagram *A*. This test also can be used with a rectangle of one reactant and a wedge of the other, especially for determining best conditions for screening tests using the reactant configuration in diagram *D*.

COMMENTS ON ONE-DIMENSIONAL DOUBLE ELECTROIMMUNODIFFUSION

These tests can be performed in media other than agar or agarose. The first electroimmunodiffusion tests were effected by Macheboeuf *et al.* in 1953 on filter paper (cf. also Lang, 1955). Nakamura published a book in 1966 on "cross-electrophoresis" in which he described several kinds of such tests carried out with filter paper. Electroprecipitation on paper has been used as a routine clinical test for antithyroid precipitins (Dawkins, 1963; Watson, 1960; Watson and Whinfrey, 1958). Cellulose acetate is used in a technique called "immunotransmigration" because, due to lack of electroosmosis in this medium, antigen is precipitated when it overtakes and passes through the cloud of precipitins to it migrating more slowly in the same direction (Zydeck *et al.*, 1966; cf. also Zydeck *et al.*, 1965a; Webster, 1965; Zydeck, 1970; Saravis and Bonacker, 1970). Transmigration is said to be four times as sensitive as a comparable immuno-diffusion test in cellulose acetate.

Polyacrylamide electroimmunodiffusion can be performed as a modi-fication of disc electrophoresis using an arrangement like that in diagram *B*, Fig. 6.21 (Fitschen, 1963). For example, rabbit antiserum was mixed into the spacer gel, and radiolabeled human growth hormone antigen was used in the sample gel. As the latter migrated electrophoretically through the former, it complexed with it. These complexes were detected and could also be quantitated, whether visible or not, by an increased concentration of radioactivity detected with a scintillation counter (see also Louis-Ferdinand and Blatt, 1967).

Single and double diffusion tests were popular for several years be-fore enough was learned about them to identify secondary precipitation (see Chapter 1) and thus to provide an undistorted estimate of their capacity to resolve genuinely different antigen–antibody precipitates. Although secondary precipitation was noticed in double electroimmuno-diffusion tests by Libich (1959), it has not been studied sufficiently for adequate definition of guidelines to its identification in these tests. Con-sequently, although the resolution of double electroimmunodiffusion tests appears to be excellent (Jameson, 1968; Assem *et al.*, 1965), it has yet to be adequately compared with that of good double diffusion plate tests (see Zydeck *et al.*, 1966).

The sensitivity of double electroimmunodiffusion does seem to be superior to that of comparable immunodiffusion tests. In electroimmuno-diffusion, all of each reactant is employed, whereas in most immunodif-fusion tests much of each reactant is lost by diffusion to the surrounding medium. However, because of this, together with the rapidity and con-tinued migration of reactants during development of an electroimmuno-diffusion test, this sensitivity depends critically on using nearly optimal proportions of reactants and, especially, on using sufficient antibody (Merétey, 1969; Jameson, 1968, 1969b). With appropriate precautions, electroimmunodiffusion tests readily have detected as little as 16 ng (Ragetli and Weintraub, 1964) or 10 ng (Culliford, 1964) of antigen without auxiliary aids.

Two-Dimensional Double Electroimmunodiffusion

This technique is related to one-dimensional double electroimmuno-diffusion as immunoelectrophoresis is to double diffusion tests. That is, before antigen and antibodies are allowed to react with each other, a mixture of one of the two is first fractionated electrophoretically; then the resulting fractions are electrophoresed, instead of being allowed only to diffuse, against a front of the opposing reactant moving in the opposite direction (Crowle and Hu, 1965; Bon and Swanborn, 1965; see Fig. 6.5).

BASIC TECHNIQUE

On an agarose-coated double-width microscope slide, cast a thin layer of 1% agarose in pH 8.2 barbital buffer, ionic strength 0.025, cut and charge a well with antigen mixture as in agarose immunoelectrophoresis, and electrophorese the mixture also as in immunoelectrophoresis. Then apply a strip of antiserum 5 mm away from the path of primary electrophoresis and parallel to it using filter paper soaked with antiserum, Mylar film as described previously, or a mixture of antiserum–agarose in a trough cut in the agarose. If antiserum is applied using filter paper or Mylar, allow it to diffuse into the gel for 45 minutes at room temperature in a humid atmosphere. Return the antiserum-charged slide to the electrophoresis chamber but at 90 degrees to its original position, and electrophorese as in one-dimensional double electroimmunodiffusion. The result will be a pattern of arcs of precipitate resembling that seen in classic immunoelectrophoresis, except that they will be staggered somewhat from anode to cathode of the primary run because of the faster migration of the more anodic components (Fig. 6.22). Some antigens with the mobility of immunoglobulins will not be detected by this basic technique. But they could be by using a variation in arrangement of re-

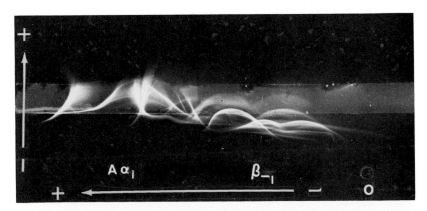

Fig. 6.22. Two-dimensional double electroimmunodiffusion of human serum using a rabbit antiserum. Performed on a double-width microscope slide in 1% agarose and barbital buffer of pH 8.2 and ionic strength 0.05, the test was completed and the pattern of precipitin arcs well developed after primary electrophoresis (horizontally) for 1.5 hours and secondary electrophoresis (vertically) for 50 minutes. The opaque stripe across the center of this photograph is the trough which was filled with antiserum–agarose mixture before the beginning of secondary electrophoresis.

actants in agarose resembling that used for the same purpose in two-dimensional single electroimmunodiffusion (see Fig. 6.16F).

Agar originally was (Bon and Swanborn, 1965; Crowle and Hu, 1965) used for two-dimensional double electroimmunodiffusion; but agarose is a more versatile medium. With agar, a buffer of pH 8.6 is better than the frequently used pH 8.2 buffer because it will moderate electroosmotic migration of the precipitins somewhat. Ideally, buffer, medium, and type of antiserum should be chosen so that only the precipitins will migrate cathodically; agarose used at pH 8.2 with rabbit antiserum therefore closely approaches the ideal. A double-width microscope slide is suggested because it is easier to use for secondary electrophoresis in most varieties of electrophoresis apparatus than one of single width, but if the distance between electrode vessels can be shortened sufficiently a single-width slide will provide comparable results.

The lengths and intensities of primary and secondary electrophoresis are determined empirically. Conditions of electrophoresis usually employed for immunoelectrophoresis and for one-dimensional double electroimmunodiffusion generally will yield satisfactory results.

Two-dimensional double electroimmunodiffusion so far has found little utility. One of the two papers known to describe it mentions only that it can resolve different antigens better than its one-dimensional counterpart (Bon and Swanborn, 1965). It might therefore be useful for investigating Liesegang-like precipitation in electroimmunodiffusion. The other paper reported its being utilized to determine the relative electrophoretic mobility of a purified antituberculosis immunizing antigen because the precipitins available against this antigen were unable in conventional immunoelectrophoresis to form a coherent arc of precipitate (Crowle and Hu, 1965). The technique therefore is more sensitive than conventional immunoelectrophoresis in detecting antigens with lower isoelectric pH than their antibodies, especially when the antibodies are inefficient precipitins, and it could be expected also to detect fast migrating and/or diffusing antigens better than conventional immunoelectrophoresis. The antituberculosis immunizing antigen, for instance, was found to have 1.87 times the anodic mobility of human serum albumin in agar and a mean molecular weight of approximately 20,000 (Crowle and Hu, 1965). This antigen also was detected in two-dimensional double electro-"immuno"-diffusion by using 6,9-diamino-2-ethoxyacridine (Ethodin, Rivanol) to precipitate it instead of antiserum.

Since this technique has been used so little, its potential application is difficult to predict. Any description of technical variations that might be made of it would mostly be speculative. Therefore, no more can be written at present than that it probably can be used in variations of reactant positioning similar to those depicted in Fig. 5.15 for its close relative, classic immunoelectrophoresis.

Electroimmunodiffusion currently is at a stage in development and application similar to that of immunoelectrophoresis in 1954. The contributions to immunochemistry and biology made by immunoelectrophoresis since that date are widely recognized and appreciated. Difficult as it is to imagine, during coming years electroimmunodiffusion almost certainly will overshadow immunoelectrophoresis considerably in both capabilities and accomplishments.

Chapter 7

Ancillary Immunodiffusion Techniques

The principal techniques of immunodiffusion have been discussed in Chapters 3, 4, 5, and 6. This chapter describes both variations in these techniques which extend their utility, and less familiar methods in immunodiffusion which can be used as alternative and sometimes better means of solving some special problem in immunochemical analysis. Like electroimmunodiffusion, some of these methods may develop into unexpectedly powerful analytic tools; others may remain no more than technical curiosities; still others probably will become standard alternatives to the immunochemist's already extensive repertoire of investigative procedures.

Alternative Methods for Detecting Antigen–Antibody Reactions

Most immunodiffusion techniques utilize antigen–antibody precipitation as a direct sign of antigen–antibody reaction. But other manifestations of such reaction can be employed, including agglutination, cell immobilization, cell lysis, or interference with any of these reactions or with specific precipitation itself.

Agglutination in Immunodiffusion Tests

SURFACE AGGLUTINATION

Figure 7.1 illustrates an immunoelectrophoretic technique for determining the electrophoretic mobility of agglutinins, specifically hemagglutinins, using surface agglutination (Hanson *et al.,* 1960).

403

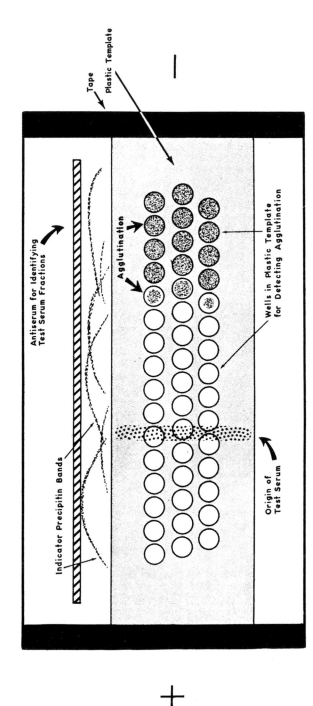

Fig. 7.1. An immunoelectrophoretic method developed by Hanson and colleagues (1960) for determining the immunoelectrophoretic mobility of agglutinins. Tapes and plastic template are positioned after preliminary electrophoresis of test serum, for the second stage of the experiment in which agglutinins are located as to their electrophoretic positions in the agar gel under the template. See text for details.

A wide slab of agar is used for electrophoresis of a human antiserum, and parallel to the axis of fractionation there is the usual trough to receive indicator reactant (antiserum to human serum) after electrophoresis. However, the origin for the human antiserum being electrophoresed is wider than usual so that separated fractions will spread over a wide area of agar. After electrophoresis, a Plexiglas template is laid upon the agar, and each of numerous wells drilled through it in two long, parallel rows corresponding to the axis of electrophoresis is charged with antigen (e.g., a suspension of red blood cells). The trough, meanwhile, is charged with antiserum to human serum in order to identify, by the usual precipitin arcs seen in immunoelectrophoresis, the separated constituents of antiserum. If hemagglutinins happen to be in the agar under a given template hole, they diffuse up into the small quantity of saline placed in this hole in a special, short preincubation period and agglutinate the red blood cells that have been added to the hole after this preincubation. By correlating the location of wells showing hemagglutination with the analytic immunoelectrophoretic pattern which identifies antiserum fractions under any particular well, one can determine which antiserum fraction is responsible for hemagglutinating activity. Isoagglutinins in human blood and colostrum were identified by a slight variation of this technique as being of similar γ_1- to β_1-globulin mobility (Hanson, 1964).

This method also has been used to determine the electrophoretic mobilities of bacterial agglutinins (Raunio and Kaarsalo, 1962). *Escherichia coli* H agglutinins, for instance, were found to be γ_2-globulins, whereas agglutinins for O and K antigens were detected in γ_1, and γ_1-to-β_1 regions, respectively. The technique can be improved by overfilling the wells in the template so that the fluid of bacterial suspension bulges above them. Then the template and electropherogram are inverted together and incubated. Agglutination will develop within the bulging droplets of suspension as though they were concave bottoms of small agglutination tubes (Raunio and Kaarsalo, 1962). In addition to making reactions easier to observe, this modification also permits use of more dilute antiserum and yields improved resolution between agglutinins of closely associated electrophoretic mobilities. With slight variations this form of immunoelectrophoresis should be adaptable to any of the many different kinds of direct and indirect agglutination and agglutination–inhibition test.

There is a simplified alternative to this technique not requiring any template (Angevine *et al.*, 1966). Cold hemagglutinins were located as γ_1-globulins in an agar electropherogram of an antiserum by soaking the electropherogram in a 2% suspension of human erythrocytes for 1 hour,

very gently removing it from this suspension, and then observing its surface for an area of adhering red blood cells where agglutination had
occurred.

INTRAGEL AGGLUTINATION

As was indicated in Chapter 1, migration of molecules or particles
much larger than serum macroglobulins through agar gels once was
thought to be improbable; but newer evidence indicates that it does
occur. Thus, under the electron microscope, precipitin bands in agar
double diffusion tests have been seen to consist of antibody molecules
complexed with virus particles (Blair *et al.*, 1966), and electroimmunodiffusion tests for precipitins (agglutinins) to various different viruses
have become commonplace (Chapter 6). Hence, several aspects of antigen agglutination practiced classically in liquid media can be adapted
to immunodiffusion tests in semisolid medium. By using 0.5% agar gel,
Milgrom and Loza (1967) were able to perform "hemagglutination"
double diffusion tests with erythrocyte stromata in place of whole
erythrocytes, and "flocculation" tests with suspended lipoidal antigens
and syphilis sera or antibrain antisera. They could distinguish between M
and N human erythrocytes and between sheep and bovine erythrocytes.
They compared antigens with small lateral diffusion in their immunodiffusion agglutination tests indirectly, by reacting two antisera against one
antigen instead of using the more conventional arrangement of two antigens against one antiserum (Chapter 4).

This intragel agglutination technique could be used for passive hemagglutination tests and similar assays for either antigen or antibody which
might be or might become attached to such carriers as erythrocytes.
Milgrom and Loza detected rabbit antibodies to human red blood cells
by reacting human erythrocyte stromata in a hemagglutination double
diffusion plate test with goat antirabbit immunoglobulin antiserum
(Milgrom and Loza, 1967).

Immunoimmobilization

A form of agglutination test using living, motile bacteria has been described for typing *Salmonella* organisms by their surface antigens (Mohit,
1968). The culture of organisms to be tested is inoculated aseptically to
the center of a petri dish of motility agar, a 0.3% nutrient gel within which
these bacteria can both multiply and spread from their inoculation site
by the action of their flagella. Paper discs impregnated with different
antiflagellar antisera are placed at even intervals in a circle around and

some distance away from the inoculation site. When the outward-spreading motile bacteria encounter a homologous antiserum diffusing radially toward them, they will become immobilized in a semicircular line resembling an arc of precipitate in a double diffusion plate test.

In addition to being useful for easy, economical screening of bacterial serotypes, this technique can also be used like a double diffusion comparison test for studying antigenic relationships between two different cultures of bacteria. Furthermore, since bacteria not reacting with an antiserum will migrate beyond the line of immobilization formed by bacteria that do react with it, immunoimmobilization is a convenient way of isolating different antigenic phases of bacteria.

Lysis and Complement Fixation

Lysis of erythrocytes suspended in agar or agarose can be used to detect antibodies directly (hemolysins) or indirectly (complement fixation, passive hemolysis) and to study complement. Analogs of single and double diffusion plate tests and of immunoelectrophoresis have been devised to employ this effect. Hemolysin can be titrated by mixing a 2% suspension of rabbit erythrocytes with an equal volume of appropriately diluted complement, and mixing this 1:1 with warm 1% agar. The mixture is poured into a petri dish and allowed to gel. Wells cast in this gel are charged with different dilutions of hemolysin, and after appropriate incubation the diameter of hemolysis in the gel is measured in the same manner as the diameter of a disc of precipitate in a conventional single diffusion plate (Milgrom and Millers, 1963; Hiramoto *et al.*, 1971). Complement can be quantitated similarly by suspending a mixture of erythrocytes and heat-inactivated hemolysin in the agar and filling the wells cast in the agar with various dilutions of complement.

The interaction of complement and hemolysin can be observed in a double diffusion plate version of these tests (Milgrom and Millers, 1963) in which the final concentration of erythrocytes in 0.5% agar is 1% and the wells are filled with heat-inactivated hemolysin and complement. The petri dishes are incubated for 70 hours at 4°C and then for 2 hours more at 37°C. Complement and hemolysin intermingling between the two wells will produce a faint zone of clearing (hemolysis) in the agar gel, which becomes somewhat more obvious with additional standing for 2 to 3 hours more at room temperature. If the agar in which the reactions have occurred is dried under filter paper, and the paper is removed before drying is quite complete, the area of lysis will be white on the paper in a surrounding area colored red with hemoglobin (Rybák *et al.*, 1963).

This in-agar[1] lysis technique also can be employed to detect "natural" hemolysins as well as antibodies to substances either naturally or artificially attached to erythrocytes (Rybák et al., 1963; Rybák and Petáková, 1964). Whether the lysin is an antibody or an enzyme, antibodies to it can be identified by a lysis-inhibition variant of this method (Thompson and Lackmann, 1970). Although not usually thought of as such, the complement-fixation test is a lysis inhibition test. It is executed by mixing 4% sheep erythrocytes with an equal volume of 50% complement, mixing this combination 1:1 with 1% agar, and casting this mixture in a petri dish to form a layer no thicker than 2 mm. Antigen and antiserum are mixed separately with warm agar and added to their respective wells cast in the erythrocyte-charged agar. The plates are held at 4°C for 18 hours, and then the agar surface is flooded with heat-inactivated 2.5% hemolysin. This is followed by additional incubations for 1 hour at 4°C, and for 15 to 40 minutes at 37°C until lysis is complete throughout the petri dish. Where complement has been fixed by antigen–antibody reaction, there will be a corresponding zone in the gel lacking lysis (Milgrom and Millers, 1963).

Lysis and complement-fixation tests should be adaptable to most variations of immunodiffusion techniques described in previous chapters. As an example, a reversed immunoelectrophoresis test has been described in which rabbit serum containing hemolysin was electrophoresed through erythrocyte-containing agar, and a trough alongside the path of electrophoresis was filled with guinea pig complement (Milgrom and Loza, 1966). The electrophoretic locations of two classes of rabbit hemolytic antibodies were revealed by development of two arcs of hemolysis; one was identified as a γ_G-globulin by reaction simultaneously with goat antiserum to rabbit serum placed in a trough on the opposite side of the electropherogram, where it formed an arc of precipitate as in conventional immunoelectrophoresis (Fig. 7.2). In a two-step alternative to this technique, antiserum can be electrophoresed in paper, successive strips of the resulting paper electropherogram can be cut and transferred to agar gel containing erythrocytes and complement, antibodies potentially present in a strip can be eluted into the gel by placing a drop of saline on each strip of paper, and the lytic effect of these antibodies can be detected by corresponding zones of lysis (Goreczky, 1959). This tech-

---

[1] These tests were described before agarose became readily available. Some agars have anticomplementary properties and must be specially treated before use to eliminate these properties (Milgrom and Loza, 1966), but good grades of agarose can be employed without this complication.

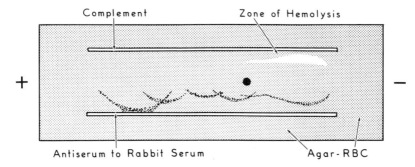

Fig. 7.2. Immunoelectrophoretic location of rabbit hemolytic antibodies using sheep erythrocyte-charged agar, complement, and antiserum to rabbit serum. The latter detects various constituents of the rabbit antiserum, including immunoglobulins. Complement locates the hemolysins by acting with them to form a zone of lysed erythrocytes which corresponds to the immunoelectrophoretic distribution of the rabbit immunoglobulin having hemolytic activity. (Adapted from Milgrom and Loza, 1966.)

nique also is applicable to other indicator media, like suspensions of living bacteria instead of erythrocytes, and it can be used in reverse to measure inhibitors such as antilysins (Goreczky, 1959).

The precipitation-enhancing effect of complement for some kinds of antibody has been mentioned (cf. Chapter 1). If it is strong enough, it can be exploited for an unconventional complement-fixation test. Thus, some guinea pig antisera precipitate hapten-specific complexes only with the help of the C_1 component of complement. This characteristic was used to study the susceptibility of this component in sera from different species of animals to various treatments (Paul and Benacerraf, 1966). Complement has been used to enhance aggregation of antigen–antibody complexes in cellulose acetate after one-dimensional single electroimmunodiffusion (Saravis and Bonacker, 1970). It also can be detected by precipitin band bending (see following section) when this depends on the presence of complement (Paul and Benacerraf, 1966). Both of these effects could be used for indicators of complement fixation.

An indirect but very sensitive way of detecting fixation of complement or any other substance to precipitates of antigen and antibody is to wash these precipitates thoroughly and then inject them into an appropriate animal to stimulate its formation of precipitins to the fixed constituents (Gengozian and Doria, 1964). This method is especially useful when the nature of the fixed components is unknown, and for producing analytic reagents to specifically detect this fixation.

Precipitin Band Bending

Antigen or antibodies unable independently to develop visible precipitation in an immunodiffusion test, because of being too dilute or too inefficient, sometimes can be detected, and the sensitivity of immunodiffusion tests increased considerably, by bending effects that they can have on the tip of a band of precipitate being formed by an immunologically related antigen–antibody system (Heiner, 1958). This phenomenon is fundamentally the same as Ouchterlony's reaction of identity (see Chapter 4). To utilize it, the test reactant must be placed in such a position on the immunodiffusogram that it can diffuse into the area of precipitation between wells charged with reference antigen and precipitins and thereby deform the precipitin band during its development (Wilson *et al.*, 1962; cf. Fig. 4.18). Maximal sensitivity is achieved in a precipitin band bending test when reference antigen and antiserum are adjusted to produce the weakest discernible band of precipitate, one that may not even be visible until it has been stained (Casman *et al.*, 1969). As little as 10 ng of antigen per milliliter thus can be detected.

Although the bending of a precipitin band in one of these tests usually is interpreted as due to the presence of cross-reactive antigen or antiserum, more precisely this bending only signifies that the solution effecting it contains something that promotes antigen–antibody precipitation. Sometimes this will not be one of the primary reactants. It could be a coprecipitin like guinea pig complement (Paul and Benacerraf, 1966). Inhibition tests (see below) can be used to determine whether bending is due to a cofactor or to a primary reactant.

Inhibition Tests

Some forms of immunodiffusion inhibition test have been mentioned in preceding chapters, with descriptions of standard techniques. Thus, the migration of one reactant can be inhibited by adding the other reactant to it at its origin, or by placing the other reactant in its path of migration. The classic example is Björklund's intragel specific absorption (Björklund, 1952a). In this, antigen added to agar gel specifically prevents diffusion of corresponding precipitins from an antiserum well in a double diffusion plate but does not affect diffusion of unrelated precipitins. With small variations, such as described below, this technique can be used as an indirect way of detecting antigens and antibodies, being especially useful when these are unable to precipitate visibly.

Precipitins deprived of precipitating capacity by papain digestion can be detected in immunodiffusion by mixing them with antigen in its origin and thus decreasing the concentration of antigen free to diffuse and to form a visible precipitate (Kulberg and Tarkhanova, 1961; Shivers and Metz, 1962; Kjellén, 1965). If the nonprecipitating antibodies are mixed with a quantity of antigen adjusted to be just sufficient to precipitate with a reference antiserum, precipitation will be prevented (Ray and Kadull, 1964). Functionally univalent antigens (i.e., haptens) can be detected similarly, except that they are added to a reference antiserum diluted to minimal precipitating capacity (Malley *et al.*, 1964; Dandliker *et al.*, 1965). The hapten can first be conjugated to some immunologically indifferent macromolecular carrier to increase its effectiveness in preventing diffusion of antibodies which will react with it (Paul and Benacerraf, 1966). Conversely, using such a conjugate as an artificially multivalent antigen may be necessary to obtain the visible precipitation which inhibition by the monovalent hapten is intended to prevent (Josephson *et al.*, 1962).

Precipitin-inhibition tests can be used to detect and to quantitate intact nonprecipitating antibodies, and therefore all antibodies against a given antigen, whether precipitins or not (Patterson, Chang, and Pruzansky, 1964; Jameson, 1969b). The simple technique illustrated in Fig. 7.3 has been used for this purpose to help diagnose farmer's lung disease (Jameson, 1969b). In it, the presence of any antibodies in a test antiserum prevents the nearly minimal quantity of antigen mixed with this antiserum from diffusing against an equally minimal quantity of standard precipitating antiserum, and precipitation is prevented. Visibly striking inhibition of double diffusion precipitation has been reported for dog

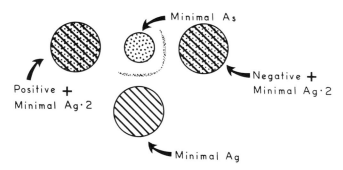

Fig. 7.3. Precipitation-inhibition test for detecting antibodies whether they themselves are precipitins or not. The antiserum to be tested is mixed with twice the minimal amount of antigen required to form a visible precipitin band with a minimal amount of reference precipitating antiserum. If the test antiserum contains no antibodies ("negative"), the reaction between reference precipitating antiserum and antigen mixed with test antiserum is not inhibited; if the test antiserum contains antibodies ("positive"), these antibodies react with antigen with which they have been mixed and prevent its precipitating with reference antiserum. (Adapted from Jameson, 1969b.)

antisera to bovine serum albumin (Patterson *et al.*, 1964a) and to ragweed antigen (Patterson *et al.*, 1965b). These antisera were used in wells adjacent to wells filled with rabbit precipitins to these antigens. Lateral growth of the precipitin bands formed by the rabbit antibodies was abruptly interrupted in areas where dog antibodies had diffused.

Quantitative data can be obtained from precipitation-inhibition tests in several ways. One of the more obvious is to add graded quantities of absorbing antigen to a constant amount of antiserum and to note the corresponding decrease in precipitation (Gussoni, 1964); or various concentrations of antisera can be mixed with a constant minimal amount of antigen (Ray and Kadull, 1964). Test variations like these have been used for reliable, sensitive determinations of antibodies in immunizations to numerous bacteria, viruses, and fungi (Ray and Kadull, 1964, 1965); they measure C-reactive protein simply and accurately (Langlois *et al.*, 1963; Shay and Ray, 1965).

Another way to use inhibition tests quantitatively is to label antigen, such as with radioactivity, and then to measure the degree of competition between it and unlabeled antigen in an unknown sample for combination with antibodies. Human growth hormone was quantitated in polyacrylamide electroimmunodiffusion by measuring its capacity to prevent known quantities of radiolabeled human growth hormone from binding with antibodies in a standard antiserum. The quantity of unlabeled hormone present was inversely proportional to the quantity of labeled hormone bound (Fitschen, 1963).

Auxiliary Indicators for Antigen–Antibody Reaction

Any property of antigen or of antibody advertising its presence can be employed in immunodiffusion tests to detect antigen–antibody reactions. This property may be natural, or it can be introduced artificially. The type of reactant marker most frequently used in immunodiffusion tests is radioactivity. It greatly increases their sensitivity and versatility (Minden *et al.*, 1966).

Radioimmunodiffusion

Although now widely and regularly practiced, radioimmunodiffusion is as much a technological newcomer as electroimmunodiffusion, having been employed for scarcely more than a dozen years. The reason for its rapid and successful adaption to various kinds of immunodiffusion test has been the simplicity of radioautography, in which radioactive bands of precipitate placed on a photographic emulsion accurately record their own presence (Rejnek and Bednařík, 1960). Radioautography effects considerable amplification, for a few antigen–antibody complexes which cannot be seen, stained, or otherwise detected directly will create a visible photographic image by the cumulative reducing effects that their prolonged radioactive bombardment has on the silver salts of the photographic emulsion. With this amplification, tenths of a nanogram of reactant can be detected by radioimmunodiffusion and radioimmunoelectrophoresis (Fitschen, 1963; Hunter and Greenwood, 1964; Rhodes, 1960).

The simplest form of radioimmunodiffusion employs radiolabeled antigen for some purpose like detecting its precipitation when the antigen–antibody complexes formed are too few to be seen (Patterson, 1961; Patterson *et al.*, 1962; Yagi *et al.*, 1962), or identifying one antigen among many in an immunoelectropherogram (Rejnek and Bednařík, 1960; Raynaud *et al.*, 1965; Clausen *et al.*, 1963). Hormones, vitamins, and other relatively simple and often nonantigenic substances also can be detected by making them radioactive and then mixing them with serum in which there are antigenic carriers which they will combine with and be precipitated with by appropriate antibodies. The simpler substances can be studied in this manner (Aly and Gillich, 1960), and so can their carriers. At least two plasma carriers, one an α_1-globulin, were identified for vitamin B_{12} in this manner (Hall and Finkler, 1963). A substance was found in gastric juice and in saliva which could bind this vitamin but which was absent from serum (Gräsbeck *et al.*, 1963). There are two such binders in normal gastric juice; the absence of one of these from juice of patients with pernicious anemia is diagnostic (Simons and Gräsbeck, 1963). Thyroxin binds to ρ-prealbumin in human serum and therefore is useful as a radioactive indicator for this antigen (Burtin and Grabar, 1967). Interestingly, this binding occurs in tris–maleate or phosphate buffers but not in a barbital buffer. Transferrin is the most prominent carrier in serum of iron; consequently radioactive iron is an excellent label for it (Keutel, 1960; Slopek *et al.*, 1965b).

The course and characteristics of the manufacture of certain antigens can be followed in selected organs by culturing pieces or homogenates of them *in vitro* in a medium containing radioactive components which will be incorporated into them as they are produced. The liver was identified thus as a principal site for α-fetoprotein synthesis in human beings and rats, but its manufacture of this antigen was observed to decline rapidly after birth (Gitlin and Boesman, 1967). Ferritin manufacture was studied similarly in rat liver slices (Saddi and Von der Decken, 1964).

Frequently the quantity of antigen produced by cultured cells, or its quantity in some other kind of sample, is so small that it will not produce a sufficiently compact arc of radioactivity to register recognizably in a radioimmunoelectropherogram (Fig. 7.4A). This difficulty is surmounted by using "carrier radioimmunoelectrophoresis" in which all the radioactive reactant is concentrated into a single, sharp band of precipitate, and in which there is the added benefit of identifying the radioactive antigen with a corresponding visible precipitate in an immunoelectropherogram (Asofsky and Thorbecke, 1961; Hochwald *et al.*, 1961; Grumbach and Kaplan, 1962; Silverstein *et al.*, 1963; Figs. 7.4B, 7.4C). In this technique, the sample and its trace of radioactive antigen (e.g., serum complement) are electrophoresed with a mixture of antigens known to contain enough of this same antigen (e.g., whole serum) to precipitate

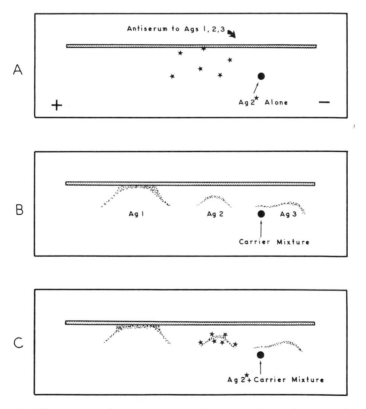

Fig. 7.4. Diagrams explaining carrier radioimmunoelectrophoresis. The concentration of radioactive antigen 2 is too small in immunoelectropherogram *A* to produce a compact zone of radioactivity with appropriate antiserum. But when it is mixed with a carrier solution of antigens containing a high enough concentration of antigen 2 to precipitate (*B*), then radioactive antigen 2 coprecipitates with carrier antigen to form a precipitin band with well localized radioactivity (*C*).

with appropriate antiserum. The resulting electropherogram then is developed with antiserum as in conventional immunoelectrophoresis, whereupon the tracer radioactive antigen coprecipitates with its nonradioactive "carrier" analog. The latter supplies the physical bulk for development of a compact, visible precipitate, and the former reveals its presence by making this visible precipitate radioactive. Then, the arc of radioactivity registering on a radioautogram can be matched with a corresponding visible (stained) arc on the original immunoelectropherogram, and the presence and nature of the radiolabeled antigen can be ascertained. A difficulty sometimes encountered in using this otherwise excellent technique is that a trace radiolabeled substance may not be the same as the antigen with which it precipitates but only have an affinity for it (Thiele and Stark, 1970).

The idea of specifically involving a trace of radioactive reactant in development of a conventional visible arc of antigen–antibody precipitate was altered somewhat to devise an indirect radioimmunodiffusion which possibly is the most sensitive and specific technique available to detect antibodies (Samloff and Barnett, 1967; Minden *et al.*, 1966). Its basis is that a class of immunoglobulins can be precipitated as antigen by an antiserum and yet retain its own capacity to act as antibodies and complex with radiolabeled antigen. For example, IgE antibodies (reagins) to ragweed in man are important in causing hay fever, but they cannot be detected by ordinary immunodiffusion tests because they are not precipitins. However, they can be detected by reacting a human serum containing them against rabbit precipitins to IgE, and then infusing radiolabeled ragweed antigen through the precipitate of IgE and rabbit antibody (Dolovich *et al.*, 1970). This precipitate thereby will acquire radioactivity as the labeled ragweed allergen complexes with precipitated IgE reagins to it.

This technique has been used in double diffusion tests (Berger *et al.*, 1967; Roth *et al.*, 1964; Heiner and Rose, 1970a,b), single diffusion tests (Heiner *et al.*, 1970), and immunoelectrophoresis (Yagi *et al.*, 1963b; Goodman *et al.*, 1964), and it should be equally applicable to electroimmunodiffusion (cf. Zwaan, 1963; Fitschen, 1963; Hunter and Greenwood, 1962). It has different variations (Fig. 7.5). In the one-step method, the immunoglobulin containing nonprecipitating antibodies that are to be detected is allowed to diffuse against a mixture of precipitins for it together with radioactive antigen which will complex with its antibodies as they form the visible precipitate[2] (Yagi *et al.*, 1962, 1963b;

---

[2] Actually, visible precipitation is unnecessary. Development of antigen–antibody complexes sufficiently large to become immobilized within the gel being used will suffice (Dolovich *et al.*, 1970; Samloff and Barnett, 1967; Patterson, 1961).

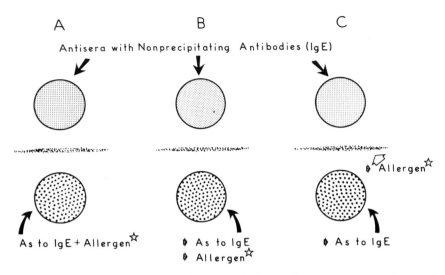

Fig. 7.5. Three varieties of radioimmunodiffusion showing detection of reactions between nonprecipitating antibodies of IgE class with the aid of precipitins to these antibodies (e.g., rabbit precipitins to human IgE) and radioactive allergen with which these antibodies are reactive. A is a one-step method; B and C are two-step methods as indicated.

Fig. 7.5A). In a two-step method the immunoglobulin is reacted with its precipitins, and the radioactive antigen then is used as a "chaser" added to the well originally charged with the precipitins (Dolovich *et al.*, 1970; Yagi *et al.*, 1963b; Fig. 7.5B). In a second two-step method, radiolabeled antigen is diffused into the area of precipitation from the surface of the gel (Fahey *et al.*, 1964; Fig. 7.5C). The two-step methods are better than the one-step method because, in the latter, if the antibodies being detected are precipitins, and they are being diffused against a mixture of both radioactive antigen which they can precipitate and antibodies which can precipitate them, the resulting two simultaneously occurring processes of precipitation which are different and yet involve a common component can interfere with each other and the interpretation of results (Biguet and Tran Van Ky, 1966). But the two-step method using a chaser of radioactive antigen diffusing from what was originally the source of anti-immunoglobulin precipitins may not be able to detect all the antibodies in a test antiserum if the concentration of radioactive antigen is too low to cross the barrier of the first antibody-containing precipitate which it encounters (Samloff and Barnett, 1967). Then the two-step technique using radioactive antigen diffusing into the gel from its surface is better.

Not only can indirect radioimmunodiffusion detect any kind of antibody, it can also identify its immunoglobulin type (Yagi *et al.*, 1963); it can follow the rise and decline of different immunoglobulin classes of antibody being manufactured by an animal to a given antigen. For instance, four different classes of mouse immunoglobulin were identified by radioimmunoelectrophoresis as having antibody activity to hemocyanin (Fahey *et al.*, 1964). Rabbits were found to begin producing both 19 S and 7 S antibodies simultaneously to various protein antigens (Freeman and Stavitsky, 1966), although they are frequently thought to make 19 S antibodies first and only later to make 7 S antibodies. Antipolio virus antibodies in adult human beings were identified by this technique in both IgA and IgG classes of serum immunoglobulin (Ainbender *et al.*, 1965). Polio immunization usually results in a predominantly IgG response, but even after repeated immunizations one individual was found to make only IgM antibodies (Philipson *et al.*, 1966). Radioimmunoelectrophoresis also has been employed to detect antigen-binding activity in fragments of degraded antibodies (Onoue *et al.*, 1964).

Radioimmunodiffusion techniques can be used for quantitation. As little as 0.16 ng of bovine serum albumin nitrogen could be detected in an early quantitative technique in which a band of precipitate entrapping radioactive antigen was cut from the surrounding gel, washed, and analyzed in a scintillation counter (Patterson, 1961). Recently, a two-step form of radial single diffusion has been described for quantitating antigen or antibody as well as identifying the immunoglobulin class of antibody being measured (Heiner *et al.*, 1970). Wells in the agar of a conventional radial diffusion plate charged with antiserum to a selected class of immunoglobulin are filled with antisera to be tested. After discs of precipitate have developed from the one class of immunoglobulin in the antisera being precipitated, and the plates subsequently have been washed free of nonprecipitated materials, these wells are filled anew with radioactive antigen and reincubated as before. As the radioactive antigen diffuses out through the disc of precipitated immunoglobulin, it is bound in proportion to the quantity and quality of antibodies constituting this immunoglobulin, and this binding is measured by photometric scanning (see Chapter 2) of radioautographs made from these radial diffusion plates.

Inhibition tests such as those described in the preceding section of this chapter also are applicable to radioimmunodiffusion. For example, insulin or growth hormone in human sera can be quantitated by mixing the sera with a standard antiserum and a known quantity of radioactive antigen and observing the degree of interference in binding of the radioactive antigen by the antiserum effected by the hormone in the test sera

(Hunter and Greenwood, 1962). This interference was detected by a transmigration test (see Chapter 6), and was sensitive to 1 μg of hormone per milliliter.

Enzymoimmunodiffusion

As has been mentioned, any readily recognized property of a constituent of antigen–antibody complexes can serve as an auxiliary indicator of these complexes in immunodiffusion tests. Enzyme activity is one such property.

This characteristic is used most directly when the antigen itself is an enzyme (or is labeled with enzyme; see next section), and antigen–antibody complexes therefore exhibit enzymatic activity. Many examples are cataloged by Uriel (1963). The utility of enzymes as indicators of antigen–antibody complexing is most dramatically illustrated when they are used to detect invisible or nonstainable antigen–antibody aggregates. There are several examples. An invisible aggregate of human red cell lysate carbonic anhydrase with its antibodies which could not be detected by a conventional protein stain was made visible by the anhydrase converting a cobalt indicator to black cobalt sulfide (Micheli, 1965). A trace precipitate of cereal amylase and its antibodies too insignificant to be stained was detected by a starch hydrolysis reaction (Daussant and Grabar, 1966). An invisible, unstainable aggregate of chicken serum esterase was revealed by the esterase acting upon an appropriate substrate (Kaminski, 1966), and complexes of antibody and lactic dehydrogenase were detected similarly (Nace, 1963). Five different arcs of antigen–antibody reaction could be detected in immunoelectropherograms of rat bone marrow by the effects of their respective enzymes, when there were no corresponding visible arcs of precipitate (Beernink et al., 1965).

In the examples given above, as well as in most forms of enzymoimmunodiffusion, the arc of antigen–antibody aggregate is subjected to direct test for the enzyme suspected of being present; and this is possible because most antibodies to enzymes do not neutralize their biological activities (cf. Chapter 2). But sometimes it is more convenient to study enzyme antigens by the physical or biochemical inhibition that can be exerted against them by antibodies under appropriate circumstances. For example, by precipitating an enzyme, antibodies can limit its diffusion and consequently its effect on appropriate substrate added to the medium. For a recent application of this venerable technique, egg yolk was used in agar to detect lipase and, correspondingly, antiserum to lipase (Lunbeck and Tirunarayanan, 1970). In a similar experiment, both IgG$_2$ and IgG$_1$ antibodies were shown to neutralize the antibiotic colicin when *Escherichia coli* growth was used as an indicator, although only the former class of antibody was a good precipitin (Tsao and Goebel, 1969; see Fig. 7.6). Both classes of antibody had less cross-neutralizing effects against a heterologous than against the homologous colicin. This experiment shows that the affected antigen need not be visibly precipitated to be inactivated, that different classes of antibody can have similar inhibitory effect without necessarily causing the same serologic effect, and that suppressive effects on biochemical activities need not be restricted to experiments solely with enzymes.

Enzyme substrates can be incorporated in agar or agarose without materially interfering with diffusion or electrophoresis. This makes various immunodiffusion tests for enzymes useful in immunoelectrophoresis and electroimmunodiffusion as well. One example was given above in the section on lysins and complement fixation in which reversed immuno-

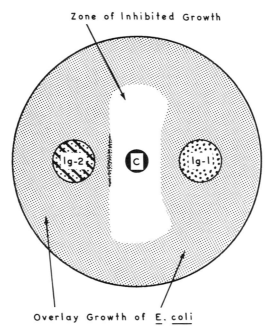

Zone of Inhibited Growth

Overlay Growth of E. coli

Fig. 7.6. Detecting nonprecipitating antibodies by their capacity to neutralize an antibiotic. The antibiotic (colicin) was placed in a small central well in nutrient agar gel, two larger wells were charged, respectively, with Ig$_1$ and Ig$_2$ antibodies to colicin, and the surface of the gel was inoculated with *Escherichia coli*. Colicin inhibited bacterial growth in a zone limited on opposite sides by the two species of antibodies, only one of which (the Ig$_2$) also was able to precipitate the antibiotic. (Adapted from Tsao and Goebel, 1969.)

electrophoresis performed in erythrocyte-containing agar identified im-munoglobulin classes of hemolytic antibodies. In another example, fibrin-charged agar was used for immunoelectrophoresis to locate and compare proteolytic enzyme inhibitors in plasmin and leukocyte extracts (Her-mann and Miescher, 1965). By matching zones of inhibited fibrinolysis with arcs of precipitate in the immunoelectrophoretic pattern forming in the fibrin–agar mixture, some of the proteases of leukocytes were shown to be antigenically different from those in plasmin.

Enzymes also can be used in immunodiffusion-like tests as substitutes for antiserum. For instance, bee venom phospholipase reacts with fresh human serum α and β lipoproteins and was employed to precipitate them selectively (Barker et al., 1966).

Other Indicators for Antigen–Antibody Reaction

Some enzymes can be coupled to antigens or antibodies (cf. Avrameas and Uriel, 1966) to make many of the indicator reactions discussed above as widely applicable as radiolabeling for immunodiffusion reactions. Although not so sensitive as radioactivity or enzyme labeling, fluoro-immunodiffusion has advantages of directness and rapidity. With fluo-rescein isothiocyanate labeling, fluoroimmunoelectrophoresis has been employed to detect and identify antibody classes, to reveal nonprecipitat-ing antigen–antibody reactions, and to localize combining sites on dif-ferent fragments of antibodies (Ghetie, 1967; Cebra and Goldstein, 1965).

Fluorescent-labeled immunologic reactants are frequently used for microscopy. These reactants tend to be difficult to make, by conventional chemical and physical methods, to the degree of specificity often desired. A preparatory fluoroimmunodiffusion technique developed by Nace not only illustrates use of this kind of test but also merits special mention as a potentially powerful preparatory immunochemical technique (Nace et al., 1960; Dray et al., 1963b). Antiserum against antigens in a tissue extract is prepared and labeled with fluorescein. The antiserum is reacted in immunodiffusion or in immunoelectrophoresis with the tissue extract, whereupon several bands of fluorescent precipitate will form. By pre-liminary investigation, one of these bands can have been identified as the antigen ultimately to be located by fluorescence microscopy in sec-tions of tissue. This band of precipitate, which consists of antigen and fluorescence-labeled antibody specific for it, is cut from the agar gel. The piece of agar containing the band is washed and minced and then is placed on the section of tissue which is to be examined microscopically. Next, the precipitate is dissociated in situ with alkali or acid, whereupon the freed fluorescent antibodies diffuse into the tissue. Then, the tissue section is washed and its pH restored to neutral; the dissociated fluorescent antibodies recombine with antigen including that within the section itself and thus label it specifically wherever it is anatomically. After subsequent additional washing to remove remnants of agar and complexes of antibody with nontissue components, the tissue section can be examined routinely by fluorescence microscopy.

Related to fluorescence microscopy conceptually is electron microscopy in which electron-dense markers like ferritin are used in place of fluorescence (Borek and Silverstein, 1961; Vogt and Kopp, 1964). Ferritin also is used to label antigen and antibodies in immunodiffusion tests, although for the slightly different reason that, because it is rich in iron, it can be detected by the sensitive and simple Prussian blue color reaction (cf. Bazin, 1967). Ferritin can be used either as the antigen itself (Patterson *et al.*, 1965a) or as a label for other reactants (Hsu *et al.*, 1963).

Dye-labeled (e.g., with hematoxylin) antibodies have been used in double diffusion plates to detect otherwise invisible antigen–antibody complexing (Katsh and Matchael, 1962), and in the original description of paper immunochromatography hematoxylin was used to make the bacterial antigen suspension visible and its reaction with antiserum in paper readily perceived (Castaneda, 1950).

Novel Varieties of Immunodiffusion

A few years ago electroimmunodiffusion would have been considered a novel immunodiffusion technique—that is, a technological curiosity with prospects of only occasional specialized application. But by its frequent use currently it is graduating from being novel to being prescriptive. The techniques described below may or may not become more than technological curiosities; but each has uses and characteristics which make it worth knowing.

Two-Dimensional Immunoelectrophoresis

In one form of this technique, the mixture of antigens to be analyzed is electrophoresed on a square slide of agar or agarose first in one direction and then in a second direction at right angles to the first (Blanc, 1959). If the electropherogram then is fixed and stained for proteins, it will show an electrophoretic separation of antigens similar to that following electrophoresis in just one dimension, except that this pattern will extend across the plate diagonally. To complete the immunoelectrophoretic technique, the electropherogram is not stained. Instead, troughs are cut in the gel parallel to, or sometimes at a slight angle to, the anticipated train of separated antigens and are charged with antiserum; arcs of precipitate then develop as in conventional immunoelectrophoresis. This form of two-dimensional immunoelectrophoresis is said to provide somewhat better resolution than classic one-dimensional immunoelectrophoresis (Blanc, 1959).

Two alternative, possibly more informative two-dimensional immunoelectrophoresis techniques are described by Yokoyama and Carr (1962) and illustrated in Figs. 7.7 and 7.8. One might be termed, rather cumbersomely, "two-dimensional single diffusion immunoelectrophoresis," because after electrophoresis in two succeeding dimensions the separated antigens are precipitated as discs, as in single diffusion tests, under a filter paper overlay of antiserum (Fig. 7.7). Although the other is a double-diffusion technique, it is not the same as that described in the

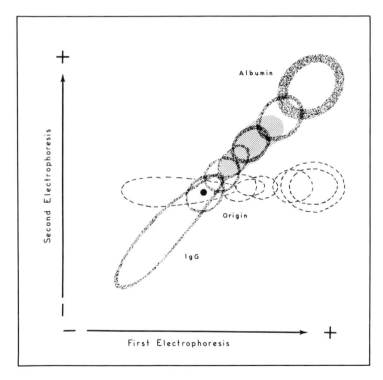

Fig. 7.7. A form of two-dimensional single diffusion immunoelectrophoresis. Antigen mixture is electrophoresed on a square plate of gel from a central origin first horizontally and then vertically. Then the gel is covered with antiserum-saturated filter paper, and antibodies diffusing into the gel from the surface precipitate corresponding antigens at their various locations in a diagonally oriented pattern otherwise generally resembling that of one-dimensional single diffusion immunoelectrophoresis (cf. Figs. 5.7 and 5.8). (Redrawn from Yokoyama and Carr, 1962.)

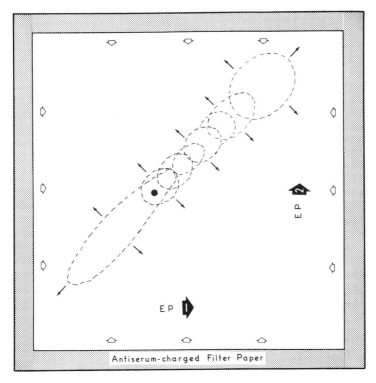

Fig. 7.8. A form of two-dimensional double diffusion immunoelectrophoresis. Antigen mixture, placed in an origin near the center of a square plate of gel, is electrophoresed first horizontally and then vertically. Then four strips of filter paper charged with antiserum are placed along the edges of the plate so that the various outward-diffusing antigens will be precipitated by corresponding inward-diffusing antibodies. (Redrawn from Yokoyama and Carr, 1962.)

preceding paragraph because, as is shown in Fig. 7.8, antigens and antibodies begin diffusing toward each other at 45 degrees, as in a gradient double diffusion test (see Chapter 4), instead of face to face. A potentially valuable application of this as yet relatively unexamined technique would be simultaneous multiantigenic analysis of the precipitins in two polyvalent antisera, the top and bottom strips of filter paper being impregnated with one antiserum and the side strips with the other.

The information obtainable from two-dimensional immunoelectrophoresis can be increased by performing primary and secondary electrophoreses under different conditions. Thus, antigens of different molecular size but similar electrophoretic mobility can be separated from each other during the second electrophoresis by using a higher concentration of agar (Raymond, 1964) or a sieving medium like polyacrylamide

(Wright *et al.*, 1970), and distinctions by differences in pH titration curves can be seen if the buffer pH for the second electrophoresis is changed (Raymond, 1964).

Immunochromatography

This technique resembles immunoelectrophoresis except that original separation of antigens is chromatographic instead of electrophoretic (Carnegie and Pacheco, 1964). Currently, immunochromatography is generally inferior to and more cumbersome than immunoelectrophoresis, but it is a valuable alternative for special problems like differentiating reactants by molecular weight, analyzing simple mixtures not easily separated by electrophoresis, or examining solvent and substrate conditions that are to be scaled up for preparatory chromatography. It may prove unexpectedly valuable when chromatography is used in place of primary electrophoresis in electroimmunodiffusion tests. In its simplest form, immunochromatography can provide rapid, easy, and economical field tests for antigen–antibody reaction (De Banchero, 1962).

IMMUNOGELFILTRATION

As in immunoelectrophoresis, any of several media can be used for primary separation of the antigens later to be detected by precipitation with their antibodies in semisolid medium. If the antigen fractionation is effected in some way peculiar and characteristic to the chromatographic medium employed, then it can be named accordingly. Hence, the technique of passing the antigen solution through a gel filtration medium has been named "gel immunofiltration" (Grant and Everall, 1965) or "immunogelfiltration" (Hanson *et al.*, 1966a,b; Agostoni, *et al.*, 1967).

Grant and Everall (1965, 1966) have described a method employing superfine Sephadex G-200 using apparatus very similar to that of immunoelectrophoresis in which there is no need to transfer chromatographically separated antigens to agar for analysis. After thin-layer gel filtration has been completed on a glass plate of 20 × 10-cm dimensions, this plate is placed on a diagram to serve as a pattern for antiserum troughs which are to be formed, and a moat which is to be made around the entire reaction area for isolating it from the surrounding slurry of Sephadex. The troughs and moat are "cut" by following the diagram through the slurry with a Pasteur pipet attached to a water aspirator. After antiserum has been added to the antiserum troughs, the plate is kept at room temperature in a damp box for 24 hours for precipitation to develop. Then, a sheet of cellulose acetate is laid upon the delicate slurry of Sephadex for protection, and the immunofiltration pattern can be washed and stained by careful use of routine techniques. Figure 7.9 shows a diagram of results which can be obtained.

Buffers used for immunogelfiltration generally must be different from those used for immunoelectrophoresis to provide good results. For instance, a buffer used with Sephadex should have a high ionic strength to minimize protein–Sephadex interactions (see Appendix IV). Antigens are separated from each other in immunogelfiltration by molecular size, and so for mixtures of smaller antigens such as might be found in urine another grade of medium will be better than Sephadex G-200 (Grant and Everall, 1966). Thus, Sephadex G-75 has been used in a variation of this technique described below for demonstrating micromolecular paraproteinemia (Vergani and Agostoni, 1967).

Because the Grant-Everall technique is performed in a slurry rather than in a gel, it is delicate. Using a print-off transfer of separated antigens to a different medium in which antigen–antibody reaction subsequently will develop is technically easier. Agostoni *et al.* (1967) obtained excellent results by applying a strip of moistened, blotted cellulose acetate to the surface of the slurry after thin-layer filtration and allowing separated antigens to diffuse into the membrane for 10 minutes. Then, they removed the membrane, cleaned off the clinging Sephadex particles, applied antiserum with strips of filter paper as is sometimes done in cellulose acetate immunoelectrophoresis (see Chapter 5), and allowed antigen–antibody precipitation to develop under mineral oil. Subsequent washing and staining, by cellulose acetate immunoelectrophoresis techniques, revealed immunofiltration patterns with better resolution and sensitivity than were obtained when antigen–antibody precipitation was developed directly in the slurry.

Another variety of immunogelfiltration avoids the delicacy of developing precipitin arcs in Sephadex slurry alone by removing all the slurry

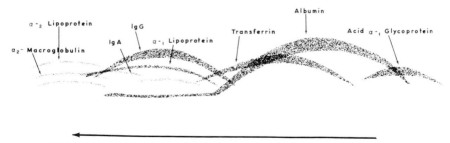

Buffer flow; increasing mobility; increasing molecular size

Fig. 7.9. Diagram illustrating immunogelfiltration of human serum and showing that the various antigens segregate principally by molecular size. (Redrawn from Grant and Everall, 1966.)

around a strip through which antigens have moved and been separated and then carefully running molten agar first around and then over this strip (Hanson et al., 1966a,b). After the agar has gelled, troughs are cut parallel to the now embedded strip of Sephadex and charged with antiserum, and the immunochromatogram is developed like an immunoelectropherogram. The utility of immunogelfiltration performed in this manner is illustrated by its capacity to detect lyophilization-induced polymerization of human growth hormone by a drawn-out skewing of its precipitin arc in contrast with a symmetrical, compact arc formed by fresh hormone (Hanson et al., 1966b).[3]

IMMUNOCHROMATOGRAPHY USING OTHER MEDIA

Only Sephadex has been used by more than one laboratory in the double immunodiffusion chromatographic analog of immunoelectrophoresis, probably because it is easy to employ and provides readily understood simple separations.[4] However, other media separating antigens by different means can be employed, as was originally demonstrated in the 1964 invention of immunochromatography by Carnegie and Pacheco. These investigators used DEAE–Sephadex and CM-Sephadex in comparative separations of dog serum.

SIMPLE IMMUNOCHROMATOGRAPHY

This term is used for lack of a better one to indicate those varieties of chromatography in which the effect of antigen–antibody complexing is detected by fixation of the complexes to the supporting medium (Castaneda, 1950, 1953; Stöss, 1957). As chromatographic solvent flows past the area of fixation, nonreacting constituents of antiserum and of the antigen mixture are washed away while the complexes remain immobilized. This technique resembles transmigration electroimmunodiffusion (Chapter 6) except that no electrophoresis is applied.

---

[3] This observation obviously suggests that a most powerful technique for future exploitation will be "two-dimensional single chromatographic electroimmunodiffusion," analogous to its purely electrophoretic counterpart as described in Chapter 6, in which antigens will first be separated by gel filtration chromatography and then electrophoresed at right angles to the chromatographic separation into antiserum-charged agarose. Conversely, a mixture of antigens could be electrophoresed first, then chromatographed in a second dimension (cf. Hanson et al., 1966a), and finally detected by an overlay of antiserum as in two-dimensional immunoelectrophoresis described earlier in this chapter. Potential variations on these compound immunodiffusion techniques are legion, and their terminology, already awkward, may become forbidding.

[4] Different kinds of gel filtration media, like Bio-Gel polyacrylamide beads, should be equally as useful as Sephadex.

Since optimal results are obtained when the supporting medium does not react nonspecifically with any of the reagents, paper made of fiber-glass is better than ordinary cellulose (Stöss, 1957). This has been used to detect antibody reaction with both soluble (protein) and insoluble (bacterial) antigens. A minute drop of antigen–antiserum mixture is applied to the paper, and buffer solution is allowed to ascend by capillary attraction. After appropriate development, the paper is stained for proteins without preliminary washing; a positive reaction is clearly evident from retention of a well-defined, intense spot of antigen–antibody complexes at the point of their application. This technique is rapid, economical, readily adaptable to field work employing minimal equipment, and sensitive enough to detect less than 100 ng of antigen (Stöss, 1957). Typically, the method employed is as follows.

Glass fiber paper sheets (S and S Glasfaserpapier No. 6), 1 × 8 cm, are washed in 5% Tween 80 and then dried at 80°C and kept over silica gel until used. The purpose of this treatment is to diminish nonspecific reactant adsorption. Antigen and antiserum are mixed and allowed to stand for 2 hours at 37°C. A paper strip is hung free in the air, and a 0.02- to 0.04-ml sample of mixture is applied 2 cm from the lower edge of the paper with a capillary pipet without making any mechanical impression on the paper. Immediately, and without drying, the strip is placed upright in a 2.5-cm-diameter vial 4 cm high with its lower end dipping into the chromatographing solution, a barbital buffer of pH 8.6 and ionic strength 0.1. Its stiffness supports it upright, and since a large upper portion is exposed to air it will draw up solvent rapidly. Development is finished within 1 hour at room temperature, and the paper is subjected to routine staining for proteins (cf. Chapter 2; De Banchero, 1962). This technique has been used for rapid (ca. 4 hours), specific diagnosis of foot-and-mouth disease (De Banchero, 1962).

Other kinds of paper and variations in technique can be used. As originally described, immunochromatography was performed on ordinary filter paper (Castaneda, 1950) with results good enough to provide a convenient diagnostic test for brucellosis (Castaneda, 1953). Amberlite-impregnated paper has been used in descending chromatography to detect antibodies to insulin and glucagon in antisera from several species of animal (Kologlu *et al.*, 1963). Antigen fixation was noted to be almost linearly proportional in this test to the concentration of specific antibody. The nature of cellulose nitrate to adsorb certain antigens is employed in another variety of immunochromatography in which the antigen-impregnated cellulose nitrate will hold back chromatographic migration of antibody-containing immunoglobulins but not immunoglobulins lacking antibody to the adsorbed antigen (Přistoupil *et al.*, 1967). Paradoxically, the opposite effect has been employed in a technique called "chromato-electrophoresis" (Yalow and Berson, 1960). Small quantities of insulin adsorb to filter paper and remain at the origin in paper electrophoresis as detected, for instance, by radioscanning. But if the insulin is mixed with a serum containing antibodies, these combine with it, prevent its adsorption, and permit it to migrate away from the origin during electrophoresis. An antigen-inhibition variation of this technique can be used to detect and quantitate nonlabeled antigen.

Immunosedimentation

Immunosedimentation is a two-step technique for analyzing antigens in which a mixture is ultracentrifuged on a sucrose gradient, and then samples are taken from successive levels of the gradient and their antigens are detected by single diffusion immunoelectrophoresis (Cordoba *et al.*, 1965, 1966). Electrophoretic mobility and sedimentation coefficient data can be obtained simultaneously for the various antigens present in a mixture by this technique.

As originally described, the technique is as follows: a 0.1- to 0.2-ml sample of antigen solution is layered on a 9 to 45% sucrose gradient and centrifuged at 100,000 g for 18 hours at 4°C. After centrifugation, the bottom of the centrifuge tube is pierced, and 25 successive samples are taken and transferred to a row of 25 wells cut in a line across a plate of agar gel cast as for immunoelectrophoresis. The plate is electrophoresed, also as in immunoelectrophoresis, and then the electrophoresed antigens are precipitated by an overlay of antiserum (i.e., single diffusion immunoelectrophoresis). The overlay is applied by covering the electropherogram after electrophoresis with warm agar and, when this has gelled, flooding this in turn with antiserum. Precipitation is allowed to develop for 48 hours (Córdoba *et al.*, 1966). Other techniques for applying the antiserum also should work—for example, using an overlay of filter paper (Yokoyama and Carr, 1962), working the antiserum into the surface with a glass rod (Afonso, 1966b) or a glass tube (Firestone and Aronson, 1969), or applying it with Mylar film. A diagrammatic representation of results obtained with immunosedimentation of human serum is presented in Fig. 7.10.

This technique might be simplified by effecting ultracentrifugation in a medium containing acrylamide and photopolymerizers, so that after centrifugation the gradient could be gelled. Then, this gel could be used in two-step immunoelectrophoretic or electroimmunodiffusion analyses (Córdoba *et al.*, 1966).

Two-step double diffusion or immunoelectrophoretic analyses of mix-

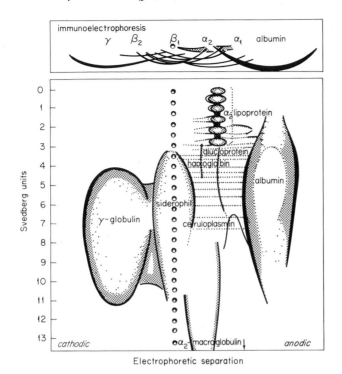

Fig. 7.10. Diagram comparing immunosedimentation (large square) with immuno-electrophoresis (upper rectangle) of human serum. (Courtesy of Córdoba *et al.*, 1965.)

tures of antigens fractionated by column chromatography (Woods *et al.*, 1962) have been fairly common, but analyzing chromatographed antigens by single diffusion immunoelectrophoresis, as described here for immunosedimentation, or by electroimmunodiffusion apparently has not. As Fig. 7.10 shows, electrophoretic analyses provide good resolution of the separated antigens and additional comprehensive information about their physicochemical characteristics.

Immunorheophoresis

The accelerating effect that localized gel drying can have on development of immunodiffusion reactions has been mentioned in previous chapters (e.g., Chapters 2 and 4). It probably has been used by several workers without formal acknowledgment in their published technical descriptions. But sometimes its beneficial effect has been mentioned. For instance, macro double diffusion plate tests used for detecting antithyroid precipitins to diagnose autoimmune thyroiditis yielded results faster when their agar gel had been slightly dehydrated (Anderson *et al.*, 1962a). Leaving off the lid of the petri dish for a few hours hastened absorption of the reactants from their wells by the gel.

Now this effect has been exploited not only to accelerate immuno-diffusion reactions, but also to increase their sensitivity. The principle of this technique, called "immunorheophoresis" (Van Oss and Bronson, 1969), is to perform a double diffusion plate test or immunoelectro-phoresis in a vessel with a cover just slightly above the developing im-munodiffusogram and with a slot cut in this cover above the area of gel between two reactants. The result (Fig. 7.11) will be that locally low humidity directly beneath this slot will cause a corresponding area of gel to dry more rapidly than elsewhere in the immunodiffusogram. In turn, this will attract water and, with it, reactants so that they will meet sooner and in higher concentration than in conventional immunodiffu-sion. As currently used, immunorheophoresis is approximately threefold as sensitive as comparable immunodiffusion (Van Oss and Bronson, 1969).

The end effect of this technique is very similar to that of double elec-troimmunodiffusion (see Chapter 6) and, incidentally, should be used with analogous interpretative precautions. However, it can be employed with a wider variety of buffers, and it can be applied without regard to the relative isoelectric points of the reactants.

This technique probably can be miniaturized by a simple adaptation of template microimmunodiffusion (see Chapter 4), in which the template is modified by cutting a slot in it between reactant wells. Conceivably, a long template with many pairs of wells and accompanying midway slots could be used for multiple, rapid screening tests entirely analogous

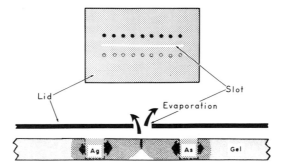

Fig. 7.11. Diagrams illustrating immunorheophoresis. A slot in the cover over the developing immunorheophoretogram permits localized evaporation of water from the agar gel. Water moving from other portions of the gel to replace that lost carries reactants with it thus enhancing the rapidity and sensitivity of what other-wise would be an ordinary double diffusion plate test.

to double electroimmunodiffusion which recently has become so popular for detecting hepatitis-associated antigen (Chapter 6). But unlike electroimmunodiffusion, immunorheophoresis would require no electrophoresis apparatus and could be used more simply and inexpensively.

Several of the techniques described in this chapter might have been thought bizarre, impractical, or even impossible by early users of immunodiffusion. It will be most interesting, therefore, to see what yet unimagined varieties of immunodiffusion may be developed in the future and whether, when the overall history of this analytic technique can be written some time many years hence, it will record that by 1972 all the most important techniques in immunodiffusion had been invented and described, at least on a rudimentary basis.

Chapter 8

History

Although a form of immunodiffusion test first was described in 1905 (Bechhold, 1905), in practice this technique received only passing attention for the next 40 years, to become popularly employed only after its rediscovery in 1946. The history of immunodiffusion, then, is divisible into a period of blind infancy before 1946 and a period of phenomenal maturation in following years. Its first period is interesting particularly for the examples it gives of great opportunities lost through misinterpretation and of how a technique may fail to receive general acceptance until an atmosphere favoring its utilization has developed.

The first immunodiffusion test appears to have been described by a chemist, H. Bechhold, interested more in colloidal precipitation in gels than in antigen–antibody reactions. In his paper of 1905, he describes an experiment in which he incorporated rabbit antiserum to goat serum in 1% gelatin, poured this mixture into test tubes, gelled it in an icebox, and then overlaid this gel with goat serum for the purpose of studying a type of precipitation differing from that he could obtain with inorganic chemicals. After a time, two heavy but distinct precipitate bands appeared in his tubes, but the possibility that each might have been formed by independent goat serum antigens did not occur to him. A later paper (Bechhold and Ziegler, 1906) shows that his interest still rested in the physics of diffusion and precipitation; in this paper he reported the effects that various additives to gelatin and to agar had on the diffusion rate of such substances as methylene blue through the gelatin and agar.

Arrhenius in 1907 saw the possibilities of using diffusion through gels to fractionate complex mixtures of antigens, but he did not use his ideas to develop any form of immunodiffusion test. He and Madsen allowed diphtheria or tetanus toxins, or their respective antibodies, to diffuse into

433

gelatin gels in test tubes for 1 to 4 weeks. Then they removed these gels, sectioned them, and analyzed them at various levels for separated reactants. These workers did not in any instance report using antigen and antibody together for reaction in one tube. In 1920, a primitive single diffusion tube test was devised by Nicolle *et al.* for quantitating antitoxin against tetanus or diphtheria toxins. After incorporating toxin in gelatin in a series of tubes, they overlaid the gelatin in each tube with samples from a serial dilution of the antiserum to be tested and then observed whether or not a precipitate formed near the interface within 2 hours. This test was devised, simply, as a possible improvement on similar tests in aqueous media then also being developed. In 1927, Reiner and Kopp made observations similar to those of Bechhold.

The early 1930's saw the first significant practical use of immunodiffusion tests and foreshadowed, although unrecognizably to contemporaries, the developments to come a decade later which would establish this technique as a potent analytic tool. During this period, the single diffusion plate test was employed successfully in several laboratories as a method for identifying bacteria. The unknown microorganism was cultured on agar containing antiserum specific for a known bacterial genus, species, group, or type. If a halo or band of precipitate formed around a colony planted on such agar by reaction of antiserum with antigen diffusing from the colony, then the inoculated bacterium was similar to that against which the antiserum had been prepared. G. F. Petrie must be given credit for originating this technique which he described in a paper published in 1932. Although this paper shows that he understood some of the mechanisms of antigen–antibody precipitation in agar gels, as did his predecessors, the idea that multiple halos might indicate multiple independent precipitates apparently remained dormant. He fully realized the specificity of the halos, for he showed that pneumococci and meningococci could be typed serologically with this technique. Associated with reaction specificity, and equally important in making immunodiffusion tests useful, is the so-called "reaction of identity" which is seen between precipitate bands formed by identical antigens. Petrie (1932) observed in his single diffusion plates that, if the areas of antigen diffusion from two adjacent bacterial colonies of the same serologic type (and therefore producing the same antigen) overlapped, the normally closed halos that should form around each colony now remained open where they faced each other and coalesced to form a figure 8 (Fig. 8.1). He understood that this mutual halo interference indicated serologic identity of the involved precipitating systems. Unfortunately, more than a dozen years passed before this basic observation was exploited again. Petrie described

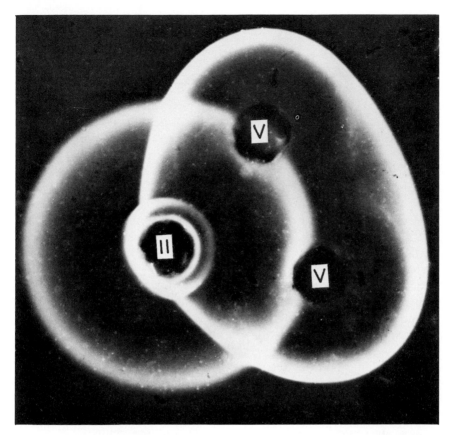

Fig. 8.1. A single diffusion microscope slide test in which horse antiserum to human serum was used in the agar at a 1:10 dilution, 0.5% human serum Cohn Fraction V was used to fill two wells, and 1.0% human serum Cohn Fraction II was employed to fill the third. A single halo is formed by human serum albumin antigen in Fraction V, and the serologic identity of this antigen in the two wells charged with V is evident from the mutual interference and fusion of halos formed by each well into a flat oval of precipitate. Since neither the inner nor the outer of the two halos originating from the well charged with Fraction II is affected by the albumin halo, they are antigenically dissimilar.

differences in the types of halo that were produced by rabbit and horse antisera, and stated that, because it formed very broad halos, the former was unsatisfactory for analytic work in his plate technique. He came close to explaining this difference in type of precipitate, perhaps foreseeing that later single diffusion tests would be used to differentiate precipitating-type from flocculating-type antibodies. A much briefer paper was published by Sia and Chung in the same year. They had developed independently the same single diffusion plate method and also found it reliable for identifying pneumococcal types.

Papers published in the following years by other experimenters confirmed Petrie's findings and recorded successful applications of this technique. In 1933, Maegraith used it to detect rough variants of meningococcus strains, variants that lacked capsular type-specific antigen. In the same year, Kirkbride and Cohen described before the national meeting of the Society of American Bacteriologists how they employed Petrie's method successfully to categorize bacteria, particularly meningococci and gonococci. In 1934, Maegraith and Adelaide reported that this technique enabled them to detect and type meningococci in spinal fluid, a development of considerable practical importance in the days when, for lack of an effective therapeutic drug, meningitis was treated with type-specific antiserum. Pittman and co-workers (1938) confirmed that Petrie's test could be used to type meningococci. They also found it a useful method for quantitating antibody content in antiserum by the intensity of the precipitin halos that appeared, and reported that titers obtained by this single diffusion test correlated well with protective antibody titers determined by mouse protection tests.

Three years before Oudin began publishing descriptions of his work with single diffusion tube tests in which, at last, multiple precipitin bands were recognized and shown to be due to multiple simultaneously precipitating antigen–antibody systems, Petrie, in collaboration with Steabben (1943), used his single diffusion plate to help identify a number of bacteria antigenically, among these members of the genus *Clostridium*. When these workers observed multiple halos forming in their plates, they still interpreted them as probably a form of periodic or Liesegang precipitation. Although they may have been partly correct in this interpretation, the important point is that even by 1942 no one seemed to recognize as a possibility the simultaneous occurrence of multiple antigen–antibody precipitates in a single test; Arrhenius' early idea of fractionating antigen and antibody mixtures by differential diffusion through semisolid media still remained latent.

Hanks in 1935 applied the type of test devised by Nicolle *et al.* (1920) to test the potency of small quantities of guinea pig antisera, but he did not attempt to use the single diffusion tube test for qualitative analyses, nor did he impute to it any essential properties lacking in the usual tests with aqueous medium. In 1940, Brown might have stumbled upon the qualitative utility of single diffusion tube tests had she not been interested primarily in Liesegang precipitation and assumed that any multiple precipitates which she saw in her experiments were of this type. She set up tests in which horse and rabbit antiserum were incorporated in 3% gelatin, and corresponding SSS and C substance antigens obtained from pneumococci were layered above. Photographs that she took of her tubes leave no doubt that she was observing in a given tube simultaneous formation of different specific precipitates corresponding to distinct antigen–antibody systems, but she overlooked this interpretation, stating rather that these tubes showed examples of rhythmic precipitation similar to the Liesegang phenomenon, which she originally had set out to study.

This then prevalent dogmatic idea that multiple precipitate bands merely were rhythmic precipitates formed by one antigen–antibody system all at once was challenged and overthrown by Jacques Oudin (1946) employing the same type of single diffusion tube test which previous experimenters had used but with different notions. Thus, although his technique was not new, his fresh and deeper interpretations led him to establish immunodiffusion in its present standing and form— an analytic technique for mixed antigen–antibody systems of unsurpassed resolution and specificity, and of great reliability. From his initial observations he developed the basic tenets of immunodiffusion reactions which still hold true. Thus, he showed that concentrated antigen, layered over dilute agar-gelled antiserum in a tube, will diffuse into the antibody column forming a percipitin band which appears to migrate down the column in proportion to the antigen's initial concentration, to its diffusion coefficient, and inversely to the antibody concentration. A crude antigen used against its antiserum, he found, forms multiple lines corresponding to its multiple precipitating systems which precipitate and move independently of each other, unless one of the antigens tends to cross-react with the other. He showed that in this situation formation of precipitin bands and their interpretation becomes somewhat more complex.

Having published preliminary evidence on the utility of single diffusion tests, Oudin set out over succeeding years in the 1940's to verify and elaborate his original findings, in particular to develop theoretical bases for interpreting single diffusion tube test results. He noted such points as (1) the positive correlation between precipitate intensity and antibody concentration in the lower agar layer, (2) the fact that sudden incubation temperature changes may cause appearance of artifacts (e.g., formation of secondary precipitates by a single antigen–antibody system)—and that these usually have distinguishing characteristics differentiating them from primary precipitates, (3) the fact that in tests set up by his method Liesegang bands never formed, and (4) how the presence of a cross-reacting antigen can influence the formation of precipitate by the homologous antigen (Oudin, 1947, 1948a,b, 1949).

These published experiments of Oudin employed only single diffusion. Agar double diffusion precipitin techniques were being developed independently in Sweden and in England by Ouchterlony and Elek, respectively, who both published their first findings in 1948 (Ouchterlony, 1948a,b; Elek, 1948). Interestingly, both experimenters developed their methods largely as tests for diphtheria bacillus toxigenicity. The following year, Elek (1949a) elaborated on his previous account of his technique which was based on the principle that, if antigen and antibody are allowed to diffuse into a common meeting ground from sources set at right angles to each other (e.g., impregnated filter paper strips in the form of an L), each antigen–antibody precipitating system will flocculate in an individual plane to form a precipitate band uninfluenced by any bands formed by other systems. In this paper, he described some of the technique's applications, and discussed how it functioned relative to contemporary theoretical understanding of classic precipitin tests in aqueous media; he pointed out particular advantages it had over these. Elek published one more paper in 1949 on diphtheria bacillus virulence (1949b) and two in 1950 (1950a,b) on staphylococcus antigens, but then he turned to other problems not connected with double diffusion tests or their mechanisms. Establishment of basic theories for double diffusion plate tests, aside from Elek's first 1949 paper, must be acknowledged as Ouchterlony's accomplishment. In addition to two reports in 1949 on using double diffusion precipitin techniques for toxigenicity tests (1949a,b), he also published a series of three papers on the mechanisms and theory of these precipitin tests in agar gel (1949c,d,e). Moreover, his interest in immunodiffusion has continued in succeeding years (Ouchterlony, 1968).

Once the reliability and remarkable analytic acuity of immunodiffusion tests had been established by Oudin, Ouchterlony, and Elek, other experimenters were quick to begin applying these tests to their own problems, to use them for studying the mechanisms of antigen–antibody reaction, and to adapt and refine them. The trickle of publications mentioning use of immunodiffusion has grown to a flood. By the end of the first 60 years of this century, scarcely a thousand such papers had been published. But in the seventh decade of this century the use of immunodiffusion has burgeoned so much that currently more than that many papers are published yearly, although of course nearly all only refer to the technique fleetingly as a commonplace analytic tool which the authors chose to employ.

Probably only one other advance in immunodiffusion techniques has been as important as their original popularization. This was development of immunoelectrophoresis. It greatly increased the resolution of immunodiffusion tests and the amount of information that they could yield, and it showed that reactants could be moved about in semisolid media by forces other than just diffusion. This latter realization, together with proof that antigen and antibodies could precipitate while actually being electrophoresed, laid the conceptual groundwork for development and acceptance of such compound techniques as electroimmunodiffusion and immunochromatography.

A two-step form of immunoelectrophoresis was first described in 1952 by M. D. Poulik, who electrophoresed purified diphtheria toxoid on filter paper, embedded the toxoid under a layer of agar, and then laid upon the gelled agar a second piece of filter paper soaked with antiserum so that precipitin arcs formed between the paper strips in the agar gel. In 1949, Gordon and co-workers had described zone electrophoresis in agar gels, and in 1953 Grabar and Williams modified agar zone electrophoresis to develop what has become the classic one-step method for immunoelectrophoresis, in which electrophoresis and subsequent double diffusion precipitation reactions are both performed in the same slab of agar. The word "immunoelectrophoresis" was used first in technical papers by Williams and Grabar (1955a) and by Martin du Pan *et al.* (1955), who reported on its utility in analyzing human serum antigens.

Immunoelectrophoresis has been improved technically and its value greatly extended by applying to it specific staining and indicator techniques usually adapted from known histological methods. Experiments performed by Uriel and Scheidegger and reported in 1955 showed that serum constituents which were electrophoresed in agar could be stained readily, and a year later these experiments led to the classic publication by Uriel and Grabar (1956a) describing methods for detecting proteins, lipids, phospholipids, and glycoproteins in immunoelectropherograms.

This paper, however, was not the first to have described methods for staining precipitin bands in agar. Björklund had shown in 1954 (1954a,b) that polysaccharide antigens in double diffusion plate precipitates could be stained specifically either with mucicarmine or with basic fuchsin. Korngold and Lipari (1955a) reported, but without procedural details, that with then-current techniques for paper electropherograms they could stain the lipids in antibody-precipitated β lipoprotein bands of double diffusion plates using Sudan black B and oil red O.

An important advance in immunoelectrophoresis was made when it was miniaturized by Scheidegger (1955). His modification for carrying it out on microscope slides simplified the equipment and techniques needed, considerably shortened the time required for all steps in the method (e.g., electrophoresis, double diffusion reaction development, staining), and instituted great savings of reactants. It also helped motivate miniaturization of other varieties of immunodiffusion.

Analogous variations in methods for setting up other kinds of immunodiffusion test have been numerous. Some have proved to be particularly useful. Use of a double diffusion tube technique first was reported in 1951 by Pope *et al.*, who give credit for its invention to C. L. Oakley. Since this method first was fully described two years later by Oakley and Fulthorpe (1953), it sometimes bears their names. The technique later was miniaturized by Preer (1956). In 1954, Jennings and Malone reported using a double diffusion gradient technique in which the reaction area had a triangular shape. One of the chief advantages of their innovation was that, by the shape of the reaction arena and the type of immunodiffusion cell employed, reactants could be used very effectively, being able only to diffuse toward their immunologic reaction centers. One year after Scheidegger had miniaturized immunodiffusion plates, Grasset *et al.* (1956) did the same for the double diffusion test. Their technique was also very simple: melted agar was poured on a microscope slide, depot holes were punched in this agar after it had gelled, and the depots were charged with the minute quantities of reactants required. The next year, in 1957, Wadsworth in Sweden described a more efficient semi-miniaturization of the double diffusion test in which reactants were fed into very thin sheets of agar gel on lantern slide glass plates from plastic matrices. In this country, this technique soon afterward was fully miniaturized for use on microscope slides (Crowle, 1958c).

For several years, immunodiffusion precipitate patterns were recorded permanently only by photography or drawing. Most commonly today, the precipitin test is preserved like a histological specimen. Gell appears to have reported earliest an effort at such preservation (1955b). He showed that the agar gel in which the precipitin reactions had occurred could be washed, mounted on a lantern slide, dried, and finally preserved with a coating of protective plastic. In the following year, Rondle and Carman (1956) published a short communication on a method for washing, staining, drying, and preserving double diffusion precipitin tests carried out in petri dishes. They used either a negative stain (toluidin blue) or, with better results, naphthol black and Congo red positive stains; and they preserved their dried, stained agar with clear plastic coatings or by mounting it under glass. It is the classic 1956 contribution of Uriel and Grabar mentioned above (1956a), however, which seems to have been the root of most methods now used for permanently preserving original immunodiffusion patterns.

Specific precipitates may occur in immunodiffusion tests which are so faint as to be invisible, impossible to photograph, and perhaps not amenable to revelation by special enhancement or staining techniques. It is in such a situation as this that autoradiography could excel, since immunologic fixation of a radioactive (labeled) antigen in agar could be detected by the ability of this antigen's invisible band of aggregate to record its own image on photosensitive material. Prolonged exposure of the photosensitive film and labeling with a strongly radioactive substance could extend the sensitivity of immunodiffusion considerably through autoradiography. However, this technique has made its most valuable contributions not by increasing the sensitivity of immunodiffusion techniques but rather by greatly broadening their capabilities for qualitative analyses. This capacity was evident even in what appears to be the first description of a radioimmunodiffusion technique in which Scheidegger and Buzzi in 1957 showed that myeloma Bence-Jones proteins are fragments of γ-globulins.

The groundwork for development of what ultimately may prove to be the single most powerful variety of immunodiffusion, namely electroimmunodiffusion,[1] was laid in 1953 when Macheboeuf and co-workers demonstrated that antigen and antibody could be brought together for precipitation in filter paper by electrophoresis itself, and in 1956 and 1959 when first Crowle and later Bussard and Huet confirmed this finding and extended it to use in agar gels. These were double electroimmunodiffusion tests. In 1960, Ressler described primitive forms of one- and two-dimensional single electroimmunodiffusion tests (1960a,b). Yet, it has not been until the 1970's that the potentialities of electroimmunodiffusion have begun to be recognized, as experimenters pushing older immunodiffusion and immunoelectrophoresis tests to their limits have begun to search for still more effective analytic techniques.

During the past decade, some other compound varieties of immunodiffusion have been described. But they are too new or untried for adequate perspective of their importance to have developed yet. Therefore, they are described historically in Chapter 7.

Until recently agar was unchallenged as the medium most often used for immunodiffusion. But it has several flaws, most notably reactivity with many different kinds of antigens, and strong electroosmotic effects on substances being electrophoresed through it. Reintroduction to the immunologic community of a constituent of agar—agarose, which lacks these undesirable properties—and a description of a practical way of making agarose from agar therefore were historically important contributions made by Hjertén in 1961. Neither agar nor agarose has much potential for separating antigens from each other by molecular sieving during electrophoresis or chromatography. Starch gels have, but starch

---

[1] The word "electroimmunodiffusion" was coined in 1966 by Hartley *et al.* "Immunodiffusion" apparently was first used by Condsen and Kohn in 1959.

gels so far have not been satisfactory media for development of antigen–antibody precipitation. Hence, demonstration that polyacrylamide gels can be used for zone electrophoresis had special significance in the development of immunodiffusion techniques, because these gels do have excellent capabilities for molecular sieving but, unlike starch, they also excellently support and exhibit antigen–antibody precipitation. This demonstration was made by Ornstein and Davis in 1959 (cf. Ornstein, 1964). The first description of polyacrylamide as a medium for immunodiffusion, specifically for immunoelectrophoresis of human serum, was published two years later in the first edition of this book (Crowle, 1961). As is detailed in Chapter 5, further practical advances, now being made in using polyacrylamide gels for immunodiffusion tests, closely parallel earlier advances made with agar in miniaturization, washing, staining, and preserving the gels.

The history of immunodiffusion still is in the making. There are many minor but important contributions to it which have not been described in this chapter; there are others which, though appearing to be minor, eventually may be judged as major but cannot yet be for lack of perspective. Therefore, though of historical interest, these various contributions have been detailed in preceding chapters, particularly in Chapters 6 and 7, where they can be given more ample discussion and have not had to be judged critically and perhaps unfairly.

References

Aalund, O., Osebold, J. W., and Murphy, F. A. (1965). *Arch. Biochem. Biophys.* **109,** 142–149.

Aas, K. (1966). *Int. Arch. Allergy Appl. Immunol.* **29,** 453–469.

Abbood Al-Hilly, J. N. (1969). *Amer. J. Vet. Res.* **30,** 1877–1880.

Abelev, G. I. (1960). *Bull. Eksperim. Biol. Med.* (*Trans.*) **49,** 118–120.

Abramoff, P., and LaVia, M. F. (1970). "Biology of the Immune Response," 492 pp. McGraw-Hill, New York.

Abramson, H. A., Moyer, L. S., and Gorin, M. H. (1942). "Electrophoresis of Proteins," 341 pp. Reinhold, New York.

Ackers, G. K., and Steere, R. L. (1962). *Biochim. Biophys. Acta* **59,** 137–149.

Adamson, D. M., and Cozad, G. C. (1966). *J. Bacteriol.* **92,** 887–891.

Adler, F. L. (1956a). *J. Immunol.* **76,** 217–227.

Adler, F. L. (1956b). *Fed. Proc.* **15,** 580–581.

Affronti, L. F. (1959). *Amer. Rev. Tuberc. Pulm. Dis.* **79,** 284–295.

Afifi, F., Besson, R., Boivin, P., and Fauvert, R. (1964). *Rev. Fr. Etud. Clin. Biol.* **9,** 541–544.

Afonso, E. (1964a). *Clin. Chim. Acta* **10,** 192.

Afonso, E. (1964b). *Clin. Chim. Acta* **10,** 114–122.

Afonso, E. (1966a). *Clin. Chim. Acta* **13,** 107–112.

Afonso, E. (1966b). *Clin. Chim. Acta* **14,** 195–198.

Agostoni, A., Vergani, C., and Lomanto, B. (1967). *J. Lab. Clin. Med.* **69,** 522–529.

Agostoni, A., Vergani, C., and Stabilini, R. (1970). *Progr. Immunobiol. St.* **4,** 149–151.

Ainbender, E., Berger, R., Hevizy, M. M., Zepp, H. D., and Hodes, H. L. (1965). *Proc. Soc. Exp. Biol. Med.* **119,** 1166–1169.

Aitken, I. D., Syme, A., and Chalmers, J. W. (1969). *Res. Vet. Sci.* **10,** 523–529.

Aladjem, F. (1964). *J. Immunol.* **93,** 682–695.

Aladjem, F. (1966). *Nature* (*London*) **209,** 1003–1005.

Aladjem, F., and Campbell, D. H. (1957). *Nature* (*London*) **179,** 203–204.

Aladjem, F., and Lieberman, M. (1952). *J. Immunol.* **69,** 117–130.

Aladjem, F., and Palmiter, M. T. (1965). *J. Theor. Biol.* **8,** 8–21.

Aladjem, F., Jaross, R. W., Paldino, R. L., and Lackner, J. A. (1959). *J. Immunol.* **83,** 221–231.

Aladjem, F., Klostergaard, H., Taylor, R. W. (1962). *J. Theor. Biol.* **3,** 134–145.

443

Aladjem, F., Paldino, R. L., Perrin, R., and Chang, F.-W. (1968). *Immunochemistry* **5**, 217–252.

Albert, A., and Johnson, P. (1961). *Biochem. J.* **81**, 669–671.

Albin, R. J., Soanes, W. A., Bronson, P., and Witebsky, E. (1970a). *J. Reprod. Fert.* **22**, 573–574.

Albin, R. J., Soanes, W. A., and Gonder, M. J. (1970b). *Urol. Int.* **25**, 511–539.

Albutt, E. C. (1966). *J. Med. Lab. Technol.* **23**, 61–82.

Alexander, A. E., and Johnson, P. (1949). "Colloid Science," Vol. 2, pp. 556–837. Oxford Univ. Press, London and New York.

Alexander, J. W., and Moncrief, J. A. (1966). *J. Trauma* **6**, 539–547.

Allen, P. Z., Sirisinha, S., and Vaughan, J. H. (1965). *J. Immunol.* **95**, 918–928.

Allerhand, J., Karelitz, S., Penbharkkul, S., Ramos, A., and Isenberg, H. D. (1963). *Pediatrics* **62**, 85–92.

Allison, A. C., and Humphrey, J. H. (1959). *Nature (London)* **183**, 1590–1592.

Allison, A. C., and Humphrey, J. H. (1960). *Immunology* **3**, 95–106.

Almássy, Ch. (1964). *Progr. Immunobiol. Std.* **1**, 209–212.

Almeida, J. D., and Goffe, A. P. (1965). *Lancet* ii, 1205–1207.

Almeida, J. D., Stannard, L. M., and Pennington, T. H. (1965). *Arch. Gesamte Virusforsch.* **17**, 330–334.

Alper, C. A., and Johnson, A. M. (1969). *Vox Sang.* **17**, 445–452.

Alpert, E., Monroe, M., and Schur, P. H. (1970). *Lancet* i, 1120.

Alter, H. J., Holland, P. V., and Purcell, R. H. (1971). *J. Lab. Clin. Med.* **77**, 1000–1010.

Alvsaker, J. O. (1966). *Scand. J. Clin. Lab. Invest.* **18**, 227–239.

Aly, F. W., and Gillich, K. H. (1960). *Naturwissenschaften* **47**, 280.

Ambrose, E. J., and Easty, G. C. (1953). *Nature (London)* **172**, 811–813.

Ambrosius, H. (1966). *Nature (London)* **209**, 524.

Ammann, A. J., and Hong, R. (1971). *J. Immunol.* **106**, 567–569.

Anacker, R. L., and Monoz, J. (1961). *J. Immunol.* **87**, 426–432.

Anderson, J. R., Buchanan, W. W., Goudie, R. B., and Gray, K. G. (1962a). *J. Clin. Pathol.* **15**, 462–471.

Anderson, J. R., Gray, K. G., Beck, J. S., Buchanan, W. W., and McElhinney, A. J. (1962b). *Ann. Rheum. Dis.* **21**, 360–369.

Angevine C. D., Andersen, B. R., and Barnett, E. V. (1966). *J. Immunol.* **96**, 578–586.

Anonymous (1962). Lancet ii, 1042.

Antoine, B. (1962). *Rev. Fr. Etude. Clin. Biol.* **7**, 612–617.

Antoine, B., and Neveu, T. (1967). *Ann. Inst. Pasteur* **113**, 509–519.

Anzai, T., Ibayashi, J., Aldrich, H., and Carpenter, C. M. (1963). *Proc. Soc. Exp. Biol. Med.* **113**, 54–58.

Anzai, T., Sato, K., Fukuda, M., and Carpenter, C. M. (1965). *Proc. Soc. Exp. Biol. Med.* **120**, 94–98.

Aoki, S., Kashiwazaki, M., Sato, S., Watase, H., and Sakamoto, C. (1963). *Nat. Inst. Anim. Health Quart.* **3**, 175–184.

Aoki, T., and Fujinami, T. (1967). *J. Immunol.* **98**, 39–45.

Appleyard, G., Hume, V. B. M., and Westwood, J. C. N. (1965). *Ann. N. Y. Acad. Sci.* **130**, 92–104.

Arbesman, C. E., Reisman, R. E., Bonstein, H. S., and Rose, N. R. (1963). *J. Immunol.* **90**, 612–618.

Armstrong, A. S., and Sword, C. P. (1967). *J. Immunol.* **98**, 510–520.

Arnon, R., and Schechter, B. (1966). *Immunochemistry* **3**, 451–461.

Aronson, S. B., Rapp, W., Kushner, I., and Burtin, P. (1965). *Int. Arch. Allergy* **26**, 327–332.

Arrhensius, S. (1907). "Immunochemistry," 309 pp. Macmillan, New York.

Asofsky, R., and Thorbecke, G. J. (1961). *J. Exp. Med.* **114**, 471–483.

Asofsky, R., Trnka, Z., and Thorbecke, G. J. (1962). *Proc. Soc. Exp. Biol. Med.* **111**, 497–499.

Assem, E. S. K., Trotter, W. R., and Belyavin, G. (1965). *Biochim. Biophys. Acta* **100**, 163–178.

Atchley, F. O. (1964). *Dis. Colon Rectum* **7**, 191.

Atchley, F. O., Auernheimer, A. H., and Wasley, M. A. (1962). *J. Parasitol.* **48**, 229–232.

Atchley, F. O., Auernheimer, A. H., and Wasley, M. A. (1963). *J. Parasitol.* **49**, 313–315.

Atchley, W. A. (1960). *Nature (London)* **188**, 579–581.

Atchley, W. A. (1961). *Arthritis Rheum.* **4**, 471–479.

Atchley, W. A., and Bhagavan, N. V. (1962). *Science* **138**, 528–529.

Audubert, R., and de Mende, S. (1960). "The Principles of Electrophoresis," 142 pp. Macmillan, New York.

Auernheimer, A. H., and Atchley, F. O. (1962). *Amer. J. Clin. Pathol.* **38**, 548–553.

Auernheimer, A. H., Atchley, F. O., and Wasley, M. A. (1966). *J. Parasitol.* **52**, 950–953.

Augustin, R. (1955). *Quart. Rev. Allergy Appl. Immunol.* **9**, 504–560.

Augustin, R. (1957). *Int. Arch. Allergy* **11**, 153–169.

Augustin, R. (1959a). *Immunology* **2**, 148–169.

Augustin, R. (1959b). *Immunology* **2**, 230–251.

Augustin, R., and Hayward, B. J. (1955). *Int. Arch. Allergy* **6**, 154–168.

Augustin, R., and Hayward, B. J. (1960). *Nature (London)* **187**, 129–130.

Augustin, R., and Hayward, B. J. (1961). *Immunology* **4**, 450–472.

Augustin, R., and Hayward, B. J. (1962). *Immunology* **5**, 424–460.

Augustin, R., Hayward, B. J., and Spiers, J. A. (1958). *Immunology* **1**, 67–80.

Aurand, L. W., Brown, J. W., and Lecce, J. G. (1963). *J. Dairy Sci.* **46**, 1177–1182.

Auscher, C., and Guinand, S. (1964). *Clin. Chim. Acta* **9**, 40–48.

Avrameas, S., and Uriel, J. (1966). *C. R. Acad. Sci. Paris* **262**, 2543–2545.

Backhausz, R. (1970). *Progr. Immunobiol. Std.* **4**, 17–21.

Baer, H., Godfrey, H., Maloney, C. J., Norman, P. S., and Lichtenstein, L. M. (1970). *J. Allergy* **45**, 347–354.

Baisden, L. A., and Tromba, F. G. (1967). *J. Parasitol.* **53**, 100–104.

Balayan, M. S. (1960). *Vopr. Virusol.* **5**, 297–303.

Balbinder, E., and Preer, J. R., Jr. (1959). *J. Gen. Microbiol.* **21**, 156–167.

Balozet, L. (1959). *Arch. Inst. Pasteur Algér.* **37**, 292–296.

Balozet, L. (1960). *Arch. Inst. Pasteur Algér.* **38**, 465–471.

Baltimore Biological Laboratory, Inc. (1960). Brochure on "K Agar."

Banach, T. M., and Hawirko, R. Z. (1966). *J. Bacteriol.* **92**, 1304–1310.

Bancroft, J. B. (1962). *Virology* **16**, 419–427.

Bao-Linh, D., Hermann, G., and Grabar, P. (1963). *Bull. Soc. Chim. Biol.* **46**, 255–269.

Bao-Linh, D., Hermann, G., and Grabar, P. (1964). *Ann. Inst. Pasteur* **106**, 670–678.

Baram, P., and Mosko, M. M. (1962). *J. Allergy* **33**, 498–506.

Barandun, S., Stampfli, K., Spengler, G. A., and Riba, G. (1959). *Helv. Med. Acta* **26**, 203–367.

Barber, C., and Taga, S. (1964). *Arch. Roum. Pathol. Exp. Microbiol.* **23**, 391–400.

Barber, C., Stamatescu-eustatziu, S., Tulpan, G., and Petrovici, A. (1960). *J. Hyg. Epidemiol. Microbiol. Immunobiol.* **4**, 379–383.

Barber, C., Lazar, I., and Meitert, E. (1966a). *Pathol. Microbiol.* (*Basel*) **29**, 84–94.

Barber, C., Vladoianu, I. R., and Dimache, Gh. (1966b). *Immunology* **11**, 287–296.

Barboriak, J. J., Sosman, A. J., and Reed, C. E. (1965). *J. Lab. Clin. Med.* **65**, 600–604.

Barbu, E., and Dandeu, J.-P. (1963). *C. R. Acad. Sci. Paris* **256**, 1166–1168.

Barbu, E., Quash, G., and Dandeu, J.-P. (1963). *Ann. Inst. Pasteur* **105**, 849–865.

Bargob, I., Cleve, H., and Hartmann, F. (1958). *Deut. Arch. Klin. Med.* **204**, 708–720.

Barker, S. A., Mitchell, A. W., Walton, K. W., and Weston, P. D. (1966). *Clin. Chim. Acta* **13**, 582–596.

Barnes, G. W., Soanes, W. A., Mamrod, L., Gonder, M. J., and Shulman, S. (1963). *J. Lab. Clin. Med.* **61**, 578-591.

Barrett, J. T. (1965). *Immunology* **8**, 129–135.

Barrett, J. T., and Thompson, L. D. (1965). *Immunology* **8**, 136–143.

Barrett, J. T., Dunlap, D. L., and Evans, R. T. (1963). *Amer. J. Med. Technol.* **29**, 245–246.

Bartel, A. H., and Campbell, D. H. (1959). *Arch. Biochem. Biophys.* **82**, 232–234.

Bartfeld, H. (1960). *J. Lab. Clin. Med.* **56**, 303–309.

Bartfeld, H., and Kelly, R. (1968). *J. Immunol.* **100**, 1000–1005.

Barth, W. F., Asofsky, R., Liddy, T. J., Tanaka, Y., Rowe, D. S., and Fahey, J. L. (1965). *Amer. J. Med.* **39**, 319–334.

Bashkaev, I. S., and Rozenbaum, G. I. (1964). *Trans. Suppl.* **23**, 355–357.

Batchelor, F. R., Dewdney, J. M., Weston, R. D., and Wheeler, A. W. (1966). *Immunology* **10**, 21–33.

Baughn, R. E., and Freeman, B. A. (1966). *J. Bacteriol.* **92**, 1298–1303.

Baumstark, J. S. (1967). *Arch. Biochem. Biophys.* **118**, 619–630.

Bazin, H. (1966). *Ann. Inst. Pasteur* **111**, 544–550.

Bazin, H. (1967). *Ann. Inst. Pasteur* **112**, 162–172.

Beaumont, J. L., Jacotot, B., Beaumont, V., Warnet, J., and Vilain, C. (1965). *Rev. Fr. Hematol.* **5**, 507–517.

Bechhold, H. (1905). *Z. Phys. Chem.* **52**, 185–199.

Bechhold, H., and Ziegler, J. (1906). *Z. Phys. Chem.* **56**, 105–121.

Beck, J., and Uzan, A. (1965). *Pathol. Biol.* (*Paris*) **13**, 969–973.

Becker, E. L. (1953). *Fed. Proc.* **12**, 717–722.

Becker, E. L., and Munoz, J. (1949a). *J. Immunol.* **63**, 173–181.

Becker, E. L., and Munoz, J. (1949b). *Proc. Soc. Exp. Biol. Med.* **72**, 287–289.

Becker, E. L., and Neff, J. C. (1958). *J. Chem. Phys.* **55**, 334–339.

Becker, E. L., and Neff, J. C. (1959). *J. Immunol.* **83**, 571–581.

Becker, E. L., Munoz, J., Lapresle, C., and LeBeau, L. J. (1951). *J. Immunol.* **67**, 501–511.

Becker, W. (1969). *Immunochemistry* **6**, 539–546.

Becker, W., Schwick, H. G., and Störiko, K. (1969). *Clin. Chem.* **15**, 649–660.

Beckman, L., Hirschfeld, J., and Söderberg, U. (1961). *Acta Pathol. Microbiol. Scand.* **51**, 132–140.

Bednařík, T. (1966). *Clin. Chim. Acta* **14**, 645–653.

Bednařík, T. (1967). *Clin. Chim. Acta* **15**, 172–174.
Beernink, K. D., and Steward, J. P. (1967). *Immunology* **12**, 207–218.
Beernink, K. D., Courcon, J., and Grabar, P. (1965). *Immunology* **9**, 377–389.
Beiser, S. M., Dworetzky, M., Smart, K. M., and Baldwin H. S. (1958). *J. Allergy* **29**, 44–47.
Belicetta, V. F., Markham, A. E., Peniston, Q. P., and McCarthy, J. L. (1949). *J. Amer. Chem. Soc.* **71**, 2879.
Belyavin, G., and Trotter, W. R. (1959). *Lancet* i, 648–652.
Benaš, A. (1962). *Nature (London)* **195**, 1194.
Benaš, A. (1963). *Biochim. Biophys. Acta* **71**, 562–567.
Benaš, A. (1967). *Clin. Chim. Acta* **15**, 541.
Benedict, A. A., Hersh, R. T., and Larson, C. (1963). *J. Immunol.* **91**, 795–802.
Benjamin, D. C., and Weimer, H. E. (1963). *J. Immunol.* **91**, 331–338.
Bennett, J. P., and Boursnell, J. C. (1962). *Biochim. Biophys. Acta* **63**, 382–397.
Ben-Or, S., and Bell, E. (1965). *Develop. Biol.* **11**, 184–201.
Bent, D. F., Rosen, H., Levenson, S. M., Lindberg, R. B., and Ajl, S. J. (1957). *Proc. Soc. Exp. Biol. Med.* **95**, 178–181.
Bentz, M. (1971). Personal communication.
Berenbaum, M. C., Kitch, G. M., and Cope, W. A. (1962). *Nature (London)* **193**, 81–82.
Berg, K. (1963). *Acta Pathol. Microbiol. Scand.* **59**, 369–382.
Berg, K. (1964). *Sangre* **9**, 24–30.
Berg, K. (1965a). *Vox Sang.* **10**, 222–224.
Berg, K. (1965b). *Vox Sang.* **10**, 513–527.
Berg, K., and Bearn, A. G. (1966). *J. Exp. Med.* **123**, 379–397.
Berg, K., and Egeberg, O. (1965). *Nature (London)* **206**, 312–313.
Berg, O., and Dencker, S. J. (1962). *Acta Pathol. Microbiol. Scand.* **54**, 434–438.
Bergdoll, M. S., Surgalla, M. J., and Dack, G. M. (1959). *J. Immunol.* **83**, 334–338.
Berger, R., Ainbender, E., Hodes, H. L., Zepp, H. D., and Hevizy, M. M. (1967). *Nature (London)* **214**, 420–422.
Berglund, G. (1962a). *Int. Arch. Allergy* **21**, 193–206.
Berglund, G. (1962b). *Brit. J. Haematol.* **8**, 204–214.
Berglund, G. (1963a). *Int. Arch. Allergy* **22**, 1–10.
Berglund, G. (1963b). *Int. Arch. Allergy* **22**, 65–72.
Bergrahm, B. (1960). *Nature (London)* **185**, 242–243.
Berman, L. D., and Sarma, P. S. (1965). *Nature (London)* **207**, 263–265.
Bernfeld, P., and Wan, J. (1963). *Science* **142**, 678–679.
Berrod, J., Larrat, J., Sandor, G., and Sureau, B. (1964). *Nature (London)* **202**, 407–408.
Betsuyaku, T., Yachi, A., Fukuda, M., Anzai, T., Wada, T., and Carpenter, C. M. (1964). *Proc. Soc. Exp. Biol. Med.* **115**, 267–271.
Betts, A., and Sewall, E. L. (1965). *Amer. J. Clin. Pathol.* **43**, 535–538.
Beutner, E. H., Sepulveda, M. R., and Barnett, E. V. (1968) *Bull. WHO* **39**, 587–606.
Bezkorovainy, A., Zschocke, R., and Grohlich, D. (1970). *J. Immunol.* **104**, 648–655.
Bideau, J., and Masseyeff, R. (1964). *Bull. Soc. Pathol. Exot.* **57**, 1231–1236.
Bier, M. (1967). "Electrophoresis, Theory, Methods and Applications," 553 pp. Academic Press, New York.
Biguet, J., and Tran Van Ky, P. (1966). *Rev. Immunol. Paris* **30**, 165–171.
Biguet, J., Havez, R., and Tran Van Ky, P. (1959). *C. R. Acad. Sci. Paris* **249**, 895–897.

Biguet, J., Capron, A., and Tran Van Ky, P. (1962a). *Ann. Inst. Pasteur* **103**, 763–777.

Biguet, J., Capron, A., Tran Van Ky, P., and d'Haussy, R. (1962b). *C. R. Acad. Sci. Paris* **254**, 3600–3602.

Biguet, J., d'Haussy, R., Capron, A., Tran Van Ky, P., and Aubry, M. (1962c). *Bull. Soc. Pathol. Exot.* **55**, 845–855.

Biguet, J., Tran Van Ky, P., Capron, A., and Fruit, J. (1962d). *C. R. Acad. Sci. Paris* **254**, 3768–3770.

Biguet, J., Tran Van Ky, P., Havez, R., and Andrieu, S. (1962e). *Ann. Inst. Pasteur* **102**, 328–338.

Biguet, J., Tran Van Ky, P., Andrieu, S., and Fruit, J. (1964). *Ann. Inst. Pasteur* **107**, 72–97.

Biguet, J., Capron, A., Tran Van Ky, P., and Rose, F. (1965a). *Rev. Immunol. Paris* **29**, 233–240.

Biguet, J., Tran Van Ky, P., Andrieu, S., and Degaey, R. (1965b). *Sabouraudia* **4**, 148–157.

Billingham, R. E., and Brent, L. (1959). *Phil. Trans.* B **242**, 439–477.

Billingham, R. E., Brent, L., and Medawar, P. B. (1956). *Phil. Trans.* B **239**, 357–412.

Bini, L., and Polosa, T. (1960). *Sang.* **31**, 865–869.

Bird, G. W. G. (1961). *Experientia* **17**, 408–410.

Bird, R., and Jackson, D. (1959). *J. Clin. Pathol.* **12**, 373–374.

Birkinshaw, V. J., Randall, S. S., and Risdall, P. C. (1962). *Nature (London)* **193**, 1089–1090.

Biserte, G., Havez, R., Hayem, A., and Laturaze, J. (1960). *C. R. Acad. Sci. Paris* **250**, 418–420.

Biserte, G., Havez, R., Samaille, J., Desmet, G., and Waroquier, R. (1964). *Biochim. Biophys. Acta* **93**, 361–373.

Bishop, J. O. (1963). *J. Gen. Microbiol.* **30**, 271–280.

Björklund, B. (1952a). *Proc. Soc. Exp. Biol. Med.* **79**, 319–324.

Björklund, B. (1952b). *Proc. Soc. Exp. Biol. Med.* **79**, 324–328.

Björklund, B. (1953a). *Atti Congr. Int. Microbiol. 6th Congr.* **2**, 344.

Björklund, B. (1953b). *Int. Arch. Allergy* **4**, 340–359.

Björklund, B. (1953c). *Int. Arch. Allergy* **4**, 379–414.

Björklund, B. (1954a). *Proc. Soc. Exp. Biol. Med.* **85**, 438–441.

Björklund, B. (1954b). *Int. Arch. Allergy* **5**, 293–298.

Björklund, B. (1956). *Int. Arch. Allergy* **8**, 179–192.

Björklund, B., and Berengo, A. (1954). *Acta Pathol. Microbiol. Scand.* **34**, 79–86.

Björklund, B., and Björklund, V. (1957). *Int. Arch. Allergy* **10**, 153–184.

Björling, H. (1963). *Vox Sang.* **8**, 641–659.

Black, M. M., Lillick, L. C., and Chabon, A. (1962). *Amer. J. Clin. Pathol.* **37**, 159–161.

Blair, P. B., Weiss, D. W., and Pitelka, D. R. (1966). *J. Nat. Cancer Inst.* **37**, 261–277.

Blanc, B. (1959). *Bull. Soc. Chim. Biol.* **41**, 891–899.

Blaney, D. J., and Mandrea, E. (1962). *J. Invest. Dermatol.* **38**, 53–54.

Block, R. J., Durrum, E. L., and Zweig, G. (1955). "Paper Chromatography and Paper Electrophoresis," 484 pp. Academic Press, New York.

Bloemendal, H. (1967). "High Resolution Techniques in Electrophoresis—Theory,

Methods and Applications" (M. Bier, ed.), 379–422. Academic Press, New York.

Blostein, R., and Rutter, W. J. (1963). *J. Biol. Chem.* **238,** 3280–3285.

Blumberg, B. S. (1963). *Ann. N. Y. Acad. Sci.* **103,** Art. 2, 1052–1057.

Blumberg, B. S., Dray, S., and Robinson, J. C. (1962). *Nature (London)* **194,** 656–658

Blumberg, B. S., Alter, H. J., Riddell, N. M., and Erlandson, M. (1964). *Vox Sang.* **9,** 128–145.

Bocci, V. (1962). *J. Chromatogr.* **8,** 218–226.

Bock, K. R. (1966). *Ann. Appl. Biol.* **57,** 131–140.

Bodman, J. (1959). *Clin. Chim. Acta* **4,** 103–109.

Bodmer, A. (1969). *Pathol. Microbiol.* **33,** 257–273.

Bodon, L. (1955). *Acta Vet. Acad. Sci. Hung.* **5,** 157–159.

Boerma, F. W. (1956). *J. Pathol. Bacteriol.* **72,** 515–518.

Boerma, F. W., and Huisman, T. H. J. (1964). *J. Lab. Clin. Med.* **63,** 264–278.

Boerma, F. W., Huisman, T. H. J., and Mandema, E. (1960). *Clin. Chim. Acta* **5,** 564–570.

Boffa, G. A., and Fine, J. M. (1962). *Rev. Fr. Etude. Clin. Biol.* **7,** 822–828.

Boffa, G. A., Zakin, M. M., Drilhon, A., Jacquot-Armand, Y., Amouch, P., and Fine, J. M. (1965). *C. R. Soc. Biol.* **159,** 2317.

Boffa, G. A., Fine, J. M., Drilhon, A., and Amouch, P. (1967). *Nature (London)* **214,** 700–702.

Boivin, P., Hartmann, L., and Fauvert, R. (1959). *Rev. Fr. Etude Clin. Biol.* **4,** 799–808.

Bojalil, L. F., and Zamora, A. (1963). *Proc. Soc. Exp. Biol. Med.* **113,** 40–43.

Bon, W. F. (1966). *Clin. Chim. Acta* **13,** 535–537.

Bon, W. F., and Swanborn, P. L. (1963). *Chem. Weekblad.* **59,** 72.

Bon, W. F., and Swanborn, P. L. (1965). *Anal. Biochem.* **11,** 16–22.

Bonilla-Soto, O., Rose, N. R., and Arbesman, C. E. (1961). *J. Allergy* **32,** 246–270.

Boquet, P., Izard, Y., Jouannet, M., and Meaume, J. (1966). *Ann. Inst. Pasteur* **111,** 719–732.

Boquet, P., Izard, Y., Meaume, J., and Jouannet, M. (1967). *Ann. Inst. Pasteur* **112,** 213–235.

Borek, F., and Silverstein, A. M. (1961). *J. Immunol.* **87,** 555–561.

Bornstein, P., and Oudin, J. (1964). *J. Exp. Med.* **120,** 655–676.

Boudin, G., Lewin, J., Dalloz, J. C., and Hillion, P. (1963). *Rev. Neurol. (Paris)* **109,** 499–512.

Boulanger, P., Bannister, G. L., and Greig, A. S. (1961). *Can. J. Comp. Med.* **25,** 113–120.

Boulet, P., Izarn, P., Mirouze, J., Barjon, P., Robinet, M., and Jaffiol, Cl. (1960). *Rev. Med. Souisse Roumande* **80,** 303–307.

Bowman, B. H. (1967). *In* "High Resolution Techniques in Electrophoresis—Theory, Methods and Applications" (M. Bier, ed.), pp. 157–212. Academic Press, New York.

Bowman, T., and Weinhold, A. R. (1963). *Nature (London)* **200,** 599–600.

Boyack, J. R., and Gidding, J. C. (1963). *Arch. Biochem. Biophys.* **100,** 16–25.

Boyce, W. H., King, J. S., Jr., and Fielden, M. L. (1962). *J. Clin. Invest.* **41,** 1180–1189.

Boyd, J. B., and Mitchell, H. K. (1965). *Anal. Biochem.* **13,** 28–42.

450 REFERENCES

Boyd, W. C. (1966). "Fundamentals of Immunology," 4th ed., 773 pp. Wiley (Interscience), New York.

Boyle, W., Davies, D. A. L., and Haughton, G. (1963). *Immunology* 6, 499–510.

Brand, K. G. (1965). *Nature (London)* 206, 1164–1165.

Brand, K. G., and Chiu, S. Y. (1966). *Nature (London)* 212, 44–46.

Brandriss, M. W., Smith, J. W., and Steinman, H. G. (1965). *J. Immunol.* 94, 696–704.

Branham, S. E., Hiatt, C. W., Cooper, A. D., and Riggs, D. B. (1959). *J. Immunol.* 82, 397–408.

Braun, H. J., and Aly, F. W. (1969). *Clin. Chim. Acta* 26, 588–590.

Brewer, J. M. (1967). *Science* 156, 256–257.

Bridges, R. A., and Good, R. H. (1959). *J. Lab. Clin. Med.* 54, 794.

Brill, N., and Brönnestam, R. (1960). *Acta Odontol. Scand.* 18, 95–100.

Briner, W. W., Riddle, J. W., and Cornwell, D. G. (1959). *Proc. Soc. Exp. Biol. Med.* 101, 784–786.

Briscoe, W. A., Kueppers, F., Davis, A. L., and Bearn, A. G. (1966). *Amer. Rev. Resp. Dis.* 94, 529–539.

Brishammar, S., Hjertén, S., and v. Hofsten, B. (1961). *Biochim. Biophys. Acta* 53, 518–521.

Broberger, O., and Perlmann, P. (1959). *J. Exp. Med.* 110, 657–674.

Brodie, H. D., and Ryckman, R. E. (1967). *J. Med. Entomol.* 4, 497–517.

Brönnestam, R., and Hallberg, T. (1965). *Acta Med. Scand.* 117, 385–392.

Brookbank, J. W., and Heisler, M. R. (1963). *J. Bacteriol.* 85, 509–515.

Brown, F., and Crick, J. (1959). *J. Immunol.* 82, 444–447.

Brown, F., and Graves, J. H. (1959). *Nature (London)* 183, 1688–1689.

Brown, R. (1940). *Proc. Soc. Exp. Biol. Med.* 45, 93–95.

Brown, R. M., Jr., and Bold, H. C. (1964). Phycological Studies. Univ. of Texas Publ. No. 6417, pp. 1–213.

Brown, R. M., Jr., and Lester, R. N. (1965). *J. Phycol.* 1, 60–65.

Brown, W. R. (1971). *J. Lab. Clin. Med.* 77, 326–334.

Brummerstedt-Hansen, E. (1961). *Acta Vet. Scand.* 2, 254–266.

Brummerstedt-Hansen, E. (1962). *Acta Vet. Scand.* 3, 245–255.

Brummerstedt-Hansen, E. (1967). "The Serum Proteins of the Pig. An Immunoelectrophoretic Study," 169 pp. Munksgaard, Copenhagen.

Brummerstedt-Hansen, E., and Hirschfeld, J. (1961). *Acta Vet. Scand.* 2, 317–322.

Burger-Girard, N. (1964). *Schweiz. Med. Wochenschr. Nr. 1* 94, 23–26.

Buri, J. F., Eyquem, A., and Pocidalo, J. J. (1964). *Presse Med.* 72, 81–86.

Burrell, R. G., Clayton, C. W., Gallegly, M. E., and Lilly, V. G. (1966). *Phytopathology* 56, 422–426.

Burstein, M. (1963). *Nouv. Rev. Fr. Hematol.* 3, 139–148.

Burstein, M. (1967). *Rev. Fr. Etude. Clin. Biol.* 12, 68–71.

Burstein, M. (1969). *Rev. Fr. Etude. Clin. Biol.* 19, 918–921.

Burstein, M., and Fine, J. M. (1964a). *Rev. Fr. Etude. Clin. Biol.* 9, 978–983.

Burstein, M., and Fine, J. M. (1964b). *Rev. Fr. Etude. Clin. Biol.* 9, 420–423.

Burstein, M., and Fine, J. M. (1964c). *Rev. Fr. Etude. Clin. Biol.* 9, 1075–1077.

Burtin, P. (1954). *Bull. Soc. Chim. Biol.* 36, 1021–1028.

Burtin, P. (1959a). *Clin. Chim. Acta* 4, 72–78.

Burtin, P. (1959b). *Ann. Inst. Pasteur* 97, 325–339.

Burtin, P., and Gendron, M. C. (1971). *Immunochemistry* 8, 423–429.

Burtin, P., and Grabar, P. (1954). *Bull. Soc. Chim. Biol.* 36, 335–345.

Burtin, P., and Grabar, P. (1967). *In* "High Resolution Techniques in Electrophoresis—Theory, Methods and Applications" (M. Bier, ed.), pp. 110–156. Academic Press, New York.

Burtin, P., and Kourilsky, R. (1959). *Ann. Inst. Pasteur* **97**, 148–170.

Burtin, P., and Pocidalo, J. (1954a). *C. R. Acad. Sci. Paris* **238**, 1628–1630.

Burtin, P., and Pocidalo, J. (1954b). *Presse Med.* **62**, 1072–1074.

Burtin, P., Grabar, P., Boussier, G., and Jayle, M. F. (1954). *Bull. Soc. Chim. Biol.* **36**, 1029–1035.

Burtin, P., Fauvert, R., and Grabar, P. (1955a). *Semaine Hôp.* **31**, 1–2.

Burtin, P., Hartmann, L., Fauvert, R., and Grabar, P. (1955b). *C. R. Acad. Sci. Paris* **241**, 339–341.

Burtin, P., Guilbert, B., and Buffe, D. (1966). *Clin. Chim. Acta* **13**, 675–677.

Burtin, P., Hartmann, L., Heremans, J., Scheidegger, J. J., Westendorp-Boerma, F., Wieme, R., Wunderly, Ch., Fauvert, R., and Grabar, P. (1957). *Rev. Fr. Etude. Clin. Biol.* **2**, 161–177.

Burtin, P., Hartmann, L., Fauvert, R., and Grabar, P. (1956). *Rev. Fr. Etude. Clin. Biol.* **1**, 17–28.

Bussard, A. (1954). *C. R. Acad. Sci. Paris* **239**, 1702–1704.

Bussard, A. (1958). Résumé, VII° Congr. Int. Microbial., p. 152.

Bussard, A., and Huet, J. (1959). *Biochim. Biophys. Acta* **34**, 258–260.

Bussard, A., and Perrin, B. (1955). *J. Lab. Clin. Med.* **46**, 689–701.

Bustamante, V. (1957). *Bull. Soc. Chim. Biol. Suppl. I* **39**, 155–160.

Butler, J. E., and Leone, C. A. (1968). *Comp. Biochem. Physiol.* **25**, 417–426.

Butler, V. P., Jr., Tanenbaum, S. W., and Beiser, S. M. (1965). *J. Exp. Med.* **121**, 19–38.

Buttery, S. (1959). *Nature (London)* **183**, 686–687.

Cabello, J., Prajoux, V., and Plaza, M. (1965). *Biochim. Biophys. Acta* **105**, 583–593.

Callaghan, O. H., and Goldfarb, A. R. (1962). *J. Immunol.* **89**, 612–622.

Campbell, D. H., Garvey, J. S., Cremer, N. E., and Sussdorf, D. H. (1970). "Methods in Immunology" 454 pp. Benjamin, New York.

Carey, J., and Warner, N. L. (1964). *Nature (London)* **203**, 198–199.

Carlisle, H. N., Hinchliffe, V., and Saslaw, S. (1962). *J. Immunol.* **89**, 638–644.

Carnegie, P. R., and Pacheco, G. (1964). *Proc. Soc. Exp. Biol. Med.* **117**, 137–141.

Carrel, S., Theilkaes, L., Skvaril, S., and Barandun, S. (1969). *J. Chromatogr.* **45**, 483–486.

Carter, B. C., and Harris, T. N. (1967). *Immunology* **12**, 75–88.

Casman, E. P., and Bennett, R. W. (1964). *Appl. Microbiol.* **12**, 363–367.

Casman, E. P., and Bennett, R. W. (1965). *Appl. Microbiol.* **13**, 181–189.

Casman, E. P., Bennett, R. W., Dorsey, A. E., and Stone, J. R. (1969). *Health Lab. Sci.* **6**, 185–198.

Castañeda, M. R. (1950). *Proc. Soc. Exp. Biol. Med.* **73**, 46–49.

Castañeda, M. R. (1953). *Proc. Soc. Exp. Biol. Med.* **83**, 36–39.

Castelnuovo, G., and Morellini, M. (1962a). *Ann. Ist. Carlo Forlanini* **22**, 1–20.

Castelnuovo, G., and Morellini, M. (1962b). *Ann. Ist. Carlo Forlanini* **22**, 189–194.

Castelnuovo, G., and Morellini, M. (1962c). *Ann. Ist. Carlo Forlanini* **22**, 195–198.

Castelnuovo, G., Gaudiano, A., Morellini, M., Penso, G., and Polizzi-Sciarrone, M. (1959). *Ann. Ist. Carlo Forlanini*, **19**, 1–18.

Castelnuovo, G., Gaudiano, A., Morellini, M., Penso, G., and Rossi, C. (1960). *Ren. Inst. Super. San.* **23**, 1222–1233.

Castelnuovo, G., Bellezza, G., Duncan, M. E., and Asselineau, J. (1964). *Ann. Inst. Pasteur* **107**, 828–844.

Castro, G. A., and Fairbairn, D. (1969). *J. Parasitol.* **55**, 59–66.

Castronova, E., Mills, W. J., and Fishkin, B. (1969). *Amer. J. Clin. Pathol.* **51**, 802–803.

Catsimpoolas, N. (1969). *Immunochemistry* **6**, 501–502.

Catsimpoolas, N. (1970). *Clin. Chim. Acta* **27**, 365–366.

Cawley, L. P. (1969). "Electrophoresis and Immunoelectrophoresis," 360 pp. Little, Brown, Boston, Massachusetts.

Cawley, L. P., Eberhardt, L., and Schneider, D. (1965a). *J. Lab. Clin. Med.* **65**, 342–354.

Cawley, L. P., Eberhardt, L., and Wiley, J. L. (1965b). *Vox Sang.* **10**, 116–125.

Cawley, L. P., Schneider, D., and Eberhardt, L. (1966). *Vox Sang.* **11**, 81–89.

Cayeux, Ph. (1962). *Ann. Inst. Pasteur* **103**, 23–31.

Cebra, J. J., and Goldstein, G. (1965). *J. Immunol.* **95**, 230–245.

Centeno, E., Shulman, S., Milgrom, F., and Witebsky, E. (1964). *Immunology* **8**, 160–169.

Centeno, E., Shulman, S., Gonder, M. J. and Soanes, W. A. (1965). *J. Lab. Clin. Med.* **65**, 706–712.

Centifanto, Y. M., and Kaufman, H. E. (1971). *J. Immunol.* **107**, 608–609.

Ceppellini, R., Dray, S., and Edelman, G. (1964). *Bull. WHO* **30**, 447–450.

Ceska, M. (1969a). *J. Immunol.* **103**, 100–106.

Ceska, M. (1969b). *Biochim. Biophys. Acta* **177**, 625–628.

Ceska, M., and Grossmüller, F. (1968). *Experientia* **15**, 391–392.

Chan, Y. C. (1965). *Nature (London)* **206**, 116–117.

Chaparas, S. D., and Baer, H. (1964). *Amer. Rev. Resp. Dis.* **90**, 87–96.

Chapman, J. S. (1961). *Ann. Int. Med.* **55**, 918–924.

Chapple, P. J., Bowen, E. T. W., and Lewis, N. D. (1963). *J. Hyg.* **61**, 373–383.

Chen, B. L., and Ely, C. A. (1968). *Proc. Soc. Exp. Biol. Med.* **127**, 1251–1254.

Chisiu, N. St. (1966). *Rev. Roum. Biochim.* **3**, 311–317.

Chiu, S. Y., Baker, P. J., and Brand, K. G. (1967). *J. Immunol.* **98**, 806–810.

Chodirker, W. B., and Tomasi, T. B., Jr. (1963). *Science* **142**, 1080–1081.

Chordi, A., and Kagan, I. G. (1964). *J. Immunol.* **93**, 439–445.

Chordi, A., Walls, K. W., and Kagan, I. G. (1964). *J. Immunol.* **93**, 1034–1044.

Chrambach, A., and Rodbard, D. (1971). *Science* **172**, 440–451.

Christian, C. L. (1963). *J. Exp. Med.* **118**, 827–844.

Christian, C. L. (1970). *Immunology* **18**, 457–466.

Christian, C. L., Hatfield, W. B., and Chase, P. H. (1963). *J. Clin. Invest.* **42**, 823–829.

Cier, J. F., Manuel, Y., and Lacour, J. R. (1963). *C. R. Soc. Biol.* **157**, 1623.

Cinader, B. (1968). "Regulation of the Antibody Response," 400 pp. Thomas, Springfield, Illinois.

Cinader, B., Whipple, H. E., and Silverzweig, S. (1963). *Ann. N. Y. Acad. Sci.* **103**, Art. 2, 493–1154.

Claman, H. N., and Merrill, D. (1964). *J. Lab. Clin. Med.* **64**, 685–693.

Claman, H. N., Merrill, D. A., and Hartley, T. F. (1967). *J. Allergy* **40**, 151–159.

Clarke, H. G. M., and Freeman, T. (1966). *Protides Biol. Fluids* **14**, 503–509.

Clarke, H. G. M., and Freeman, T. (1968). *Clin. Sci.* **35**, 403–413.

Clarke, J. T. (1964). *Ann. N. Y. Acad. Sci.* **121**, Art. 2, 428–436.

Clarkson, M. J. (1963). *Immunology* **6**, 156–168.

Clausen, J. (1963). *Sci. Tools* **10**, 29.

Clausen, J., and Heremans, J. (1960). *J. Immunol.* **84**, 128–134.

Clausen, J., Krogsgaard, A. R., and Quaade, F. (1962). *J. Infect. Dis.* **111**, 128–134.

Clausen, J., Gjedde, F., and Jørgensen, K. (1963). *Proc. Soc. Exp. Biol. Med.* **112**, 778–781.

Cleve, H. (1958). *Z. Rheumaforsch.* **17**, 250–361.

Cleve, H., and Bearn, A. G. (1961). *Amer. J. Hum. Genet.* **13**, 372–378.

Cleve, H., Prunier, J. H., and Bearn, A. G. (1963). *J. Exp. Med.* **118**, 711–726.

Cline, L. J. (1967). Doctoral dissertation, Dept. Microbiol., Univ. Colorado School Medicine.

Codd, A. A., Hale, J. H., Selkon, J. B., and Ingham, H. R. (1968). *Brit. J. Exp. Pathol.* **49**, 365–370.

Coffino, P., Laskov, R., and Scharff, M. D. (1970). *Science* **167**, 186–188.

Coggins, L., and Heuschele, W. P. (1966). *Amer. J. Vet. Res.* **27**, 485–488.

Cohen, J. J., Myers, J., Rose, B., and Goodfriend, L. (1964). *Can. J. Biochem.* **42**, 1787–1792.

Cohen, J. O., Newton, W. L., Cherry, W. B. and Updyke, E. L. (1963). *J. Immunol.* **90**, 358–367.

Cohen, S. (1963). *Nature (London)* **197**, 253–255.

Coleman, A. W. (1963). *J. Protozool.* **10**, 141–148.

Coleman, R. M., and deSa, L. M. (1964). *Nature (London)* **204**, 397–398.

Collins-Williams, C., Trachyk, S. J., Toft, B., and Moscarello, M. (1967). *Int. Arch. Allergy* **31**, 94–103.

Colover, J., Feinberg, J. G., Temple, A., and Tooley, M. (1963). *J. Clin. Pathol.* **16**, 370–374.

Conner, R. M. (1970). *Rev. Sci. Instrum.* **41**, 875–876.

Consden, R., and Kohn, J. (1959). *Nature (London)* **183**, 1512–1513.

Cooper, W. C., Halbert, S. P., and Manski, W. J. (1963). *Invest. Ophthalmol.* **2**, 369–377.

Corcos, J. M., and Ovary, Z. (1965). *Proc. Soc. Exp. Biol. Med.* **119**, 142–148.

Córdoba, F., Gonzalez, C., and Rivera, P. (1965). *Nature (London)* **205**, 565–567.

Córdoba, F., Gonzalez, C., and Rivera, P. (1966). *Clin. Chim. Acta* **13**, 611–625.

Cornillot, P., Bourrillon, R., Michon, J., and Got, R. (1963). *Biochim. Biophys. Acta* **71**, 89–96.

Correni, E. (1964). *Naturwissenschaften* **2**, 51.

Couffer-Kaltenbach, J., and Perlmann, P. (1961). *J. Biophys. Biochem. Cytol.* **9**, 93–104.

Coulson, E. J., and Jackson, R. H. (1962). *Arch. Biochem. Biophys.* **97**, 378–382.

Courtice, F. C. (1967). *In* "High Resolution Techniques in Electrophoresis—Theory, Methods and Applications" (M. Bier, ed.), pp. 241–310. Academic Press, New York.

Cowan, K. M. (1966a). *J. Immunol.* **97**, 647–653.

Cowan, K. M. (1966b). *Amer. J. Vet. Res.* **27**, 1217–1227.

Cowan, K. M., and Graves, J. H. (1968). *Virology* **34**, 544–548.

Cowan, K. M., and Trautman, R. (1965). *J. Immunol.* **94**, 858–867.

Creyssel, R., and Richard, G. B. (1966). *Acta Med. Scand. Suppl.* **445**, 171–177.

Creyssel, R., Manuel, Y., Richard, G. B., and Fine, J. M. (1962). *Rev. Fr. Etude. Clin. Biol.* **7**, 253–259.

Creyssel, R., Richard, G., Manuel, Y., Silberzahn, P., and Betuel, H. (1964). "Protides of the Biological Fluids" (H. Peeters, ed.), pp. 161–164. Elsevier, Amsterdam.

Crockson, R. A. (1963). *J. Clin. Pathol.* **16**, 287–289.

Croissile, Y. (1959). *C. R. Acad. Sci. Paris* **249**, 1712–1714.

Croisille, Y. (1962). *C. R. Soc. Biol.* **156**, 1221–1225.

Cross, T., and Spooner, D. F. (1963). *J. Gen. Microbiol.* **33**, 275–282.

Crowle, A. J. (1954). A Study of the Immunizing Factors of the Tubercle Bacillus, Dissertation, 140 pp. Stanford Univ., Stanford, California.

Crowle, A. J. (1956). Unpublished experiments.

Crowle, A. J. (1956). *J. Lab. Clin. Med.* **48**, 642–648.

Crowle, A. J. (1958a). *J. Immunol.* **81**, 194–198.

Crowle, A. J. (1958b). *Int. Arch. Allergy* **12**, 215–222.

Crowle, A. J. (1958c). *J. Lab. Clin. Med.* **52**, 784–787.

Crowle, A. J. (1960a). *Int. Arch. Allergy* **16**, 113–125.

Crowle, A. J. (1960b). *J. Lab. Clin. Med.* **55**, 593–604.

Crowle, A. J. (1960c). *Ann. Rev. Microbiol.* **14**, 161–176.

Crowle, A. J. (1961). "Immunodiffusion," 333 pp. Academic Press, New York.

Crowle, A. J. (1963). *J. Asthma Res.* **1**, 11–38.

Crowle, A. J. (1971). *In* "Methods in Immunology and Immunochemistry" (C. A. Williams and M. W. Chase, eds.), Vol. 3, pp. 357–364. Academic Press, New York.

Crowle, A. J. (1972). *Exp. Physiol. Biochem.* **6**, 183–200.

Crowle, A. J., and Hu, C. C. (1965). *Tubercle* **46**, 214–223.

Crowle, A. J., and Hu, C. C. (1967). *Proc. Soc. Exp. Biol. Med.* **126**, 729–731.

Crowle, A. J., and Lueker, D. C. (1961a). Unpublished experiments.

Crowle, A. J., and Lueker, D. C. (1961b). *Nature (London)* **192**, 50–52.

Crowle, A. J., and Lueker, D. C. (1962). *J. Lab. Clin. Med.* **59**, 697–704.

Crowle, A. J., Lueker, D. C., and Gaskill, H. S., Jr. (1963). *Nature (London)* **199**, 623–624.

Crumpton, M. J., and Davies, D. A. L. (1956). *Proc. Roy. Soc.* **145**, 109–134.

Cruse, J. M. (1966). *Proc. Soc. Exp. Biol. Med.* **121**, 833–838.

Cuadrado, R. R. (1966). *J. Immunol.* **96**, 892–897.

Cuadrado, R. R., and Casals, J. (1967). *J. Immunol.* **98**, 314–320.

Culliford, B. J. (1964). *Nature (London)* **201**, 1092–1094.

Cummings, N. A., and Franklin, E. C. (1965). *J. Lab. Clin. Med.* **65**, 8–17.

D'Addabbo, A. (1963). *Med. Clin. Sper.* **13**, 331–344.

D'Amelio, V., Mutolo, V., and Barbarino, A. (1963a). *Exp. Cell Res.* **29**, 1–16.

D'Amelio, V., Mutolo, V., and Piazza, E. (1963b). *Exp. Cell Res.* **31**, 499–507.

Dameshek, W. (1963). *Blood* **21**, 243–245.

Damian, R. T. (1966). *Exp. Parasitol.* **18**, 255–265.

Dandliker, W. B., Halbert, S. P., Florin, M. C., Alonso, R., and Schapiro, H. C. (1965). *J. Exp. Med.* **122**, 1029–1048.

Daniel, T. M., and Wisnieski, J. J. (1970). *Amer. Rev. Resp. Dis.* **101**, 762–764.

Darbyshire, J. H., and Pereira, H. G. (1964). *Nature (London)* **201**, 895–897.

Darcy, D. A. (1955). *Nature (London)* **176**, 643–644.

Darcy, D. A. (1957). *Brit. J. Cancer* **11**, 137–147.

Darcy, D. A. (1960). *Immunology* **3**, 325–335.

Darcy, D. A. (1961). *Nature (London)* **191**, 1163–1165.

Dardas, T. J., and Mallmann, V. H. (1966). *J. Bacteriol.* **92**, 76–81.

Dasgupta, A., and Cunliffe, A. C. (1970). *Clin. Exp. Immunol.* **6**, 891–898.
Da Silva, L. C., and Ferri, R. G. (1965a). *Rev. Inst. Med. Trop. Sao Paulo* **7**, 1–6.
Da Silva, L. C., and Ferri, R. G. (1965b). *Rev. Inst. Med. Trop. Sao Paulo* **7**, 7–10.
Daufi, L., and Rondell, P. (1969). *Proc. Soc. Exp. Biol. Med.* **131**, 1353–1356.
Daussant, J., and Grabar, P. (1966). *Ann. Inst. Pasteur* **110**, 79–83.
David-West, T. S. (1966). *J. Pathol. Bacteriol.* **92**, 477–489.
Davies, D. R., Spurr, E. D., and Versey, J. M. B. (1970). *Biochem. J.* **118**.
Davis, B. J. (1964). *Ann. N. Y. Acad. Sci.* **121**, Art. 2, 404–427.
Dawkins, B. F. (1963). *N. Z. J. Med. Lab. Technol.* **17**, 40.
Dayton, D. H., Jr., Small, P. A., Jr., Chanock, R. M., Kaufman, H. E., and Tomasi, T. B., Jr. (eds.), (1971). "The Secretory Immunologic System," 544 pp. U. S. Govt. Printing Office, Washington, D. C. 0-402-006.
De Araujo, W. C., Varah, E., and Mergenhagen, S. E. (1963). *J. Bacteriol.* **86**, 837–844.
De Banchero, E. P. (1962). *Rev. Invest. Ganad.* **14**, 159–184.
Debray-Sachs, M., and Sachs, Ch. (1962a). *Ann. Biol. Clin.* **20**, 937–949.
Debray-Sachs, M., and Sachs, Ch. (1962b). *Rev. Fr. Etude. Clin. Biol.* **7**, 927–937.
DeCarvalho, S. (1960). *J. Lab. Clin. Med.* **56**, 333–341.
DeCarvalho, S. (1964). *Nature (London)* **203**, 1186–1188.
DeCarvalho, S., Rand, H. J., and Uhrick, J. R. (1962). *Exp. Mol. Pathol.* **1**, 96–103.
DeCarvalho, S., Uhrick, J., and Rand, H. J. (1962). *Nature (London)* **194**, 1275–1276.
DeCarvalho, S., Lewis, A. J., Rand, H. J., and Uhrick, J. R. (1964). *Nature (London)* **204**, 265–266.
Deckers, C. (1967). *Symp. Ser. Immunobiol. Std.* **4**, 31–36.
Deckers, C., and Abelev, G. I. (1963). *Protides Biol. Fluids* **10**, 312–315.
Deckers, C., and Maisin, J. (1963). *Nature (London)* **197**, 397.
Deeb, B. J., and Kenny, G. E. (1967). *J. Bacteriol.* **93**, 1416–1424.
DeGroat, A., Anastassiadis-Aries, U. E., and White, M. F. (1964). *Amer. J. Clin. Pathol.* **41**, 441–447.
Deicher, H. R. G., Holman, H. R., and Kunkel, H. G. (1959). *J. Exp. Med.* **109**, 97–114.
Del Giacco, G. S., and Luporini, G. (1962). *Boll. I.S.M.* **41**, 138–143.
De Muralt, G. (1962). *Helv. Med. Acta Suppl.* **42 29**, 1–160.
Dencker, S. J. (1963). *Acta Neurol. Scand. Suppl. 4* **39**, 317–322.
Dencker, S. J., and Swahn, B. (1961). *Lunds Univ. Årsskrift* **57**, 1–54.
Denis, H. (1964). *J. Embryol. Exp. Morphol.* **12**, 197–217.
Dennis, E. G., Hornbrook, M. M., and Ishizaka, K. (1964). *J. Allergy* **35**, 464–471.
De Oliveria, H. L. (1958). *Int. Arch. Allergy* **12**, 356–360.
Depelchin, A. (1964). *Rev. Immunol. (Paris)* **28**, 15–35.
Depieds, R., Cartouzou, G., Lissitzky, S., Gignoux, H., and Gignoux, D. (1962). *C. R. Soc. Biol.* **156**, 1450.
Depieds, R., Cartouzou, G., Lissitzky, S., and Gignoux, H. (1963). *Rev. Fr. Etude. Clin. Biol.* **8**, 653–661.
DePree, A. L., Little, J., and Langman, J. (1964). *Arch. Ophthalmol.* **72**, 660–666.
De Repentigny, J., Sonea, S., and Frappier, A. (1964). *J. Bacteriol.* **88**, 444–448.
De Sequeira, O. A. (1967). *Virology* **31**, 314–322.
Deutsch, H. F. (1964). *J. Immunol.* **93**, 879–885.
De Vaux Saint-Cyr, C., and Hermann, G. (1963). *Rev. Fr. Etude. Clin. Biol.* **8**, 445–454.

456   REFERENCES

De Vaux Saint-Cyr, C., Hermann, G., and Talal, N. (1963). *Rev. Fr. Etude. Clin. Biol.* **8**, 241–249.

DeVillez, E. J. (1964). *Anal. Biochem.* **9**, 485–586.

Di Capua, R. A. (1966). *J. Exp. Zool.* **162**, 1–13.

Di Ferrante, N. (1964). *Science* **143**, 250–252.

Dike, G. W. R. (1960). *J. Clin. Pathol.* **13**, 87–89.

Dimmock, N. J. (1967). *Virology* **31**, 338–353.

Dimmock, N. J. (1969). *Virology* **39**, 224–234.

Dineen, J. K. (1963). *Nature (London)* **197**, 471–472.

Dirksen, E. R. (1964). *Exp. Cell Res.* **36**, 256–269.

Distler, J., and Roseman, S. (1964). *Proc. Nat. Acad. Sci. USA* **51**, 897–905.

Dobson, C. (1966). *J. Parasitol.* **52**, 1037–1038.

Dobson, C. (1967). *J. Parasitol.* **57**, 201–219.

Dodin, A. (1963). *Ann. Inst. Pasteur* **105**, 1098–1107.

Dodin, A., Ratovondrahety, J. P. M., and Richaud, J. (1965). *Ann. Inst. Pasteur* **109**, 128–137.

Döhner, L. (1970). *Pathol. Microbiol. (Basel)* **35**, 338–347.

Doležalová, V., Brada, Z., and Kočent, A. (1965). *Biochim. Biophys. Acta* **107**, 294–306.

Dolovich, J., Tomasi, T. B., Jr., and Arbesman, C. E. (1970). *J. Allergy* **45**, 286–294.

Doniach, D., and Roitt, I. M. (1957). *J. Clin. Endocrinol. Metab.* **17**, 1293–1304.

Doniach, D., and Roitt, I. M. (1959). "Immunopathology, 1st International Symposium, Basel/Seelisberg, 1958," pp. 168–179. Schwabe, Basel.

Dony, J., and Muyldermans, H. (1970). *Progr. Immunobiol. Stand.* **4**, 395–405.

Dorrington, K. J., and Tanford, C. (1970). *Advan. Immunol.* **12**, 333–382.

Downe, A. E. R. (1962). *Can. J. Zool.* **40**, 957–967.

Downe, A. E. R. (1963). *Science* **139**, 1286–1287.

Dray, S. (1960). *Fed. Proc.* **19**, 205.

Dray, S. (1962). *Nature (London)* **195**, 677–680.

Dray, S. (1963). *Proc. 11th Int. Congr. Genet. The Hague* 165–180.

Dray, S., Lieberman, R., and Hoffman, H. A. (1963a). *Proc. Soc. Exp. Biol. Med.* **113**, 509–513.

Dray, S., Young, G. O., and Gerald, L. (1963b). *J. Immunol.* **91**, 403–415.

Dreesman, G., Larson, C., Pinckard, R. N., Groyon, R. M., and Benedict, A. A. (1965). *Proc. Soc. Exp. Biol. Med.* **118**, 292–296.

Drouhet, E., Segretain, G., Pesle, G., and Bidet, L. (1963). *Ann. Inst. Pasteur* **105**, 597–604.

Duclaux, J. (1936). *Actual Sci. Ind.* **350**, 1–50.

Dudman, W. F. (1964a). *Nature (London)* **201**, 995–997.

Dudman, W. F. (1964b). *J. Bacteriol.* **88**, 782–794.

Dudman, W. F. (1965a). *Phytopathology* **55**, 635–639.

Dudman, W. F. (1965b). *J. Immunol.* **95**, 704–717.

Dudman, W. F., and Brockwell, J. (1968). *Aust. J. Agr. Res.* **19**, 739–747.

Dufour, D., and Noël, H. P. (1964). *Laval Med.* **35**, 279–281.

Dufour, D., and Tremblay, A. (1964). *Rev. Can. Biol.* **23**, 501–503.

Dufour, D., Tremblay, A., and Lemieux, S. (1965). *Rev. Fr. Etude. Clin. Biol.* **11**, 89–92.

Dumonde, D. C., Al-Askari, S., Lawrence, H. S., and Thomas, L. (1963). *Nature (London)* **198**, 598.

Dupouey, P. (1963). *Ann. Inst. Pasteur* **105**, 949–970.

Dupouey, P., and Maréchal, J. (1966). *Ann. Inst. Pasteur* 110, 888–911.
Duquesnoy, R. J. (1966). *Life Sci.* 5, 1605–1610.
Durand, M., and Schneider, R. (1962a). *Arch. Inst. Pasteur Tunis* 39, 137–151.
Durand, M., and Schneider, R. (1962b). *Arch. Inst. Pasteur Tunis* 39, 153–163.
Durand, M., and Schneider, R. (1963). *Arch. Inst. Pasteur Tunis* 40, 91–95.
Durieux, J., and Kaminski, M. (1956). *Bull. Soc. Chim. Biol.* 38, 1445–1456.
Dusanic, D. G., and Lewert, R. M. (1966). *J. Infect. Dis.* 116, 270–284.
Easty, G. C. (1954). *Discuss. Faraday Soc.* 18, 364.
Easty, G. C., and Ambrose, E. J. (1957). *J. Exp. Biol.* 34, 60–70.
Easty, G. C., and Mercer, E. H. (1958). *Immunology* 1, 353–364.
Ebel, D. (1955). *Int. Arch. Allergy* 7, 75–91.
Edelman, I. S., and Bryan, W. P. (1960). *J. Amer. Chem. Soc.* 82, 1491–1494.
Egdahl, R. H., Cress, H., and Mannick, J. A. (1962). *Nature (London)* 196, 183–184.
Ehrlich, G., Halbert, S. P., and Manski, W. (1962). *J. Immunol.* 89, 391–399.
Eiguer, T., and Staub, A. M. (1966). *Ann. Inst. Pasteur* 110, 707–726.
Elek, S. D. (1948). *Brit. Med. J.* 1, 493–496.
Elek, S. D. (1949a). *Brit. J. Exp. Pathol.* 30, 484–500.
Elek, S. D. (1949b). *J. Clin. Pathol.* 2, 250–258.
Elek, S. D., and Levy, E. (1950a). *J. Pathol. Bacteriol.* 62, 541–554.
Elek, S. D., and Levy, E. (1950b). *Brit. J. Exp. Pathol.* 31, 358–368.
Elevitch, F. R., Aronson, S. B., Feichtmeir, T. V., and Enterline, M. L. (1966). *Amer. J. Clin. Pathol.* 46, 692–697.
Ellis, H. A., and Gell, P. G. H. (1958). *Nature (London)* 181, 1667–1668.
Ellner, P. D., and Green, S. S. (1963a). *J. Bacteriol.* 86, 604–605.
Ellner, P. D., and Green, S. S. (1963b). *J. Bacteriol.* 86, 1084–1097.
El-Marsafy, M. K., and Abdel-Gaward, Z. (1962). *Experientia* 18, 240–243.
El-Sharkawy, T. A., and Huisingh, D. (1971). *Infect. Immunity* 3, 711.
Emmart, E. W., Bates, R. W., Condliffe, P. G., and Turner, W. A. (1963). *Proc. Soc. Exp. Biol. Med.* 114, 754–763.
Emmart, E. W., Spicer, S. S., Turner, W. A., and Henson, J. G. (1962). *Exp. Cell Res.* 26, 78–97.
Engelberg, J. (1959). *J. Immunol.* 82, 467–470.
Engelhardt, N. V., Khramkova, N. I., and Postnikova, Z. A. (1963). *Neoplasma* 9, 133–142.
Escribano, M. J. (1962). *C. R. Acad. Sci. Paris* 255, 409–411.
Escribano, M. J., and Grabar, P. (1966). *Ann. Inst. Pasteur* 110, 84–88.
Espinosa, E., and Insunza, I. (1962). *Proc. Soc. Exp. Biol. Med.* 111, 174–177.
Epstein, W. V., and Tan, M. (1962). *J. Lab. Clin. Med.* 60, 125–137.
Eyquem, A., Jouanne, C., and Landrein, S. (1966). *Ann. Inst. Pasteur* 110, 89–94.
Eyster, M. E., Nachman, R. L., Cristenson, W. N., and Engle, R. L., Jr. (1966). *J. Immunol.* 96, 107–111.
Fahey, J. L., and Barth, W. F. (1965). *Proc. Soc. Exp. Biol. Med.* 118, 596–600.
Fahey, J. L., and Goodman, H. (1964). *Science* 143, 588–590.
Fahey, J. L., and Horbett, A. P. (1959). *J. Biol. Chem.* 234, 2645–2651.
Fahey, J. L., and McKelvey, E. M. (1965). *J. Immunol.* 94, 84–90.
Fahey, J. L., and McLaughlin, C. (1963). *J. Immunol.* 91, 484–497.
Fahey, J. L., Wunderlich, J., and Mishell, R. (1964). *J. Exp. Med.* 120, 223–242.
Fahey, J. L., Barth, W., and Ovary, Z. (1965). *J. Immunol.* 94, 819–823.
Fairbrother, F., and Mastin, H. (1923). *J. Chem. Soc.* 123, 1412–1424.

Fasel, J., and Scheidegger, J. J. (1960). *Gastroenterologia* **94**, 236–250.

Fasella, P., Baglioni, C., and Turano, C. (1957). *Experientia* **13**, 406–407.

Faure, J. P. (1963). *C. R. Acad. Sci. Paris* **256**, 295–297.

Faure, R., Fine, J. M., Saint-Paul, M., Eyquem, A., and Grabar, P. (1955). *Bull. Soc. Chim. Biol.* **37**, 783–796.

Fayet, M. T., Mackowiak, C., Camand, R., and Leftheriotis, E. (1957). *Ann. Inst. Pasteur* **92**, 466–472.

Fedida, M. (1960). *C. R. Acad. Sci. Paris* **250**, 3425–3427.

Feinberg, J. G. (1956). *Nature (London)* **178**, 1406.

Feinberg, J. G. (1957). *Int. Arch. Allergy* **11**, 129–152.

Feinberg, J. G. (1961). *Nature (London)* **192**, 985–986.

Feinberg, J. G. (1962). *Nature (London)* **194**, 307–308.

Feinberg, J. G. (1963). *J. Clin. Pathol.* **16**, 282–284.

Feinberg, J. G., and Grant, R. A. (1957). *Biochem. J.* **65**, 40 P.

Feinberg, J. G., and Grayson, H. (1959). *Nature (London)* **183**, 987.

Feinberg, J. G., and Temple, A. (1962). *Int. Arch. Allergy* **22**, 274–293.

Feinberg, J. G., Goldsmith, K. L. G., and Kekwick, R. A. (1964). *J. Clin. Pathol.* **17**, 690–692.

Feinberg, M. P., Mann, L. T., Jr., and Blatt, W. F. (1965). *Amer. J. Clin. Pathol.* **44**, 177–181.

Feinstein, A., and Rowe, A. J. (1965). *Nature (London)* **205**, 147–149.

Felsenfeld, O., Decker, W. J., Wohlhieter, J. A., and Rafyi, A. (1965). *J. Immunol.* **94**, 805–817.

Fernelius, A. L. (1966). *J. Immunol.* **96**, 488–494.

Ferri, R. G. (1960). *Selecta Chim.* **19**, 99–107.

Ferri, R. G. (1961). *Ann. Microbiol., Suppl.,* **9**, 11–22.

Ferri, R. G., and Cossermelli, W. (1964a). *Rev. Fr. Etude. Clin. Biol.* **9**, 128–133.

Ferri, R. G., and Cossermelli, W. (1964b). *Rev. Fr. Etude. Clin. Biol.* **9**, 134–138.

Ferris, T. G., Easterling, R. E., and Budd, R. E. (1962a). *Amer. J. Clin. Pathol.* **38**, 383–387.

Ferris, T. G., Easterling, R. E., and Budd, R. E. (1962b). *Blood* **19**, 479–482.

Ferris, T. G., Easterling, R. E., and Budd, R. E. (1963). *Amer. J. Clin. Pathol.* **39**, 193–197.

Fessel, W. J. (1963a). *Nature (London)* **197**, 1307.

Fessel, W. J. (1963b). *Proc. Soc. Exp. Biol. Med.* **113**, 446–449.

Fey, H. (1960). *Milchwissenschaften* **15**, 105–107.

Fey, H., and Margadant, A. (1961). *Pathol. Microbiol. (Basel)* **24**, 970–976.

Fey, H., Hauser, H., and Messerli, W. (1960). *Schweiz. Arch. Tierheilkd.* **102**, 285–296.

Filitti-Wurmser, S., and Hartman, L. (1962a). *Bull. Soc. Chim. Biol.* **44**, 725–733.

Filitti-Wurmser, S., and Hartman, L. (1962b). *Bull. Soc. Chim. Biol.* **44**, 919–949.

Filitti-Wurmser, S., Jugon, M. P., and Hartman, L. (1958). *Rev. Fr. Etude. Clin. Biol.* **3**, 1080–1083.

Finck, H. (1965). *Biochim. Biophys. Acta* **111**, 208–220.

Fine, J. M. (1968). *Ann. Biol.* **7**, 597–604.

Fine, J. M., and Battistini, A. (1960). *Experientia* **16**, 57–59.

Fine, J. M., and Drilhon, A. (1963). *C. R. Soc. Biol.* **157**, 1937.

Fine, J. M., and Drilhon, A. (1964). *C. R. Soc. Biol.* **158**, 1307.

Fine, J. M., Boffa, G. A., and Zajdela, F. (1962a). *C. R. Acad. Sci. Paris* **255**, 1045–1047.

Fine, J. M., Mouray, H., and Moretti, J. (1962b). *Clin. Chim. Acta* 7, 346–354.

Fine, J. M., Boffa, G. A., and Drilhon, A. (1963). *Proc. Soc. Exp. Biol. Med.* 114, 651–654.

Fine, J. M., Boffa, G. A., and Drilhon, A. (1964). *C. R. Soc. Biol.* 158, 2021.

Finger, I. (1964). *Nature* (*London*) 203, 1035–1039.

Finger, I., and Heller, C. (1963). *J. Mol. Biol.* 6, 190–202.

Finger, I., Heller, C., and Smith, J. P. (1963). *J. Mol. Biol.* 6, 182–189.

Fink, M. A., and Cowles, C. A. (1965). *Science* 150, 1723–1725.

Fink, M. A., Sibal, L. R., Wivel, N. A., Cowles, C. A., and O'Conner, T. E. (1969). *Virology* 37, 605–614.

Fireman, P., Vannier, W. E., and Goodman, H. C. (1963). *J. Exp. Med.* 117, 603–620.

Firestone, H. J., and Aronson, S. B. (1969). *Tech. Bull. Regist. Med. Technol.* 39, 217–224.

Fisher, J. P. (1965). *J. Invest. Dermatol.* 44, 43–50.

Fiset, L. G. (1962). *Immunology* 5, 580–594.

Fitschen, W. (1963). *Biochem. J.* 88, 13 P.

Flandre, O., and Damon, M. (1961). *Rev. Fr. Etude. Clin. Biol.* 6, 717–718.

Fleischmajer, R., and Krol, S. (1967). *J. Invest. Dermatol.* 48, 359–363.

Flocks, R. H., Bandhaur, K., Patel, C., and Begley, B. J. (1962). *J. Urol.* 87, 475–478.

Flodin, P., and Killander, J. (1962). *Biochim. Biophys. Acta* 63, 403–410.

Fodor, O., Barbarino, F., Iaina, A., and Tragor, S. (1962). *Acta Gastroenterol. Belg.* 25, 901–905.

Ford, R. E. (1964). *Phytopathology* 54, 615–616.

Forsgren, A., and Sjöquist, J. (1966). *J. Immunol.* 97, 822–827.

Forsgren, M. (1966). *Acta Pathol. Microbiol. Scand.* 66, 262–263.

Fox, A. S., Yoon, S. B., and Mead, C. G. (1962). *Proc. Nat. Acad. Sci. USA* 48, 546–561.

Fox, E. N. (1963). *J. Bacteriol.* 85, 536–540.

Fox, I., Knight, W. B., and Bayona, I. G. (1963). *J. Allergy* 34, 196–202.

Fox, I., Bayona, I. G., Umpierre, C. C., and Morris, J. M. (1967). *J. Parasitol.* 53, 402–405.

François, J., and Rabaey, M. (1963). *Exp. Eye Res.* 2, 196–202.

François, J., Rabaey, M., Wieme, R. J., and Kaminski, M. (1956). *Amer. J. Ophthalmol.* 42, 577–584.

Francq, J. C., Eyquem, A., Podliachouk, L., and Jacqueline, F. (1959). *Ann. Inst. Pasteur* 96, 413–419.

Franklin, E. C. (1962a). *Nature* (*London*) 195, 392–394.

Franklin, E. C. (1962b). *Proc. Soc. Exp. Biol. Med.* 109, 338–342.

Franklin, E. C., Lowenstein, J., Bigelow, B., and Meltzer, M. (1964). *Amer. J. Med.* 37, 332–350.

Frederick, J. F. (1964). *Ann. N. Y. Acad. Sci.* 121, Art. 2, 305–650.

Freeman, M. J., and Stavitsky, A. B. (1966). *J. Immunol.* 95, 981–990.

Freeman, V. J. (1950). *Pub. Health Rep.* (*U. S.*) 65, 875–882.

Freimer, E. H. (1963). *J. Exp. Med.* 117, 377–399.

Freimer, E. H., Krause, R. M., and McCarty, M. (1959). *J. Exp. Med.* 110, 853–874.

Frey, J., Hoa, N., Gras, J., Henry, J. C., and Gudefin, Y. (1965). *Science* 150, 751–752.

Frick, E., and Scheid-Seidel, L. (1957). Z. Ges. Exp. Med. 129, 221–246.

Friedman, H. (1971). Immunological tolerance to microbial antigens. Ann. N. Y. Acad. Sci. 181, 315 pp.

Friesen, H., Irie, M., and Barrett, R. J. (1962). J. Exp. Med. 115, 513–525.

Froman, S., Edgington, T. S., Will, D. W., Scammon, L., Faber, D. R., and Eckmann, B. H. (1964). Amer. J. Clin. Pathol. 42, 340–345.

Fromm, G., Langheld, I., and Wurziger, J. (1964). Arch. Hyg. Bakteriol. 148, 244–260.

Fujio, H., Kishigushi, S., Noma, Y., Skinka, S., Saiki, Y., and Amano, T. (1958). Biken J. 1, 138–156.

Fujio, H., Nowa, Y., and Amano, T. (1959). Biken J. 2, 35–49.

Fultz, S. A., and Sussman, A. S. (1966). Science 152, 785–787.

Furminger, I. G. S. (1964). Biochim. Biophys. Acta 90, 521–533.

Furminger, I. G. S. (1965). J. Pathol. Bacteriol. 89, 337–342.

Gabridge, M. G., and Newman, J. P. (1971). Appl. Microbiol. 21, 147–148.

Gajos, E. (1970). Experientia 26, 1007–1008.

Gallien, C. L., Foulgoc, M. T. C. L., and Fine, J. M. (1966). C. R. Acad. Sci. Paris 263, 2040–2042.

Garb, S., Stein, A. A., and Sims, G. (1962). J. Immunol. 88, 142–152.

Gargani, G., and Guerra, M. (1962). Boll. I. S. M. 41, 227–235.

Gavrilesco, K., Courcon, J., Hillion, P., Uriel, J., Lesin, J., and Grabar, P. (1955). Bull. Soc. Chim. Biol. 37, 803–807.

Gazzaniga, P. P., Lipari, M., and Sonnino, F. R. (1965). J. Pathol. Bacteriol. 90, 682–685.

Gell, P. G. H. (1955a). J. Clin. Pathol. 8, 269–275.

Gell, P. G. H. (1955b). Biochem. J. 59, viii.

Gell, P. G. H. (1957). J. Clin. Pathol. 10, 67–71.

Gendon, I. Z. (1958). J. Microbiol. Epidemiol. Immunobiol. (U.S.S.R.) 29, 416–423.

Gengozian, N. (1959). J. Immunol. 83, 173–183.

Gengozian, N., and Doria, G. (1964). J. Immunol. 93, 426–432.

Gengozian, N., Makinodan, T., and Carter, R. R. (1962). J. Immunol. 88, 426–433.

Ghetie, V. (1967). Immunochemistry 4, 467–473.

Ghosh, S. N., and Mukerjee, S. (1961). Ann. Biochem. Exp. Med. 21, 183–190.

Gibb, B., Becker, I., Zahn, I., and Scheibe, E. (1968). Z. Immuns-forsch. 134, 417–423.

Gijsels, H. (1963). Gerfaut 54, 16–28.

Gilder, R. S. (1963). Med. Biol. Illus. 13, 231–235.

Gillert, K. E. (1958). Blut 4, 8–13.

Gilman, A. M., Nisonoff, A., and Dray, S. (1964). Immunochemistry 1, 109–120.

Gimpl, F., and Weissfeiler, J. (1962). Acta Microbiol. Hung. 9, 175–181.

Girard, M. L. (1963). Presse Med. 71, 2628–2630.

Gispen, R. (1955). J. Immunol. 74, 134–141.

Gitlin, D., and Boesman, M. (1967). J. Clin. Invest. 46, 1010–1016.

Gitlin, D., Hitzig, W. H., and Janeway, C. A. (1956). J. Clin. Invest. 35, 1199–1204.

Glass, C. B. J. (1967). In "High Resolution Techniques in Electrophoresis—Theory, Methods and Applications" (M. Bier, ed.), pp. 311–377. Academic Press, New York.

Glasstone, S. (1950). "The Elements of Physical Chemistry," 695 pp. Van Nostrand–Reinhold, Princeton, New Jersey.

Glenchur, H., Seal, U. S., Zinneman, H. H., and Hall, W. H. (1962). J. Lab. Clin. Med. 59, 220–230.

Glenn, W. G. (1956a). School Aviation Med., USAF, Rep. No. 56-116.

Glenn, W. G. (1956b). *J. Immunol.* **77,** 189–192.

Glenn, W. G. (1958a). School Aviation Med., USAF, Rep. No. 58-133.

Glenn, W. G. (1958b), in "Serological and Biochemical Comparisons of Proteins (W. H. Cole, ed.), pp. 71–91. Rutger Univ. Press, New Brunswick, New Jersey.

Glenn, W. G. (1959a). School Aviation Med., USAF, Rep. No. 58-134.

Glenn, W. G. (1959b). *Aerospace Med.* **30,** 576–579.

Glenn, W. G. (1959c). *Med. Tech. Bull.* **10,** 101–104.

Glenn, W. G. (1960). *Fed. Proc.* **19,** 204.

Glenn, W. G. (1961a). School of Aerospace Med., USAF, Rep. No. 62-1, pp. 1–6, Dec.

Glenn, W. G. (1961b). School of Aerospace Med., USAF, Rep. No. 62-2, pp. 1–7, Dec.

Glenn, W. G. (1961c). School of Aerospace Med., USAF, Rep. No. 62-3, pp. 1–10, Dec.

Glenn, W. G. (1961d). School of Aerospace Med., USAF, Rep. No. 62-4, pp. 1–7, Dec.

Glenn, W. G. (1962a). *J. Immunol.* **88,** 535–539.

Glenn, W. G. (1962b). *J. Immunol.* **88,** 540–544.

Glenn, W. G. (1962c). *J. Immunol.* **88,** 545–550.

Glenn, W. G. (1963). Lectures in Aerospace Medicine, School of Aerospace Med., USAF, Feb., Brooks Air Force Base, Texas.

Glenn, W. G. (1968). *Aeromed. Rev.* 1-68, 1–47.

Glenn, W. G., and Becker, R. E. (1969). *Tex. Rep. Biol. Med.* **27,** 997–1004.

Glenn, W. G., and Garner, A. C. (1956). School Aviation Med., USAF, Rep. No. 56-92.

Glenn, W. G., and Garner, A. C. (1957). *J. Immunol.* **78,** 395–400.

Glenn, W. G., and Marable, I. W. (1957). School Aviation Med., USAF, Rep. No. 58-10.

Glenn, W. G., and Marable, I. W. (1967). *Appl. Microbiol.* **15,** 1505–1506.

Glenn, W. G., Lanchantin, G. F., Mitchell, R. B., and Marable, I. W. (1958a). *Tex. Rep. Biol. Med.* **16,** 320–332.

Glenn, W. G., Lanchantin, G. F., Mitchell, R. B., and Marable, I. W. (1958b). School Aviation Med., USAF, Rep. No. 58-32.

Glenn, W. G., King, A. H., and Marable, I. W. (1959). School Aviation Med., USAF, Rep. No. 59-32.

Glenn, W. G., Prather, W. E., and Jaeger, H. A. (1963). Serological Museum, Bull. No. 29, 2-3. Rutgers Univ., New Brunswick, New Jersey.

Glenn, W. G., Prather, W. E., and Jaeger, H. A. (1965). School Aviation Med., TR-65-1, pp. 1–7, May.

Gleye, M., and Sandor, G. (1965). *Ann. Inst. Pasteur* **109,** 24–29.

Glueck, H. I., and Hong, R. (1965). *J. Clin. Invest.* **44,** 1866–1881.

Glynn, A. A., and Parkman, R. (1964). *Immunology* **7,** 724–729.

Gocke, D. J., and Howe, C. (1970). *J. Immunol.* **104,** 1031–1032.

Godzińska, H. (1966). *Arch. Immunol. Ther. Exp.* **14,** 263–274.

Godzińska, H., Osińska, M., and Slopek, S. (1970). *Arch. Immunol. Ther. Exp.* **18,** 305–314.

Goetinck, P. F., and Pierce, J. G. (1966). *Arch. Biochem. Biophys.* **115,** 277–290.

Göing, H., and Micke, H. (1962). *Z. Immuns-forsch.* **124,** 315–324.

Gold, L. (1964). *Nature (London)* **202,** 889–890.

Gold, P., and Freedman, S. O. (1965a). *J. Exp. Med.* **121,** 439–462.

Gold, P., and Freedman, S. O. (1965b). *J. Exp. Med.* **122,** 467–481.

Gold, R., Rosen, F. S., and Weller, T. H. (1969). *Amer. J. Trop. Med. Hyg.* **18,** 545–552.

Goldfarb, A. R., and Callaghan, O. H. (1961). *Int. Arch. Allergy* **19,** 86–93.

Goldfarb, A. R., Bhattacharya, A. K., and Kaplan, M. (1959). *Int. Arch. Allergy* **15,** 165–171.

Goldin, M., and Glenn, A. (1964a). *J. Clin. Pathol.* **17,** 268–270.

Goldin, M., and Glenn, A. (1964b). *J. Bacteriol.* **87,** 227–228.

Goldin, M., and McMillen, S. (1963). *Amer. Rev. Resp. Dis.* **87,** 592–593.

Goldstein, I. J., and So, L. L. (1965). *Arch. Biochem. Biophys.* **111,** 407–414.

Gombert, J. (1969). *Rev. Fr. Etude. Clin. Biol.* **14,** 921–924.

Gomes da Costa, S. F., Filipe da Silva, J. A., Chaves, F. J. Z. C., and Crespo, E. V. M. (1962). *Clin. Chim. Acta* **7,** 247–254.

Gooding, G. V., Jr. (1966). *Phytopathol. Notes* 1310–1311.

Gooding, G. V., Jr., and Powers, H. R., Jr. (1965). *Phytopathology* **55,** 670–674.

Goodman, H. C., Exum, E. D., and Robbins, J. (1964). *J. Immunol.* **92,** 843–853.

Goodman, J. W. (1963). *Science* **139,** 1292–1293.

Goodman, M. (1962). *Hum. Biol.* **34,** 104–150.

Goodman, M., and Riopelle, A. J. (1963). *Nature (London)* **197,** 259–261.

Goodman, M., Ramsey, D. S., Simpson, W. L., and Brennan, M. J. (1957). *J. Lab. Clin. Med.* **50,** 758–768.

Gordon, A. H., and Eastoe, J. E. (1964). "Practical Chromatographic Techniques," 200 pp. Newnes, London.

Gordon, A. H., Keil, B., and Sebesta, K. (1949). *Nature (London)* **164,** 498.

Goreczky, L. (1959). *Schweiz. Z. Pathol. Bakteriol.* **22,** 500–505.

Gotschlich, E., and Stetson, C. A. (1960). *J. Exp. Med.* **111,** 441–451.

Götz, H., and Scheiffarth, F. (1957). *Z. Immuns.-forsch.* **114,** 72–84.

Goudie, R. B., Anderson, J. R., and Gray, K. G. (1959). *Immunology* **4,** 309–321.

Goudie, R. B., Horne, C. H. W., and Wilkinson, P. C. (1966). *Lancet* **ii,** 1224–1226.

Goullet, Ph. (1964). *Experientia* **20,** 1–3.

Grabar, P. (1954). *Bull. Soc. Chim. Biol.* **36,** 65–77.

Grabar, P. (1955a). *Ann. Acad. Sci. Fennicae Ser. A. II* **60,** 401–405.

Grabar, P. (1955b). *Arch. Sci. Biol. (Bologna)* **39,** 589–592.

Grabar, P. (1955c). *Zentr. Bakteriol., Parasitenk, Atb. I Orig.* **164,** 15–24.

Grabar, P. (1957a). *Bull. Soc. Chim. Biol. Suppl. I* **39,** 3–9.

Grabar, P. (1957b). *Proc. Eur. Brewery Convention* 147–154.

Grabar, P. (1957c). *Ann. N. Y. Acad. Sci.* **69,** 591–607.

Grabar, P. (1958). *Advan. Protein Chem.* **13,** 1–33.

Grabar, P. (1959a). *Methods Biochem. Anal.* **7,** 1–38.

Grabar, P. (1959b). *Ann. Inst. Pasteur* **97,** 613–625.

Grabar, P. (1960). *Triangle* **4,** 185–196.

Grabar, P., and Burtin, P. (1955a). *Bull. Soc. Chim. Biol.* **37,** 797–802.

Grabar, P., and Burtin, P. (1955b). *Presse Med.* **63,** 804–805.

Grabar, P., and Burtin, P. (1959). *Sang.* **4,** 1–6.

Grabar, P., and Courcon, J. (1958). *Bull. Soc. Chim. Biol.* **40,** 1993–2003.

Grabar, P., and Williams, C. A., Jr. (1953). *Biochim. Biophys. Acta* **10,** 193–194.

Grabar, P., and Williams, C. A., Jr. (1955). *Biochim. Biophys. Acta* **17,** 67–74.

Grabar, P., Séligmann, M., and Bernard, J. (1954). *C. R. Acad. Sci. Paris* **239,** 920–922.

Grabar, P., Séligmann, M., and Bernard, J. (1955a). *Ann. Inst. Pasteur* **88**, 548–562.

Grabar, P., Fauvert, R., Burtin, P., and Hartmann, L. (1955b). *C. R. Acad. Sci. Paris* **241**, 262–264.

Grabar, P., Fauvert, R., Burtin, P., and Hartmann, L. (1956a). *Rev. Fr. Etude. Clin. Biol.* **1**, 175–186.

Grabar, P., Nowinski, W. W., and Genereaux, B. D. (1956b). *Nature (London)* **178**, 430.

Grabar, P., Burtin, P., and Séligmann, M. (1958). *Rev. Fr. Etude. Clin. Biol.* **3**, 41–47.

Grabar, P., Benhamou, N., and Daussant, J. (1962a). *Arch. Biochem. Biophys. Suppl.* **1**, 187–199.

Grabar, P., Courcon, J., Barnes, D. W. H., Ford, C. E., and Micklem, H. S. (1962b). *Immunology* **5**, 673–686.

Grabar, P., Courcon, J., and Wostmann, B. S. (1962c). *J. Immunol.* **88**, 679–682.

Grabar, P., Toucas, M., and Bonnefoi, A. (1962d). *Ann. Inst. Pasteur* **103**, 751–762.

Grabar, P., Pisi, E., Courcon, J., and Lespinats, G. (1964). *Ann. Inst. Pasteur* **107**, 749–763.

Grabner, W., Morhard, E., and Berg, G. (1968). *Z. Klin. Chem. Klin. Biochem.* **6**, 478–480.

Graf, L., and Rapport, M. M. (1965). *Int. Arch. Allergy* **28**, 171–177.

Grant, G. H. (1959). *J. Clin. Pathol.* **12**, 510–517.

Grant, G. H., and Everall, P. H. (1965). *J. Clin. Pathol.* **18**, 654–659.

Grant, G. H., and Everall, P. H. (1966). *Protides Biol. Fluids Proc. Colloq.* **14**, 321–326.

Grappel, S. F., Blank, F., and Bishop, C. T. (1967). *J. Bacteriol.* **93**, 1001–1008.

Gräsbeck, R., Simons, K., and Sinkkonen, I. (1963). *Protides Biol. Fluids Proc. Colloq.* **11**, 242–244.

Grasset, E., Pongratz, E., and Brechbuhler, T. (1956). *Ann. Inst. Pasteur* **91**, 162–186.

Grasset, E., Bonifas, V., and Pongratz, E. (1958). *Proc. Soc. Exp. Biol. Med.* **97**, 72–77.

Grasset, N. (1962a). *Ann. Inst. Pasteur* **103**, 911–917.

Grasset, N. (1962b). *Ann. Inst. Pasteur* **103**, 917–920.

Graves, J. H. (1960). *Amer. J. Vet. Res.* **21**, 691–693.

Graves, J. H., Cowan, K. M., and Trautman, R. (1964). *J. Immunol.* **92**, 501–506.

Gray, A. R. (1961). *Immunology* **4**, 253–261.

Gregg, J. H. (1961). *Develop. Biol.* **3**, 757–766.

Greenspan, I., Brown, E. R., and Schwartz, S. O. (1963). *Blood* **21**, 717–728.

Greenwald, J. H., Nelson, R. P., Markowitz, A. S., Grossman, A., Kushner, D. S., and Armstrong, S. H., Jr. (1962). *Clin. Res.* **10**, 216 (Abstract).

Greuter, W., and Bütler, R. (1963). *Vox Sang.* **8**, 308–316.

Grey, H. M. (1967). *J. Immunol.* **98**, 811–819.

Grieble, H. G., Courcon, J., and Grabar, P. (1965). *J. Lab. Clin. Med.* **66**, 216–231.

Griffin, R. M. (1965). *J. Comp. Pathol.* **75**, 223–231.

Griffiths, B. W., Sparkes, B. G., and Greenberg, L. (1965). *Can. J. Biochem.* **43**, 1915–1917.

Groc, W. (1970). *Clin. Chim. Acta* **30**, 365–368.

Grogan, R. G., Taylor, R. H., and Kimble, K. A. (1964). *Phytopathology* **54**, 163–166.

Grossberg, A. L., Chen, C. C., Rendina, L., and Pressman, D. (1962). *J. Immunol.* **88**, 600–603.

Grubb, A. (1970). *Scand. J. Clin. Lab. Invest.* **26**, 249–255.

Grumbach, M. M., and Kaplan, S. L. (1962). In "Ciba Foundation Colloquim on Endrocrinology," Vol. 14, Immunoassay of Hormones, pp. 63–102. Churchill, London.

Grumbach, M. M., Kaplan, S. L., and Solomon, S. (1960). *Nature (London)* **185**, 170–172.

Grunbaum, B. W., Zec, J., and Durrum, E. L. (1963). *Microchem. J.* **7**, 41–53.

Grzybek-Hryncewicz, K., Ładosz, J., Kubis, K., and Ślopek, S. (1964). *Arch. Immunol. Ther. Exp. (Warz)* **12**, 676–682.

Guillon, J. C., Vallée, A., and Renault, L. (1962). *Ann. Inst. Pasteur* **103**, 921–924.

Guillon, J. C., Renault, L., Rafstedt, G., and Perrault, C. (1963). *Rec. Med. Vet.* **134**, 635–640.

Gundersen, W. B. (1959). *Acta Pathol. Microbiol. Scand.* **47**, 65–74.

Gussoni, C. (1962). *Amer. Rev. Resp. Dis.* **85**, 248–257.

Gussoni, C. (1964). *Int. Arch. Allergy* **24**, 1–16.

Habeeb, A. F. S. A. (1963). *Can. J. Microbiol.* **9**, 863–869.

Hackl, H. (1962). *Arch. Hyg. Bakteriol.* **146**, 385–387.

Hadden, D. R., and Prout, T. E. (1964). *Nature (London)* **202**, 1342–1343.

Haferland, W. (1963). *Z. Immuns.-Forsch.* **125**, 464–469.

Halbert, S. P., and Ehrlich, G. (1962). *Invest. Ophthalmol.* **1**, 233–243.

Halick, P., and Seegers, W. H. (1956). *Amer. J. Physiol.* **187**, 103–106.

Hall, C. A., and Finkler, A. E. (1963). *Biochim. Biophys. Acta* **78**, 233–236.

Hallermann, W., and Stürner, K. H. (1963). *Blut* **9**, 185–187.

Halpern, B., Young, J. J., Dolkart, J., Armour, P. D., III, and Dolkart, R. E. (1967). *J. Lab. Clin. Med.* **69**, 467–471.

Halpern, B. N., Binaghi, R., Liacopoulos, P., Parlebas, M., and Jacob, M. (1961). *Bull. Soc. Chim. Biol.* **43**, 1141–1154.

Hamilton, R. I. (1965). *Virology* **26**, 153–154.

Hamilton, R. I., and Ball, E. M. (1966). *Virology* **30**, 661–672.

Hanks, J. H. (1935). *Immunology* **28**, 95–104.

Hannestad, K. (1969). *Ann. N. Y. Acad. Sci.* **168**, Art. 1, 63–75.

Hannouz, M. (1965). *Pathol. Microbiol.* **28**, 139–146.

Hansen, A., and Clausen, J. (1964). *Clin. Chim. Acta* **9**, 370–375.

Hanson, L. Å. (1959). *Int. Arch. Allergy* **14**, 279–290.

Hanson, L. Å. (1962). *Acta Pathol. Microbiol. Scand.* **54**, 328–334.

Hanson, L. Å. (1964). *Int. Arch. Allergy* **25**, 76–82.

Hanson, L. Å., and Johansson, B. (1959a). *Int. Arch. Allergy* **15**, 245–256.

Hanson, L. Å., and Johansson, B. (1959b). *Int. Arch. Allergy* **15**, 257–269.

Hanson, L. Å., and Johansson, B. (1959c). *Experientia* **15**, 377.

Hanson, L. Å., and Johansson, B. G. (1962). *Int. Arch. Allergy* **20**, 65–79.

Hanson, L. Å., and Nillson, L. Å., (1962). *Acta Pathol. Microbiol. Scand.* **56**, 409–414.

Hanson, L. Å., Raunio, V., and Wadsworth, C. (1960). *Experientia* **16**, 327–329.

Hanson, L. Å., Johansson, B. G., and Rymo, L. (1966a). *Clin. Chim. Acta* **14**, 391–398.

Hanon, L. Å., Roos, P., and Rymo, L. (1966b). *Nature (London)* **212**, 948–949.

Hanson, L. Å., Holmgren, J., Jodal, U., and Kaijser, B. (1971). *Clin. Exp. Immunol.* **8**, 573–580.

Hantschel, H., and Bergmann, H. (1965). *Arch. Exp. Veterinärmed.* **19,** 157–163.

Harboe, M., Osterland, C. K., Mannik, M., and Kunkel, H. G. (1962). *J. Exp. Med.* **116,** 719–738.

Hargreave, F. E., Pepys, J., Longbottom, J. L., and Wraith, D. G. (1966). *Lancet* **i,** 445–449.

Harrington, J. C., Fenton, J. W., II, and Pert, J. H. (1971). *Immunochemistry* **8,** 413–421.

Harris, G., and Fairley, G. H. (1962). *Clin. Chim. Acta* **7,** 416–424.

Harris, H., and Robson, E. B. (1963). *Vox Sang.* **8,** 348–355.

Harris, T. N., Harris, S., and Ogburn, C. A. (1955). *Proc. Soc. Exp. Biol. Med.* **90,** 39–45.

Hartley, T. F., Merrill, D. A., and Claman, H. N. (1966). *Arch. Neurol.* **15,** 472–479.

Hartman, R. J. (1947). "Colloid Chemistry," 2nd ed., 572 pp. Houghton, Boston, Massachusetts.

Hartmann, L., and Toilliez, M. (1957). *Rev. Fr. Etude. Clin. Biol.* **2,** 197–199.

Hartmann, L., Burtin, P., Grabar, P., and Fauvert, R. (1956). *C. R. Acad. Sci. Paris* **243,** 1937–1939.

Hartmann, L., Cornet, A., Bignon, J., and Ollier, M. P. (1964). *Arch. Mal. App. Dig. Mal. Nutr.* **53,** 413–426.

Hase, T. (1964). *Clin. Chem.* **10,** 62–68.

Hasenclever, H. F., and Mitchell, W. O. (1964). *J. Immunol.* **93,** 763–771.

Haupt, H., and Heide, K. (1964). *Clin. Chim. Acta* **10,** 555–558.

Haurowitz, F. (1968). "Immunochemistry and the Biosynthesis of Antibodies," 301 pp. Wiley (Interscience), New York.

Havez, R., and Biserte, G. (1959a). *Clin. Chim. Acta* **4,** 334–339.

Havez, R., and Biserte, G. (1959b). *Clin. Chim. Acta* **4,** 694–700.

Havez, R., Bonte, M., and Moschetto, Y. (1965). *Bull. Soc. Chim. Biol.* **47,** 223–238.

Hawkes, J. G., and Lester, R. N. (1968). *Ann. Bot.* **32,** 165–186.

Hawkins, J. D. (1965). *Immunology* **9,** 107–117.

Hay, D. (1962). *Nature (London)* **196,** 995.

Hayashida, T., and Grunbaum, B. W. (1962). *Endocrinology* **71,** 734–739.

Hayward, B. J., and Augustin, R. (1957). *Int. Arch. Allergy* **11,** 192–205.

Hegenauer, J. C., and Nace, G. W. (1965). *Biochim. Biophys. Acta* **111,** 334–336.

Heide, K., Haupt, H., and Schultze, H. E. (1964). *Nature (London)* **201,** 1218–1219.

Heide, V. K. (1961). *Bibl. Haematol.* **12,** 245–259.

Heimer, R., Levin, F. M., Primack, A., Corcos, J. M., and Nosenzo, C. (1962). *J. Immunol.* **89,** 382–390.

Heiner, D. C. (1958). *Pediatrics* **22,** 616–627.

Heiner, D. C. (1959). *Amer. J. Dis. Childhood* **98,** 673–674.

Heiner, D. C., and Kevy, S. V. (1956). *New England J. Med.* **254,** 629–636.

Heiner, D. C., and Rose, B. (1970a). *J. Immunol.* **104,** 691–697.

Heiner, D. C., and Rose, B. (1970b). *J. Allergy* **45,** 30–42.

Heiner, D. C., Sears, J. W., and Kniker, W. T. (1962). *Amer. J. Dis. Childhood* **103,** 634–654.

Heiner, D. C., Hague, G. M., and Rose, B. (1970). *Clin. Exp. Immunol.* **6,** 773–787.

Heitefuss, R., Buchanan-Davidson, D. J., and Stahmann, M. A. (1959). *Arch. Biochem. Biophys.* **85,** 200–208.

Hekman, A., and Rümke, P. (1969). *Fert. Steril.* **20,** 312–323.

Heller, P., Yakulis, V. J., and Zimmerman, H. J. (1959). *Proc. Soc. Exp. Biol. Med.* **101**, 509–513.

Heller, P., Yakulis, V. J., and Josephson, A. M. (1962). *J. Lab. Clin. Med.* **59**, 401–411.

Hellsing, K. (1969). *Biochem. J.* **112**, 483–487.

Hellsing, K., and Laurent, T. C. (1964). *Acta Chem. Scand.* **18**, 1303–1304.

Helms, C. M., and Allen, P. Z. (1970). *Immunochemistry* **7**, 401–412.

Henney, C. S., and Ishizaka, K. (1969). *J. Immunol.* **103**, 56–61.

Henson, J. B. (1964). *Amer. J. Vet. Res.* **25**, 1706–1711.

Herbert, W. J. (1967). *Immunochemistry* **4**, 143–150.

Herbert, W. J. (1968). *Immunology* **14**, 301–318.

Herbeuval, R., Duheille, J., Bellut, F., and Bellut, M. (1964). *C. R. Soc. Biol.* **158**, 890.

Heremans, J. F. (1959). *Clin. Chim. Acta* **4**, 639–646.

Heremans, J., and Vaerman, J. P. (1958). *Clin. Chim. Acta* **3**, 430–434.

Heremans, J. F., Heremans, M. Th., and Schultze, H. E. (1959b). *Clin. Chim. Acta* **4**, 96–102.

Heremans, M. Th., Vaerman, J. P., and Heremans, J. F. (1959a). *Protides Biol. Fluids* **7**, 396–403.

Heremans, J. F., Vaerman, J. P., and Vaerman, C. (1963). *J. Immunol.* **91**, 11–17.

Hermann, G. (1959). *Clin. Chim. Acta* **4**, 116–123.

Hermann, G. (1970). *Progr. Immunobiol. Std.* **4**, 422–425.

Hermann, G., and Miescher, P. A. (1965). *Int. Arch. Allergy* **27**, 346–354.

Hermann, G., Talal, N., De Vaux St. Cyr, C., and Escribano, J. (1963). *J. Immunol.* **90**, 257–264.

Hermans, P. E., McGuckin, W. F., McKenzie, B. F., and Bayrd, E. D. (1960). *Proc. Mayo Clinic* **35**, 792–807.

Herndon, B. L., and Ringle, D. A. (1967). *Nature (London)* **213**, 624–625.

Herrick, H. E., and Lawrence, J. M. (1965). *Anal. Biochem.* **12**, 400–402.

Herrmann, W. P. (1961). *Arch. Klin. Exp. Dermol.* **212**, 452–459.

Herrmann, W. P., and Hermann, G. (1969). *Arch. Klin. Exp. Dermol.* **234**, 100–116.

Hersh, R. T., and Benedict, A. A. (1966). *Biochim. Biophys. Acta* **115**, 242–244.

Heymann, W., Hackel, D. B., and Hunter, J. L. P. (1960). *Fed. Proc.* **19**, 195.

Hill, C. W., Greer, W. E., and Felsenfeld, O. (1967). *Psychosom. Med.* **29**, 279–283.

Hill, R. J. (1968). *Immunochemistry* **5**, 185–202.

Hillemanns, H. G., and Urbaschek, B. (1962). *Z. Immuns.-Forsch.* **123**, 503–521.

Hillyer, G. V. (1969). *Exp. Parasitol.* **25**, 376–381.

Hillyer, G. V., and Frick, L. P. (1967). *Exp. Parasitol.* **20**, 321–325.

Hinsdill, R. D., and Goebel, W. F. (1964). *Ann. Inst. Pasteur* **107**, 54–66.

Hiramoto, R., McGhee, J. R., Hurst, D. C., and Hamlin, N. M. (1971). *Immunochemistry* **8**, 355–365.

Hirata, Y., and Blumenthal, H. T. (1962). *J. Lab. Clin. Med.* **60**, 194–211.

Hirose, S.-I., and Osler, A. G. (1967). *J. Immunol.* **98**, 618–637.

Hirschfeld, J. (1959a). *Acta Pathol. Microbiol. Scand.* **47**, 160–168.

Hirschfeld, J. (1959b). *Acta Pathol. Microbiol. Scand.* **47**, 169–172.

Hirschfeld, J. (1959c). *Acta Pathol. Microbiol. Scand.* **46**, 229–238.

Hirschfeld, J. (1960a). *Nature (London)* **187**, 164–165.

Hirschfeld, J. (1960b). *Acta Pathol. Microbiol. Scand.* **49**, 255–269.

Hirschfeld, J. (1960c). *Nature (London)* **187**, 126–129.

Hirschfeld, J. (1960d). *Sci. Tools* 7, 18–25.

Hirschfeld, J. (1962). *Progr. Allergy* 6, 155–186.

Hirschfeld, J. (1963). *Sci. Tools* 10, 45.

Hirschfeld, J., and Heiken, A. (1963). *Amer. J. Human Genet.* 15, 19–23.

Hirschfeld, J., and Lunell, N. O. (1962). *Nature (London)* 196, 1220.

Hirschfeld, J., and Nilsson, B. A. (1962). *Acta Pathol. Microbiol. Scand.* 56, 471–477.

Hirschfeld, J., and Söderberg, U. (1960). *Experientia* 16, 198–199.

Hirsch-Marie, H., and Burtin, P. (1963). *Rev. Fr. Etude. Clin. Biol.* 8, 145–155.

Hirsch-Marie, H., and Burtin, P. (1964). *Rev. Fr. Etude. Clin. Biol.* 9, 518–520.

Hitzig, W. H. (1961). *Int. Arch. Allergy* 19, 284–311.

Hitzig, W. H., Scheidegger, J. J., Butler, R., Gugler, E., and Hässig, A. (1959). *Helv. Med. Acta* 26, 142–151.

Hjertén, S. (1961). *Biochim. Biophys. Acta* 53, 514–517.

Hjertén, S. (1962). *Biochim. Biophys. Acta* 62, 445–449.

Hochster, R. M., and Cole, S. E. (1967). *Can. J. Microbiol.* 13, 569–572.

Hochwald, G. M., and Thorbecke, G. J. (1962). *Proc. Soc. Exp. Biol. Med.* 109, 91–95.

Hochwald, G. M., Thorbecke, G. J., and Asofsky, R. (1961). *J. Exp. Med.* 114, 459–470.

Hodgins, H. O., Ridgway, G. J., and Utter, F. M. (1965). *Nature (London)* 208, 1106–1107.

Hodgkin, W. E., Giblett, E. R., Levine, H., Bauer, W., and Motulsky, A. G. (1965). *J. Clin. Invest.* 44, 486–493.

Hokama, Y., Coleman, M. K., and Riley, R. F. (1965). *J. Immunol.* 95, 156–161.

Holland, N. H., and Holland, P. (1965). *Nature (London)* 207, 1307–1308.

Holland, N. H., Hong, R., Davis, N. C., and West, C. D. (1962). *J. Pediatr.* 61, 181–195.

Holländer, L. P., Franz, J., and Berde, B. (1966). *Experientia* 22, 325.

Holm, S. E. (1965). *Int. Arch. Allergy* 26, 34–43.

Holme, T., and Edebo, L. (1965). *Acta Pathol. Microbiol. Scand.* 65, 287–294.

Hornung, M., and Arquembourg, R. C. (1965). *J. Immunol.* 94, 307–316.

Horowitz, M. I., Martinez, L., and Murty, V. L. N. (1964). *Biochim. Biophys. Acta* 83, 305–317.

Horsfall, F. L., Jr., and Goodner, K. (1935). *J. Exp. Med.* 62, 485–503.

Howe, C., Avrameas, S., De Vaux St. Cyr, C., Grabar, P., and Lee, L. T. (1963). *J. Immunol.* 91, 683–692.

Howe, C., Lee, L. T., Harboe, A., and Haukenes, G. (1967). *J. Immunol.* 98, 543–557.

Hruby, S., Alvord, E. C., and Shaw, C. M. (1969). *Int. Arch. Allergy* 36, 599–611.

Hsu, K. C., Rifkind, R. A., and Zabriskie, J. B. (1963). *Science* 142, 1471–1473.

Hughes, D. E., and Watson, D. H. (1965). *Nature (London)* 207, 495–497.

Hughes-Jones, N. C. (1963). *Brit. Med. Bull.* 19, 171–177.

Hukuhara, T., and Hashimoto, Y. (1966). *J. Invertebr. Pathol.* 8, 234–239.

Huneeus-Cox, F. (1964). *Science* 143, 1036–1037.

Hunter, A. G. (1969). *J. Reprod. Fert.* 20, 413–418.

Hunter, A. G., and Hafs, H. D. (1964). *J. Reprod. Fert.* 7, 357–365.

Hunter, W. M., and Greenwood, F. C. (1962). *Biochem. J.* 85, 39–40.

Hunter, W. M., and Greenwood, F. C. (1964). *Biochem. J.* 91, 43–56.

Huntley, C. C. (1963). *Pediatrics* 31, 123–129.

Huntley, C. C., and Lyerly, A. (1963). *Pediatrics* 31, 130–133.

Huntley, C. C., and Moreland, A. (1963). *Amer. J. Trop. Med. Hyg.* **12**, 204–208.

Hurlimann, J. (1963). *Helv. Med. Acta* **30**, 126–155.

Hurwitz, E., Fuchs, S., and Sela, M. (1965). *Biochim. Biophys. Acta* **111**, 512–521.

Hutchison, J. G. P. (1962). *J. Clin. Pathol.* **15**, 185–186.

Hyde, R. M., Bennett, A. J., and Garb, S. (1965). *Int. Arch. Allergy* **28**, 271–279.

Hyodo, H., and Uritani, I. (1965). *J. Biochem.* **57**, 161–166.

Hyslop, N. E., Jr., and Stone, S. H. (1969). *J. Immunol.* **102**, 751–762.

Ibrahim, A. N., and Sweet, B. H. (1970). *Proc. Soc. Exp. Biol. Med.* **135**, 23–29.

Innella, F. P., and Redner, W. J. (1965). *Transfusion* **5**, 78–81.

Innella, F., Pansegrau, M. L., and Redner, W. J. (1961). *Amer. J. Clin. Pathol.* **36**, 322–327.

Inoue, T. (1957). *Ann. Tuberc.* **8**, 1–8.

Irunberry, J., and Pilo-Moron, E. (1965a). *Arch. Inst. Pasteur Algerie* **43**, 106–115.

Irunberry, J., and Pilo-Moron, E. (1965b). *Ann. Inst. Pasteur* **108**, 378–383.

Ishizaka, K., Dennis, E. G., and Hornbrook, M. (1964). *J. Allergy* **35**, 143–148.

Ishizaka, K., Ishizaka, T., and Hornbrook, M. M. (1966). *J. Immunol.* **97**, 75–85.

Ishizaka, K., Ishizaka, T., and Hornbrook, M. M. (1967). *J. Immunol.* **98**, 490–501.

Ishizaka, T., Campbell, D. H., and Ishizaka, K. (1960). *Proc. Soc. Exp. Biol. Med.* **103**, 5–9.

Isliker, H. C. (1953). *Ann. N. Y. Acad. Sci.* **57**, 225.

Isliker, H. C. (1957). *Advan. Protein Chem.* **12**, 387–463.

Isojima, S., and Stepus, S. (1959). *Int. Arch. Allergy* **15**, 350–359.

Itagaki, K., and Tsubokura, M. (1963). *Jap. J. Vet. Sci.* **25**, 119–125.

Itakura, K. (1963). *Gann* **54**, 93–104.

Itano, A. (1933). *Ber. Ohara Inst. Landwirt. Forsch. Kurashiki* **6**, 59–72; from *Chem. Abstr.* **28**, 3846 (1934).

Iványi, J., and Valentová, V. (1966). *Folia Biol. (Prague)* **12**, 36–48.

Iványi, J., Valentová, V., and Černý, J. (1966). *Folia Biol. (Prague)* **12**, 157–167.

Iverius, P. H., and Laurent, T. C. (1967). *Biochim. Biophys. Acta* **133**, 371–373.

Jackson, D. S., Sandberg, L. B., and Cleary, E. G. (1966). *Nature (London)* **210**, 195–196.

Jackson, R. (1964). *J. Biol. Photogr. Ass.* **32**, 13–17.

Jacotot, B., Nguyen-Trong, T., and Beaumont, J. L. (1965). *Rev. Fr. Hematol.* **5**, 777–779.

Jacquot-Armand, Y., Boffa, G. A., and Fine, J. M. (1962). *C. R. Acad. Sci. Paris* **255**, 590–592.

Jaffé, W. G., and Hannig, K. (1965). *Arch. Biochem. Biophys.* **109**, 80–91.

James, K., Johnson, G., and Fudenberg, H. H. (1966). *Clin. Chim. Acta* **14**, 207–214.

Jameson, J. E. (1968). *J. Clin. Pathol.* **21**, 376–382.

Jameson, J. E. (1969a). *J. Clin. Pathol.* **22**, 515–518.

Jameson, J. E. (1969b). *J. Clin. Pathol.* **22**, 519–526.

Jenkins, P. A., and Pepys, J. (1965). *Vet. Rec.* **77**, 464–466.

Jennings, R. K. (1953). *J. Immunol.* **70**, 181–186.

Jennings, R. K. (1954a). *J. Bacteriol.* **67**, 559–564.

Jennings, R. K. (1954b). *J. Bacteriol.* **67**, 565–570.

Jennings, R. K. (1956). *J. Immunol.* **77**, 156–164.

Jennings, R. K. (1958). *J. Lab. Clin. Med.* **51**, 152–162.

Jennings, R. K. (1959a). *J. Immunol.* **83**, 237–245.

Jennings, R. K. (1959b). Unpublished papers.

Jennings, R. K. (1959c). Unpublished papers.
Jennings, R. K. (1959d). Unpublished papers.
Jennings, R. K., and Kaplan, M. A. (1962). *Ann. Allergy* **20**, 15–28.
Jennings, R. K., and Malone, F. (1954). *J. Immunol.* **72**, 411–418.
Jennings, R. K., and Malone, F. (1955). *Brit. J. Exp. Pathol.* **36**, 1–7.
Jensen, J., and Hyde, M. O. (1963). *Science* **141**, 45–46.
Jensen, K. (1965). *Scand. J. Clin. Lab. Invest.* **17**, 192–194.
Jensh, R. P., and Brent, R. L. (1969). *Appl. Microbiol.* **18**, 280–281.
Jirka, M., and Masopust, J. (1963). *Biochim. Biophys. Acta* **71**, 217–218.
Jochim, M. M., and Chow, T. L. (1969). *Amer. J. Vet. Res.* **30**, 33–41.
John, V. T. (1965). *Virology* **27**, 121–123.
Johnson, A. E. (1967). *J. Bacteriol.* **93**, 1476–1477.
Johnson, C. M., and Westwood, J. C. N. (1968). *Can. J. Microbiol.* **14**, 53–60.
Johnson, C. M., Westwood, J. C. N., and Beaulieu, M. (1964). *Nature (London)* **204**, 1321–1322.
Johnston, S. L., and Allen, P. Z. (1968). *J. Immunol.* **100**, 942–945.
Jones, D. (1970). *Clin. Chim. Acta* **29**, 551–556.
Jones, J. H., and Marshall, R. J. (1960). *J. Clin. Pathol.* **13**, 532.
Jones, V. E., and Cunliffe, A. C. (1961). *Nature (London)* **192**, 136–138.
Jordan, F. T. W., and Chubb, R. C. (1962). *Res. Vet. Sci.* **3**, 245–255.
Jordan, W. C., and White, W. (1965). *Amer. J. Med. Technol.* **31**, 169–174.
Josephson, A. S. (1964). *Arch. Environ. Health* **8**, 143–146.
Josephson, A. S., and Lockwood, D. W. (1964). *J. Immunol.* **93**, 532–539.
Josephson, A. S., Franklin, E. C., and Ovary, Z. (1962). *J. Clin. Invest.* **41**, 588–593.
Jouannet, M. (1968). *Toxicon* **5**, 191–199.
Jutisz, M., Cummins, T., and Legault-démare, J. (1957). *Biochim. Biophys. Acta* **23**, 173–180.
Kabat, E. A. (1958). *In* "Serological and Biochemical Comparisons of Proteins" (W. H. Cole, ed.), pp. 92–112. Rutgers Univ. Press, New Brunswick, New Jersey.
Kabat, E. A. (1967). *In* "Methods in Immunology and Immunochemistry" (C. A. Williams and M. W. Chase, eds.), Vol. I, pp. 224, 335. Academic Press, New York.
Kabat, E. A. (1968). "Structural Concepts in Immunology and Immunochemistry," 310 pp. Holt, New York.
Kagan, I. G. (1961). *Proc. Helminth. Soc.* **28**, 97–102.
Kagan, I. G. (1963). *J. Parasitol.* **49**, 773–798.
Kagan, I. G., and Norman, L. (1961). *Amer. J. Trop. Med. Hyg.* **10**, 727–734.
Kagan, I. G., Jeska, E. L., and Gentzkow, C. J. (1958). *J. Immunol.* **80**, 400–406.
Kagen, L. J. (1965). *Proc. Soc. Exp. Biol. Med.* **119**, 985–988.
Kaivola, S., Kiistala, U., and Axelson, E. (1962). *Ann. Med. Exp. Biol. Fenn.* **40**, 419–422.
Kalf, G. F., and White, T. G. (1963). *Arch. Biochem. Biophys.* **102**, 39–47.
Kaliss, N. (1969). *Int. Rev. Exp. Pathol.* **8**, 241–276.
Kaminski, M. (1954a). *Bull. Soc. Chim. Biol.* **36**, 279–288.
Kaminski, M. (1954b). *Bull. Soc. Chim. Biol.* **36**, 289–293.
Kaminski, M. (1954c). *Biochim. Biophys. Acta* **13**, 216–223.
Kaminski, M. (1954d). *Bull. Soc. Chim. Biol.* **36**, 79–84.
Kaminski, M. (1955a). *J. Immunol.* **75**, 367–376.
Kaminski, M. (1955b). *Actes Colloq. Diffusion Montpellier* pp. 1–14.

Kaminski, M. (1957a). *Ann. Inst. Pasteur* **93**, 102–122.
Kaminski, M. (1957b). *Ann. Inst. Pasteur* **92**, 802–816.
Kaminski, M. (1957c). *Bull. Soc. Chim. Biol. Suppl. I* **39**, 85–104.
Kaminski, M. (1960). *Ann. Inst. Pasteur* **98**, 51–60.
Kaminski, M. (1962). *Immunology* **5**, 322–332.
Kaminski, M. (1965). *Progr. Allergy* **9**, 79–157.
Kaminski, M. (1966). *Nature (London)* **209**, 723–725.
Kaminski, M., and Durieux, J. (1954). *Bull. Soc. Chim. Biol.* **36**, 1037–1051.
Kaminski, M., and Durieux, J. (1956). *Exp. Cell Res.* **10**, 590–618.
Kaminski, M., and Gajos, E. (1962). *Rev. Fr. Etude. Clin. Biol.* **7**, 959–962.
Kaminski, M., and Gajos, E. (1965). *Bull. Soc. Chim. Biol.* **47**, 829–832.
Kaminski, M., and Ligouzat, B. (1964). *C. R. Acad. Sci. Paris* **258**, 2705–2706.
Kaminski, M., and Meffroy-Biget, A. M. (1961). *C. R. Acad. Sci. Paris* **252**, 1527–1529.
Kaminski, M., and Nouvel, J. (1952). *Bull. Soc. Chim. Biol.* **34**, 11–20.
Kaminski, M., and Ouchterlony, Ö. (1951). *Bull. Soc. Chim. Biol.* **33**, 758–770.
Kaminski, M., and Tanner, C. E. (1959). *Biochim. Biophys. Acta* **33**, 10–21.
Kantor, F. S., and Cole, R. M. (1959). *Proc. Soc. Exp. Biol. Med.* **102**, 146–150.
Kaplan, M. E., Zalusky, R., Remington, J., and Herbert, V. (1963). *J. Clin. Invest.* **42**, 368–382.
Kaplan, M. H., and Svec, K. H. (1964). *J. Exp. Med.* **119**, 651–666.
Kaplan, S. L., and Grumbach, M. M. (1962). *Nature (London)* **196**, 336–338.
Karjala, S. A., and Nakayama, Y. (1959). *Clin. Chim. Acta* **4**, 369–373.
Karlsson, B. W. (1965). *Ark. Zool.* **18**, 33–50.
Karlsson, B. W. (1966). *Acta Pathol. Microbiol. Scand.* **67**, 83–101.
Kasper, C. B., and Deutsch, H. F. (1963). *J. Biol. Chem.* **238**, 2343–2350.
Kasukawa, R., Calkins, E., and Milgrom, F. (1966). *J. Immunol.* **97**, 260–266.
Katsh, S. (1967). *Advan. Obstet. Gynecol.* **1**, 478–483.
Katsh, S., and Matchael, J. (1962). *Nature (London)* **194**, 1186–1187.
Katz, J., Kantor, F. S., and Herskovic, T. (1968a). *Ann. Intern. Med.* **69**, 1149–1153.
Katz, J., Spiro, H. M., and Herskovic, T. (1968b). *New England J. Med.* **278**, 1191–1194.
Kaufman, H. S. (1970). *J. Allergy* **46**, 122–124.
Kawerau, E., and Ott, H. (1961). *Exp. Eye Res.* **1**, 137–144.
Keele, D. K., Remple, J., Bean, J., and Webster, J. (1962). *J. Clin. Endocrinol. Metab.* **22**, 287–299.
Keimowitz, R. I. (1964). *J. Lab. Clin. Med.* **63**, 54–59.
Kelen, A. E., Hathaway, A. E., and McLeod, D. A. (1971). *Can. J. Microbiol.* **17**, 993–1000.
Kelleher, P., and Villee, C. (1962). *Biochim. Biophys. Acta* **59**, 252–254.
Keller, R. (1966). *J. Immunol.* **96**, 96–106.
Kemp, W. G., and Fazekas, L. J. (1966). *Can. J. Bot.* **44**, 1261–1265.
Kenny, J. F., Boesman, M. I., and Michaels, R. H. (1967). *Pediatrics* **39**, 202–213.
Kenrick, K. G. (1969). *Tech. Bull. Regist. Med. Technol.* **39**, 278–280.
Keutel, H. J. (1960). *Klin. Wochenschr.* **38**, 768.
Keutel, H. J. (1964). *Ann. N. Y. Acad. Sci.* **121**, Art. 2, 484–489.
Keutel, H. J., Hermann, G., and Licht, W. (1959). *Clin. Chim. Acta* **4**, 665–673.
Keutel, H. J., Ammons, C. R., Jr., and Boyce, W. H. (1964). *Invest. Urol.* **2**, 22–29.
Keyser, J. (1964). *Anal. Biochem.* **9**, 249–252.
Khramkova, N. I., and Abelev, G. I. (1963). *Neoplasma* **10**, 2, 121–216.

King, E. P., Frobisher, M., Jr., and Parsons, E. I. (1949). *Amer. J. Public Health* **39**, 1314–1320.

King, S., and Meyer, E. (1963). *J. Bacteriol.* **85**, 186–190.

King, T. P., Norman, P. S., and Connell, J. T. (1964). *Biochemistry* **3**, 458–468.

Kirkbride, M. B., and Cohen, S. M. (1934). *Amer. J. Hyg.* **20**, 444–453.

Kirst, R. (1966). *Z. Klin. Chem.* **3**, 134–135.

Kistner, S. (1959). *Acta Chem. Scand.* **13**, 1149–1158.

Kithier, K., Houštěk, J., Masopust, J., and Rádl, J. (1966). *Nature (London)* **212**, 414.

Kjellén, L. (1965). *Immunology* **8**, 557–565.

Kleczkowski, A. (1957). *J. Exp. Microbiol.* **16**, 405–417.

Kleczkowski, A. (1965). *Immunology* **8**, 170–181.

Klein, F., Haines, B. W., Mahlandt, B. G., and Lincoln, R. E. (1963). *J. Immunol.* **91**, 431–437.

Klein, P., and Opferkuch, W. (1963). *Int. Arch. Allergy* **22**, 388–398.

Klinman, N. R., Rockey, J. H., and Karush, F. (1964). *Science* **146**, 401–403.

Klinman, N. R., Rockey, J. H., Frauenberger, G., and Karush, F. (1966). *J. Immunol.* **96**, 587–595.

Klite, P. D. (1965). *J. Lab. Clin. Med.* **66**, 770–787.

Klontz, G. W., Svehag, S. E., and Gorham, J. R. (1962). *Arch. Ges. Virusforsch.* **12**, 259–268.

Klopstock, A., Haas, R., and Rimon, A. (1963). *Fert. Steril.* **14**, 530–534.

Kobayashi, M., Stahmann, M. A., Rankin, J., and Dickie, H. A. (1963). *Proc. Soc. Exp. Biol. Med.* **113**, 472–476.

Koenig, R. (1970). *J. Gen. Virol.* **7**, 257–261.

Kohn, J. (1957). *Nature (London)* **180**, 986–987.

Kohn, J. (1958). *Clin. Chim. Acta* **3**, 450–454.

Kohn, J. (1960). *Protides Biol. Fluids* **8**, 315–318.

Kohn, J. (1961). *Protides Biol. Fluids* **9**, 120–122.

Kohn, J. (1967). *Int. Symp. Immunolog. Methods Biolog. Standardizat. Royaumont 1965; Symp. Ser. Immunobiol. Std.* **4**, 17–24.

Kohn, J. (1970). *Methods Med. Res.* **12**, 243–260.

Kohn, J. (1971). *In* "Methods in Immunology and Immunochemistry" (C. A. Williams and M. W. Chase, eds.), Vol. 3, pp. 273–279. Academic Press, New York.

Kologlu, Y., Wiesel, L. L., Positano, V., and Anderson, G. E. (1963). *Proc. Soc. Exp. Biol. Med.* **112**, 518–523.

Kölsch, E. (1967). *J. Immunol.* **98**, 854–859.

Komárková, A., and Kořínek, J. (1959). *J. Lab. Clin. Med.* **54**, 707–711.

Kořínek, J. (1964). *Folia Biol.* **10**, 45–49.

Kořínek, J., and Paluska, E. (1959). *Z. Immuns.-Forsch.* **117**, 60–69.

Korngold, L. (1956a). *J. Immunol.* **77**, 119–122.

Korngold, L. (1956b). *Fed. Proc.* **15**, 597–598.

Korngold, L. (1957). *Ann. N. Y. Acad. Sci.* **69**, 681–697.

Korngold, L. (1963a). *Int. Arch. Allergy* **23**, 268–280.

Korngold, L. (1963b). *Anal. Biochem.* **6**, 47–53.

Korngold, L., and Lipari, R. (1955a). *Science* **121**, 170–171.

Korngold, L., and Lipari, R. (1955b). *Cancer Res.* **15**, 159–161.

Korngold, L., and Lipari, R. (1956a). *Cancer* **9**, 183–192.

Korngold, L., and Lipari, R. (1956b). *Cancer* **9**, 262–272.

Korngold, L., and Van Leeuwen, G. (1957a). *J. Exp. Med.* **106**, 467–476.
Korngold, L., and Van Leeuwen, G. (1957b). *J. Exp. Med.* **106**, 477–484.
Korngold, L., and Van Leeuwen, G. (1957c). *J. Immunol.* **78**, 172–177.
Korngold, L., and Van Leeuwen, G. (1958). *Fed. Proc.* **17**, 521.
Korngold, L., and Van Leeuwen, G. (1959a). *J. Exp. Med.* **110**, 1–8.
Korngold, L., and Van Leeuwen, G. (1959b). *Int. Arch. Allergy* **15**, 278–290.
Korngold, L., and Van Leeuwen, G. (1961). *Int. Arch. Allergy* **19**, 271–283.
Korngold, L., and Van Leeuwen, G. (1962). *Int. Arch. Allergy* **21**, 99–110.
Korngold, L., Van Leeuwen, G., and Brener, J. L. (1959). *J. Lab. Clin. Med.* **53**, 517–524.
Kovaleva, V. V. (1958). *J. Microbiol. Epidemiol. Immunobiol.* (*U.S.S.R.*) **29**, 129–132.
Kraft, S. C., Rothberg, R. M., and Kriebel, G. W., Jr. (1970). *J. Immunol.* **104**, 528–529.
Krascheninnikow, S., and Jeska, E. L. (1961). *Immunology* **4**, 282–288.
Krauel, K. K., and Ridgway, G. J. (1963). *Int. Arch. Allergy* **23**, 246–253.
Krause, U., and Raunio, V. (1967). *Acta Pathol. Microbiol. Scand.* **71**, 328–332.
Krauss, S., and Sarcione, E. J. (1964). *Biochim. Biophys. Acta* **90**, 301–308.
Kristoffersen, T. (1969). *Acta Pathol. Microbiol. Scand.* **77**, 717–726.
Krogh, H. K. (1970). *Int. Arch. Allergy* **37**, 104–112.
Krøll, J. (1968a). *Scand. J. Clin. Lab. Invest.* **22**, 79–81.
Krøll, J. (1968b). *Scand. J. Clin. Lab. Invest.* **22**, 112–114.
Krøll, J. (1968c). *Scand. J. Clin. Lab. Invest.* **21**, 187–189.
Krøll, J. (1969a). *Scand. J. Clin. Lab. Invest.* **23**, 227–230.
Krøll, J. (1969b). *Scand. J. Clin. Lab. Invest.* **24**, 55–60.
Krøll, J. (1970). *Protides Biol. Fluids* **17**, 529–532.
Krøll, J. (1971). *Protides Biol. Fluids* **18**, 539–541.
Krøll, J., and Thambiah, R. (1970). *Protides Biol. Fluids* **17**, 533–536.
Krøll, J., Jensen, K. A., and Lyngbye, J. (1970). *Methods Clin. Chem.* **1**, 131–139.
Kronman, B. S. (1965). *J. Immunol.* **95**, 13–18.
Kronvall, C., and Williams, R. C., Jr. (1971). *Immunochemistry* **8**, 477–580.
Kruyt, H. R. (1949). "Colloid Science," 753 pp. Elsevier, Amsterdam.
Krywienczyk, J. (1962). *J. Insect Pathol.* **4**, 185–191.
Kubes, V. (1965). *Rev. Col. Médico Gualemala* **16**, 55–70.
Kubo, R. T., and Benedict, A. A. (1969). *J. Immunol.* **103**, 1022–1028.
Kueppers, F., Briscoe, W. A., and Bearn, A. G. (1964). *Science* **146**, 1678–1679.
Kulberg, A. J., Tarkhanova, I. A., and Khramkova, N. I. (1961). *Folia Biol.* **7**, 213–216.
Kulberg, A. Y., and Tarkhanova, I. A. (1961). *J. Hyg. Epidemiol. Microbiol. Immunol.* **5**, 444–453.
Kumar, S., Loken, K. I., Kenyon, A. J., and Lindorfer, R. K. (1962). *J. Exp. Med.* **115**, 1107–1115.
Kunin, C. M., and Tupasi, T. (1970). *Proc. Soc. Exp. Biol. Med.* **133**, 858–861.
Kunkel, H. G., Mannik, M., and Williams, R. C. (1963). *Science* **140**, 1218–1219.
Kunter, E. (1963). *Zentralbl. Bakteriol.* **188**, 190–194.
Kurata, Y., and Okada, S. (1966). *Int. Arch. Allergy* **29**, 495–509.
Kurata, Y., Watanabe, Y., Okada, S., and Fukuyama, Y. (1969). *Int. Arch. Allergy* **35**, 392–401.
Kurnick, N. B. (1955). *Stain Technol.* **30**, 213–230.
Kushner, I., and Kaplan, M. H. (1961). *J. Exp. Med.* **114**, 961–974.

References 473

Kushner, I., Rapp, W., and Burtin, P. (1964). *J. Clin. Invest.* **43**, 1983–1993.
Kwa, H. G., Van Der Bent, E. M., Feltkamp, C. A., Rümke, PH., and Bloemendal, H. (1965). *Biochim. Biophys. Acta* **111**, 447–465.
Kuwert, E., and Niedieck, B. (1965). *Nature (London)* **207**, 991–992.
Lachmann, P. J. (1962). *Immunology* **5**, 687–705.
Lacko, L., Kořínek, J., and Burger, M. (1959). *Clin. Chim. Acta* **4**, 800–806.
Lacour, F., Harel, J., Harel, L., and Hermet, J. (1962a). *C. R. Acad. Sci. Paris* **255**, 1161–1163.
Lacour, F., Harel, J., Harel, L., and Nahon, E. (1962b). *C. R. Acad. Sci. Paris* **255**, 2322–2324.
Lahti, A., Saukkonen, J., Vainio, T., and Allas, Y. (1963a). *Acta Pathol. Microbiol. Scand.* **58**, 517–520.
Lahti, A., Saukkonen, J., Vainio, T., and Allas, Y. (1963b). *Acta Pathol. Microbiol. Scand.* **59**, 124–128.
Lakin, J. D., Patterson, R., and Pruzansky, J. J. (1967). *J. Immunol.* **98**, 745–756.
Lambotte, R. (1963). *C. R. Soc. Biol.* **157**, 1849.
Lambotte, R., and Salmon, J. (1962). *C. R. Soc. Biol.* **156**, 530.
Lamy, M., Frézal, J., Polonovski, J., Druez, G., and Rey, J. (1963). *Pediatrics* **31**, 277–289.
Landay, M. E., Wheat, R. W., Conant, N. F., and Lowe, E. P. (1967). *J. Bacteriol.* **93**, 1–6.
Lang, N. (1955). *Klin. Wochschr.* **33**, 29–30.
Lang, N., and Hoeffgen, B. (1963). *Protides Biol. Fluids* **11**, 377–384.
Lange, C. F., Poulos, A., and Dubin, A. (1966). *Clin. Chim. Acta* **14**, 311–319.
Langlois, C., Shulman, S., and Arbesman, C. E. (1963a). *J. Allergy* **34**, 235–241.
Langlois, C., Shulman, S., and Arbesman, C. E. (1963b). *J. Allergy* **34**, 385–393.
Langlois, C., Shulman, S., and Arbesman, C. E. (1965). *J. Allergy* **36**, 109–120.
Lannigan, R., and McQueen, E. G. (1962). *Brit. J. Exp. Pathol.* **43**, 549–555.
Lapresle, C. (1955). *Ann. Inst. Pasteur* **89**, 654–665.
Lapresle, C. (1959). *Ann. Inst. Pasteur* **97**, 626–635.
Lapresle, C., and Durieux, J. (1957a). *Ann. Inst. Pasteur* **92**, 62–73.
Lapresle, C., and Durieux, J. (1957b). *Bull. Soc. Chim. Biol.* **39**, 833–841.
Lapresle, C., and Durieux, J. (1958). *Ann. Inst. Pasteur* **94**, 38–48.
Lapresle, C., and Grabar, P. (1957). *Rev. Fr. Etude. Clin. Biol.* **2**, 1025–1037.
Lapresle, C., Webb, T., Kaminski, M., and Campagne, M. (1959a). *Bull. Soc. Chim. Biol.* **41**, 695–706.
Lapresle, C., Kaminski, M., and Tanner, C. E. (1959b). *J. Immunol.* **82**, 94–102.
Larkey, B. J., and Belko, J. S. (1959). *Clin. Chem.* **5**, 566–568.
Laron, Z., and Assa, S. (1962a). *Nature (London)* **194**, 491–492.
Laron, Z., and Assa, S. (1962b). *Acta Endocrinol.* **40**, 311–320.
Laron, Z., and Assa, S. (1963). *Nature (London)* **197**, 299–300.
Larson, T. L., and Feinberg, R. (1954). *Science* **120**, 426.
Laterre, E. C., and Heremans, J. F. (1963). *Clin. Chim. Acta* **8**, 220–226.
Laudel, A. F., Grunbaum, B. W., and Kirk, P. L. (1962). *Science* **137**, 862–864.
Laufer, H. (1963). *Ann. N. Y. Acad. Sci.* **103**, Art. 2, 1137–1154.
Laurell, C. B. (1965a). *Anal. Biochem.* **10**, 358–361.
Laurell, C. B. (1965b). *Scand. J. Clin. Lab. Invest.* **17**, 271–274.
Laurell, C. B. (1965c). *Scand. J. Clin. Lab. Invest.* **17**, 297–298.
Laurell, C. B. (1966). *Anal. Biochem.* **15**, 45–52.
Laurin, S. (1964). *Union Méd. Can.* **93**, 28–31.

Lawrence, M. (1964). *Amer. J. Med. Technol.* **30**, 209–221.

Lawrence, S. H., and Melnick, P. J. (1961). *Proc. Soc. Exp. Biol. Med.* **107**, 998–1001.

Lawrence, S. H., and Shean, F. C. (1962). *Science* **137**, 227–228.

Lawrence, T. G., Jr., and Williams, R. C., Jr. (1967). *J. Exp. Med.* **125**, 233–248.

Lebedev, A. D., and Tsilinskii, I. I. (1958). *J. Microbiol. Epidemiol. Immunobiol.* (*U.S.S.R.*) **29**, 685–693.

Lederer, M. (1955). "An Introduction to Paper Electrophoresis and Related Methods," 206 pp. Elsevier, Amsterdam.

Lee, K. P., and Olson, C. (1969). *Amer. J. Vet. Res.* **30**, 725–731.

Lee, M. (1965). *Pediatrics* **35**, 247–253.

Leise, E. M., and Evans, C. G. (1965). *Proc. Soc. Exp. Biol. Med.* **120**, 310–313.

Lemcke, R. M. (1965). *J. Gen. Microbiol.* **38**, 91–100.

Leonard, C. G., and Thorne, C. B. (1961). *J. Immunol.* **87**, 175–188.

Leone, C. A. (1964). "International Conference on Taxonomic Biochemistry, Physiology, and Serology," 728 pp. Ronald Press, New York.

Lerner, E. M., II, Bloch, K. J., and Dray, S. (1963). *Proc. Soc. Exp. Biol. Med.* **114**, 270–273.

Leskowitz, S. (1963). *J. Immunol.* **90**, 98–106.

Lester, R. N. (1965). *Ann. Bot. N.S.* **29**, 609–624.

Lester, R. N., Alston, R. E., and Turner, B. L. (1965). *Amer. J. Bot.* **52**, 165–172.

Levitt, J., and Polson, A. (1964). *J. Hyg.* **62**, 239–256.

Levy, G., and Polonovski, J. (1958). *Bull. Soc. Chim. Biol.* **40**, 1293–1298.

Levy, R. I., and Fredrickson, D. S. (1965). *J. Clin. Invest.* **44**, 426–441.

Levy, R. I., Fredrickson, D. S., and Laster, L. (1966). *J. Clin. Invest.* **45**, 531–541.

Libich, M. (1959). *Folia Biol.* **5**, 71–81.

Lichter, E. A. (1964). *Proc. Soc. Exp. Biol. Med.* **116**, 555–557.

Lichter, E. A. (1967). *J. Immunol.* **98**, 139–142.

Lichter, E. A., and Dray, S. (1964). *J. Immunol.* **92**, 91–99.

Lieberman, P., Ricks, J., Chakrin, L. W., Wardell, J. R., Jr., and Patterson, R. (1970). *Proc. Soc. Exp. Biol. Med.* **135**, 713–716.

Lieberman, R., and Dray, S. (1964). *J. Immunol.* **93**, 584–594.

Lim, S. D., and Fusaro, R. M. (1962). *J. Invest. Dermatol.* **39**, 303–306.

Lim, S. D., and Fusaro, R. M. (1963). *J. Invest. Dermatol.* **40**, 173–176.

Limbosch, J. M., Robyn, Cl., Heuse-Henry, J., and Hubinont, P. O. (1966). *Vox Sang.* **11**, 504–511.

Lind, A. (1959). *Int. Arch. Allergy* **14**, 264–278.

Linscott, W. D. (1963). *Science* **142**, 1170–1172.

Liu, C. T., and McCrory, W. W. (1958). *J. Immunol.* **81**, 492–498.

Liu, C. T., Das, B. R., and Maurer, P. H. (1967). *Immunochemistry* **4**, 1–10.

Liu, P. V. (1961a). *J. Gen. Microbiol.* **24**, 145–153.

Liu, P. V. (1961b). *J. Bacteriol.* **81**, 28–35.

Liu, P. V. (1961c). *Amer. J. Clin. Pathol.* **36**, 471–473

Loewi, G, and Muir, H. (1965). *Immunology* **9**, 119–127.

Löfkvist, T., and Sjöquist, J. (1962). *Acta Pathol. Microbiol. Scand.* **56**, 295–304.

Löfkvist, T., and Sjöquist, J. (1963). *Int. Arch. Allergy* **23**, 289–305.

Lohss, F., and Kallee, E. (1959). *Clin. Chim. Acta* **4**, 127–133.

Lomanto, B., and Vergani, C. (1967). *Clin. Chim. Acta* **15**, 169–171.

Long, C. F., and Silverman, P. H. (1965). *J. Econ. Entomol.* **58**, 1070–1074.

Long, K. R., and Top, F. H. (1964). *Amer. Rev. Resp. Dis.* **89**, 49–54.

Long, P. L., and Pierce, A. E. (1963). *Nature (London)* **200**, 426–427.

Longbottom, J. L., and Pepys, J. (1964). *J. Pathol. Bacteriol.* **88**, 141–151.

Longbottom, J. L., Pepys, J., and Clive, F. T. (1964). *Lancet* **i**, 588–589.

Longsworth, L. G. (1967). *In* "High Resolution Techniques in Electrophoresis—Theory, Methods and Applications" (M. Bier, ed.), pp. xv–xviii. Academic Press, New York.

Loriewicz, Z., Huianicka, E., and Weinrauder, H. (1957). *Acta Microbiol. Polon.* **6**, 311–320.

Losnegard, N., and Oeding, P. (1963). *Acta Pathol. Microbiol. Scand.* **58**, 493–500.

Louis-Ferdinand, R., and Blatt, W. F. (1967). *Clin. Chim. Acta* **16**, 259–266.

Lueker, D. C., and Crowle, A. J. (1963). *Int. Arch. Allergy* **23**, 65–80.

Lundbeck, H., and Tirunarayanan, M. O. (1970). *Progr. Immunobiol. Std.* **4**, 417–421.

Lunde, M. N., and Diamond, L. S. (1969). *Amer. J. Trop. Med. Hyg.* **18**, 1–6.

Luz, A. Q., and Todd, R. H. (1964). *Amer. J. Dis. Childhood* **108**, 479–486.

Lyster, R. L. J., Jenness, R., Phillips, N. I., and Sloan, R. E. (1966). *Comp. Biochem. Physiol.* **17**, 967–971.

Macheboeuf, M., Rebeyrotte, P., Dubert, J., and Brunerie, M. (1953). *Bull. Soc. Chim. Biol.* **35**, 334–345.

Mackiewicz, S., and Fenrych, W. (1961). *Amer. Rheum. Dis.* **20**, 265–273.

Mackler, B., Erickson, R. J., Davis, S. D., Mehl, T. D., Sharp, C., Wedgweed, R. J., Palmer, G., King, T. E. (1968). *Arch. Biochem. Biophys.* **125**, 40–45.

MacPherson, C. F. C. (1962). *Can. J. Biochem. Physiol.* **40**, 1811–1818.

MacPherson, C. F. C., and Cosgrove, J. B. R. (1961). *Can. J. Biochem. Physiol.* **39**, 1567–1574.

MacPherson, C. F. C., and Saffran, M. (1965). *J. Immunol.* **95**, 629–634.

Macy, N. E., O'Sullivan, M. B., and Gleich, G. J. (1968). *Proc. Soc. Exp. Biol. Med.* **128**, 1098–1102.

Maddison, S. E. (1965). *Exp. Parasitol.* **16**, 224–235.

Madoff, M. A., and Weinstein, L. (1962). *J. Bacteriol.* **83**, 914–918.

Maegraith, B. G. (1933). *Brit. J. Exp. Pathol.* **14**, 227–235.

Maegraith, B. G., and Adelaide, M. B. (1934). *Lancet* **i**, 17–19.

Mage, M. G., and Harrison, E. T. (1966). *Arch. Biochem. Biophys.* **113**, 709–717.

Makinodan, T., Gengozian, H., and Canning, R. E. (1959). *Science* **130**, 1419.

Makonkawkeyoon, S., and Haque, R. U. (1970). *Anal. Biochem.* **36**, 422–427.

Malkiel, S., and Hargis, B. J. (1962). *J. Allergy* **33**, 494–497.

Malley, A., Campbell, D. H., and Heimlich, E. M. (1964). *J. Immunol.* **93**, 420–425.

Mancini, G., Carbonara, A. O., and Heremans, J. F. (1965). *Immunochemistry* **2**, 235–254.

Mancini, G., Nash, D. R., and Heremans, J. F. (1970). *Immunochemistry* **7**, 261–264.

Maniatis, G. M., Steiner, L. A., and Ingram, V. M. (1969). *Science* **165**, 67–69.

Mankiewicz, E. (1958). *Can. J. Microbiol.* **4**, 565–570.

Mannik, M. (1967). *J. Immunol.* **99**, 899–906.

Mannik, M., and Kunkel, H. G. (1962). *J. Exp. Med.* **116**, 859–877.

Mannik, M., and Kunkel, H. G. (1963). *J. Exp. Med.* **117**, 213–230.

Mansa, B. (1962). *Acta Pathol. Microbiol. Scand.* **55**, 250–254.

Mansa, B., and Kjems, E. (1965). *Acta Pathol. Microbiol. Scand.* **65**, 303–310.

Mansi, W. (1958). *Nature (London)* **181**, 1289–1290.

Manski, W. (1969). "On the Biological Basis of Organ-Specific Cross-Reactions of

Tissue Antigens." *Int. Convoc. Immunol. Buffalo, New York* pp. 19–26. Karger, Basel.

Manski, W., Auerbach, T. P., and Halbert, S. P. (1960). *Amer. J. Ophthalmol.* **50**, 985–990.

Manski, W. J., Halbert, S. P., and Auerbach, T. P. (1961). *Arch. Biochem. Biophys.* **92**, 512–524.

Mäntyjärvi, R. (1965). *Acta Pathol. Microbiol. Scand.* **65**, 581–586.

Mäntyjärvi, R., and Arvilomni, H. (1964). *Acta Pathol. Microbiol. Scand.* **61**, 653–654.

Marbrook, J., and Matthews, R. E. F. (1966). *Virology* **28**, 219–228.

Marchal, G., Adida, J., and Fine, J. M. (1964). *Nouv. Rev. Fr. Hematol.* **4**, 365–373.

Mardiney, M. R., Jr., and Müller-Eberhard, H. J. (1965). *J. Immunol.* **94**, 877–882.

Margolis, F., and Feigelson, P. (1964). *Biochim. Biophys. Acta* **90**, 117–125.

Markowitz, A. S. (1963). *J. Bacteriol.* **85**, 495–496.

Markowitz, H. (1964). *J. Bacteriol.* **87**, 232.

Marquardt, J., Holm, S. E., and Lycke, E. (1964). *Proc. Soc. Exp. Biol. Med.* **116**, 112–116.

Marquevielle, J. (1957). "Research on the Role Exercised by Serum Lipids on the Antigen-antibody Precipitation Reaction," 128 pp. Drouillard, Bordeau, France.

Marsh, J., and Whereat, A. F. (1959). *J. Biol. Chem.* **234**, 3196–3200.

Martin, E., Scheidegger, J. J., Grabar, P., and Williams, C. A., Jr. (1954). *Bull. Acad. Suisse Sci. Med.* **10**, 193–198.

Martin du Pan, R., Scheidegger, J. J., Pongratz, E., and Roulet, H. (1955). *Arch. Fr. Pediatr.* **12**, 243–250.

Martin du Pan, R., Wenger, P., Koechli, S., Scheidegger, J. J., and Roux, J. (1959). *Clin. Chim. Acta* **4**, 110–115.

Masseyeff, R. (1960). *Rev. Fr. Etude. Clin. Biol.* **5**, 471–475.

Masseyeff, R., and Josselin, J. (1965). *Bull. Mem. Faculté Pharm. Dakar* **13**, 100–104.

Masseyeff, R. F., and Zisswiller, M. C. (1969). *Anal. Biochem.* **30**, 180–189.

Masseyeff, R., Camerlynck, P., and Hocquet, P. (1960). *C. R. Soc. Biol.* **154**, 1571.

Masseyeff, R., Godet, R., and Gombert, J. (1963). *C. R. Soc. Biol.* **157**, 167.

Masson, P., Heremans, J. F., and Prignot, J. (1964). *Experientia* **21**, 604.

Masson, P. L., Carbonara, A. O., and Heremans, J. F. (1965a). *Biochim. Biophys. Acta* **107**, 485–500.

Masson, P. L., Heremans, J. F., and Prignot, J. (1965b). *Biochim. Biophys. Acta* **111**, 466–478.

Mata, L. J. (1963). *J. Immunol.* **91**, 151–162.

Mata, L. J., and Weller, T. H. (1962). *Proc. Soc. Exp. Biol. Med.* **109**, 705–709.

Mato, M., Aikawa, E., and Kishi, K. (1964). *Exp. Cell Res.* **34**, 427–439.

Mattern, P., Duret, J., and Pautrizel, R. (1963). *C. R. Acad. Sci. Paris* **256**, 820–822.

Mattern, P., Masseyeff, R., and Taufflieb, R. (1966). Personal communication.

Matthews, P. R. J. (1958). *J. Med. Lab. Technol.* **15**, 95–101.

Maurer, P. H. (1962). *J. Immunol.* **88**, 330–338.

Maurer, P. H. (1963a). *Ann. N. Y. Acad. Sci.* **103**, Art. 2, 549–580.

Maurer, P. H. (1963b). *J. Immunol.* **90**, 493–505.

Maurer, P. H., Subrahmanyam, D., Katchalski, E., and Blout, E. R. (1959). *J. Immunol.* **83**, 193–197.

Maurer, P. H., Gerulat, B. F., and Pinchuck, P. (1963a). *J. Immunol.* **90**, 381–387.

Maurer, P. H., Gerulat, B. F., and Pinchuck, P. (1963b). *J. Immunol.* **90**, 388–392.

Maximescu, P., and Saragea, A. (1964). *Microbiol. Parazitol. Epidemiol.* (*Bucur*) **9**, 169–172.

May, J. R., and Rawlins, G. A. (1962). *J. Clin. Pathol.* **15**, 186–188.

McCluskey, R. T., Miller, F., and Benacerraf, B. (1962). *J. Exp. Med.* **115**, 253–273.

McCormick, W. F. (1963). *Amer. J. Clin. Pathol.* **39**, 485–491.

McCracken, G. H., Jr., Chen, T. C., Hardy, J. B., and Tzan, N. (1969). *J. Pediatr.* **74**, 378–382.

McCrone, J. D., and Netzloff, M. L. (1965). *Toxicon* **3**, 107–110.

McCully, K. A., Mok, C. C., and Common, R. H. (1962), *Can. J. Biochem. Physiol.* **40**, 937–952.

McDonald, H. J. (1955). "Ionography," 268 pp. Yearbook Publ., Chicago, Illinois.

McDonald, H. J., and Rebeiro, L. P. (1959). *Clin. Chim. Acta* **4**, 458–459.

McDonald, L. W., and Duhig, J. T. (1965). *Int. Arch. Allergy* **27**, 27–34.

McDuffie, F. C., Kabat, E. A., Allen, P. Z., and Williams, C. A., Jr. (1959). *J. Immunol.* **81**, 48–64.

McFarlin, D. E., Strober, W., Wochner, R. D., and Waldmann, T. A. (1965). *Science* **150**, 1175–1177.

McGhie, J. R., Hurst, D. C., Hamlin, N. M., and Hiramoto, R. N. (1971). *Immunochemistry* **8**, 367–373.

McGregor, I. A., Hall, P. J., Williams, K., and Hardy, C. L. S. (1966). *Nature* (*London*) **210**, 1384–1386.

McIlwain, H. (1938). *Brit. J. Exp. Pathol.* **19**, 411–416.

McIvor, B. C., and Moon, H. D. (1959). *J. Immunol.* **82**, 328–331.

McNeill, D., and Meyer, K. F. (1965). *J. Immunol.* **94**, 778–784.

McPherson, T. A., and Carnegie, P. R. (1968). *J. Lab. Clin. Med.* **72**, 824–831.

McWright, C. G., and Wright, G. L., Jr. (1970). *Bact. Proc.* **91**, M112.

Mead, T. H. (1962). *J. Gen. Microbiol.* **27**, 415–426.

Medgyesi, G., and Koch, Fr. (1964). *Klin. Wochenschr.* **42**, 939–942.

Meffroy-Biget, A. M. (1966). *C. R. Acad. Sci. Paris* **263**, 583–585.

Meffroy-Biget, A. M. (1967a). *C. R. Acad. Sci. Paris* **264**, 1949–1952.

Meffroy-Biget, A. M. (1967b). Personal communication.

Meffroy-Biget, A. M. (1967c). Personal communication.

Meffroy-Biget, A. M. (1967d). *J. Chim. Phys. Phys.-Chim. Biol.* **64**, 899–900.

Meffroy-Biget, A. M. (1968). *J. Chim. Phys. Phys.-Chim. Biol.* **65**, 993–1005.

Mehl, J. W., O'Connell, W., and DeGroot, J. (1964). *Science* **145**, 821–822.

Melartin, L., and Blumberg, B. S. (1966). *Nature* (*London*) **210**, 1340–1341.

Mengoli, H. F., and Watne, A. L. (1966). *Nature* (*London*) **212**, 481–483.

Merétey, K. (1969). *Experientia* **25**, 407–408.

Merrill, D., Hartley, T. F., and Claman, H. N. (1967). *J. Lab. Clin. Med.* **69**, 151–159.

Merrill, D. A., Kohler, P. F., and Singleton, J. W. (1971). *J. Allergy* **47**, 315–320.

Merskey, C., Johnson, A. J., Pert, J. H., and Wohl, H. (1964). *Blood* **24**, 701–715.

Messineo, L. (1964). *Arch. Biochem. Biophys.* **108**, 471–478.

Metianu, T., and Sudi, L. (1969). *Rev. Immunol.* **33**, 323–332.

Metz, C. B., Hinsch, G. W., and Anika, J. L. (1968). *J. Reprod. Fertil.* **17**, 195–198.

Metzgar, R. S. (1964). *J. Immunol.* **93**, 176–182.

Metzger, J. F., and Smith, C. W. (1962). *Proc. Soc. Exp. Biol. Med.* **110**, 903–906.

Meyer, T. S., and Lamberts, B. L. (1965). *Biochim. Biophys. Acta* **107**, 144–145.

Michael, J. G., and Massell, B. F. (1965). *J. Lab. Clin. Med.* **65**, 322–328.

Micheli, A. (1963). *Experientia* **19**, 138–139.

Micheli, A. (1965). *Enzymol. Biol. Clin.* **5**, 175–178.

Micheli, A., and Aebi, H. (1965). *Rev. Fr. Etude. Clin. Biol.* **10**, 431–433.

Micheli, A., and Buzzi, C. (1965). *Biochim. Biophy. Acta* **96**, 533–534.

Middleton, G. K., Jr., Cramblett, H. G., Moffett, H. L., Black, J. P., and Shulen-berger, H. (1964). *J. Bacteriol.* **87**, 1171–1176.

Midgley, A. R., Jr., Pierce, G. B., Jr., and Weigle, W. O. (1961). *Proc. Soc. Exp. Biol. Med.* **108**, 85–89.

Migita, S., and Putnam, F. W. (1963). *J. Exp. Med.* **117**, 81–104.

Milgrom, F., and Loza, U. (1966). *J. Immunol.* **96**, 415–423.

Milgrom, F., and Loza, U. (1967). *J. Immunol.* **98**, 102–109.

Milgrom, F., and Millers, R. (1963). *Vox Sang.* **8**, 537–548.

Milgrom, F., and Witebsky, E. (1962). *Immunology* **5**, 46–66.

Milgrom, F., Tuggac, Z. M., and Witebsky, E. (1963). *Immunology* **6**, 105–118.

Milgrom, F., Campbell, W. A., and Witebsky, E. (1964a). *Proc. Soc. Exp. Biol. Med.* **115**, 165–169.

Milgrom, F., Tuggac, M., Campbell, W. A., and Witebsky, E. (1964b). *J. Immunol.* **92**, 82–90.

Milgrom, F., Tuggac, Z. M., and Witebsky, E. (1964c). *J. Immunol.* **93**, 902–909.

Milgrom, F., Tuggac, Z. M., and Witebsky, E. (1965). *J. Immunol.* **94**, 157–163.

Miller, C. A., and Anderson, A. W. (1971). *Infect. Immun.* **4**, 126–129.

Miller, H. T., and Feeney, R. E. (1964). *Arch. Biochem. Biophys.* **108**, 117–124.

Miller, J. K. (1965). *Immunology* **9**, 521–528.

Miller, R. L., and Heckly, R. J. (1959). *J. Lab. Clin. Med.* **54**, 333–334.

Millman, I., Ziegenfuss, J. F., Jr., Raunio, V., London, W. T., Sutnick, A. I., and Blumberg, B. S. (1970). *Proc. Soc. Exp. Biol. Med.* **133**, 1426–1431.

Minden, P., Reid, R. T., and Farr, R. S. (1966). *J. Immunol.* **96**, 180–187.

Moghissi, K., Neuhaus, O. W., and Stevenson, C. S. (1960). *J. Clin. Invest.* **39**, 1358–1363.

Mohit, B. (1968). *J. Bacteriol.* **96**, 160–164.

Mohos, S. C. (1966). *Brit. J. Exp. Pathol.* **47**, 76–81.

Mok, C. C., and Common, R. H. (1964). *Can. J. Biochem.* **42**, 1119–1131.

Mollaret, P., Delay, J., Burtin, P., and Lemperiere, T. (1956). *Arch. Biol. Med.* **14**, 1–5.

Molnár, K., and Berczi, I. (1965). *Z. Immuns.-Forsch.* **129**, 263–267.

Monier, J. Cl. (1963). *Pathol. Biol.* **11**, 1413–1416.

Moore, J. M. (1961). *J. Clin. Pathol.* **14**, 533–535.

Morard, J. C., Halpern, B. N., and Robert, L. (1963). *C. R. Acad. Sci. Paris* **256**, 1169–1172.

Mori, T. (1953). *Advan. Carbohyd. Chem.* **8**, 315–350.

Morrill, J. B., Norris, E., and Smith, S. D. (1964). *Acta Embryol. Morpholog. Exp.* **7**, 155–166.

Morris, R. S., Spies, J. R., and Coulson, E. J. (1965). *Arch. Biochem. Biophys.* **110**, 300–302.

Morse, J. H. (1968). *Immunology* **14**, 713–724.

Morse, J. H., and Heremans, J. F. (1962). *J. Lab. Clin. Med.* **59**, 891–897.

Morse, S. I. (1963). *J. Exp. Med.* **117**, 19–26.

Morton, J. I., and Deutsch, H. F. (1958). *J. Biol. Chem.* **231**, 1119–1127.

Morton, W., and Dodge, H. J. (1963). *Amer. Rev. Resp. Dis.* **88**, 264–266.

Motet, D. (1964). *Rev. Roum. Biochim.* **1**, 321–325.

Motet, D. (1965). *Rev. Roum. Biochim.* **2**, 37–44.
Moudgal, N. R., and Li, C. H. (1961). *Arch. Biochem. Biophys.* **95**, 93–98.
Moy, P., Sinha, M., Sinha, D., and Furth, J. (1964). *Proc. Soc. Exp. Biol. Med.* **116**, 643–646.
Muckle, T. J. (1964). *Nature (London)* **203**, 773–774.
Mull, J. D., Peters, J. H., and Nichols, R. L. (1970). *Infect. Immun.* **2**, 489–494.
Muller, M., Fontaine, G., Muller, P., and Donazzan, M. (1958a). *Lille Med.* **3**, 218–223.
Muller, M., Fontaine, G., and Muller, P. (1958b). *Lille Med.* **3**, 773–776.
Muller, M., Fontaine, G., and Muller, P. (1959). *Lille Med.* **4**, 150–153.
Muller, W., Klein, N., and Matthes, M. (1958). *Z. Rheumaforsch.* **17**, 226–233.
Müller-Beissenhirtz, W., and Keller, H. (1966). *Clin. Chim. Acta* **13**, 95–99.
Müller-Eberhard, H. J., and Biro, C. E. (1963). *J. Exp. Med.* **118**, 447–466.
Müller-Eberhard, H. J., and Nilsson, U. (1960). *J. Exp. Med.* **111**, 217–234.
Müller-Eberhard, H. J., Nilsson, U., and Aronsson, T. (1960). *J. Exp. Med.* **111**, 201–215.
Munoz, J. (1957). *Proc. Soc. Exp. Biol. Med.* **95**, 757–759.
Munoz, J. (1959). *Anal. Chem.* **31**, 981–985.
Munoz, J., and Becker, E. L. (1950). *J. Immunol.* **65**, 47–58.
Munoz, J., and Becker, E. L. (1952). *J. Immunol.* **68**, 405–412.
Muraschi, T. F., and Tompkins, V. N. (1963). *J. Infect. Dis.* **113**, 151–154.
Muraschi, T. F., Lindsay, M., and Bolles, D. (1965). *J. Infect. Dis.* **115**, 100–104.
Murchio, J. C. (1960). *J. Biol. Photogr. Ass.* **28**, 65–68.
Murphy, F. A., Osebold, J. W., and Aalund, O. (1965). *Arch. Biochem. Biophys.* **112**, 126–136.
Murray, E. S., O'Connor, J. M., and Gaon, J. A. (1965). *J. Immunol.* **94**, 734–740.
Murray, K. (1962). *Biochim. Biophys. Acta* **59**, 211–212.
Murray, R. F., Jr., and Blumberg, B. S. (1965). *Nature (London)* **208**, 357–359.
Murty, D. K., and Hanson, L. E. (1961). *Amer. J. Vet. Res.* **22**, 274–278.
Mutolo, V., and D'Amelio, V. (1962). *Experientia* **18**, 556.
Mutolo, V., D'Amelio, V., and Piazza, E. (1965). *Exp. Cell Res.* **37**, 597–607.
Myers, J., Frei, J. V., Cohen, J. J., Rose, B., and Richter, M. (1966). *Immunology* **11**, 155–162.
Myers, W. L., and Hanson, R. P. (1962). *Amer. J. Vet. Res.* **23**, 896–899.
Nace, G. W. (1963). *Ann. N. Y. Acad. Sci.* **103**, Art. 2, 980–988.
Nace, G. W., and Alley, J. W. (1961). *J. Biol. Photogr. Ass.* **29**, 125–133.
Nace, G. W., Suyama, T., and Smith, N. (1961). *Symp. Germ Cells Develop.* pp. 564–603. Fusi di L. Ripa e Figli., Pavia, Italy.
Nachkov, D., and Nachkova, O. (1959). *Bull. Soc. Chim. Biol.* **41**, 159–171.
Nachman, R. L. (1965). *Blood* **25**, 703–711.
Nagler, A. L., Kochwa, S., and Wasserman, L. R. (1962). *Proc. Soc. Exp. Biol. Med.* **111**, 746–749.
Nagy, L. K. (1967). *Immunology* **12**, 463–474.
Nakamura, S. (1966). "Cross Electrophoresis—its Principle and Applications," 194 pp. Elsevier, New York.
Nakamura, S., Hosoda, T., and Ueta, T. (1959a). *Proc. Jap. Acad.* **34**, 742–746.
Nakamura, S., Takeo, K., Katuno, A., and Tominaga, S. (1959b). *Clin. Chim. Acta* **4**, 893–900.
Nakane, P. K., and Pierce, G. B., Jr. (1967). *J. Cell Biol.* **33**, 307–318.
Nariuchi, H., Usui, M., and Matuhasi, T. (1970). *Jap. J. Exp. Med.* **40**, 15–22.

Nash, D. R., and Heremans, J. F. (1969). *Immunology* 17, 685–694.

Nash, D. R., and Schwab, J. H. (1968). *J. Immunol.* 100, 252–258.

Nash, D. R., Crabbé, P. A., Bazin, H., Eyssen, H., and Heremans, J. F. (1969). *Experientia* 25, 1094–1096.

Nash, D. R., Scolari, L., and Heremans, J. F. (1970). *Immunochemistry* 7, 265–274.

Nasz, I., Cserba, I., and Rozsa, K. (1967). *Z. Immuns.-Forsch.* 134, 225–234.

Navalkar, R. G., Norlin, M., and Ouchterlony, Ö. (1964). *Int. Arch. Allergy* 25, 105–113.

Naylor, G. R. E., and Adair, M. E. (1962). *Nature (London)* 194, 838–840.

Nedjalkov, St., and Yomtov, M. (1965). *Z. Immuns.-Forsch.* 128, 105–116.

Neff, J. C., and Becker, E. L. (1956). Walter Reed Army Inst. Res. Rep. 147–56, 12 pp.

Neff, J. C., and Becker, E. L. (1957a). *Fed. Proc.* 16, 427.

Neff, J. C., and Becker, E. L. (1957b). *J. Immunol.* 78, 5–10.

Nelken, D., and Nelken, E. (1962). *Immunology* 5, 595–602.

Nelson, T. L., Stroup, G., and Weddell, R. (1964). *Amer. J. Clin. Pathol.* 42, 237–244.

Németh, I. (1964). *Zentralbl. Bakteriol.* 192, 126–132.

Nerstrøm, B. (1963a). *Acta Genet.* 13, 30–43.

Nerstrøm, B. (1963b). *Acta Pathol. Microbiol. Scand.* 57, 495–496.

Nerstrøm, B. (1964). *Acta Pathol. Microbiol. Scand.* 60, 540–548.

Nerstrøm, B., and Jensen, J. S. (1963). *Acta Pathol. Microbiol. Scand.* 58, 257–263.

Nerstrøm, B., Mansa, B., and Frederiksen, W. (1964). *Acta Pathol. Microbiol. Scand.* 61, 474–482.

Neuzil, E., and Masseyeff, R. (1958). *C. R. Soc. Biol.* 152, 599.

Neuzil, E., and Masseyeff, R. (1959). *Bull. Soc. Med. Afr. Noire Langue Fr.* 4, 111–138.

Neuzil, E., Masseyeff, R., Gombert, J., and Tanguy, U. (1963). *Bull. Soc. Chim. Biol.* 45, 1125–1144.

Newton, J. W., and Levine, L. (1959). *Arch. Biochem. Biophys.* 83, 456–471.

Nicoli, J., and Jolibois, C. (1964). *Ann. Inst. Pasteur* 107, 374–383.

Nicoli, J., Jolibois, C., Bordas, J., and Demarchi, J. (1964). *Ann. Inst. Pasteur* 107, 453–457.

Nicolle, M., Cesari, E., and Debains, E. (1920). *Ann. Inst. Pasteur* 34, 596–599.

Niedieck, B. (1967). *Z. Immuns.-Forsch.* 132, 139–146.

Niedieck, B., and Palacois, O. (1965). *Z. Immuns.-Forsch.* 129, 234–243.

Niedieck, B., Kuwert, E., Palacois, O., and Drees, O. (1965). *Ann. N. Y. Acad. Sci.* 122, 266–276.

Nielsen, J. C., Nerstrøm, B., and Felbo, M. (1963). *Acta Pathol. Microbiol. Scand.* 58, 264–271.

Nigam, P. C., and Musgrave, A. J. (1964). *Can. J. Zool.* 42, 1041–1048.

Nilsson, L. Å., and Hanson, L. Å. (1962a). *Acta Pathol. Microbiol. Scand.* 54, 335–340.

Nilsson, L. Å., and Hanson, L. Å. (1962b). *Acta Pathol. Microbiol. Scand. Suppl.* 154, 255–257.

Nordenfelt, E., Lindholm, T., and Dahlquist, E. (1970). *Acta Pathol. Microbiol. Scand. Sect. B* 78, 692–700.

Nordin, A. A., Cosenza, H., and Sell, S. (1970). *J. Immunol.* 104, 495–501.

Norkrans, B., and Bertrandsson, K. (1962). *Acta Pathol. Microbiol. Scand.* 55, 255–256.

Norkrans, B., and Wahlström, L. (1962). *Acta Pathol. Microbiol. Scand.* 56, 451–458.

Norman, L., and Kagan, I. G. (1966). *J. Immunol.* 96, 814–821.

Notkins, A. L., Mergenhagen, S. E., Rizzo, A. A., Scheele, C., and Waldmann, T. A. (1966). *J. Exp. Med.* 123, 347–364.

Nussenzweig, V., and Benacerraf, B. (1964). *J. Exp. Med.* 119, 409–423.

Nussenzweig, V., and Benacerraf, B. (1966). *J. Immunol.* 97, 171–176.

Oakley, C. L. (1954). *Disc. Faraday Soc.* 18, 358–364.

Oakley, C. L., and Fulthorpe, A. J. (1953). *J. Pathol. Bacteriol.* 65, 49–60.

O'Connor, G. R. (1957). *A. M. A. Arch. Ophthol.* 57, 52–57.

Oeding, P., and Haukenes, G. (1963). *Acta Pathol. Microbiol. Scand.* 57, 438–450.

Oehme, J., and Schwick, G. (1961). *Vox Sang.* 6, 435–450.

Ohi, Y. (1962). *Jap. J. Zool.* 13, 383–393.

Ohlson, M. (1963). *Acta Pathol. Microbiol. Scand.* 57, 494–495.

Okada, T. S. (1965). *Exp. Cell Res.* 39, 591–603.

Okada, T. S., and Sato, A. G. (1963a). *Nature (London)* 197, 1216–1217.

Okada, T. S., and Sato, A. G. (1963b). *Exp. Cell Res.* 31, 251–265.

Okubo, H. (1965). *Proc. 10th Congr. Int. Soc. Blood Transf. Stockholm, 1964,* pp. 62–65. Karger, Basel.

Olins, D. E., and Edelman, G. M. (1962). *J. Exp. Med.* 116, 635–651.

Olitski, A. L., and Berakha, L. (1962). *Pathol. Microbiol.* 25, 859–870.

Olitski, A. L., and Godinger, D. (1962). *Boll. Ist. Serol. Milano* 41, 362–376.

Olitski, A. L., and Godinger, D. (1963). *Boll. Ist. Serol. Milano* 42, 213–232.

Oliver-González, J., and Levine, D. M. (1962). *Amer. J. Trop. Med. Hyg.* 11, 241–244.

Olson, G. B., and Wostmann, B. S. (1964). *Proc. Soc. Exp. Biol. Med.* 116, 914–918.

Omland, T. (1963a). *Acta Pathol. Microbiol. Scand.* 59, 341–356.

Omland, T. (1963b). *Acta Pathol. Microbiol. Scand.* 59, 507–520.

O'Neill, C. H. (1964). *Exp. Cell Res.* 35, 477–496.

Onoue, K., Yagi, Y., Stelos, P., and Pressman, D. (1964). *Science* 146, 404–405.

Orlans, E. (1960). *Immunology* 5, 306–321.

Orlans, E., and Rose, M. E. (1965). *Immunology* 8, 193–205.

Orlans, E., Rose, M. E., and Marrack, J. R. (1961). *Immunology* 4, 262–277.

Orlans, E., Rose, M. E., and Clapp, K. H. (1962). *Immunology* 5, 656–665.

Ornstein, L. (1964). *Ann. N. Y. Acad. Sci.* 121, Art. 2, 321–349.

Osawa, S., and Yabuuchi, E. (1965). *C. R. Soc. Biol.* 159, 275.

Osserman, E. F. (1959). *J. Immunol.* 84, 93–97.

Osserman, E. F., and Lawlor, D. P. (1966). *J. Exp. Med.* 124, 921–952.

Osterland, C. K., and Chaplin, H., Jr. (1966). *J. Immunol.* 96, 842–848.

Osterland, C. K., Miller, E. J., Karakawa, W. W., and Kruase, R. M. (1966). *J. Exp. Med.* 123, 599–614.

Osunkoya, B. O., and Williams, A. I. O. (1971). *Clin. Exp. Immunol.* 8, 205–212.

Otto, R. (1960). *Zentralbl. Bakteriol.* 177, 546–554.

Ouchterlony, Ö. (1948a). *Ark. Kemi Mineral. Geol.* 26B, 1–9.

Ouchterlony, Ö. (1948b). *Acta Pathol. Microbiol. Scand.* 25, 186–191.

Ouchterlony, Ö. (1949a). *Acta Pathol. Microbiol. Scand.* 26, 516–524.

Ouchterlony, Ö. (1949b). *Lancet* i, 346–348.

Ouchterlony, Ö. (1949c). *Acta Pathol. Microbiol. Scand.* 26, 507–515.

Ouchterlony, Ö. (1949d). *Ark. Kemi* **1**, 43–48.

Ouchterlony, Ö. (1949e). *Ark. Kemi* **1**, 55–59.

Ouchterlony, Ö. (1953). *Acta Pathol. Microbiol. Scand.* **32**, 231–240.

Ouchterlony, Ö. (1958). *Progr. Allergy* **5**, 1–78.

Ouchterlony, Ö. (1959). *Recent Progr. Microbiol.* **7**, 163–169.

Ouchterlony, Ö. (1962). *Progr. Allergy* **6**, 30–154.

Ouchterlony, Ö. (1968). "Handbook of Immunodiffusion and Immunoelectrophoresis," 215 pp. Ann Arbor Sci. Publ., Ann Arbor, Michigan.

Ouchterlony, Ö., Ericsson, H., and Neumuller, C. (1950). *Acta Med. Scand.* **138**, 76–79.

Oudin, J. (1946). *C. R. Acad. Sci. Paris* **222**, 115–116.

Oudin, J. (1947). *Bull. Soc. Chim. Biol.* **29**, 140–148.

Oudin, J. (1948a). *Ann. Inst. Pasteur* **75**, 30–51.

Oudin, J. (1948b). *Ann. Inst. Pasteur* **75**, 109–129.

Oudin, J. (1949). *C. R. Acad. Sci. Paris* **228**, 1890–1892.

Oudin, J. (1952). *Methods Med. Res.* **5**, 335–378.

Oudin, J. (1954). *Disc. Faraday Soc.* **18**, 351–357.

Oudin, J. (1955). *Ann. Inst. Pasteur* **89**, 531–555.

Oudin, J. (1956a). *C. R. Acad. Sci. Paris* **242**, 2489–2490.

Oudin, J. (1956b). *C. R. Acad. Sci. Paris* **242**, 2606–2608.

Oudin, J. (1957). *In* "Symposium on Protein Structure" (A. Neuberger, ed.), pp. 298–301. Methuen, London.

Oudin, J. (1958a). *Congr. Int. Microbiol. 7th Stockholm.*

Oudin, J. (1958b). *J. Immunol.* **81**, 376–388.

Oudin, J. (1960a). *C. R. Acad. Sci. Paris* **250**, 770–772.

Oudin, J. (1960b). *J. Immunol.* **84**, 143–151.

Oudin, J. (1961). *Biochem. Biophys. Res. Commun.* **5**, 358–361.

Oudin, J. (1962). *C. R. Acad. Sci. Paris* **254**, 2877–2879.

Oudin, J. (1971). *In* "Methods in Immunology and Immunochemistry" (C. A. Williams and M. W. Chase, eds.), pp. 118–138. Academic Press, New York.

Ozaki, M., Higashi, Y., Saito, H., An, T., and Amano, T. (1966). *Biken J.* **9**, 201–213.

Ozato, K., and Okada, T. S. (1963). *Nature (London)* **197**, 1310–1311.

Ozerol, N. H., and Silverman, P. H. (1969). *J. Parasitol.* **55**, 79–87.

Page, C. O., Jr., and Remington, J. S. (1967). *J. Lab. Clin. Med.* **69**, 634–650.

Palmer, E. L., Martin, M. L., Hierholzer, J. C., and Ziegler, D. W. (1971). *Appl. Microbiol.* **21**, 903–906.

Paluska, E. (1963). *Z. Immuns.-Forsch.* **125**, 381–394.

Paluska, E., and Kořínek, J. (1960). *Z. Immuns.-Forsch.* **119**, 244–257.

Pandey, R., and Pathak, R. C. (1966). *Indian J. Exp. Biol.* **4**, 20–22.

Paniker, C. K. J., and Kalra, S. L. (1962). *Indian J. Med. Res.* **50**, 686–689.

Papaconstantinou, J., Resnik, R. A., and Saito, E. (1962). *Biochim. Biophys. Acta* **60**, 205–216.

Papermaster, B. W., Condie, R. M., and Good, R. A. (1962). *Nature (London)* **196**, 355–357.

Pappagianis, D., Lindsey, N. J., Smith, C. E., and Saito, M. T. (1965). *Proc. Soc. Exp. Biol. Med.* **118**, 118–122.

Parikh, G., and Shechmeister, I. L. (1964). *Virology* **22**, 177–185.

Parikh, G. C., Koike, H., and Shechmeister, I. L. (1965). *Appl. Microbiol.* **13**, 122–123.

Parker, W. C., and Bearn, A. G. (1962). *J. Exp. Med.* **115**, 83–105.

Parks, J. J., Leibowitz, H. M. I., and Maumenee, A. E. (1961). *J. Immunol.* **87**, 199–204.

Parlebas, J., and Robert, L. (1963). *C. R. Acad. Sci. Paris* **256**, 323–325.

Parnas, J. (1963). *Zentralbl. Bakteriol.* **188**, 230–241.

Parnas, J., Burdzy, K., and Cegielka, M. (1961a). *Bull. Acad. Polan. Sci.* **9**, 289–294.

Parnas, J., Burdzy, K., and Cegielka, M. (1961b). *Z. Immuns.-Forsch.* **121**, 383–394.

Parnas, J., Burdzy, K., and Cegielka, M. (1961c). *Bull. Acad. Polan. Sci.* **9**, 295–298.

Parnas, J., Burdzy, K., and Cegielka, M. (1963). *Zentralbl. Veterinarmed.* **10**, 575–588.

Parnes, V. A. (1957). *Bull. Exp. Biol. Med.* **44**, 1408–1412.

Partlett, R. C. (1961). *Amer. Rev. Resp. Dis.* **84**, 589–591.

Pasieka, A. E., Guerin, L. F., and Mitchell, C. A. (1970). *Can. J. Mircobiol.* **16**, 1153–1159.

Pastewka, J. V., Ness, A. T., and Peacock, A. C. (1966). *Clin. Chim. Acta* **14**, 219–226.

Patnode, R. A., Allin, R. C., and Carpenter, R. L. (1966). *Amer. J. Clin. Pathol.* **45**, 398–401.

Patterson, R. (1961). *J. Lab. Clin. Med.* **57**, 657–660.

Patterson, R., Pruzansky, J. J., and Feinberg, S. M. (1962). *J. Allergy* **33**, 236–244.

Patterson, R., Chang, W. W. Y., and Pruzansky, J. J. (1964a). *Immunology* **7**, 150–157.

Patterson, R., Colwell, J. A., Gregor, W. H., and Cary, E. (1964b). *J. Lab. Clin. Med.* **64**, 399–411.

Patterson, R., Pruzansky, J. J., and Janis, B. (1964c). *J. Immunol.* **93**, 51–58.

Patterson, R., Suszko, I. M., and Pruzansky, J. J. (1965a). *Proc. Soc. Exp. Biol. Med.* **118**, 307–311.

Patterson, R., Tennenbaum, J. I., Pruzansky, J. J., and Nelson, V. L. (1965b). *J. Allergy* **36**, 138–146.

Paul, W. E., and Benacerraf, B. (1966). *J. Immunol.* **95**, 1067–1073.

Paul, W. E., Yoshida, T., and Benacerraf, B. (1970). *J. Immunol.* **105**, 314–321.

Peetoom, F., and Kramer, E. (1962). *Vox Sang.* **7**, 298–304.

Peetoom, F., Rose, N., Ruddy, S., Micheli, A., and Grabar, P. (1960). *Ann. Inst. Pasteur* **98**, 252–260.

Peetoom, F., Van Der Hart, M., and Pondman, K. W. (1964). *Vox Sang.* **9**, 85–90.

Pepys, J., and Jenkins, P. A. (1965). *Thorax* **20**, 21–35.

Pepys, J., Riddell, R. W., Citron, K. M., and Clayton, Y. M. (1962). *Thorax* **17**, 366–374.

Pepys, J., Longbottom, J. L., and Jenkins, P. A. (1964). *Amer. Rev. Resp. Dis.* **89**, 842–858.

Pepys, J., Jenkins, P. A., Lachmann, P. J., and Mahon, W. E. (1966). *Clin. Exp. Immunol.* **1**, 377–389.

Perelmutter, L., Lea, D. J., Freedman, S. O., and Sehon, A. H. (1962). *Int. Arch. Allergy* **20**, 355–367.

Perkins, D. L. (1958a). *Biochem. J.* **69**, 35 P.

Perkins, D. J. (1958b). *Biochem. J.* **69**, 45 P.

Perkowska, E. (1963). *Exp. Cell Res.* **32**, 259–271.

Perlmann, P., Couffer-Kaltenbach, J., and Perlmann, H. (1960). *J. Immunol.* **85**, 284–291.

Peterson, R. D. A., and Good, R. A. (1963). *Pediatrics* **31**, 209–221.

Petrie, G. F. (1923). *Brit. J. Exp. Pathol.* **13**, 380–394.

Petrie, G. F., and Steabben, D. (1943). *Brit. Med. J. i*, 377–379.

Petrovský, E., and Slavíková, O. (1970). *Folia Biol. (Prague)* **16**, 77–80.

Pettersson, U., and Höglund, S. (1969). *Virology* **39**, 90–106.

Philipson, L., Killander, J., and Albertsson, P. Å. (1966). *Virology* **28**, 22–34.

Piazzi, S. E. (1969). *Anal. Biochem.* **27**, 281–284.

Picard, J., Heremans, J., and Vandebroek, G. (1962). *Vox Sang.* **7**, 425–448.

Pierce, A. E. (1962). *Biochim. Biophys. Acta* **59**, 149–157.

Pierce, A. E. (1966). *Brit. Vet. J.* **122**, 3–17.

Pierce, A. E., and Feinstein, A. (1965). *Immunology* **8**, 106–123.

Pierce, A. E., Long, P. L., and Horton-Smith, C. (1962). *Immunology* **5**, 129–152.

Pierce, W. A., Jr. (1959). *J. Bacteriol.* **77**, 726–732.

Pike, R. M. (1967). *Bacteriol. Rev.* **31**, 157–174.

Pillot, J., and Dupouey, P. (1964a). *Ann. Inst. Pasteur* **106**, 456–468.

Pillot, J., and Dupouey, P. (1964b). *Ann. Inst. Pasteur* **106**, 617–627.

Pittman, M., Branham, S. E., and Sockrider, E. M. (1938). *Public Health Rep. (U. S.)* **53**, 1400–1408.

Planas, J., and De Castro, S. (1961). *Sangre* **6**, 195–204.

Plescia, O. J. (1967). *In* "Methods in Immunology and Immunochemistry" (C. A. Williams and M. W. Chase, eds.), Vol. I, pp. 175–187. Academic Press, New York.

Plescia, O. J., and Braun, W. (1967). *Advan. Immunol.* **6**, 231–253.

Plescia, O. J., Noval, J. J., Palczuk, N. C., and Braun, W. (1961). *Proc. Soc. Exp. Biol. Med.* **106**, 748–752.

Podliachouk, M., and Kaminski, M. (1964). *Ann. Inst. Pasteur* **106**, 497–501.

Pollock, M. R. (1964). *Immunology* **7**, 707–723.

Polonovski, J., Lévy, G., and Wald, R. (1958). *Bull. Soc. Chim. Biol.* **40**, 1319–1324.

Polonovski, J., Lévy, G., and Wald, R. (1959). *Ann. Inst. Pasteur* **97**, 466–472.

Polson, A. (1958). *Sci. Tools* **5**, 17–20.

Poortmans, J. (1962). *Clin. Chim. Acta* **7**, 334–345.

Pope, C. G. (1966). *Advan. Immunol.* **5**, 209–244.

Pope, C. G., and Stevens, M. F. (1958a). *Brit. J. Exp. Pathol.* **39**, 139–149.

Pope, C. G., and Stevens, M. F. (1958b). *Brit. J. Exp. Pathol.* **39**, 150–157.

Pope, C. G., and Stevens, M. F. (1959). *Brit. J. Exp. Pathol.* **40**, 410–416.

Pope, C. G., Stevens, M. F., Caspary, E. A., and Fenton, E. L. (1951). *Brit. J. Exp. Pathol.* **32**, 246–258.

Porath, J., and Ui, N. (1964). *Biochim. Biophys. Acta* **90**, 324–333.

Porter, D. D., and Dixon, F. J. (1966). *Amer. J. Vet. Res.* **27**, 335–338.

Potter, J. M., and Northey, W. T. (1962). *Amer. J. Trop. Med. Hyg.* **11**, 712–716.

Potter, M., and Kuff, E. L. (1961). *J. Nat. Cancer Inst.* **26**, 1109–1137.

Poulik, M. D. (1952). *Can. J. Med. Sci.* **30**, 417–419.

Poulik, M. D. (1953). *Can. J. Med. Sci.* **31**, 485–492.

Poulik, M. D. (1956). *Nature (London)* **177**, 982–983.

Poulik, M. D. (1959). *J. Immunol.* **82**, 502–515.

Poulik, M. D. (1963a). *Protides Biol. Fluids* **10**, 170–182.

Poulik, M. D. (1963b). *Protides Biol. Fluids* **11**, 385–387.

Poulik, M. D. (1964). *Ann. N. Y. Acad. Sci.* **121**, Art. 2, 470–483.

Poulik, M. D. (1966). *Methods Biochem. Anal.* **14**, 455–495.

Poulik, M. D., and Bearn, A. G. (1962). *Clin. Chim. Acta* **7**, 374–382.

Poulik, M. D., and Poulik, E. (1958). *Nature (London)* **181**, 354–355.

Pournaki, R., Vieuchange, J., and Lépine, P. (1963). *Bull. Acad. Nat. Med. Paris* **147**, 11–20.

Powell, S. J., Maddison, S. E., Wilmot, A. J., and Elsdon-Dew, R. (1965). *Lancet* **ii**, 602–603.

Prager, M. D., and Bearden, J. (1964). *J. Immunol.* **93**, 481–488.

Prager, S. (1956). *J. Chem. Phys.* **25**, 279–283.

Preer, J. R., Jr. (1956). *J. Immunol.* **77**, 52–60.

Preer, J. R., Jr., and Telfer, W. H. (1957). *J. Immunol.* **79**, 288–293.

Press, E. M., and Porter, R. R. (1962). *Biochem. J.* **83**, 172–180.

Pressman, D. (1967). *In* "Methods in Immunology and Immunochemistry" (C. A. Williams and M. W. Chase, eds.), p. 394. Academic Press, New York.

Pressman, D., James, A. W., Yagi, Y., Hiramoto, R., Woernley, D., and Maxwell, W. T. (1957). *Proc. Soc. Exp. Biol. Med.* **96**, 773–777.

Priolisi, A., and Giuffré, L. (1965). *Acta Haematol.* **33**, 210–219.

Přistoupil, T. I., Fričová, V., and Hruba, A. (1967). *J. Chromatogr.* **26**, 127–131.

Proctor, A. G. (1966). *J. Med. Lab. Technol.* **23**, 109–114.

Pruzanski, J. J., and Feinberg, S. M. (1962). *J. Immunol.* **88**, 256–261.

Pun, J. Y., and Lombrozo, L. (1964). *Anal. Biochem.* **9**, 9–20.

Putnam, F. W., Tan, M., Lynn, L. T., Easley, C. W., and Migita, S. (1962). *J. Biol. Chem.* **237**, 717–726.

Quash, G., Dandeu, J. P., Barbu, E., and Panijel, J. (1962). *Ann. Inst. Pasteur* **103**, 3–23.

Quinlivan, W. L. G. (1969). *Fert. Steril.* **20**, 58–66.

Rabaey, M. (1962). *Exp. Eye Res.* **1**, 310–316.

Rabinovitz, M., and Schen, R. J. (1965). *Clin. Chim. Acta* **12**, 474–476.

Rabinovitz, M., Chayen, R., Schen, R. J., and Goldschmidt, L. (1966). *Clin. Chim. Acta* **14**, 270–273.

Rabinowitz, S. B. (1964). *J. Lab. Clin. Med.* **64**, 488–494.

Rachmilewitz, E. A., Izak, G., and Nelken, D. (1963). *Blood* **22**, 566–579.

Radhakrishnamurthy, B., Chapman, K., and Berenson, G. S. (1963). *Biochim. Biophys. Acta* **75**, 276–279.

Radola, B. J. (1960a). *Bull. Acad. Pol. Sci.* **8**, 493–498.

Radola, B. J. (1960b). *Bull. Acad. Pol. Sci.* **8**, 499–503.

Radola, B. J. (1961). *Nature (London)* **191**, 382–383.

Ragetli, H. W. J., and Weintraub, M. (1964). *Science* **144**, 1023–1024.

Ragetli, H. W. J., and Weintraub, M. (1965). *Biochim. Biophys. Acta* **111**, 522–528.

Ragetli, H. W. J., and Weintraub, M. (1966). *Biochim. Biophys. Acta* **112**, 160–167.

Rakhman, E. Z. (1958). *Zh. Microbiol. Epidemiol. Immunobiol.* **29**, 1404–1410.

Ramsey, H. A. (1963). *Anal. Biochem.* **5**, 83–86.

Randall, J. E. (1958). "Elements of Biophysics," 333 pp. Yearbook, Chicago, Illinois.

Rao, S. S., and Munshi, S. R. (1963). *Experientia* **19**, 92.

Rapp, W., Aronson, S. B., Burtin, P., and Grabar, P. (1964). *J. Immunol.* **92**, 579–595.

Rappaport, I., Siegel, A., and Haselkorn, R. (1965). *Virology* **25**, 325–328.

Rapport, M. M. (1967). *In* "Methods in Immunology and Immunochemistry" (C. A. Williams and M. W. Chase, eds.), p. 187. Academic Press, New York.

Rapport, M. M., and Graf, L. (1967). *In* "Methods in Immunology and Immunochemistry" (C. A. Williams and M. W. Chase, eds.), Vol. 1, pp. 187–196. Academic Press, New York.

Rapport, M. M., and Graf, L. (1969). *Progr. Allergy* **13**, 273–331.

Rathbun, W. B., Morrison, M. A., and Fusaro, R. M. (1967). *Exp. Eye Res.* 6, 267–272.

Raunio, V. (1968). *Acta Pathol. Microbiol. Scand., Suppl. 195* 73, 38 pp.

Raunio, V., and Kaarsalo, E. (1962). *Ann. Med. Exp. Biol. Fenn.* 40, 193–197.

Rawson, A. J. (1962). *Clin. Chem.* 8, 310–317.

Rawstron, J. R., and Farthing, C. P. (1962). *J. Clin. Pathol.* 15, 153–155.

Ray, J. G., Jr., and Kadull, P. J. (1964). *Appl. Microbiol.* 12, 349–354.

Ray, J. G., Jr., and Kadull, P. J. (1965). *Appl. Microbiol.* 13, 925–930.

Ray, J. G., Jr., and Shay, D. E. (1965). *Appl. Microbiol.* 13, 297–300.

Raymond, S. (1964). *Ann. N. Y. Acad. Sci.* 121, Art. 2, 350–365.

Raymond, S., and Nakamichi, M. (1962a). *Anal. Biochem.* 3, 23–30.

Raymond, S., and Nakamichi, M. (1962b). *Clin. Chem.* 8, 471–474.

Raymond, S., and Weintraub, L. (1959). *Science* 130, 711.

Raynaud, M., and Relyveld, E. H. (1959). *Ann. Inst. Pasteur* 97, 636–678.

Raynaud, M., Relyveld, E. H., Girard, O., and Corvazier, R. (1959a). *Ann. Inst. Pasteur* 96, 129–139.

Raynaud, M., Turpin, A., Relyveld, E. H., Corvazier, R., and Girard, O. (1959b). *Ann. Inst. Pasteur* 96, 649–658.

Raynaud, M., Iscaki, S., and Mangalo, R. (1965). *Ann. Inst. Pasteur* 109, 525–551.

Read, R. B., Jr., Pritchard, W. L., Bradshaw, J., and Black, L. A. (1965). *J. Dairy Sci.* 48, 411–419.

Rebeyrotte, P., Koutsoukos, A., and Labbé, J. P. (1969). *C. R. Acad. Sci. Paris* 269, 531–534.

Rees, R. J. W., and Tee, R. D. (1962). *Brit. J. Exp. Pathol.* 43, 480–487.

Regamey, R. H., De Barbieri, A., Hennessen, W., and Perkins, F. T. (1970). *Progr. Immunobiol. Std.* 4, 707 pp.

Reimer, C. B., Phillips, D. J., Maddison, S. E., and Shore, S. L. (1970). *J. Lab. Clin. Med.* 76, 949–960.

Reiner, L., and Kopp, M. (1927). *Kolloid-Z.* 42, 335.

Reinskou, T. (1963). *Acta Pathol. Microbiol. Scand.* 59, 526–532.

Reinskou, T. (1964). *Sangre* 9, 337–341.

Reinskou, T. (1966a). *Vox Sang.* 11, 59–69.

Reinskou, T. (1966b). *Vox Sang.* 11, 70–80.

Reising, G., and Kellog, D. S., Jr. (1965). *Proc. Soc. Exp. Biol. Med.* 120, 660–663.

Reisman, R. E., Rose, N. R., and Arbesman, C. E. (1961). *J. Amer. Med. Ass.* 176, 1004–1008.

Rejnek, J. (1964). *Folia Microbiol.* 9, 299–303.

Rejnek, J., and Bednařík, T. (1960). *Clin. Chim. Acta* 5, 250–258.

Relyveld, E. H., and Efraim, S. B. (1959). *Ann. Inst. Pasteur* 97, 697–717.

Relyveld, E. H., and Raynaud, M. (1957). *Ann. Inst. Pasteur* 93, 246–250.

Relyveld, E. H., and Raynaud, M. (1959). *Ann. Inst. Pasteur* 96, 537–547.

Relyveld, E. H., and Raynaud, M. (1963). *C. R. Acad. Sci. (Paris)* 257, 802–804.

Relyveld, E. H., Turpin, A., Laffaille, A., Paris, C., and Raynaud, M. (1954). *Ann. Inst. Pasteur* 87, 301–313.

Relyveld, E. H., Grabar, P., Raynaud, M., and Williams, C. A., Jr. (1956). *Ann. Inst. Pasteur* 90, 688–696.

Relyveld, E. H., Girard, O., Corvazier, R., and Raynaud, M. (1957). *Ann. Inst. Pasteur* 92, 631–641.

Relyveld, E. H., Van Triet, A. J., and Raynaud, M. (1959). *J. Microbiol. Serol.* 25, 369–402.

Remington, J. S., and Finland, M. (1961). *Proc. Soc. Exp. Biol. Med.* 107, 765–770.
Remington, J. S., Merler, E., Lerner, A. M., Gitlin, D., and Finland, M. (1962). *Nature (London)* 194, 407–408.
Ressler, N. (1960a). *Clin. Chim. Acta* 5, 359–365.
Ressler, N. (1960b). *Clin. Chim. Acta* 5, 795–800.
Ressler, N., Kaufman, J. H., and Glas, W. W. (1962). *Clin. Chim. Acta* 7, 365–373.
Revis, G. J. (1968). *Proc. Soc. Exp. Biol. Med.* 128, 1110–1111.
Revis, G. J. (1971). *Proc. Soc. Exp. Biol. Med.* 137, 90–96.
Rhodes, J. M. (1960). *Nature (London)* 187, 793–794.
Rhodes, J. M., and Fjelde, A. (1963). *Acta Pathol. Microbiol. Scand.* 59, 456–464.
Rice, C. E. (1962). *Can. J. Comp. Med. Vet. Sci.* 26, 212–217.
Rich, L. J., and Norcross, N. L. (1969). *Amer. J. Vet. Res.* 30, 1001–1005.
Richards, C. B., and Orlans, E. (1965). *Nature (London)* 205, 92–93.
Richards, W. D., Ellis, E. M., and Wright, H. S. (1966a). *Amer. Rev. Resp. Dis.* 93, 951–952.
Richards, W. D., Ellis, E. M., Wright, H. S., and Van Deusen, R. A. (1966b). *Amer. Rev. Resp. Dis.* 93, 912–918.
Richou, R., Velu, H., and Kourilsky, R. (1959). *Rev. Immunol.* 23, 354–358.
Richter, G. W. (1967). *Exp. Mol. Pathol.* 6, 96–105.
Richter, M., Rose, B., and Sehon, A. H. (1958). *Can. J. Biochem. Physiol.* 36, 1105–1113.
Richter, M., Blumer, H., Cua-Lim, F., and Rose, B. (1962). *Can. J. Biochem. Physiol.* 40, 105–111.
Ridgway, G. J. (1962a). *Fish. Bull.* 63, 205–211.
Ridgway, G. J. (1962b). *Amer. Natur.* 96, 219–224.
Ridgway, G. J., Klontz, G. W., and Matsumoto, C. (1962). Bull. 8, Int. North Pac. Fish, Comm. 1-13.
Rife, U., Milgrom, F., and Shulman, S. (1963). *Blood* 21, 322–334.
Riley, R. F., and Coleman, M. K. (1968). *J. Lab. Clin. Med.* 72, 714–720.
Riley, R. F., Coleman, M. K., and Hokama, Y. (1965). *Clin. Chim. Acta* 11, 530–537.
Ringle, D. A., and Herndon, B. L. (1965). *J. Immunol.* 95, 966–979.
Ristic, M., and Sibinovic, S. (1964). *Amer. J. Vet. Res.* 25, 1519–1526.
Rittner, Ch. (1966). *Z. Immuns.-Forsch.* 130, 229–241.
Robbins, J. B., Mozes, E., Rimon, A., and Sela, M. (1967). *Nature (London)* 213, 1013–1014.
Robbins, J. L., Hill, G. A., Marcus, S., and Carlquist, J. H. (1963). *J. Lab. Clin. Med.* 62, 753–761.
Robbins, K. C., and Summaria, L. (1966). *Immunochemistry* 3, 29–40.
Robbins, K. C., Wu, H., Baram, P., and Mosko, M. M. (1963). *J. Immunol.* 91, 354–361.
Roberson, B. S., and Schwab, J. H. (1960). *Biochim. Biophys. Acta* 44, 436–444.
Robert, B., De Vaux Saint-Cyr, C., Robert, L., and Grabar, P. (1959). *Clin. Chim. Acta* 4, 828–840.
Robert, B., Parlebas, J., and Robert, L. (1963). *C. R. Acad. Sci. Paris* 256, 323–325.
Robertson, M. (1960). *J. Hyg.* 58, 207–213.
Robyn, C. (1965). *Rev. Belge Pathol.* 31, 334–405.
Robyn, D., Limbosch, J. M., and Hubinont, P. O. (1963). *Bull. Fed. Soc. Gynecol. Obstet.* 15, 432–438.

Roche, J., Fine, J. M., Audran, R., and Boffa, G. A. (1965). *C. R. Soc. Biol.* 159, 1521.

Rockey, J. H., Hanson, L. A., Heremans, J. F., and Kunkel, H. G. (1964). *J. Lab. Clin. Med.* 63, 205–212.

Rodkey, L. S., and Freeman, M. J. (1970). *Immunology* 19, 219–224.

Roholt, O. A., and Pressman, D. (1967). *In* "Methods in Immunology and Immunochemistry" (C. A. Williams and M. W. Chase, eds.), Vol. 1, pp. 394–396. Academic Press, New York.

Roitt, I. M., and Doniach, D. (1958a). *Lancet* ii, 1027–1033.

Roitt, I. M., and Doniach, D. (1958b). *In* "Mechanisms of Hypersensitivity," International Symposium, pp. 325–348. Little, Brown, Boston, Massachusetts.

Roitt, I. M., Campbell, P. N., and Doniach, D. (1958). *Biochem. J.* 69, 248–256.

Rolfe, U., and Sinsheimer, R. L. (1965). *J. Immunol.* 94, 18–21.

Romanovský, A. (1964). *Folia Biol. (Prague)* 10, 1–11.

Rondle, C. J. M., and Carman, B. J. (1956). *Experientia* 12, 443–447.

Rose, H. R., and Witebsky, E. (1959). *J. Immunol.* 83, 34–40.

Rose, M. E., and Long, P. L. (1962). *Immunology* 5, 79–92.

Rose, N. R., Reisman, R. E. Witebsky, E., and Arbesman, C. E. (1962). *J. Allergy* 33, 250–258.

Rose, N. R., Bonstein, H. S., Mazow, J. B., Arbesman, C. E., and Witebsky, E. (1965). *J. Immunol.* 94, 741–751.

Rosen, F. S., Charache, P., Pensky, J., and Donaldson, V. (1965). *Science* 148, 957–958.

Roth, J., Glick, S. M., Yalow, R. S., and Berson, S. A. (1964). *J. Clin. Invest.* 43, 1056–1065.

Roulet, D. L. A., Spengler, G. A., Gugler, E., Bütler, R., Ricci, C., Riva, G., and Hässig, A. (1961). *Helv. Med. Acta* 38, 1–148.

Roulet, D. L. A., Spengler, G. A., and Hässig, A. (1962). *Vox Sang.* 7, 281–297.

Rowe, D. S. (1970). *Lancet* i, 760.

Rowe, D. S., and Fahey, J. L. (1965). *J. Exp. Med.* 121, 185–199.

Rowe, J. R., Newcomer, V. D., and Wright, E. T. (1963). *J. Invest. Dermatol.* 41, 225–233.

Rowe, J. R., Landau, J. W., and Newcomer, V. D. (1965). *J. Invest. Dermatol.* 44, 237–245.

Rowen, R. (1963). *Proc. Soc. Exp. Biol. Med.* 114, 183–187.

Ruckerbauer, G. M., Appel, M., Gray, D. P., Bannister, G. L., and Boulanger, P. (1965). *Can. J. Comp. Med. Vet. Sci.* 29, 157–163.

Rudbach, J. A., and Johnson, A. G. (1962). *Proc. Soc. Exp. Biol. Med.* 111, 651–655.

Rüde, E., and Goebel, W. F. (1962). *J. Exp. Med.* 116, 73–100.

Rümke, P., and Breekveldt-Kielich, J. C. (1969). *Vox Sang.* 16, 486–490.

Ruschmann, E., Bayadal, K., and Haas, R. (1962). *Z. Immuns.-Forsch.* 123, 326–340.

Russell, B., Mead, T. H., and Polson, A. (1964). *Biochim. Biophys. Acta* 86, 169–174.

Russell, W. J. (1965). *J. Immunol.* 94, 942–949.

Russell, W. J. (1966). *J. Immunol.* 95, 1142–1146.

Rybak, M. (1959). *Clin. Chim. Acta* 4, 310–312.

Rybak, M., and Petáková, M. (1964). *Z. Immuns.-Forsch.* 127, 151–155.

Rybak, M., Petáková, M., and Simonianova, E. (1963). *Z. Immuns.-Forsch.* 125, 351–357.

Saddi, R., and Von der Decken, A. (1964). *Biochim. Biophys. Acta* **90**, 196–198.
Saint-Blancard, J., Reynier, Ch., Monteil, R., Thiercelin, P. C., and Gesteau, Ph. (1964). *Rev. Fr. Etude. Clin. Biol.* **9**, 524–529.
Salerno, A., Courcon, J., and Grabar, P. (1967). *Ann. Inst. Pasteur* **112**, 38–53.
Salmon, J. (1959). *Clin. Chim. Acta* **4**, 767–775.
Salmon, J. (1960). *Experientia* **16**, 26–27.
Salvaggio, J. E., Arquembourg, P. C., and Sylvester, G. A. (1970). *J. Allergy* **46**, 326–335.
Salvinien, J. (1957). *Bull. Soc. Chim. Biol. Suppl. 1* **39**, 11–44.
Salvinien, J., and Kaminski, M. (1955a). *C. R. Acad. Sci. Paris* **240**, 257–258.
Salvinien, J., and Kaminski, M. (1955b). *C. R. Acad. Sci. Paris* **240**, 377–378.
Samloff, I. M., and Barnett, E. V. (1967). *J. Immunol.* **98**, 558–567.
Sandor, G., and Gleye, M. (1960). *C. R. Soc. Biol.* **154**, 725–727.
Sandor, G., and Korach, S. (1966). *Ann. Inst. Pasteur* **111**, 7–27.
Sandor, G., and Orley, C. (1968). *Ann. Inst. Pasteur* **115**, 803–812.
Sandor, G., and Sandor, M. (1960). *C. R. Acad. Sci. Paris* **250**, 767–769.
Sandor, G., Orley, C., Kraus, W., and Korach, S. (1967). *Ann. Inst. Pasteur* **112**, 747–761.
Saperstein, S., Anderson, D. W., Jr., Goldman, A. S., and Kniker, W. T. (1963). *Pediatrics* **32**, 580–587.
Saravis, C. A., and Bonacker, L. (1970). *Nature (London)* **228**, 61–62.
Sarcione, E. J., and Aungst, C. W. (1962). *Blood* **20**, 156–164.
Sartorelli, A. C., Fischer, D. S., and Downs, W. G. (1966). *J. Immunol.* **96**, 676–682.
Saslaw, S., Carlisle, H. N., and Hinchliffe, V. (1962). *Amer. J. Med. Sci.* **244**, 81–91.
Sassen, A. (1965). *Clin. Chim. Acta* **11**, 288–290.
Sassen, A., Kennes, F., and Maisin, J. R. (1963). *Rev. Fr. Etude. Clin. Biol.* **8**, 366–373.
Savanat, T., and Chaicumpa, W. (1969). *Bull. WHO* **40**, 343–353.
Scanu, A., and Page, I. H. (1959). *J. Exp. Med.* **109**, 239–256.
Scanu, A., Lewis, L. A., and Page, I. H. (1958). *J. Exp. Med.* **108**, 185–196.
Schabinski, G., and Urbach, R. (1963). *Z. Immuns.-Forsch.* **125**, 405–411.
Schaebel, S. (1962). *Acta Pathol. Microbiol. Scand.* **56**, 219–222.
Scheidegger, J. J. (1955). *Int. Arch. Allergy* **7**, 103–110.
Scheidegger, J. J. (1956). *Semaine Hôp.* **32**, 2119–2127.
Scheidegger, J. J. (1957). *Bull. Soc. Chim. Biol. Suppl. 1* **39**, 45–63.
Scheidegger, J. J., and Buzzi, C. (1957). *Rev. Fr. Etude. Clin. Biol.* **2**, 895.
Scheidegger, J. J., and Roulet, H. (1955). *Praxis* **44**, 73–76.
Scheidegger, J. J., Martin, E., and Riotton, G. (1956). *Schweiz. Med. Wochenschr.* **86**, 224–225.
Scheidegger, J. J., Weber, R., and Hassig, A. (1958). *Helv. Med. Acta* **25**, 25–40.
Scheiffarth, F., and Götz, H. (1960). *Int. Arch. Allergy* **16**, 61–92.
Scheiffarth, F., Götz, H., and Soergel, K. (1957a). *Int. Arch. Allergy* **10**, 82–99.
Scheiffarth, F., Berg, G., Götz, H., and Trabulsi, L. R. (1957b). *Int. Arch. Allergy* **10**, 276–284.
Scheiffarth, F., Götz, H., and Soergel, K. (1958a). *Klin. Wochenschr.* **36**, 82–86.
Scheiffarth, F., Frenger, W., and Götz, H. (1958b). *Klin. Wochenschr.* **36**, 367–369.
Scheiffarth, F., Götz, H., and Warnatz, H. (1958c). *Clin. Chim. Acta* **3**, 535–547.
Scheiffarth, F., Götz, H., and Baigger, E. (1963). *Med. Welt* **48**, 2442–2448.
Scheller, S., and Dudziak, Z. (1962). *Arch. Immunol. Ther. Exp.* **10**, 447–458.
Schen, R. J., and Rabinovitz, M. (1966a). *Israel J. Med. Sci.* **2**, 86–87.

Schen, R. J., and Rabinovitz, M. (1966b). *Clin. Chim. Acta* **13**, 537–538.

Schen, R. J., and Rabinovitz, M. (1967a). *Clin. Chim. Acta* **15**, 209–212.

Schen, R. J., and Rabinovitz, M. (1967b). *Clin. Chim. Acta* **15**, 547–549.

Schenberg, S. (1963). *Toxicon* **1**, 67–75.

Schild, G. C., and Pereira, H. G. (1969). *J. Gen. Virol.* **4**, 355–363.

Schmidt, N. J., and Styk, B. (1968). *J. Immunol.* **101**, 210–216.

Schmidt, N. J., Dennis, J., Frommhagen, L. H., and Lennette, E. H. (1963). *J. Immunol.* **90**, 654–662.

Schmidt, N. J., Dennis, J., Lennette, E. H., Ho, H. H., and Shinomoto, T. T. (1965). *J. Immunol.* **95**, 54–69.

Schmidt, W. C. (1957). *J. Immunol.* **78**, 178–184.

Schneider, C. R., and Hertig, M. (1966). *Exp. Parasitol.* **18**, 25–34.

Schneider, R. G., and Arat, F. (1964). *Brit. J. Haematol.* **10**, 15–22.

Schneider, R. G., and Jones, R. T. (1965). *Science* **148**, 240–242.

Schneiderbaur, A., and Rettenbacher, F. (1968). *Wien. Med. Wochenschr.* **11**, 229–235.

Schricker, R. L., and Hanson, L. E. (1963). *Amer. J. Vet. Res.* **24**, 854–860.

Schubert, J. H., Lynch, H. J., Jr., and Ajello, L. (1961). *Amer. Rev. Resp. Dis.* **84**, 845–849.

Schuchardt, L. F., Munoz, J., and Verwey, W. F. (1958). *J. Immunol.* **80**, 237–242.

Schultze, H. E. (1962). *Clin. Chim. Acta* **3**, 24–33.

Schultze, H. E., and Schwick, G. (1959). *Clin. Chim. Acta* **4**, 15–25.

Schultze, H. E., Schönenberger, M., and Schwick, G. (1956). *Biochem. Z.* **328**, 267–284.

Schultze, H. E., Haupt, H., Heide, K., Möschlin, G., Schmidtberger, R., and Schwick, G. (1962a). *Z. Naturforsch.* **17**, 313–322.

Schultze, H. E., Heide, K., and Haupt, H. (1962b). *Klin. Wochenschr.* **15**, 729–732.

Schultze, H. E., Heide, K., and Haupt, H. (1963). *Nature (London)* **200**, 1103.

Schumacher, G. F. B., Strauss, E. K., and Wied, G. L. (1965). *Amer. J. Obst. Gynecol.* **91**, 1035–1049.

Schur, P. H., and Monroe, M. (1969). *Proc. Nat. Acad. Sci.* **63**, 1108–1112.

Schur, P. H., and Sandson, J. (1963). *Arthritis Rheum.* **6**, 115–129.

Schutz, J. N. (1958). *J. Biol. Photo. Ass.* **26**, 159–164.

Schwick, G., and Schultze, H. E. (1959). *Clin. Chim. Acta* **4**, 26–35.

Schwick, G., and Störiko, K. (1964). Laboratoriums Blätter, Behringwerke Ag., May, 1–64.

Searcy, R. L., and Bergquist, L. M. (1965). *Biochim. Biophys. Acta* **106**, 603–615.

Searcy, R. L., Asher, T. M., and Bergquist, L. M. (1962). *Clin. Chim.* **8**, 616–625.

Seed, J. R., and Weinman, D. (1963). *Nature (London)* **198**, 197–198.

Seeliger, H. (1955). *Z. Hyg. Infektionskrankh.* **141**, 110–121.

Seeliger, H. (1956). *J. Invest. Dermatol.* **26**, 81–93.

Seeliger, H. P. R., and Sulzbacher, F. (1956). *Can. J. Microbiol.* **2**, 220–231.

Sela, M. (1966). *Advan. Immunol.* **5**, 30–130.

Sela, M., and Fuchs, S. (1967). In "Methods in Immunology and Immunochemistry" (C. A. Williams and M. W. Chase, eds.), Vol. 1, pp. 167, 185. Academic Press, New York.

Seligmann, M. (1956). *C. R. Acad. Sci. Paris* **243**, 531–534.

Seligmann, M. (1957a). *C. R. Acad. Sci. Paris* **244**, 2192–2194.

Seligmann, M. (1957b). *Vox Sang.* **2**, 270–282.

Seligmann, M. (1958a). *Rev. Fr. Etude. Clin. Biol.* **3**, 558–580.

Seligmann, M. (1958b). *Protides Biol. Fluids* 5, 167–177.

Seligmann, M. (1959). *Proc. 1st Int. Symp. Immunopathol. Basel/Seelisberg, 1958,* pp. 402–415. Benno Schwabe, Basel.

Seligmann, M. (1961). *Colloq. 8th Congr. Eur. Soc. Haematol., Vienna. Methods Immunohaematolog. Res.* pp. 141–169. Karger, Basel.

Seligmann, M., and Grabar, P. (1958). *Rev. Fr. Etude. Clin. Biol.* 3, 1073–1075.

Seligmann, M., and Hanau, C. (1958). *Rev. Hématol.* 13, 239–248.

Seligmann, M., and Marder, V. (1965). *Nouv. Rev. Fr. Hematol.* 5, 345–354.

Seligmann, M., Grabar, P., and Bernard, G. (1955). *Sang* 26, 52–70.

Seligmann, M., Danon, F., and Fine, J. M. (1963). *Proc. Soc. Exp. Biol. Med.* 114, 482–486.

Sell, S. (1964). *J. Immunol.* 93, 122–131.

Sell, S., Park, A. B., and Nordin, A. A. (1970). *J. Immunol.* 104, 483–494.

Sen, A., Ghosh, S. N., Mukerjee, S., and Ray, J. C. (1961). *Nature (London)* 192, 893.

Serre, H., and Jaffiol, C. (1958). *Presse Méd.* 66, 2044–2047.

Sewell, M. M. H. (1964). *Immunology* 7, 671–680.

Sharon, N. (1961). *Pathol. Microbiol.* 24, 1091–1098.

Shay, D. E., and Ray, J. G., Jr. (1965). *Appl. Microbiol.* 13, 305–307.

Sherman, J. D., Adner, M. M., and Dameshek, W. (1963). *Blood* 22, 252–271.

Shivers, C. A. (1965). *Biol. Bull.* 128, 328–336.

Shivers, C. A., and James, J. M. (1967). *Immunology* 13, 547–554.

Shivers, C. A., and Metz, C. B. (1962). *Proc. Soc. Exp. Biol. Med.* 110, 385–387.

Shore, S. L., Phillips, D. J., and Reimer, C. B. (1971). *Immunochemistry* 8, 562–565.

Shulman, S. (1963). *Int. Arch. Allergy* 23, 262–267.

Shulman, S., and Bronson, P. (1969). *J. Reprod. Fert.* 18, 481–491.

Shulman, S., Hubler, L., and Witebsky, E. (1964a). *Science* 145, 815–817.

Shulman, S., Mamrod, L., Gonder, M. J., and Soanes, W. A. (1964b). *J. Immunol.* 93, 474–480.

Shulman, S., Mamrod, L., Lang, R. W., Gonder, M. J., and Soanes, W. A. (1965). *J. Reprod. Fert.* 10, 55–60.

Shulman, S., Bigelsen, F., Lang, R., and Arbesman, C. (1966a). *J. Immunol.* 96, 29–38.

Shulman, S., Lang, R., Beutner, E., and Witebsky, E. (1966b). *Immunology* 10, 289–303.

Sia, R. H. P., and Chung, S. F. (1932). *Proc. Soc. Exp. Biol. Med.* 29, 792–795.

Sibal, L. R., Fink, M. A., McCune, C. L., and Cowles, C. A. (1967). *J. Immunol.* 98, 368–373.

Silverstein, A. M., Feinberg, R., and Flax, M. H. (1958). *Fed. Proc.* 17, 535.

Silverstein, A. M., Thorbecke, G. J., Kraner, K. L., and Lukes, R. J. (1963a). *J. Immunol.* 91, 384–395.

Silverstein, A. M., Uhr, J. W., Kraner, K. L., and Lukes, R. J. (1963b). *J. Exp. Med.* 117, 799–812.

Simons, K., and Gräsbeck, R. (1963). *Clin. Chim. Acta* 8, 425–433.

Sinell, H. J., Untermann, F., and Baumgart, J. (1969). *Zentralbl. Bakteriol. Abt. I., Orig.* 210, 19–31.

Singleton, L., and Ross, G. W. (1964). *Nature (London)* 203, 1173–1174.

Sirek, O. V., and Sirek, A, (1962). *Nature (London)* 196, 1214–1215.

Sirisinha, S., and Allen, P. Z. (1965). *J. Bacteriol.* 90, 1120–1128.

Siskind, G. W. (1966). *J. Immunol.* **96**, 401–408.

Skalba, D. (1964). *Nature (London)* **204**, 894.

Škvaril, F., and Rádl, J. (1967). *Clin. Chim. Acta* **15**, 544–546.

Škvaril, F., Brummelová, V., Fragner, J., and Sindelár, J. (1970). *Progr. Immunobiol. Std.* **4**, 183–187.

Slater, R. J., Ward, S. M., and Kunkel, H. G. (1955). *J. Exp. Med.* **101**, 85–108.

Slaterus, K. W. (1961). *J. Microbiol. Serol.* **27**, 305–315.

Ślopek, S., Ładosz, J., and Crzybek-Hryncewicz, K. (1965a). *Arch. Immunol. Ther. Exp.* **13**, 324–330.

Ślopek, S., Ładosz, J., Hryncewicz, K., and Brzuchowska, W. (1965b). *Arch. Immunol. Ther. Exp.* **13**, 157–160.

Ślopek, S., Ładosz, J., Hryncewicz, K., and Brzuchowska, W. (1966). *Nature (London)* **209**, 1036.

Smibert, R. M., Davis, J. W., and Allen, R. C. (1961). *Amer. J. Vet. Res.* **23**, 460–464.

Smith, D. B. (1967). A Precipitin-Gel Analysis for Host-Parasite Relationships Demonstrated with Culture Systems of Mouse NCTC-2071 Cells and Human NCTC-3075 Cells Parasitized by *Toxoplasma gondii*, 47 pp. A dissertation, Univ. of California, Los Angeles, California.

Smith, D. B. (1968). *Anal. Biochem.* **22**, 543–545.

Smith, D. C., and Murchison, W. (1959). *J. Med. Lab. Technol.* **16**, 197–200.

Smith, D. G., and Shattock, P. M. F. (1962). *J. Gen. Microbiol.* **29**, 731–736.

Smith, D. G., and Shattock, P. M. F. (1964). *J. Gen. Microbiol.* **34**, 165–175.

Smith, E. L., and Jager, B. V. (1952). *Ann. Rev. Microbiol.* **6**, 207–228.

Smith, H., Keppie, J., Pearce, J. H., and Witt, K. (1962a). *Brit. J. Exp. Pathol.* **43**, 538–548.

Smith, H., Tozer, B. T., Gallop, R. C., and Scanes, F. S. (1962b). *Biochem. J.* **84**, 74–80.

Smith, H., Gallop, R. C., and Tozer, B. T. (1964). *Immunology* **7**, 111–117.

Smith, I. (1960). "Chromatographic and Electrophoretic Techniques," pp. 56–90. Wiley (Interscience), New York.

Smith, R. S., Longmire, R. L., Reid, R. T., and Farr, R. S. (1970). *J. Immunol.* **104**, 367–376.

Smith, R. T. (1966). *Pediatrics* **37**, 822–827.

Smithies, O. (1955). *Biochem. J.* **61**, 629–641.

Sonea, S., De Repentigny, J., and Frappier, A. (1962). *Can. J. Microbiol.* **8**, 815–818.

Sonneborn, D. R., Sussman, M., and Levine, L. (1964). *J. Bacteriol.* **87**, 1321–1329.

Sonneborn, D. R., Levine, L., and Sussman, M. (1965). *J. Bacteriol.* **89**, 1092–1096.

Soothill, J. F. (1962). *J. Lab. Clin. Med.* **59**, 859–870.

Soothill, J. F., Blainey, J. D., Neale, F. C., Fischer-Williams, M., and Melnick, S. C. (1961). *J. Clin. Pathol.* **14**, 264–270.

Sorger, G. J., Ford, R. E., and Evans, H. J. (1965). *Proc. Nat. Acad. Sci. U.S.A.* **54**, 1614–1621.

Šourek, J. (1965). *Čs. Epidemiol. Mikrobiol. Immunol.* **14**, 100–105.

Šourek, J., and Raška, K., Jr. (1963). *J. Hyg. Epidemiol. Microbiol. Immunol.* **7**, 46–54.

South, M. A., Cooper, M. D., Wollheim, F. A., Hong, R., and Good, R. A. (1966). *J. Exp. Med.* **123**, 615–627.

Speiser, P. (1964). *Ophthalmologica* **147**, 291–296.

Spiers, J. A., and Augustin, R. (1958). *Trans. Faraday Soc.* **54**, 287–295.

Sprent, J. F. A., Scott, R. S. H., and Timourian, H. (1963). *Nature* (*London*) **200**, 913.

Stahmann, M. A., Tsuyuki, H., Weinke, K., Lapresle, C., and Grabar, P. (1955). *C. R. Acad. Sci. Paris* **241**, 1528–1529.

Stahmann, M. A., Buchanan-Davidson, D. J., Lapresle, C., and Grabar, P. (1959a). *Nature* (*London*) **184**, 549–550.

Stahmann, M. A., Lapresle, C., Buchanan-Davidson, D. J., and Grabar, P. (1959b). *J. Immunol.* **83**, 534–542.

Stallybrass, F. C. (1964). *J. Pathol. Bacteriol.* **87**, 89–97.

Stallybrass, F. C. (1965). *J. Pathol. Bacteriol.* **90**, 205–211.

Steigerwald, H., Spielmann, W., Fries, H., and Grebe, S. F. (1960). *Klin. Wochenschr.* **19**, 973–980.

Stein, A. A., Manlapas, F. C., Soike, K. F., and Patterson, P. R. (1964). *J. Pediatr.* **65**, 495–500.

Steinbuch, M., and Audran, R. (1965). *Transfusion* **8**, 141–163.

Steinbuch, M., and Audran, R. (1969). *Rev. Fr. Etude. Clin. Biol.* **14**, 1054–1058.

Steinbuch, M., Audran, R., and Pejaudier, L. (1970). *C. R. Soc. Biol.* **164**, 296–301.

Stephen, J. (1961). *J. Biochem.* **80**, 578–584.

Stern, K. H. (1954). *Chem. Rev.* **54**, 79–100.

Stevens, K. R., Hafs, H. D., and Hunter, A. G. (1964). *J. Reprod. Fert.* **8**, 319–324.

Stewart-Tull, D. E. S. (1965). *Immunology* **8**, 221–222.

Stewart-Tull, D. E. S., Wikinson, P. C., and White, R. G. (1965). *Immunology* **9**, 151–160.

Stiehm, E. R. (1967). *J. Lab. Clin. Med.* **70**, 528–534.

Stobo, J. D., and Tomasi, T. B., Jr. (1967). *J. Clin. Invest.* **46**, 1329–1337.

Stoffer, H. R., Kraus, F. W., and Holmes, A. C. (1962). *Proc. Soc. Exp. Biol. Med.* **111**, 467–471.

Stollar, D., and Levine, L. (1963). *Methods Enzymol.* **6**, 848–854.

Stoop, J. W., Ballieux, R. E., and Weyers, H. A. (1962). *Pediatrics* **29**, 97–104.

Stöss, B. (1957). *Zentralbl. Bakteriol. I. Orig.* **171**, 103–116.

Strannegård, Ö. (1962). *Brit. J. Exp. Pathol.* **43**, 600–613.

Strannegård, Ö., and Lycke, E. (1964). *Acta Pathol. Microbiol. Scand.* **60**, 409–419.

Stratton, F. (1966). *Vox Sang.* **11**, 232–237.

Strauss, A. J. L., Kemp, P. G., Jr., Vannier, W. E., and Goodman, H. C. (1964). *J. Immunol.* **93**, 24–34.

Strebel, L. (1960). *Biol. Neonate.* **2**, 55–67.

Strejan, G. (1965). *Experientia* **21**, 399.

Struck, H., and Heinrich, S. (1967). *Z. Immuns.-Forsch.* **133**, 376–384.

Stuart, C. R. (1970). *Med. Biol. Illus.* **20**, 58–59.

Stuchlíková, E., Jelínková, M., and Lhotka, J. (1966). *Clin. Chim. Acta* **13**, 638–641.

Styk, B., and Hána, L. (1966). *Acta Virol.* **10**, 281–290.

Styk, B., and Hána, L. (1968). *Acta Virol.* **12**, 203–207.

Styk, B., and Schmidt, N. J. (1968). *J. Immunol.* **100**, 1223–1229.

Subrahmanyam, D., and Maurer, P. H. (1959). *J. Immunol.* **83**, 327–333.

Sulitzeanu, D. (1965). *Brit. J. Exp. Pathol.* **46**, 481–488.

Sulitzeanu, D., Bernecky, J., Yagi, Y., and Pressman, D. (1963). *Proc. Soc. Exp. Biol. Med.* **114**, 468–472.

Süllmann, H. (1964). *Clin. Chim. Acta* **10**, 569–571.

Sun, T., and Gibson, J. B. (1969). *Amer. J. Trop. Med. Hyg.* **18**, 241–252.

Suskind, S. R., Wickham, M. L., and Carsiotis, M. (1963). *Ann. N. Y. Acad. Sci.* **103**, Art. 2, 1106–1127.

Svendsen, P. J., and Axelsen, N. H. (1972). *J. Immunol. Methods* **1**, 169–176.

Svendsen, P. J., and Rose, C. (1970). *Sci. Tools* **17**, 13–17.

Svensson, S., Hammarström, S. G., and Kabat, E. A. (1970). *Immunochemistry* **7**, 413–422.

Sweet, G. H. (1971a). *Amer. Rev. Resp. Dis.* **104**, 394–400.

Sweet, G. H. (1971b). *Amer. Rev. Resp. Dis.* **104**, 401–407.

Szabo, Gy., Gergely, J., and Magyar, Zs. (1963). *Experientia* **19**, 98.

Szatalowicz, F. T. (1969). *Amer. J. Vet. Res.* **30**, 149–150.

Taketomi, T., and Yamakawa, T. (1963). *J. Biochem.* **54**, 444–451.

Tala, N., and Tomkins, G. M. (1964). *Science* **146**, 1309–1311.

Talal, N., Hermann, G., De Vaux St. Cyr, C., and Grabar, P. (1963). *J. Immunol.* **90**, 246–256.

Tan, M., and Epstein, W. V. (1963). *Science* **139**, 53–54.

Tan, M., and Epstein, W. V. (1965). *J. Lab. Clin. Med.* **66**, 344–356.

Tanaka, C. (1957). *Arch. Ophthalmol.* **58**, 850–856.

Tanner, C. E. (1963). *Exp. Parasitol.* **14**, 346–357.

Tanner, C. E., and Gregory, J. (1961). *Can. J. Microbiol.* **7**, 473–481.

Tawde, S. S., Ram, J. S., and Iyengar, M. R. (1963). *Arch. Biochem. Biophys.* **100**, 270–278.

Tayeau, F., and Faure, F. (1953). *Bull. Sté. Chim. Biol.* **35**, 1193–1199.

Tayeau, F., and Jouzier, E. (1961a). *Bull. Soc. Pharm. Bordeaux* **100**, 6–16.

Tayeau, F., and Jouzier, E. (1961b). *Bull. Soc. Pharm. Bordeaux* **100**, 120–124.

Tayeau, F., and Marquevielle, J. (1958). *Bull. Soc. Chim. Biol.* **40**, 1107–1115.

Taylor, F. B., Jr., and Staprans, I. (1966). *Arch. Biochem. Biophys.* **114**, 38–49.

Taylor-Robinson, D., Somerson, N. L., Turner, H. C., and Chanock, R. M. (1963). *J. Bacteriol.* **85**, 1261–1273.

Taylor-Robinson, D., Sobeslavský, O., and Chanock, R. M. (1965). *J. Bacteriol.* **90**, 1432–1437.

Taymor, M. L., Saravis, C., Batt, R., and Goss, D. A. (1965). *Fert. Steril.* **16**, 579–586.

Tee, D. E. H., Wang, M., and Watkins, J. (1964). *Nature (London)* **204**, 897–898.

Teichmann, B., and Vogt, R. (1964). *Naturwissenschaften* **6**, 141–142.

Telfer, W. H., and Williams, C. M. (1953). *J. Gen. Physiol.* **36**, 389–413.

Tempelis, C. H., and Lofy, M. F. (1965). *J. Immunol.* **95**, 418–421.

Tenenhouse, H. S., and Deutsch, H. F. (1966). *Immunochemistry* **3**, 11–20.

Tengerdy, R. P. (1965). *Anal. Biochem.* **11**, 272–280.

Terando, M. L., and Feir, D. (1967). *Comp. Biochem. Physiol.* **21**, 31–38.

Terr, A. I., and Bentz, J. D. (1965). *J. Allergy* **36**, 433–445.

Thiele, H. G., and Stark, R. (1970). *Z. Immuns.-Forsch.* **140**, 424–427.

Thomas, J. B., and Krywienczyk, J. (1966). *Can. Ent.* **98**, 1094–1099.

Thompson, R. A., and Lachmann, P. J. (1970). *J. Exp. Med.* **131**, 629–641.

Thomson, A. D. (1964). *Nature (London)* **201**, 422–423.

Thorbecke, G. J., and Franklin, E. C. (1961). *J. Immunol.* **87**, 753–759.

Thorpe, N. O., and Deutsch, H. F. (1966). *Immunochemistry* **3**, 317–327.

Tokumaru, T. (1965a). *J. Immunol.* **95**, 181–188.

Tokumaru, T. (1965b). *J. Immunol.* **95**, 189–195.

Tönjum, A. M. (1962). *Acta Pathol. Microbiol. Scand.* **54**, 96–98.

Torii, M., Kabat, E. A., and Bezer, A. E. (1964). *J. Exp. Med.* **120**, 13–29.

Tormo, J., and Chordi, A. (1965). *Nature* (*London*) **205**, 983–985.
Tornabene, T., and Bartel, A. H. (1962). *Tex. Rep. Biol. Med.* **20**, 683–685.
Traill, M. A. (1968). *Lab. Practice* **17**, 709.
Tran Van Ky, P., Havez, R., Biguet, J., and Leys, J. C. (1966a). *Ann. Inst. Pasteur* **110**, 86–98.
Tran Van Ky, P., Uriel, J., and Rose, F. (1966b). *Ann. Inst. Pasteur* **111**, 161–170.
Tran Van Ky, P., Vaucelle, T., Capron, A., and Biguet, J. (1967). *Ann. Inst. Pasteur* **112**, 763–771.
Tremaine, J. H., and Wright, N. S. (1967). *Virology* **31**, 481–488.
Tromba, F. G., and Baisden, L. A. (1963). *J. Parasitol.* **49**, 633–638.
Tromba, F. G., and Baisden, L. A. (1964). *Proc. Helmintholog. Soc. Washington* **31**, 10–18.
Trump, G. N. (1970). *J. Immunol.* **104**, 1267–1275.
Tsao, S., and Goebel, W. F. (1969). *J. Exp. Med.* **130**, 1313–1335.
Tsuchiya, Y., and Hong, K. C. (1965). *Tohoku J. Agr. Res.* **16**, 141–146.
Tsuchiya, T., and Tamanoi, I. (1965). *Int. J. Radiat. Biol.* **10**, 203–206.
Tsuyuki, H. (1963). *Anal. Biochem.* **6**, 203–205.
Tureen, L. L., Warecka, K., and Young, P. A. (1966). *Proc. Soc. Exp. Biol. Med.* **122**, 729–732.
Turner, M. W., and Rowe, D. S. (1964). *Immunology* **7**, 639–656.
Turpin, A., and Raynaud, M. (1959). *Ann. Inst. Pasteur* **97**, 718–732.
Turpin, A., Relyveld, E. H., Pillet, J., and Raynaud, M. (1954). *Ann. Inst. Pasteur* **87**, 185–193.
Ultmann, J. E., Feigelson, P., and Harris, S. (1962). *J. Immunol.* **88**, 113–120.
Urbach, H., and Schabinski, G. (1960). *Zentralbl. Bakteriol.* **180**, 433–441.
Uriel, J. (1957). *Bull. Soc. Chim. Biol.* **39**, 105–118.
Uriel, J. (1958a). *Bull. Soc. Chim. Biol.* **40**, 277–280.
Uriel, J. (1958b). *Clin. Lab.* **65**, 89–94.
Uriel, J. (1958c). *Clin. Chim. Acta* **3**, 17–23.
Uriel, J. (1960). *Nature* (*London*) **188**, 853–854.
Uriel, J. (1961). *Ann. Inst. Pasteur* **101**, 104–118.
Uriel, J. (1963). *Ann. N. Y. Acad. Sci.* **103**, 956–979.
Uriel, J. (1965). *Laval Méd.* **36**, 235–238.
Uriel, J. (1966). *Bull. Soc. Chim. Biol.* **48**, 969–982.
Uriel, J. (1971). *In* "Methods in Immunology and Immunochemistry" (C. A. Williams and M. W. Chase, eds.), Vol. 3, pp. 294–321. Academic Press, New York.
Uriel, J., and Avrameas, S. (1964). *Ann. Inst. Pasteur* **106**, 396–407.
Uriel, J., and Grabar, P. (1956a). *Ann. Inst. Pasteur* **90**, 427–440.
Uriel, J., and Grabar, P. (1956b). *Bull. Soc. Chim. Biol.* **38**, 1253–1269.
Uriel, J., and Grabar, P. (1961). *Anal. Biochem.* **2**, 80–82.
Uriel, J., and Scheidegger, J. J. (1955). *Bull. Soc. Chim. Biol.* **37**, 165–168.
Uriel, J., Götz, H., and Grabar, P. (1957). *Schweiz. Med. Wochenschr.* **87**, 431–434.
Uriel, J., Avrameas, S., and Grabar, P. (1963). *Protides Biol. Fluids* **11**, 355–359.
Ursing, B. (1965). *Acta Med. Scand. Suppl.* **429**, 7–99.
Vaerman, J. P., and Heremans, J. F. (1969). *Immunochemistry* **6**, 779–786.
Vaerman, J. P., Johnson, L. B., Mandy, W., and Fudenberg, H. H. (1965). *J. Lab. Clin. Med.* **65**, 18–25.
Vaerman, J. P., Lebacq-Verheyden, A. M., Scolari, L., and Heremans, J. F. (1969). *Immunochemistry* **6**, 279–285.
Valladares, Y. (1962). *Sangre* **7**, 55–107.

Vanegas Alvarado, M. E. (1961). *Rev. Ecuator. Hig. Med. Trop.* **18,** 89–108.

Van Furth, R. (1966). *Immunology* **11,** 13–18.

Van Furth, R., Schuit, H. R. E., and Hijmans, W. (1965). *J. Exp. Med.* **122,** 1173–1188.

Van Furth, R., Schuit, H. R. E., and Hijmans, W. (1966a). *Brit. J. Haematol.* **12,** 202–211.

Van Furth, R., Schuit, H. R. E., and Hijmans, W. (1966b). *Immunology* **11,** 1–11.

Vanha-Perttula, T., Hopsu, V. K., and Glenner, G. G. (1965). *Histochemie* **5,** 448–449.

Van Orden, D. E. (1968). *Immunochemistry* **5,** 497–499.

Van Orden, D. E., and Treffers, H. P. (1968a). *J. Immunol.* **100,** 659–663.

Van Orden, D. E., and Treffers, H. P. (1968b). *J. Immunol.* **100,** 664–674.

Van Oss, C. J. (1959). *Science* **129,** 1365–1366.

Van Oss, C. J. (1963). *Naturwissenschaften* **18,** 594–595.

Van Oss, C. J., and Bronson, P. M. (1969). *Immunochemistry* **6,** 775–778.

Van Oss, C. J., and Heck, Y. S. L. (1963). *Rev. Immunol. (Paris)* **27,** 27–41.

Van Oss, C. J., Dhennin, L., and Dhennin, L. (1964). *Virology* **22,** 428–430.

Van Regenmortel, M. H. V. (1959). *Biochim. Biophys. Acta* **34,** 553–554.

Van Regenmortel, M. H. V. (1967). *Virology* **31,** 467–480.

Van Riel, J., Van Sande, M., and Van Riel, M. (1971). Personal communication.

Van Slogteren, E., and Van Slogteren, D. H. M. (1957). *Ann. Rev. Microbiol.* **11,** 149–164.

Van Vreedendall, M. (1967). *Clin. Chim. Acta* **15,** 359–360.

Varandani, P. T. (1963). *Ann. N. Y. Acad. Sci.* **103,** Art. 2, 750–753.

Vaughan, J. G., Waite, A., Boulter, D., and Waiters, S. (1966). *J. Exp. Bot.* **17,** 332–343.

Vaughan, J. H., and Kabat, E. A. (1953). *J. Exp. Med.* **97,** 821–844.

Vaughan, J. H., and Kabat, E. A. (1954a). *J. Immunol.* **73,** 205–211.

Vaughan, J. H., and Kabat, E. A. (1954b). *J. Allergy* **25,** 387–394.

Vaux Saint-Cyr, C. (1959). *C. R. Acad. Sci. Paris* **248,** 2818–2820.

Vaux Saint-Cyr, C., Courcon, J., and Grabar, P. (1958). *Bull. Soc. Chim. Biol.* **40,** 579–590.

Ventruto, V., Cimino, R., and Bianchi, P. (1963). *Ann. Sclavo (Napoli)* **5,** 69–110.

Ver, B. A., Rao, S. S., and Jhala, H. I. (1962). *Indian J. Pathol. Bacteriol.* **5,** 131–136.

Vergani, C., and Agostoni, A. (1967). *Clin. Chim. Acta* **16,** 326–327.

Vergani, C., Stabilini, R., and Agostoni, A. (1967). *Immunochemistry* **4,** 233–237.

Virella, G. (1969). *Experientia* **25,** 1175–1177.

Vogt, A., and Kopp, R. (1964). *Nature (London)* **202,** 1350–1351.

Vogt, A., Kopp, R., Maass, G., and Reich, L. (1964). *Science* **145,** 1447–1448.

Von der Decken, A. (1967). *Anal. Biochem.* **18,** 444–452.

Von Muralt, G., and Gugler, E. (1959). *Helv. Med. Acta* **26,** 410–423.

Vosti, K. L., Ward, M. K., and Tigertt, W. D. (1962). *J. Clin. Invest.* **41,** 1436–1445.

Vyazov, O. E., Konyukhov, B. V., and Lishtvan, L. L. (1959). *Bull. Exp. Biol. Med.* **47,** 646–649.

Wachendörfer, G. (1965). *Zentralbl. Veterinarmed.* **12,** 55–66.

Wadsworth, C. (1957). *Int. Arch. Allergy* **10,** 355–360.

Wadsworth, C. (1962). *Int. Arch. Allergy* **21,** 131–137.

Wadsworth, C. (1963). *Int. Arch. Allergy* **23**, 103–114.

Wahl, R., Goichot, J., and Drach, G. (1965). *Ann. Inst. Pasteur* **109**, 479–486.

Wahlström, L., and Norkrans, B. (1964). *Acta Pathol. Microbiol. Scand.* **60**, 420–430.

Wallraff, E. B., Snow, I., and Wilson, S. (1965). *Proc. Soc. Exp. Biol. Med.* **119**, 914–918.

Watanabe, Y., and Felsenfeld, O. (1963). *J. Bacteriol.* **85**, 31–36.

Watanabe, Y., and Seaman, G. R. (1962). *Arch. Biochem. Biophys.* **97**, 393–398.

Watkins, D. S. (1969). *Amer. J. Med. Technol.* **35**, 162–165.

Watkins, J., Tee, D. E. H., Wang, M., and Tarlow, O. (1966). *Biochim. Biophys. Acta* **127**, 66–71.

Watson, D. (1960). *Aust. Anal. Med.* **9**, 99–102.

Watson, D., and Whinfrey, H. (1958). *Lancet* ii, 1375.

Webber, R. V., and Williams, J. W. (1963). *Ann. N. Y. Acad. Sci.* **103**, Art. 2, 643–652.

Webster, J. E. (1965). *J. Med. Lab. Technol.* **22**, 10–11.

Wedman, E. E., Richards, W. D., and Pomeroy, B. S. (1964). *Amer. Rev. Resp. Dis.* **90**, 935–943.

Wedman, E. E., Richards, W. D., and Pomeroy, B. S. (1965). *Can. J. Comp. Med. Vet. Sci.* **29**, 129–133.

Weeke, B. (1968a). *Scand. J. Clin. Lab. Invest.* **21**, 351–354.

Weeke, B. (1968b). *Scand. J. Clin. Lab. Invest.* **22**, 107–111.

Weeke, B. (1969). *Ugeskr. Laeger.* **131**, 1419–1423.

Weeke, B., and Thomsen, J. P. (1968). *Scand. J. Clin. Lab. Invest.* **22**, 165–166.

Wehmeyer, P. (1965). *Nord. Vet. Med.* **17**, 614–616.

Wei, M. M., and Stavitsky, A. B. (1967). *Immunology* **12**, 431–444.

Weigle, W. O. (1960). *Fed. Proc.* **19**, 205.

Weigle, W. O. (1961). *J. Immunol.* **87**, 599–607.

Weigle, W. O., and McConahey, P. J. (1962). *J. Immunol.* **88**, 121–127.

Weil, A. J., and Finkler, A. E. (1959). *Proc. Soc. Exp. Biol. Med.* **102**, 624–626.

Weiler, E., Melletz, E. W., and Breuninger-Peck, E. (1965). *Proc. Nat. Acad. Sci.* **54**, 1310–1317.

Weiner, L. M., Rosenblatt, M., and Howes, H. A. (1963). *J. Immunol.* **90**, 788–792.

Weiner, L. M., Macko, I., Poulik, E., and Goodman, M. (1964). *J. Immunol.* **93**, 228–231.

Weintraub, M., and Raymond, S. (1963). *Science* **142**, 1677–1678.

Weiser, R. S., Myrivik, Q. N., and Pearsall, N. N. (1969). "Fundamentals of Immunology," 363 pp. Lea and Febiger, Philadelphia, Pennsylvania.

Wenzel, F. J., and Emanuel, D. A. (1967). *Arch. Environ. Health* **14**, 385–389.

Wenzel, F. J., Emanuel, D. A., Lawton, B. R., and Magnin, G. E. (1964). *Ann. Allergy* **22**, 533–540.

West, C. D., and Hong, R. (1962). *J. Pediatr.* **60**, 430–464.

West, C. D., Hinrichs, V., and Hinkle, N. H. (1961). *J. Lab. Clin. Med.* **58**, 137–148.

Wetter, C. (1967a). *Z. Naturforsch.* **22b**, 1008–1013.

Wetter, C. (1967b). *Virology* **31**, 498–507.

Weyzen, W. W. H., and Vos, O. (1967). *Nature (London)* **180**, 288–289.

Whipple, H. E., ed. (1964). *Ann. N. Y. Acad. Sci.* **121**, Art. 2, 305–650.

White, G., and Cowan, K. M. (1962). *Virology* **16**, 209–210.

White, G., Simpson, R. M., and Scott, G. R. (1961). *Immunology* **4**, 203–205.

White, G. B. B., Lasheen, R. M., Basillie, M. B., and Turner, G. C. (1971). *J. Clin. Pathol.* **24**, 8–12.

Whiteside, R. E., and Baker, E. E. (1960). *J. Immunol.* **84**, 221–226.

Whiteside, R. E., and Baker, E. E. (1962). *J. Immunol.* **88**, 650–660.

Widra, A., McMillen, S., and Rhodes, H. J. (1968). *Mycopathol. Mycol. Acta* **36**, 353–358.

Wieme, R. J. (1955). *Bull. Soc. Chim. Biol.* **37**, 995–997.

Wieme, R. J. (1958). *Behringwerk. Mitt.* **34**, 27–37.

Wieme, R. J. (1959a). "Studies on Agar Gel Electrophoresis; Techniques—Applications," 531 pp. Arscia Uitgaven N. V. Publ., Brussels.

Wieme, R. J. (1959b). *Clin. Chim. Acta* **4**, 317–321.

Wieme, R. J. (1964). *Ann. N. Y. Acad. Sci.* **121**, Art. 2, 366–372.

Wieme, R. J., and Kaminski, M. (1955). *Bull. Soc. Chim. Biol.* **37**, 247–253.

Wieme, R. J., and Veys, E. M. (1970). *Clin. Chim. Acta* **27**, 77–86.

Wiggins, G. L., and Schubert, J. H. (1965). *J. Bacteriol.* **89**, 589–596.

Wilheim, E., and Lamm, M. E. (1966). *Nature* (*London*) **212**, 846–847.

Wilkerson, P. C., and White, R. G. (1966). *Immunology* **11**, 229–241.

Williams, C. A., and Chase, M. W., eds. (1967). "Methods in Immunology and Immunochemistry," Vol. 1, 479 pp. Academic Press, New York.

Williams, C. A., Jr. (1960). *Sci. Amer.* **202**, 130–140.

Williams, C. A., Jr., and Grabar, P. (1955a). *J. Immunol.* **74**, 158–168.

Williams, C. A., Jr., and Grabar, P. (1955b). *J. Immunol.* **74**, 397–403.

Williams, G. A., Hargis, G. K., Sidwell, C. G., and Yakulis, V. J. (1964). *Proc. Soc. Exp. Biol. Med.* **115**, 61–64.

Williams, J. (1962a). *Biochem. J.* **83**, 346–355.

Williams, J. (1962b). *Biochem. J.* **83**, 355–364.

Williams, R. C., Jr. (1964). *J. Immunol.* **93**, 850–859.

Wilson, A. T. (1964). *J. Immunol.* **92**, 431–434.

Wilson, G. S., and Miles, A. A. (1955). "Topley and Wilson's Principles of Bacteriology and Immunity," 4th ed., 2331 pp. Williams and Wilkins, Baltimore, Maryland.

Wilson, J. F., and Warren, G. (1962). *J. Clin. Pathol.* **15**, 40–43.

Wilson, J. F., Heiner, D. C., and Lahey, M. E. (1962). *J. Pediatr.* **5**, 787–800.

Wilson, M. W. (1958). *J. Immunol.* **81**, 317–330.

Wilson, M. W., and Pringle, B. H. (1954). *J. Immunol.* **73**, 232–243.

Wilson, M. W., and Pringle, B. H. (1955). *J. Immunol.* **75**, 460–469.

Wilson, M. W., and Pringle, B. H. (1956). *J. Immunol.* **77**, 324–331.

Winchester, R. J., Agnello, V., and Kunkel, H. G. (1969). *Ann. N. Y. Acad. Sci.* **168**, Art. 1, 195–203.

Winnick, T., and Goldwasser, R. (1961). *Exp. Cell Res.* **25**, 428–436.

Winter, A. J. (1966). *J. Immunol.* **95**, 1002–1012.

Witebsky, E., and Milgrom, F. (1962). *Immunology* **5**, 67–78.

Witebsky, E., and Rose, N. R. (1959). *J. Immunol.* **83**, 41–48.

Witter, R. L. (1962). *Avian Dis.* **6**, 478–492.

Wodehouse, R. P. (1953). *Ann. Allergy* **11**, 720–731.

Wodehouse, R. P. (1954a). *Ann. Allergy* **12**, 363–374.

Wodehouse, R. P. (1954b). *Int. Arch. Allergy* **5**, 337–366.

Wodehouse, R. P. (1954c). *Int. Arch. Allergy* **5**, 425–433.

Wodehouse, R. P. (1955a). *Ann. Allergy* 13, 39–52.
Wodehouse, R. P. (1955b). *Int. Arch. Allergy* 6, 65–79.
Wodehouse, R. P. (1956a). *Ann. Allergy* 14, 96–113.
Wodehouse, R. P. (1956b). *Ann. Allergy* 14, 121–138.
Wodehouse, R. P. (1957). *Ann. Allergy* 15, 527–536.
Wollheim, F. A., and Williams, R. C., Jr. (1965). *J. Lab. Clin. Med.* 66, 433–445.
Woodin, A. M. (1959). *Biochem. J.* 73, 225–237.
Woods, W. A., Weiss, R. A., and Robbins, F. C. (1962). *Proc. Soc. Exp. Biol. Med.* 111, 401–404.
Wright, D. N., and Lockhart, W. R. (1965). *J. Bacteriol.* 89, 1026–1031.
Wright, G. L., Jr., Roberts, D. B., Farrell, K. B., Murphy, E. C., Jr., and Grow, L. J. (1970). *Bacteriol. Proc.* 90, M104.
Wright, N. S., and Stace-Smith, R. (1966). *Phytopathology* 56, 944–948.
Wright, S. T. C. (1959). *Nature (London)* 183, 1282–1283.
Wunderly, C. (1957). *Experientia* 13, 421–464.
Wunderly, C. (1958a). *Clin. Chim. Acta* 3, 298–299.
Wunderly, C. (1958b). *Deut. Med. Wochenschr.* 83, 407–410.
Wunderly, C. (1959). *Naturwissenschaften* 46, 107–108.
Wunderly, C. (1960). *J. Chromatogr.* 3, 536–544.
Yagi, Y., Maier, P., and Pressman, D. (1962). *J. Immunol.* 89, 736–744.
Yagi, Y., Maier, P., Pressman, D., Arbesman, C. E., and Reisman, R. E. (1963a). *J. Immunol.* 91, 83–89.
Yagi, Y., Maier, P., Pressman, D., Arbesman, C. E., Reisman, R. E., and Lenzner, A. R. (1963b). *J. Immunol.* 90, 760–769.
Yalulis, V. J., and Heller, P. (1962). *Amer. J. Clin. Pathol.* 37, 253–256.
Yalow, R. S., and Berson, S. A. (1960). *J. Clin. Invest.* 39, 1157–1175.
Yamamoto, R., and Clark, G. T. (1966). *Vet. Rec.* 79, 95–100.
Yantorno, C., Soanes, W. A., Gonder, M. J., and Shulman, S. (1967). *Immunology* 12, 395–410.
Yogore, M. G., Jr., Lewert, R. M., and Madraso, E. D. (1965). *Amer. J. Trop. Med. Hyg.* 14, 586–591.
Yokoyama, M., and Carr, M. (1962). *Jap. J. Med. Sci. Biol.* 15, 1–8.
Yokoyama, M., and Tsuchiya, T. (1963). *Hiroshima J. Med. Sci.* 12, 65–69.
Yomtov, M., and Nedjalkov, S. (1962). *Z. Immuns.-Forsch.* 124, 211–218.
Yoshida, A., and Hedén, C. G. (1962). *J. Immunol.* 88, 389–393.
Young, J. H., and Brubaker, P. (1963). *Turtox News* 41, 275–276.
Zaman, V., and Chellappah, W. T. (1964). *Experientia* 20, 429.
Zaman, V., and Chellappah, W. T. (1965). *Experientia* 21, 297.
Zaman, V., Fernando, C. H., and Chellappah, W. T. (1963). *Experientia* 19, 106.
Zamora, A., Bojalil, L. F., and Bastarrachea, F. (1963). *J. Bacteriol.* 85, 549–555.
Zanussi, C., Invernizzi, F., Del Giacco, G. S., and Luporini, G. (1961). *Bol. Ist. Serol. Milano* 40, 1–44.
Zelkowitz, L., and Yakulis, V. (1970). *J. Lab. Clin. Med.* 76, 973–980.
Zelzer, G. (1962). *J. Hyg.* 60, 69–78.
Zimmer, J., Dub, M-Th., and Woringer, Fr. (1960). *Bull. Soc. Fr. Dermatol. Syphiligr.* 67, 329–331.
Zimmer, M. J. (1960). *Bull. Soc. Fr. Dermatol. Syphiligr.* 78, 616–618.
Zingale, S. B., Mattioli, C. A., and Elizalde, M. M. (1964). *Medicina (Buenos Aires)* 24, 132–146.

Zlotnick, A., and Landau, S. (1966). *J. Lab. Clin. Med.* **68**, 70–80.

Zlotnick, A., and Rodnan, G. P. (1962). *Proc. Soc. Exp. Biol. Med.* **109**, 742–746.

Zuckerman, A., Goberman, V., Ron, N., Spira, D., Hamburger, J., and Burg, R. (1969). *Exp. Parasitol.* **24**, 299–312.

Zwaan, J. (1963). "Immunochemical Analysis of the Eye Lens during Development," 103 pp. Rototype, Amsterdam.

Zwartouw, H. T., Westwood, J. C. N., and Harris, W. J. (1965). *J. Gen. Microbiol.* **38**, 39–45.

Zydeck, F. A. (1970). *Experientia* **26**, 88–90.

Zydeck, F. A., Muirhead, E. E., and Schneider, H. (1965a). *Nature (London)* **205**, 189–190.

Zydeck, F. A., Muirhead, E. E., and Schneider, H. (1965b). *Amer. J. Clin. Pathol.* **44**, 596–599.

Zydeck, F. A., Muirhead, E. E., and Schneider, H. (1966). *Amer. J. Clin. Pathol.* **45**, 323–328.

Glossary

The following collection of terms is peculiar to the language of immunodiffusion. It does not include the much larger number of terms which, though often used in this field, are more general and pertain to immunology and serology. The reader should consult immunology textbooks for explanation of these.

Most of the terms in this glossary have appeared previously in publication, some many times. However, a few here are being used for the first time (e.g., the verb *immunodiffuse;* the noun *electroimmunodiffusogram*). I have included these to help systematize the language and concepts of immunodiffusion, to supplant confusing and sometimes conflicting terms with words that are both descriptive and based on precedent, and to minimize the need for qualifying phrases. For example, from the precedent of *chromatogram,* meaning "pattern of substances separated by chromatography," came the noun *electropherogram;* and from this was derived *immunoelectropherogram,* meaning "pattern of precipitin arcs produced by immunoelectrophoresis." All three nouns have become commonly used. Therefore, the word *immunodiffusogram* is a logical and useful continuation in this mode of terminology, being both congruous with already established similar words and immediately meaningful to the average reader even if he has only passing acquaintance with immunodiffusion. Admittedly, this word at first may sound awkward and unpleasant to a veteran user of immunodiffusion tests, but it seemed the better choice over an alternative superficially more pleasing word like *immunogram,* because it is more explicit and descriptive.

When several terms have been invented by different investigators to describe one kind of test, I have chosen from among these that which seemed most descriptive and best associated with existing terminology,

501

and have used this term preferentially both in other sections of this book and as the word to be defined in the glossary. For example, I have used *electroimmunodiffusion* in this way as a name for tests in which antigen and antibody precipitate while being electrophoresed. In addition to being innerently descriptive, it provides a rational nomenclatural basis for relating the many otherwise confusing varieties of this type of test to each other according to terminological precedent employed to describe older immunodiffusion techniques, as was explained in Chapter 6.

Communicative accuracy depends on good terminology. I hope that by helping to provide the latter this glossary will promote the former.

Antibody: an antiserum immunoglobulin capable of reacting specifically with the antigen against which the antiserum was raised; it may or may not have the capacity to precipitate the antigen.

Antibody determinant site: the physical portion of an antibody molecule designed to recognize a corresponding ligand of the molecule of antigen with which it is reactive; there are two identical sites on most molecules of precipitin.

Antigen: a substance that can induce antibody formation and can react specifically with antibody formed in response to exposure to it.

Antigen–antibody crossed electrophoresis: equivalent to two-dimensional single electroimmunodiffusion.

Antigen determinant site: the physical portion of an antigen molecule with which an antibody molecule is built to react; *cf.* Ligand.

Chromatogram: a chromatographic pattern.

Chromatograph: to fractionate by chromatography.

Coalescence: see Reaction of identity.

Compound immunodiffusion test: one in which fractionation of one of the reactants, such as by electrophoresis or chromatography, is effected before it is allowed to react with the other immunologically.

Coprecipitin: a constituent of antiserum, usually an antibody, which enhances precipitation of antigen by the antiserum.

Countercurrent immunoelectrophoresis: equivalent to double electroimmunodiffusion, with both reactants migrating toward each other.

Counterimmunoelectrophoresis: equivalent to double electroimmunodiffusion, with both reactants migrating toward each other.

Crossing electrophoresis: equivalent to electroimmunodiffusion.

Double diffusion: an immunodiffusion test in which both antigen and antibody must diffuse into a common reaction area before precipitating.

Electroimmunodiffusion: an immunodiffusion test in which the reactants are intermingled by electrophoresis in addition to diffusion.

Electroimmunodiffusion, double: an electroimmunodiffusion test in which both reactants are being moved electrophoretically to intermingle and react.

Electroimmunodiffusion, single: an electroimmunodiffusion test in which only one of the two reactants is moved electrophoretically during their interaction.

Electroimmunodiffusogram: the pattern of precipitin bands in an electroimmunodiffusion test.

Electroosmosis: the flow of electrolyte fluid caused by passage of electric current through it while it is held within a charged medium; electroosmosis is strongly cathodic in agar gels.

Electropherogram: an electrophoretic pattern.

Electrophorese: a verb, analogous to the verb "chromatograph," indicating that something is being submitted to electrophoresis.

Electroprecipitation: a term used to describe antigen–antibody precipitation during the course of an electroimmunodiffusion test.

Electrosyneresis: equivalent to double electroimmunodiffusion, with both reactants migrating toward each other.

External reactant: in single immunodiffusion tests, or electroimmunodiffusion, the reactant that moves; *cf.* Internal reactant.

Gap: in immunodiffusion tests, an artifactual rarefaction in antigen–antibody precipitation caused by a sudden relative increase in the concentration of one reactant at its front of precipitation with the other; *cf.* Stria.

Gel immunofiltration: immunochromatography employing gel filtration for the preliminary chromatographic fractionation of one of the reactants; also called immunogelfiltration.

-gram: suffix attached to the name of an immunodiffusion test to form a word describing the pattern of precipitin bands developed in that test: e.g., immunoelectropherogram, immunodiffusogram, electroimmunodiffusogram, immunochromatogram.

H-type precipitins: precipitins with a narrow range of ratios to antigen over which they will precipitate it, and which form a precipitate with antigen readily soluble in either antigen or antibody excess; *cf.* R-type precipitins.

Immunochromatogram: the pattern of precipitin bands in an immunochromatography test.

Immunodiffuse: a verb, analogous to the verb "chromatograph," indicating that something is being submitted to analysis by immunodiffusion.

Immunodiffusion: an immunologic test, usually one of antigen–antibody precipitation, which is performed in or on an anticonvection medium so that one or the other or both of the reactants move principally by diffusion to intermingle and react.

Immunodiffusogram: the pattern of precipitin bands in an immunodiffusion test.

Immunoelectrofocusing: analogous to immunoelectrophoresis, but using electrofocusing instead of electrophoresis for preliminary fractionation of one of the reactants.

Immunoelectropherogram: the pattern of precipitin bands in an immunoelectrophoresis test.

Immunoelectrophoresis: an immunodiffusion test in which one of the reactants is electrophoresed before being allowed to diffuse against and react with the other.

Immunoelectrophoresis, reversed: an immunoelectrophoretic test in which antiserum is electrophoresed instead of antigen.

Immunogelfiltration: see Gel immunofiltration.

Immunoglobulin: any one of several antiserum constituents with presumed or demonstrable specific reactivity for the antigen used to raise the antiserum; all known immunoglobulins are γ-globulins.

Immunoosmophoresis: equivalent to double electroimmunodiffusion, with both reactants migrating toward each other.

Immunoprecipitation: specific precipitation of a substance by immunologic reaction; i.e., antigen–antibody precipitation.

Immunorheophoresis: an immunodiffusion test in which reactants are moved directionally through the reaction medium by hydrodynamic transport effected by controlled drying of appropriate areas of the medium.

Immunosedimentation: a compound immunodiffusion test in which one type of reactant is fractionated by differential centrifugation before being analyzed with the other.

Immunotransmigration: a form of double electroimmunodiffusion in which one reactant migrates through the other during electrophoresis, both traveling toward the same electrode.

Internal reactant: in single immunodiffusion or electroimmunodiffusion tests, the reactant that is stationary; *cf.* External reactant.

Ionic strength: an expression of the conductivity of an electrolyte solution; it is one-half the sum of the molality of all electrolyte ions present in the solution times the square of each one's valence.

Lectin: a plant protein that is precipitin-like in having relatively specific capacity to precipitate certain antigens.

Liesegang precipitation: secondary precipitation by a single antigen–antibody system which occurs under certain conditions in which one reactant moderately overbalances the other serologically, and the two reactants have different diffusion coefficients.

Ligand: equivalent to antigen determinant site.

One-step technique: a compound immunodiffusion test in which all steps (e.g., electrophoresis and antigen–antibody precipitation) are performed in one medium; *cf.* Two-step technique.

Ouchterlony test: a radial double diffusion plate test.

Precipitin: an immunoglobulin that specifically precipitates antigen.

Precipitinogen: an antigen that can induce an animal to form precipitins against it.

Reaction of fusion: see Reaction of identity.

Reaction of identity: joining and fusion of two precipitin bands produced by two compared reactants diffusing from separate origins and interacting simultaneously with a reference reactant and suggesting immunologic identity; reaction of fusion or coalescence.

Reaction of nonidentity: crossing of precipitin bands formed by compared reactants diffusing from different origins and reacting simultaneously with a reference reactant, indicating immunologic nonidentity.

Reaction of partial identity: joining and partial fusion of two precipitin bands produced by two compared reactants diffusing from separate origins and interacting simultaneously with a reference reactant, one or the other or both precipitin bands continuing to precipitate weakly beyond the point of joining to form a "spur"; suggests that the compared reactants cross-react serologically but are not identical.

R-type precipitins: precipitins with a broad range of ratios to antigen over which they will precipitate it, and which form a precipitate with antigen poorly soluble in antigen or, especially, in antibody excess; *cf.* H-type precipitins.

Simple diffusion: equivalent to single diffusion.

Single diffusion: an immunodiffusion test in which only one of the two reactants diffuses, the other remaining essentially immobile.

Spur: weak precipitin band extending beyond the point of joining of precipitin bands formed by two compared, related but nonidentical reactants being precipitated simultaneously by a common reference reactant more reactive with one than the other; *see* Reaction of partial identity.

Stria: in immunodiffusion tests, an artifactual intensification of precipitation caused by sudden relative decrease in the concentration of one reactant at its front of precipitation with the other; *cf.* Gap.

Two-dimensional: adjective applied to compound immunodiffusion techniques, like electroimmunodiffusion, in which one of the reactants undergoes preliminary fractionation, such as by electrophoresis or chromatography, before being exposed to the other.

Two-step technique: a compound immunodiffusion test in which the first step (e.g., electrophoresis) is performed apart from the medium in which the second step (e.g., antigen–antibody precipitation) will be effected; *cf.* One-step technique.

Appendix I

Adjuvants

Freund Adjuvants

1. Incomplete type (without mycobacteria), two formulas:
    (*a*)   3 parts light mineral oil U.S.P.
            1 part Aquaphore, Falba, or anhydrous lanolin
            4 parts physiologic phosphate buffer
    (*b*)   4 parts *n*-hexadecane
            1 part glycerol monooleate (Myverol, Distillation Products, Inc.)
            10 parts physiologic phosphate buffer
2. Complete type (with mycobacteria).

Thoroughly disperse mycobacteria (living avirulent tubercle bacilli, heat-killed virulent tubercle bacilli, *Mycobacterium butyricum,* or *M. smegmatis*) in the oil phase of incomplete-type adjuvant, before oil and water phases are emulsified, at a concentration of 7.5 mg/ml.

Emulsification of Freund's adjuvants, incomplete or complete: emulsifier (e.g., glycerol monooleate) is dissolved in oil, mycobacteria are added if complete adjuvant is to be prepared, and this oil phase is layered upon water to which antigen already has been added. The two phases are emulsified by vigorous mixing such as by pumping them in and out of a syringe and large-gauge needle, ultrasonicating or mechanically vibrating them, or intermingling them with a high-speed stirrer. Handy for the latter method is a 2½-inch box nail used as a disposable impeller in a high-speed engraving tool or dental drill. The stability of a water-in-oil emulsion, such as must be obtained for Freund adjuvants, is tested by dropping some emulsion on cold water. Stability is indicated by the drop's remaining intact.

507

Aluminum Hydroxide Adjuvant

25 ml antigen solution (e.g., human serum)
80 ml distilled water
90 ml 10% $KAl(SO_4)_2 \cdot 12\ H_2O$

Adjust pH to 6.5 with 5 N NaOH. Centrifuge the mixture, collect and wash the precipitate twice with physiologic saline containing 0.01% Merthiolate, and resuspend the washed precipitate in 100 ml of the same kind of saline. This suspension can be kept at 4°C for at least 14 days (Hirschfeld, 1960d).

Appendix II

Selected Immunodiffusion Electrolyte Solutions

(All formulas are made up to 1 liter)

1. Physiologic sodium chloride, ionic strength 0.15, pH variable.
   8.8 gm sodium chloride
2. Barbital, ionic strength 0.15,* pH 7.4.
   6.98 gm sodium barbital
   6.0 gm sodium chloride
   27 ml 1 N hydrochloric acid
3. Phosphate, ionic strength 0.15,* pH 7.4.
   12.8 gm Na_2HPO_4
   2.62 gm $NaH_2PO_4 \cdot H_2O$
4. Tris, ionic strength 0.15,* pH 7.4.
   9.3 gm 2-amino-2-(hydroxymethyl)-1,3-propanediol
   74 ml 1 N hydrochloric acid
   7.0 gm sodium chloride
5. Ethylenediamineacetic acid, ionic strength 0.15,* pH 7.4.
   15.8 gm ethylenediamine
   23.8 gm glacial acetic acid
Allow to stand for 24 hours for maximum electrolyte dissociation.
6. Sodium chloride–borate, physiologic, pH 8.
   8.8 gm sodium chloride
   2.0 gm sodium borate
Constitutes antiseptic buffer especially useful for washing immuno-diffusograms before staining.

---

* Ionic strengths have been determined by electric conductivity in comparison with physiologic sodium chloride.

Selected Immunoelectrophoresis and Electroimmunodiffusion Buffers

(All formulas are made up to 1 liter)

All-purpose formulas:
1. Barbital, ionic strength 0.025, pH 8.2.
   3.96 gm sodium barbital
   770 ml distilled water
   230 ml 0.025 N hydrochloric acid
2. Barbital–acetate, ionic strength 0.05,* pH 8.6.
   5.4 gm sodium barbital
   4.3 gm sodium acetate·3 H_2O
   58.2 ml 0.1 N hydrochloric acid
3. Phosphate, ionic strength 0.05,* pH 7.4.
   6.4 gm Na_2HPO_4
   1.3 gm $NaH_2PO_4 \cdot H_2O$

Self-sterilizing buffer especially useful for glycoproteins:
4. Borate, ionic strength 0.05,* pH 8.6.
   6.7 gm boric acid
   13.4 gm sodium borate·10 H_2O

Volatile, high-capacity buffer with strong chelating effects:
5. Ethylenediamineacetic acid, ionic strength 0.05,* pH 8.2.

* Ionic strengths have been determined by electric conductivity in comparison with physiologic sodium chloride.

2.5 gm ethylenediamine
2.4 gm glacial acetic acid
Allow to stand for 24 hours for maximum electrolyte dissociation.

Self-sterilizing buffer of high capacity, low conductivity, and strong chelating properties:
6.   EDTA–tris–borate, ionic strength 0.024,* pH 8.9.
      60.5 gm 2-amino-2-(hydroxymethyl)-1,3-propanediol
      6.0 gm ethylenediaminetetraacetic acid
      4.6 gm boric acid
Use undiluted in electrode vessels and at 75% in electropherogram, for a discontinuous buffer system (Zwaan, 1963).
7.   Barbital–citrate–oxalate, ionic strength 0.05, pH 8.3 (Bednařík, 1966).
      10.3 gm sodium barbital
      0.45 gm citric acid
      0.402 gm oxalic acid

Discontinuous buffer system providing superior resolution in the α-globulin region of human serum immunoelectropherograms (Nerstrøm, 1963a):
8.   Barbital–calcium lactate, ionic strength 0.009 (electrode vessels)* and 0.036 (agar gel),* pH 8.4.

Electrode vessel	Agar gel
1.38 gm barbituric acid	1.66 gm barbituric acid
8.76 gm sodium barbital	10.51 gm sodium barbital
0.384 gm calcium lactate	1.536 gm calcium lactate

Most of the above buffers can be used with special additives such as 0.01% thimerosal as an antiseptic, 10% sucrose to minimize dehydration of very thin gels (Elevitch et al., 1966), 7.5% glycine to suppress reassociation of dissociated antigens (Merskey et al., 1964), or 0.021 M magnesium acetate to prevent dissociation of bacterial ribonucleic acid (Quash et al., 1962).

Several of the above buffers can be used for polyacrylamide gels; a tris-glycine buffer seems generally to be favored for electrophoresis of serum antigens:
9.   Tris–glycine, ionic strength of 10% working solution 0.002,* pH 8.1 (Clarke, 1964).
      29 gm glycine
      6.0 gm 2-amino-2-(hydroxymethyl)-1,3-propanediol
      5 ml 1 N hydrochloric acid

Above stock solution is diluted to 10% original strength just before use.

10. Tris–EDTA–borate, ionic strength of 5% working solution 0.027,* pH 8.25.

   215.5 gm 2-amino-2-(hydroxymethyl)-1,3-propanediol
   18.5 gm disodium ethylenediaminetetraacetic acid
   110.1 gm boric acid

Above stock solution is diluted to 5% original strength just before use.

11. Discontinuous buffer system for starch gel immunoelectrophoresis, pH 8.5–8.6 (Korngold, 1963b).

Electrode vessels	*Starch gel*
18.5 gm boric acid	9.2 gm 2-amino-2-(hydroxymethyl)-1,3-propanediol
2.5 gm NaOH	1.05 gm citric acid, monohydrate

Appendix IV

Immunochromatography Buffers

(Both formulas made up to 1 liter)

1.   Phosphate, ionic strength 0.205,* pH 6.5, for Sephadex G-200.
     1.77 gm $NaH_2PO_4 \cdot H_2O$
     1.02 gm Na_2HPO_4
     11.7 gm NaCl
2.   Phosphate, antiseptic, ionic strength 0.19,* pH 7.2, for Sephadex gels (Grant and Everall, 1965).
     2.272 gm Na_2HPO_4
     0.544 gm KH_2PO_4
     11.7 gm NaCl
     1.0 gm sodium azide

---

* Ionic strengths have been determined by electric conductivity in comparison with physiologic sodium chloride.

Appendix V

Selected Protein Stains

1.   Triple stain, maximal sensitivity for agar or agarose gels (Crowle and Jarrett, unpublished).
      0.5 gm light green SF
      0.5 gm thiazine red R
      0.5 gm Buffalo black NBR
      5.0 gm $HgCl_2$
      100 ml 2% acetic acid
Stain microimmunodiffusion tests for 10 to 15 minutes; differentiate in 5% acetic acid.

2.   Single stain (Banach and Hawirko, 1966).
      0.5 gm Buffalo black NBR
      5.0 gm $HgCl_2$
      100 ml 5% acetic acid
Stain microimmunodiffusion tests for 10 to 15 minutes; differentiate in 5% acetic acid. The mercuric chloride acts as a mordant. Other dyes can be used in place of Buffalo black for improved photographic rendition.

The above stains can be applied to agar or agarose gels either before or after they have been dried, but they work best on undried gels. If the undried gel is 1 mm or more thick, it should be presoaked with differentiating solution before being stained. Staining and differentiating times depend on the nature and thickness of the gel (see Chapter 2). These stains also can be used for polyacrylamide gels.

3.   Double stain for cellulose acetate (Rabinowitz, 1964).
      (*a*)   0.2 gm ponceau S
              3.0 gm trichloroacetic acid
              100 ml distilled water

517

(b)   5 mg nigrosin WS
            100 ml 3% acetic acid

Stain for 15 minutes in mixture a; differentiate in 5% acetic acid. Weaker precipitin bands can subsequently be stained by 24-hour exposure to mixture b and differentiation in 2% acetic acid.

Appendix VI

Selected Lipid Stains

1.   Sudan black (Grabar, 1959a; Uriel, 1958a).
     100 ml 60% ethanol
     sufficient Sudan black B to saturate this ethanol at 37°C

Cool solution to room temperature and filter. Just before use, filter again and add 0.1 ml of 25% sodium hydroxide solution for every 50 ml of dye. Stain from a few minutes (micro techniques) to 2 hours or more (macro techniques); differentiate with 50% ethanol. Preferably apply to dried agar, but if agar has not been dried, then soak it in 60% ethanol before staining.

2.   Tetracycline hydrochloride indicator in aqueous solution for serum lipoproteins (Rabinovitz and Schen, 1965).
     20 mg tetracycline hydrochloride
     6.7 mg $ZnSO_4$
     10 ml distilled water

Perfuse into wet gel from surface. Wash with pH 8.6 electrophoresis buffer. Observe with ultraviolet light (366 nm) for fluorescent lipoproteins.

3.   Nile blue A (Crowle, 1961).
     0.1 gm Nile blue A
     100 ml 1% sulfuric acid

Boil staining mixture for 5 minutes; cool before using. Stain as required (15 to 20 minutes for micro tests), and differentiate with 1% sulfuric acid. Wash, before drying, with distilled water and then with distilled water containing 1% glycerol.

Appendix VII

Selected Polysaccharide Stains

1. Schiff reagent (Uriel and Grabar, 1956a).
   A. Solutions
      (a) 1.5 gm basic fuchsin
          500 ml boiling distilled water
          Filter at 55°C and cool to 40°C. Add
          25 ml 2 N hydrochloric acid
          3.75 gm $Na_2S_2O_5$
          Agitate to ensure rapid solution. Allow to stand
             stoppered in refrigerator for 6 hours. Add
          1.2 gm animal charcoal
   Mix vigorously for 50 seconds and filter rapidly, filtration time not exceeding 2 to 3 minutes. Store stoppered in refrigerator.
      (b) 1.0 gm periodic acid
          0.82 gm anhydrous sodium acetate
          100 ml distilled water
      (c) 0.54 gm acetic acid
          0.89 gm anhydrous sodium acetate
          10 gm hydroxylamine hydrochloride
          100 ml distilled water
      (d) 5 ml 10% $Na_2S_2O_5$
          5 ml 2 N hydrochloric acid
          90 ml distilled water
   Solution d should be made just before it is used. This also serves as the final wash bath when it contains 20% glycerol.
   B. Procedure
      Soak immunodiffusogram in c for 15 minutes.
      Wash in running water for 15 minutes.

Soak in *b* for 10 minutes.

Wash in running water for 10 minutes.

Soak in *a*, diluted immediately before use with an equal volume of distilled water, for 3 minutes.

Wash 3 times for 2 minutes each in *d*.

Wash 3 times for 1 hour each in glycerinated *d*.

Dry agar in warm air oven.

Spray with protective plastic or varnish.

2.   *p*-Phenylenediamine oxidation reaction (Grabar, 1959a; Uriel, 1958a).

    A.   Solutions

        (*a*)   1 gm periodic acid

             1.64 gm anhydrous sodium acetate

             100 ml 50% ethanol

        (*b*)   144 mg α-naphthol

             100 ml distilled water

             Dissolve with heat and then cool

        (*c*)   108 mg *p*-phenylenediamine

             100 ml distilled water

             Prepare immediately before using

        (*d*)   10% hydrogen peroxide

    B.   Procedure

Soak immunodiffusogram in *a* for 15 minutes.

Wash for 10 minutes in running water, and for 5 minutes in distilled water.

Soak in fresh mixture of $b:c:d = 5:5:1$ for 5 to 10 minutes.

Wash for 10 minutes in running water; rinse in distilled water.

Air-dry in warm oven.

Spray with protective plastic or varnish.

3.   Copper-formazan reaction (Uriel and Grabar, 1961).

    A.   Solutions

        (*a*)   1 gm periodic acid

             1.64 gm anhydrous sodium acetate

             100 ml distilled water

        (*b*)   50 mg phenylhydrazine hydrochloride

             100 ml pH 4 acetate buffer (solution *c*, below)

             Prepare no more than 24 hours before using

        (*c*)   8.2 gm sodium acetate

             2.4 gm glacial acetic acid

             100 ml distilled water

(*d*)　　100 mg Diazo blue B (*o*-dianisidine tetrazotized)
100 ml 1 *M* sodium acetate
Prepare immediately before use

(*e*)　　Saturated solution copper acetate in 1 *M* sodium acetate

B.　Procedure

Soak predried slide for 10 minutes in *a* for glycoproteins (for dextrans continue this oxidation for 3 hours).

Wash in running water for 10 minutes.

Heat *b* to from 60° to 70°C; soak slide in this at same temperature for 5 minutes.

Wash in *c* for 10 minutes.

Soak in *d* for 10 minutes.

Wash in running water for 10 minutes.

Soak in *e* for 5 minutes.

Wash for 5 minutes in running water.

Dry.

The blue-violet coloration of polyosidic substances is very stable.

Appendix VIII

Selected Nucleic Acid Stains

1. Acridine orange (Cowan and Graves, 1968).
    A. Solutions
        (a)   60 ml absolute ethanol
              30 ml chloroform
              10 ml glacial acetic acid
        (b)   1.2 ml 0.1 M citric acid
              0.8 ml 0.2 M Na_2HPO_4
              48 ml 25% methanol
        (c)   10 mg acridine orange
              100 ml solution b
              To be used for differentiating nucleic acids
        (d)   1 mg acridine orange
              100 ml solution b
              To be used for detecting nucleic acids
    B. Procedure
        Fix slide in solution a for 15 minutes at room temperature.
        Rinse with solution b.
        Stain with solution c or solution d for 10 minutes at room
            temperature.
        Wash several times with solution b for several hours.
        Rinse with distilled water, dry, examine under intense
            UV light.
        Single-stranded RNA and DNA are flame-red; double-
            stranded nucleic acids are yellow-green.
2. Pyronine Y (Kurnick, 1955).
    A. Solutions

(*a*)   12.5 ml 2% chloroform-extracted pyronine Y in
          distilled water
          7.5 ml 2% chloroform-extracted methyl green in
          distilled water
          30 ml distilled water

(*b*)   *n*-butanol

B.   Procedure

Stain predried agar for 6 minutes in solution *a*.

Blot with filter paper.

Wash twice for 5 minutes each in solution *b*.

Air-dry.

Polymerized DNA is green; depolymerized DNA or RNA
is red.

Note: pyronine Y (not pyronine B) must be used. Chloroform extraction is done by shaking aqueous solution of each stain with successive volumes of chloroform until the chloroform layer no longer extracts color from the water layer.

Appendix IX

Selected Double Stains

1. For protein and lipid (Uriel and Scheidegger, 1955).
    50 mg bromphenol blue or Buffalo black NBR
    2 ml acetic acid
    100 ml 60% ethanol saturated with oil red 0

Stain predried agar as required. Differentiate with 50% ethanol containing 1% acetic acid. If bromphenol blue version is used, expose dried slide to ammonia vapor.

2. For protein and lipid (Uriel and Scheidegger, 1955).
    50 mg azocarmine B
    2 ml acetic acid
    100 ml 60% ethanol saturated with Sudan black B

Stain predried agar as required. Differentiate with 50% ethanol containing 1% acetic acid.

Subject Index

A

Absorption
  antigenic, 106
  batch method, 106–108
  Björkelund in-agar, 108, 410
  chromatographic, 109
  dried antigen, 107
  immunophoretic, 348–349
  intragel, 106, 410
  local, 106
  quantitative, 348–349
  reversed, 106
  specific, 105
  specificity, 108
Acanthocytosis patient, 176
Acetate buffer, 53, 114, 154
  in methanol, 191
  rinse, 190–192
Acetylation, 42
Acid alcohol, 115, 191
Acid dye, 50, 113, 157
Acid phosphatase, 188
Acridine orange, 187
Acrylamide, 63
  photopolymerization, 144, 146
  polymer, 141
  polymerization, 127
  toxicity, 143
Adjuvant, 17, 19, 80–82, 502–508, *see also* specific substances
  haptens, 80
  mycobacteria, 81, 507

Adrenal gland antigen, 69
  guinea pig, 91
  rabbit, 91
Adsorption, 61
Afonso method, 355
Agar, 31, 42, 57–58, 125–126, 163–166, 176, 181, 289, 292, 311–312, 323, 332, 408
  coating, 163–166
  concentration in use, 136
  drying, 190–192
  extraction, 132
  gel making, 136–138
  gel zone electrophoresis, 102
  laboratory grade, 135
  lysis technique, 408
  making gels, 136–138
  nature of, 132–134
  pore size, 132–134
  preparation, 135
  preserving, 190–192
  properties, 132
  purification, 134–136
  slab, 405
  structure of gel, 43
  sulfate group, 42
Agaropectin, 122, 126, 134, 176, 311
Agarose, 8, 42, 57–59, 126–127, 135, 289, 292, 311, 323, 331, 339, 352, 357, 374, 377–384, 388, 394, 400
  coated microscopic slide, 239
  drying, 190–192

529

film, 165
gel making, 138–141
polyacrylamide mixture, 145, 334–335
preparation, 138–140
preserving, 190–192
solution, 141
Agglutination, 22, 35–36, 403–406
active, 35
artificial, 35
compared with precipitation, 35
definition, 35
in immunodiffusion test, 403–406
intragel, 406
natural, 35
passive, 35
surface-, 403–406
Agglutinin, 4, 16, 345
electrophoretic mobility, 403–405
in *Escherichia coli,* 405
Agglutinogen, 22
Aggregation of precipitin, spontaneous, 98–99
Agitation, thermal, 31
Albumin, 33, 52, 59, 330, 345, 362
artifact, 77
bovine, 47, 261
chicken egg, 86
human serum, 22, 23, 32, 77, 114, 122, 175, 178, 222, 225, 261, 279
Alcian blue, 186, 189
Allergy patient precipitin, 96
Alloantigen, 91
Aluminum hydroxide adjuvant, 80
Amide, 32
Amido black B, 184, 328
ε-Aminocaproic acid, 98, 121, 159
Aminopeptidase, 189
Ampholyte, 62
Amyl alcohol, 104
Amylase, 183, 188
cereal, 418
Anamnestic precipitin production, 95
Anemia, pernicious, 413
Angle double diffusion plate test, 270–272, 294–295
Aniline blue, 184
Anterior pituitary hormone, 90, 338
Antibody, 1–17
against antibodies, 76–77
agglutinating, 16

antigen equivalence, 255–257
antigen lattice, 5–7, 28, 29, 32
antigen mixing by electrophoresis, 59–61
antigen ratio, 214
antigen reaction, 3
atopic, 16
blocking, 4, 16, 20
combining site, 24, 110
complement fixing, 4, 16, 37
coprecipitating, 6
hay fever, 40, 415
iodination, 31
isolation during electroimmunodiffusion, 365–367
labeled, 40
lattice formation, 5–7, 28–29, 31–34
multiple, 217
nonprecipitating, 6, 31
response with time, 95
sink, 45
Anticonvection medium, *see* various media, Agar, Agarose, Gelatin, Polyacrylamide, etc.
Antiferritin precipitin, 91
Antigen, 3, 9, 17–22, 72–78, *see also* specific types
administration, 19, 95
analysis, 121–124
antibody affinity, 27
complexing with, 24–29
crossed electrophoresis, 361
dissociation, 25
environmental factors, 27–28
electrolyte, 27
pH, 27
salt concentration, 27
temperature, 27
equivalence, 255–257
lattice, 5–7, 28–29, 31–34
mixing by electrophoresis, 59–61
precipitation
factors, 32
primary, 24–28
secondary, 25
ratio, 214
reaction, 3, 412–421
invisible, 38–40
primary, 39
of *Aspergillus,* 9, 67